Integrated Colposcopy

Integrated Colposcopy

For colposcopists, histopathologists and cytologists

Second edition

M.C. Anderson, FRCPath, FRCOG
Reader in Gynaecological Pathology and Honorary Consultant
Department of Histopathology, University Hospital,
Queen's Medical Centre, Nottingham, UK

J.A. Jordan, MD, FRCOG
Medical Director
Birmingham Maternity Hospital, Queen Elizabeth Medical
Centre, Birmingham, UK

A.R. Morse, CFIAC
Principal Cytologist
Department of Cytology and Experimental Pathology, St Mary's
Hospital Medical School, and The Samaritan Hospital for
Women, London, UK

F. Sharp, MD, FRCOG
Professor of Obstetrics and Gynaecology
The University of Sheffield, Northern General Hospital,
Sheffield, UK

with a chapter from

A. Stafl, MD, PhD
Professor of Obstetrics and Gynaecology
Medical College of Wisconsin, Milwaukee, USA

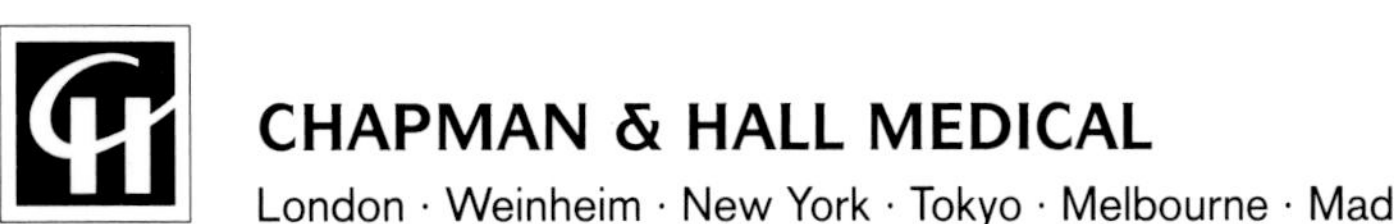

CHAPMAN & HALL MEDICAL
London · Weinheim · New York · Tokyo · Melbourne · Madras

Published by Chapman & Hall, 2–6 Boundary Row, London SE1 8HN, UK

Chapman & Hall, 2–6 Boundary Row, London SE1 8HN, UK

Blackie Academic & Professional, Wester Cleddens Road, Bishopbriggs, Glasgow G64 2NZ, UK

Chapman & Hall GmbH, Pappelallee 3, 69469 Weinheim, Germany

Chapman & Hall USA, 115 Fifth Avenue, New York, NY 10003, USA

Chapman & Hall Japan, ITP-Japan, Kyowa Building, 3F, 2-2-1 Hirakawacho, Chiyoda-ku, Tokyo 102, Japan

Chapman & Hall Australia, 102 Dodds Street, South Melbourne, Victoria 3205, Australia

Chapman & Hall India, R. Seshadri, 32 Second Main Road, CIT East, Madras 600 035, India

First edition 1992

Second edition 1996

Typeset in 10/12 Palatino by Keyset Composition, Colchester, Essex

Printed and bound in Hong Kong

ISBN 0 412 70840 X

A catalogue record for this book is available from the British Library

Library of Congress Catalog Card Number: 95-71086

Contents

Foreword

This excellent working text and atlas, written by four experts in the fields of colposcopy, histology and cytology, is timely in its appearance.

The authors have worked closely together over many years, on numerous courses given at the Royal College of Obstetricians and Gynaecologists, as well as nationally and internationally. This book is a distillation of the knowledge and expertise gained in their own clinical work and enhanced by their very extensive teaching experience. The authors are all international experts in their own right.

The text is authoritative and clear in its meaning, the complementary skills and value of cytology, histology and colposcopy are emphasized, and the excellent illustrations greatly enhance the written word.

Having had the privilege of collaborating with all four authors over the years in various capacities, and working closely with Mrs Anne Morse and Dr Malcolm Anderson over the past 20 years, it is a special honour for me to 'cap' those ties by writing the foreword for a book which deserves, and I believe will achieve, international acclaim.

George Pinker
Consultant Gynaecologist
St Mary's Hospital and
The Samaritan Hospital for Women
London

Preface

We have been organizing and teaching on colposcopy courses for many years, and this book is an attempt to put together all the information that we would like to impart on the courses if the time were available.

This volume is primarily intended for colposcopists; therefore the bulk of it covers the colposcopic appearances of the cervix in health and disease, largely in the form of an atlas. However, the book is much more than an atlas of colposcopy, as the colposcopist needs to be familiar with the factors responsible for the causation of disease and its histogenesis, as well as with the histological and cytological means of diagnosis which necessarily complement the colposcopic approach. The sections on histology and cytology have been incorporated in such a way that they will also be of value to the histologist and cytologist working alongside the colposcopist.

In addition to the basic 'core' chapters on histology, cytology, colposcopic appearances and treatment of disease of the cervix, vagina and vulva, we have also included chapters discussing policies of referral for colposcopy, setting up a colposcopy service, and training considerations. These wider issues are particularly important to everyone involved with colposcopy.

For the second edition, Adolf Stafl has joined us as a guest author, contributing Chapter 21 on cervicography. This is an area that he has personally pioneered and developed and his department in The Medical College of Wisconsin organizes cervicography tutorials for experts in colposcopy. In addition, of course, Professor Stafl is a colposcopist of international renown.

A further addition to the second edition is a chapter on anal intraepithelial disease, a logical extension of colposcopy of the lower genital tract. With the increasing use of colposcopy, the diseases of this area have become more of a problem since the first edition of the book was published.

Although our book contains elements of an atlas and a textbook, it covers more ground than either of these could. By adopting this wider approach, we believe that we have satisfied a need for a book that provides in one volume all the information required by colposcopists and those working with them.

Malcolm C. Anderson, Nottingham
Joseph A. Jordan, Birmingham
Anne R. Morse, London
Frank Sharp, Sheffield

March 1995

1. *The normal cervix*

NORMAL STRUCTURE

General features

The uterus is composed of the upper, muscular body and the lower, more fibrous cervix; the 'internal cervical os' marks the junction between the two. Approximately one half of the cervix protrudes into the vaginal vault through its anterior wall, and the other half remains supravaginal. The part of the cervix lying in the vagina is referred to as the 'portio vaginalis', or often merely as the 'portio'.

The cervix varies considerably in size and shape, depending on age and parity, but it is typically cylindrical, about 3 cm in length and 2.5 cm in diameter.

The 'external os' is an imprecise landmark, marking the point at which the cervical canal opens out into the vagina.

The 'cervical canal' connects the uterine cavity with the vaginal lumen, extending from the external to the internal os, and is flattened from front to back.

Tissue lying outside the external os is described as 'ectocervical', and inside the canal as 'endocervical'. Histopathologists tend to use the terms 'ectocervical' and 'endocervical' in a descriptive manner, to indicate original squamous or glandular tissue respectively, without taking into account its anatomical position on the cervix. This may give rise to confusion; for example, a biopsy taken from the vaginal surface of the cervix may be reported as showing endocervical tissue where eversion has occurred. The colposcopist should be aware of this frequent, but permissible, looseness of terminology.

Epithelial covering

Epithelium covering the cervix is initially of two types: squamous and columnar. It is laid down during embryological development, and is referred to as 'original' or 'native' epithelium.

SQUAMOUS EPITHELIUM

Histological appearances

The original squamous epithelium covers the ectocervix and is continuous with the vaginal epithelium. It is stratified, non-keratinizing epithelium, which is separated from the underlying stroma by a slightly undulating basal lamina.

In describing both normal and abnormal squamous epithelium, the terms 'differentiation', 'maturation' and 'stratification' are frequently used. These terms are closely interrelated in meaning, but are not quite synonymous.

Differentiation

Differentiation refers to the process in which the squamous cell becomes fully functional as a flattened, protective layer. In the skin, full differentiation involves keratinization, but in the normal cervix differentiation falls short of this. In normal epithelium, maturation and differentiation are virtually synonymous, i.e. the cells differentiate as they mature.

In abnormal epithelium, in common with other premalignant and malignant states, the term 'dif-

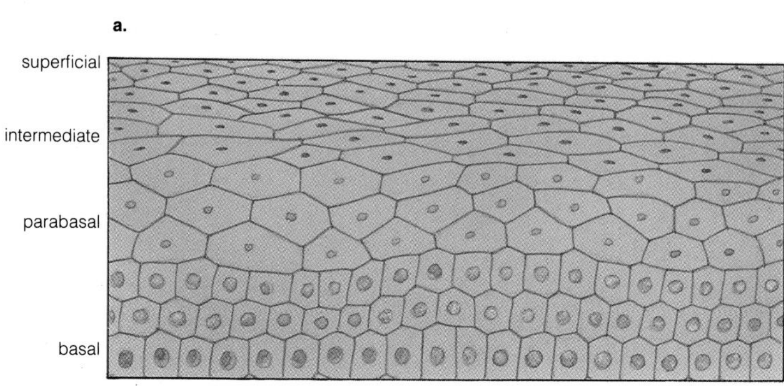

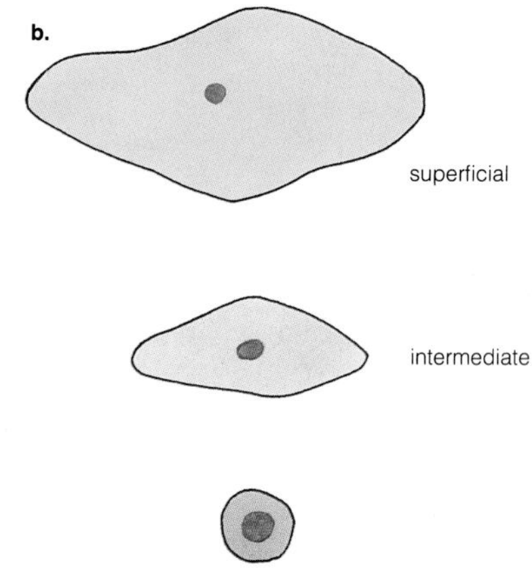

Fig. 1.1 Diagrammatic representation of (a) the histology of original cervical squamous epithelium, and (b) the cytology of normal squamous cells.

ferentiation' relates to the degree of morphological and functional similarity between abnormal and normal cells at all stages of maturation. Therefore, the equivalence of 'differentiation' with 'maturation' diminishes as the epithelium becomes more abnormal.

Maturation

Maturation is very closely related to differentiation in meaning, and characterizes the changes seen in cells as the surface of normal squamous epithelium is reached. A mature squamous cell must also show good differentiation, but an immature squamous cell may show some degree of differentiation that enables it to be recognized as squamous in type.

Stratification

Stratification is a necessary consequence of maturation and differentiation; it refers to the way in which the epithelium is divided into layers of progressively more mature and flattened cells as the surface is reached.

The processes of differentiation, maturation and stratification are illustrated in Fig. 1.1. The maturing squamous epithelium of the ectocervix has a well-defined basal layer attached to the basal lamina (Figs 1.2 and 1.3). These cells have a large nuclear cytoplasmic ratio. The parabasal cells form the next few layers, and these also have a high nuclear cytoplasmic ratio with rather basophilic cytoplasm. It is in this layer that occasional mitotic figures are normally seen.

Further maturation and differentiation (Fig. 1.4) produces the intermediate cells in which the cytoplasm is more abundant, often with a prominent space containing glycogen around the nucleus (Fig. 1.5). These cells often form a 'basket weave' pattern (see Fig. 1.2). The cytoplasm becomes more abundant

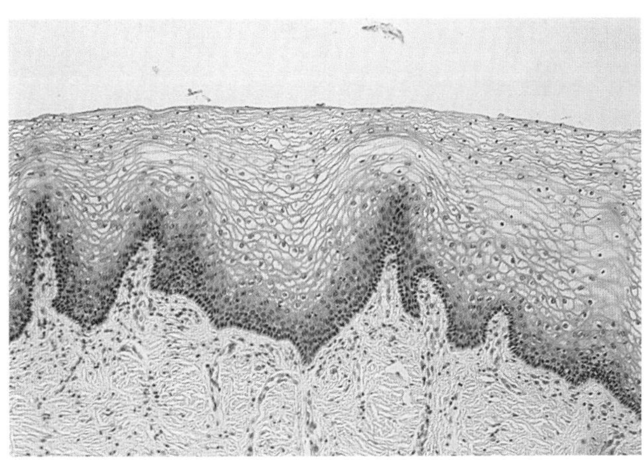

Fig. 1.2 Original squamous epithelium.

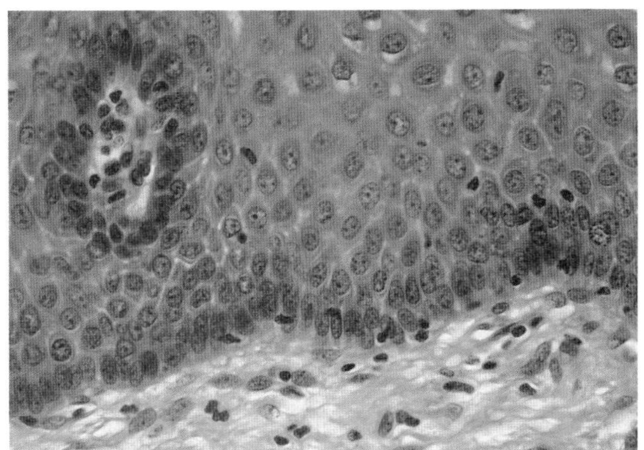

Fig. 1.3 Original squamous epithelium. Basal and parabasal layers are seen.

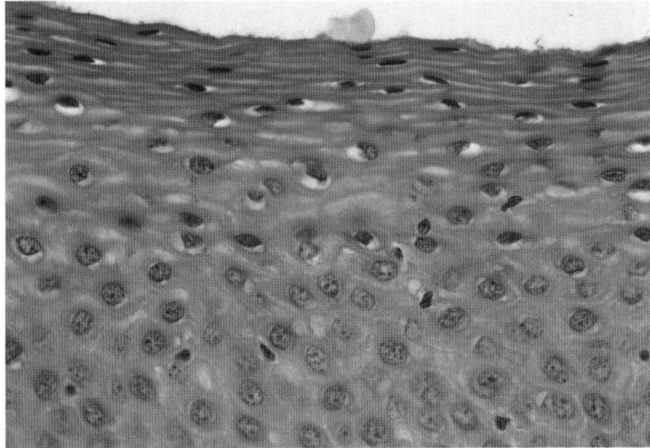

Fig. 1.4 Original squamous epithelium. Intermediate and superficial cells are seen.

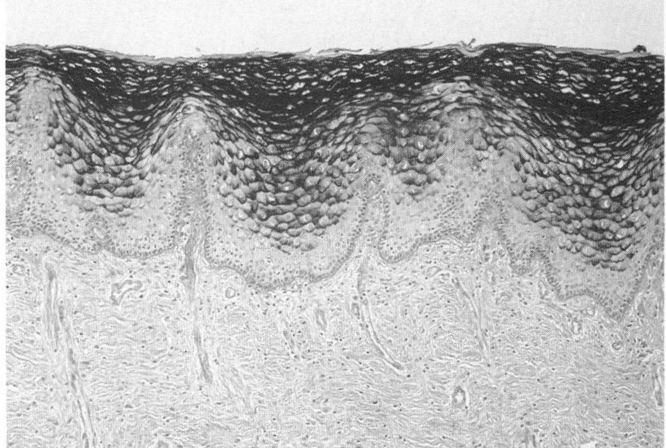

Fig. 1.5 Original squamous epithelium. This has been stained to demonstrate glycogen. Periodic acid–Schiff.

as maturation progresses, and the nucleus becomes smaller, so that cells in the intermediate zone are slightly flattened with round nuclei of moderate size, in which the chromatin pattern is readily discernible.

The intercellular 'prickles' are usually very prominent in the skin and characterize the stratum spinosum of normal skin. Although these are a diagnostic feature of squamous cell carcinoma, they are not so striking in the cervical epithelium, but may be identified in the parabasal and, with more difficulty, in the intermediate layer. Further maturation of the squamous cells produces the superficial layer of epithelium (see Fig. 1.4). This layer is composed of markedly flattened cells, with eosinophilic cytoplasm and small, slightly flattened nuclei. At this final stage of maturation the nuclei become pyknotic, small and very dense, with no nuclear structure discernible within them.

The fully mature and differentiated cell of the squamous epithelium is very flat, and its nature is probably better appreciated when the cell is seen lying flat in a cytological preparation, rather than when cut across in a histological section.

Cytological features

The cytological features of normal squamous cells closely reflect the histological appearances (Fig. 1.6). However, the overall size of the cell and size of the nucleus, together with the differential staining of the cytoplasm, are of paramount importance to the cytologist. Thus, the type of stain used, as well as the subtle variations associated with it at cellular level, is of great relevance.

The standard method for staining cytological preparations is that of Papanicolaou. Haematoxylin is used to stain the nucleus of cells blue/black. Other counterstains (EA50 and OG6) will stain the cytoplasm various hues of green to blue and pink, depending on the maturity of differentiation of the cell as a result of changes in cell metabolism and chemical reactions in the cytoplasm.

Throughout this book, all references to cytological staining and the colours observed at microscopy relate to the use of Papanicolaou stain.

Parabasal squamous cells

Parabasal squamous cells have a large nucleus which occupies approximately 80–90% of the overall cell size. The nucleus is darkly stained, with a well-defined, coarse chromatin pattern. The cytoplasm has a thick, homogeneous appearance, and stains green or blue. The cell has a rounded shape, with well-defined cell borders (Fig. 1.7).

Intermediate squamous cells

As the cell matures, the amount of cytoplasm increases in relation to cell size and also to nuclear cytoplasmic ratio. The cytoplasm retains an affinity to basophilic staining but becomes 'thinner' and more transparent, characteristically staining pale blue. It

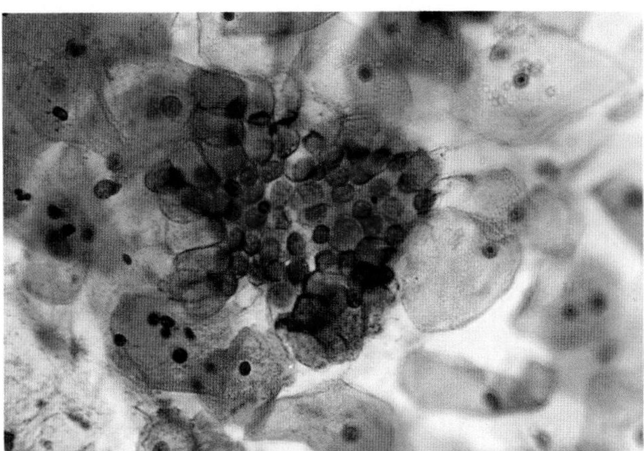

Fig. 1.6 A normal cervical smear appearance, with a mixture of superficial and intermediate squamous cells. A small sheet of endocervical glandular cells can be seen at the centre.

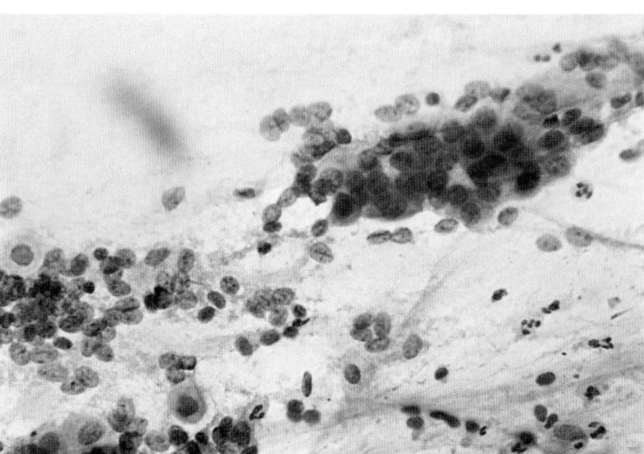

Fig. 1.7 Atrophic pattern. The smear consists of regular-sized parabasal cells, many of which have shed their cytoplasm and consist of bare nuclei.

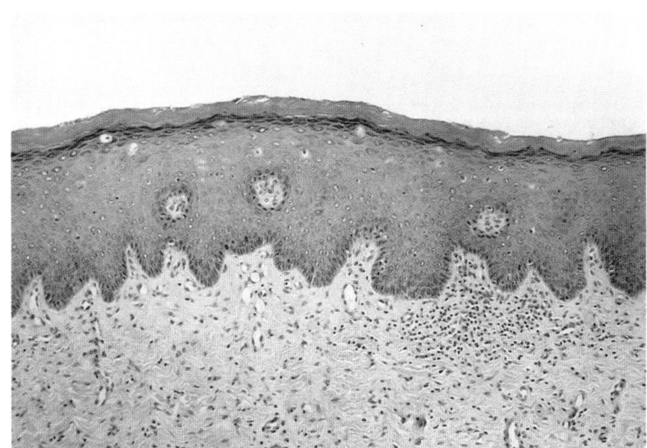

Fig. 1.8 Prolapse. The original squamous epithelium is showing hyperkeratosis with a prominent granular layer.

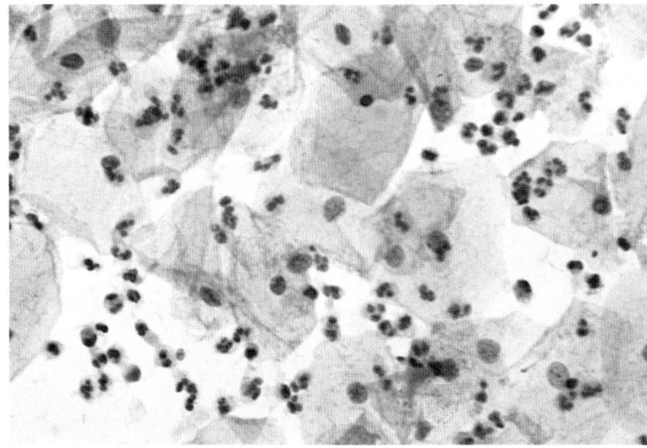

Fig. 1.9 Prolapse. The atrophic pattern is usually retained, with parabasal cells predominating. Random superficial squamous cells are present, which sometimes show marked keratinization.

may show a well-defined region around the nucleus, which stains yellow; this denotes the presence of glycogen.

The nucleus of the intermediate squamous cell is round, with an obvious chromatin structure; however, this is pale stained and finely granular, not showing the hyperchromasia and coarseness associated with the parabasal cell.

Superficial squamous cells

As maturation progresses, squamous cells from the superficial layers of the epithelium become larger, with a pink-staining, almost transparent, cytoplasm. The cells are flattened, with angled edges suggesting a polyhedral shape. The nuclei are very small and dense, with no visible chromatin structure, and are referred to as pyknotic.

Keratinization is not a normal occurrence in the cervix, and maturation of normal squamous epithelial cells is arrested at this point. However, when genital prolapse occurs, keratinization may be seen on a section, along with some thickening of the epithelium (Fig. 1.8). The keratinized superficial cells are often readily recognized with cytology (Fig. 1.9).

Hormonal response

The squamous epithelium of the cervix is responsive to hormonal stimuli, and is dependent on oestrogen for full development. If oestrogen is deficient, or its effects are counteracted by high levels of progesterone, full maturation does not take place and cells at the surface of the epithelium do not become fully differentiated.

Following the menopause, the cells do not mature beyond the parabasal stage. As a result, the epithelium becomes atrophic, i.e. thin and composed of cells that have a relatively high nuclear cytoplasmic ratio, with virtually no flattening as the surface is reached (Fig. 1.10). Glycogen is absent, as maturation does not reach the intermediate cell stage. A rather similar appearance is seen during the late stages of pregnancy, and even more markedly in the postpartum period.

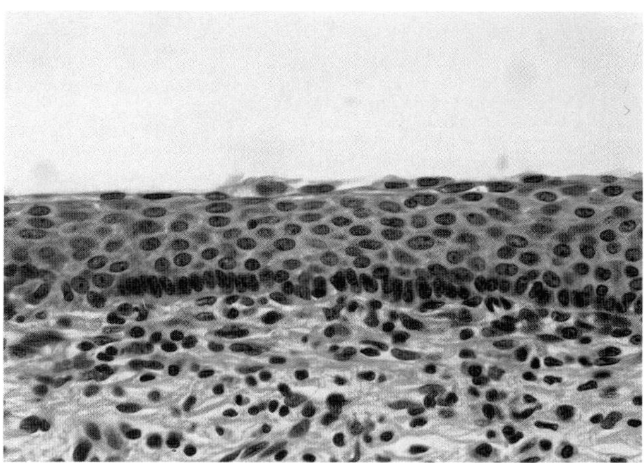

Fig. 1.10 Postmenopausal squamous epithelium.

The cyclical changes are best observed in vaginal smears, but they are also seen in normal cervical smears. The most striking change is an alteration of the ratio of superficial to intermediate squamous cells during the normal menstrual cycle. These basic changes can be measured by the karyopyknotic index (KPI): this represents the percentage of superficial squamous cells with pyknotic nuclei, to intermediate cells (parabasal cells are excluded), based on a minimum count of 200 cells.

Oestrogen effect/proliferation

Following menstruation, the proportion of superficial squamous to intermediate squamous cells rises towards midcycle; the smear is dominated by superficial squamous cells, although a few intermediate cells are still seen (normal range KPI: 80–90%). At this time, the cells are nicely displayed in flat sheets, with a clean background and few polymorphs (Fig. 1.11).

Secretory changes and progesterone effect

After ovulation, the effect of oestrogen suppression by progesterone is reflected in the increasing proportion of intermediate to superficial cell types. At this time, cells tend to clump together in large clusters, with poorly differentiated cell borders or folded and curled edges (Fig. 1.12). There is an increase

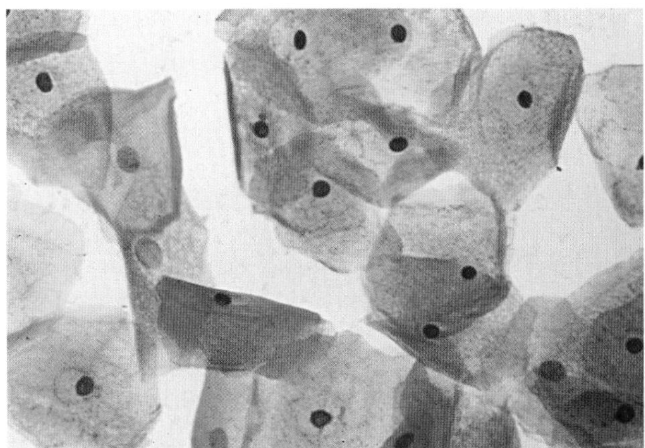

Fig. 1.11 Superficial squamous cells at midcycle. A fully developed oestrogen effect is seen with a clean background.

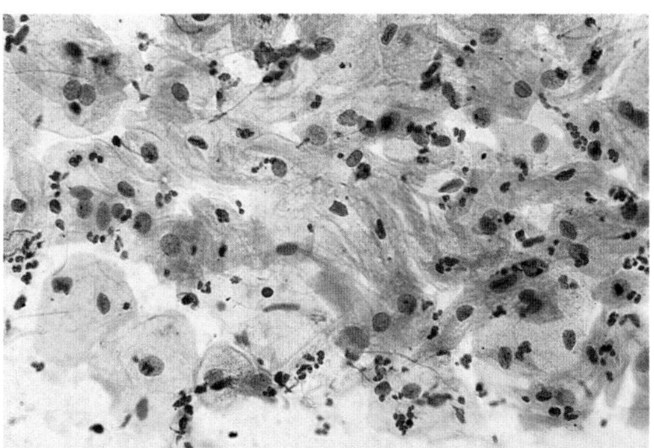

Fig. 1.12 Day 19 of the menstrual cycle. The intermediate cells are showing clumping and folding, with occasional glycogenated cells. Some polymorphonuclear leucocytes are present.

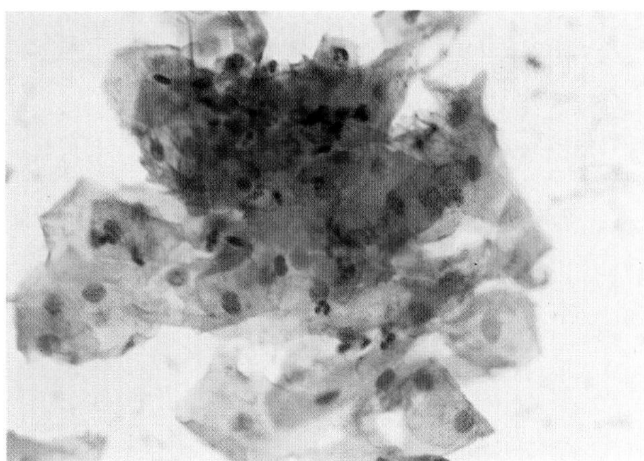

Fig. 1.13 Day 24 of the menstrual cycle. Clumping and folding of the cells are more pronounced features. There are numerous polymorphonuclear leucocytes and cell debris in the background. The appearance is untidy, and can often render the smear unsatisfactory for assessment.

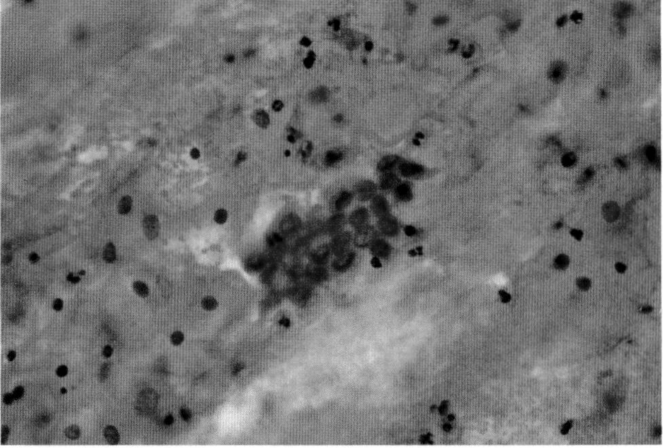

Fig. 1.14 Menstrual pattern. Small groups of comparatively darkly stained endometrial cells in a bloodstained background. This appearance often makes a reliable cytological assessment impossible.

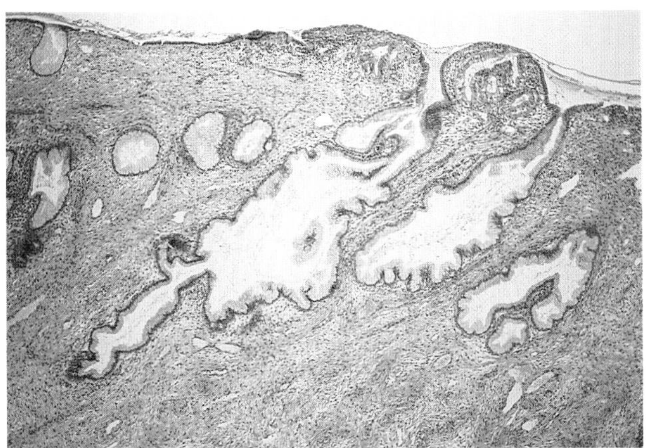

Fig. 1.15 Endocervical crypts.

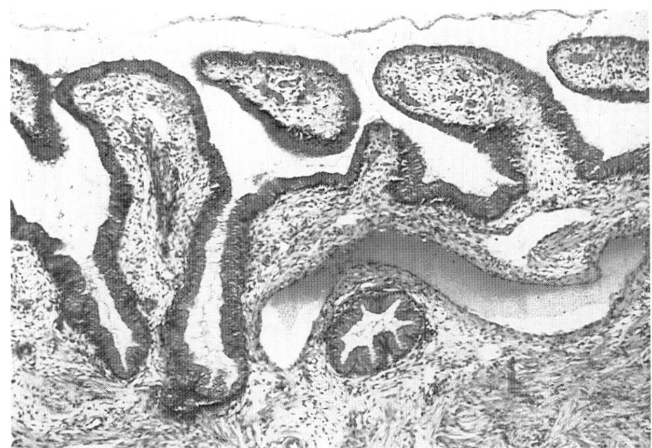

Fig. 1.16 Endocervical villi. Note the 'picket-fence' appearance

in background debris and polymorphs (Fig. 1.13), which may make a cellular assessment difficult, if not impossible, and also unreliable.

Menstrual appearances

A smear taken during menstruation consists mainly of red blood cells, with small groups of darkly staining endometrial cells (Fig. 1.14). Predictably, the squamous cell detail is often obscured, making the specimen unacceptable for a reliable assessment. The optimal time for taking a smear is midcycle. Therefore, if possible, arrangements for smear tests should be made with this in mind.

Postmenopausal atrophic pattern

In the postmenopausal woman, the cervical smear pattern is composed almost entirely of parabasal and low intermediate cell types, with no cyclical changes and rarely any endocervical glandular cells (see Fig. 1.7).

A similar pattern may be seen postpartum, although the presence of squamous metaplasia, endocervical glandular cells and regenerative changes are frequently noted, making possible a distinction from atrophy of the postmenopausal type.

COLUMNAR EPITHELIUM

Histological appearances

Architectural features

The caudal limit of the field of endocervical epithelium is the original squamocolumnar junction. At its cephalic extreme, the endocervical epithelium merges (through a zone of isthmic endometrium several millimetres in length) with endometrial epithelium of the lower part of the uterine body. The columnar epithelium of endocervix lines the cervical canal, forms crypts that pass deep into the substance of the cervix, and develops into papillary projections protruding into the lumen of the canal.

Endocervical crypts may extend as far as 1 cm from the surface of the cervix, but usually they are much more superficial (Fig. 1.15). Although often loosely termed 'glands', their structure is not that of a true gland in that there is no duct leading to acini. Endocervical crypts are elongated, branching tunnels, and are lined by the same epithelium which lines the canal on the surface.

The endocervical epithelium is not a simple, flattened surface, and particularly in the few millimetres immediately above the squamocolumnar junction it forms multiple papillary projections. Colposcopically, these 'grape-like' villi are the hallmark of endocervical tissue (see Chapter 7). Each villus is covered by a single layer of columnar epithelium, and has a core of superficial endocervical stroma containing a single vessel (Fig. 1.16).

Cellular features

In the normal, unaltered state, the endocervical epithelium is a single layer of tall, columnar cells with regular basal nuclei, giving 'a picket fence' appearance (Fig. 1.17). The cytoplasm contains finely dispersed mucin (Fig. 1.18). Goblet cells are not characteristic of endocervical epithelium. Some ciliated cells are normally present. Not uncommonly, areas of tubal metaplasia are seen in the endocervi-

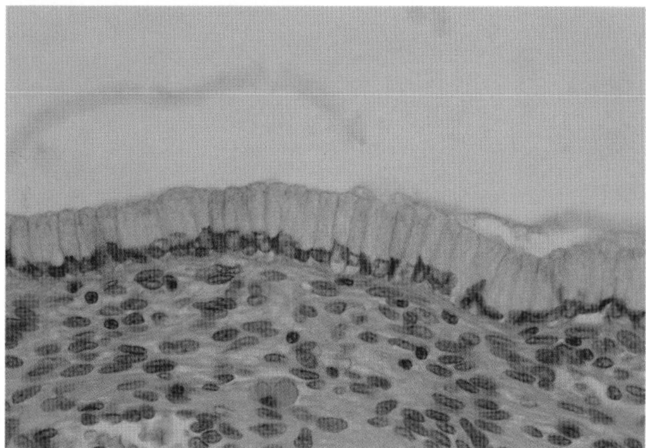

Fig. 1.17 Original columnar epithelium.

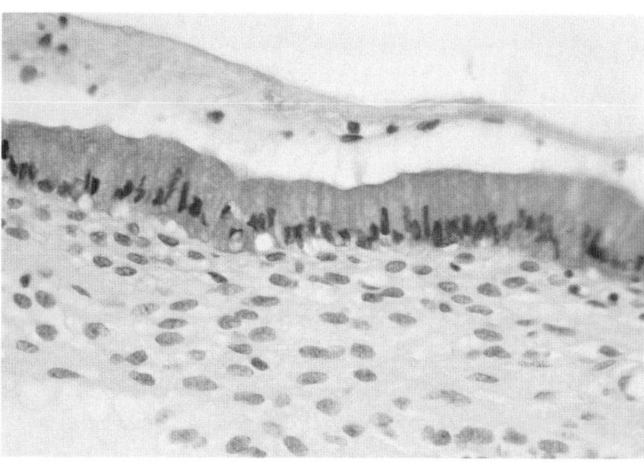

Fig. 1.18 Original columnar epithelium. This has been stained with Alcian blue to show mucin.

cal crypts. Developmentally, this may well be heterotopia rather than metaplasia, and care must be taken not to confuse its appearance with that of glandular atypia. Epithelium of endometrial type may sometimes also be seen in the cervix. (These features are discussed in greater detail in Chapter 11.)

Cytological features

Glandular cells of endocervical origin are loosely referred to by cytologists as endocervical cells (Figs 1.19 and 1.20). In general, these cells are easily identified, particularly since they frequently occur in small groups and sheets, although occasionally whole villi may be seen (Fig. 1.21).

The nuclei are basophilic and darkly stained with a prominent but finely granular chromatin structure, sometimes with chromocentres or small nucleoli. The nuclei are basally located in a cylindrically shaped cell. The cytoplasm stains a rather pale blue/grey (although occasionally pink hues can be seen), and is finely vacuolated with poorly defined cell borders.

Endocervical cells are approximately five times the size of lymphocytes, and somewhat smaller than mature squamous cells. When seen end-on, they appear round with a small rim of pale blue/grey cytoplasm. A differential diagnosis between parabasal and endocervical cells may be difficult.

CERVICAL POLYPS

Cervical polyps are extremely common, and consist of a localized overgrowth of endocervical tissue. Most are symptomless, but sometimes they present with irregular vaginal bleeding.

The polyp is composed of the lamina propria of the endocervix, with surface epithelium and underlying crypts. The surface epithelium may be ulcerated, and the underlying tissue may then take on the features of granulation tissue; this is often seen with symptomatic polyps. When the surface epithelium is present, it very often shows squamous metaplasia of varying degrees of maturity. Moreover, the superficial stroma is commonly infiltrated by inflammatory cells, with plasma cells being predominant among them.

Associated with squamous metaplasia, a polyp is frequently found to contain dilated endocervical crypts. Sometimes it may be composed solely of a few mucus-filled cysts covered by a layer of metaplastic squamous epithelium.

Endocervical polyps must be distinguished from polyps arising in the endometrium, and also from fibroid polyps, both of which may extend into the endocervical canal and protrude through the external os. It must also be remembered that cervical intraepithelial neoplasia can affect the surface epithelium of a polyp, usually in association with this condition involving another area of the transformation zone. However, sometimes the polyp may bear the only recognizable cervical intraepithelial neoplasia.

Stroma

The stroma of the cervix is fibromuscular. Layers nearest to the surface are predominantly composed of rather loose fibrous tissue, with muscle lying deeper, beyond the field of the more superficial

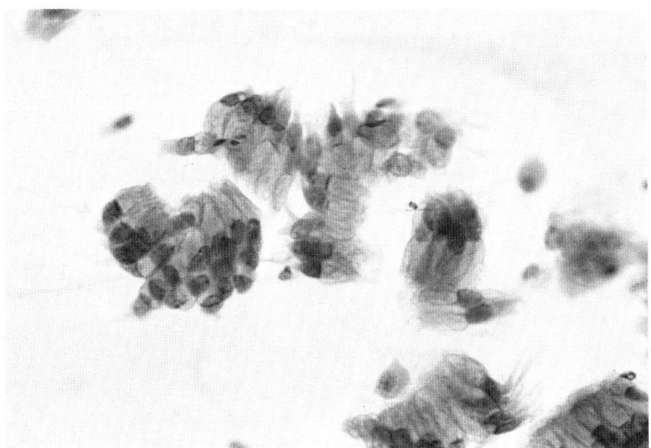

Fig. 1.19 Endocervical glandular cells. These are showing palisading with a typically columnar shape and basally located nuclei. The cytoplasm is finely vacuolated.

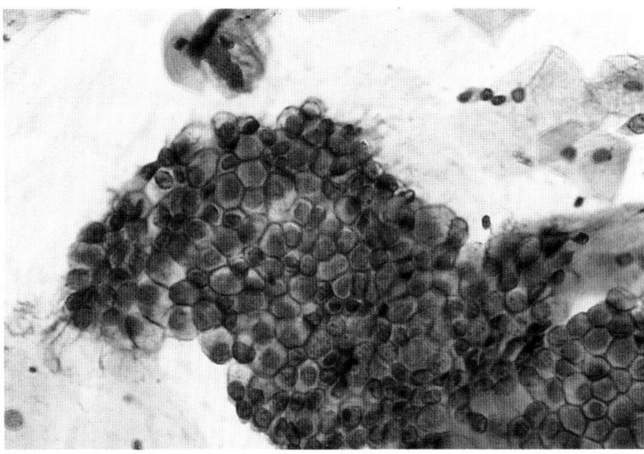

Fig. 1.20 A nicely displayed clump of endocervical cells. The typical 'honeycomb' appearance of the cells is seen when viewed end-on. Some cells at the edge of the group are of a characteristic, cylindrical shape.

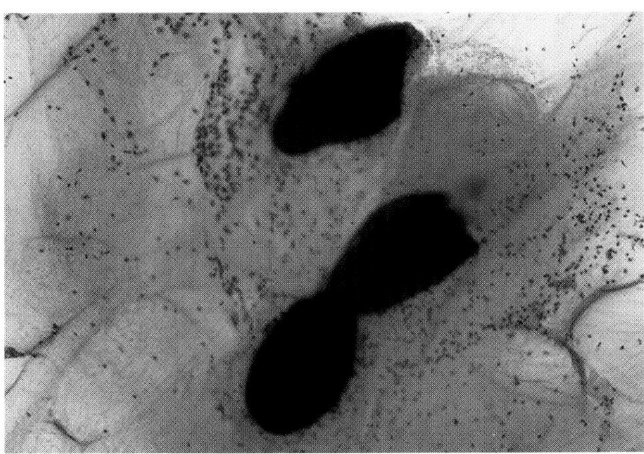

Fig. 1.21 Endocervical villus. Cytologically, this is seen as a darkly stained, dense cluster of cells. The columnar cells on the surface can be seen at higher magnification, but the core of the villus is composed of stromal cells.

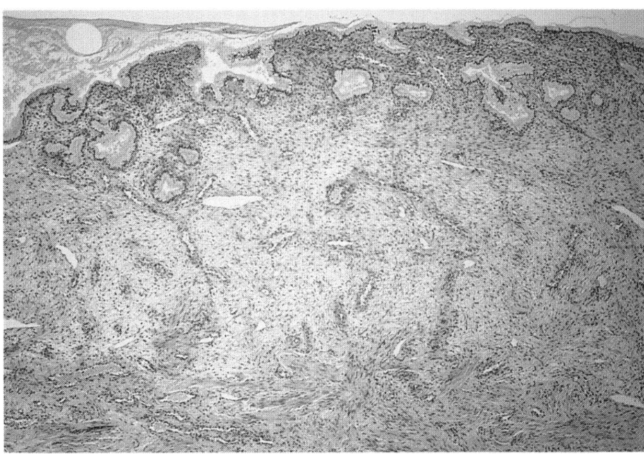

Fig. 1.22 Endocervix showing stroma. The deep, denser, muscular layer is seen at the bottom of the field.

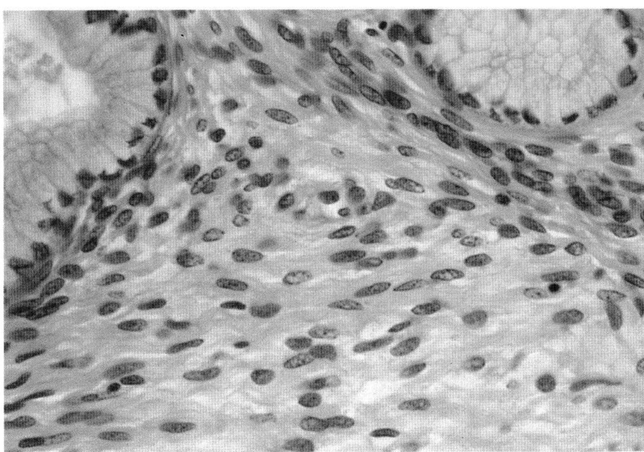

Fig. 1.23 Endocervical stroma. Typical spindle cells are seen.

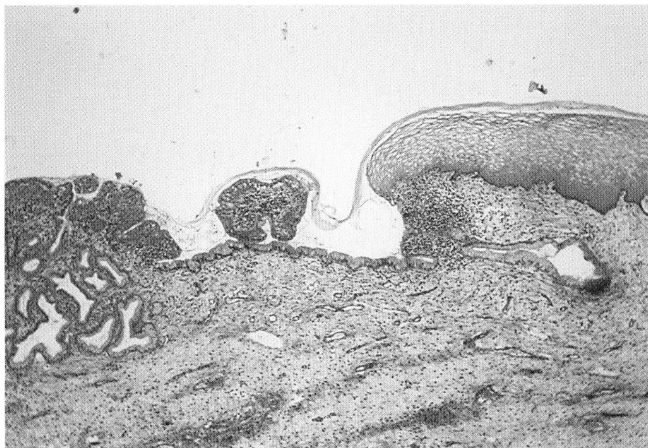

Fig. 1.24 Squamocolumnar junction. This shows a sparse, chronic inflammatory infiltrate in the superficial stroma.

crypts (Figs 1.22 and 1.23). Muscular tissue is more superficial beneath the ectocervical squamous epithelium than in the endocervix.

Several small blood vessels are present in the cervical stroma, forming a subepithelial plexus beneath the columnar epithelium. Those, together with the vessels within the endocervical villi, contribute to the formation of characteristic abnormal vascular patterns of mosaic and punctation (for the colposcopic appearances, see pages 90–93).

The superficial cervical stroma almost invariably contains an infiltrate of inflammatory cells, usually plasma cells and lymphocytes, particularly in the region of the squamocolumnar junction (Fig. 1.24). Unless extreme, this infiltrate should not be considered pathological; it represents the response to a continuous low-grade stimulation by a variety of antigenic factors.

TRANSFORMATION ZONE

Squamocolumnar junction

Ideally, the squamocolumnar junction would be situated at the external os (Fig. 1.25), so that squamous epithelium lies on the ectocervix, and columnar epithelium lines the canal. This seems to be what the two types of epithelium are best suited for. However, in the great majority of women this is not the configuration encountered; it is this deviation from the 'ideal' anatomy of the cervix that is the starting point of a chain of events that may eventually lead to invasive squamous cell carcinoma.

Hormonal changes

At the time of puberty and during adolescence, the female genital tract enlarges in response to increasing levels of ovarian hormones and continuing stimulation by the physiological levels that are soon reached. This increase in size is most apparent in the body of the uterus, but the cervix also enlarges and alters in shape; the most significant element of this alteration is an eversion which appears to be concomitant with a 'rolling out' of the ectocervical component (this process is illustrated by comparing Figs 1.25 and 1.26).

Development of the transformation zone

The process of eversion causes a change in the position of cervical epithelium, so that epithelium initially lining the lower part of the cervical canal is now situated on the vaginal portion of the cervix (see Fig. 1.26). When viewed with a vaginal speculum, a red area is seen to surround the external cervical os,

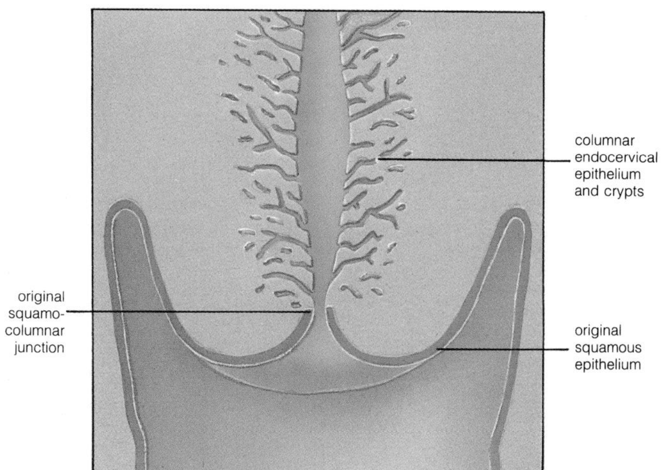

Fig. 1.25 'Ideal' cervix. The squamocolumnar junction is situated at the external cervical os. The arrows show the direction of the movement that takes place as a result of the increase in bulk of the cervix during adolescence.

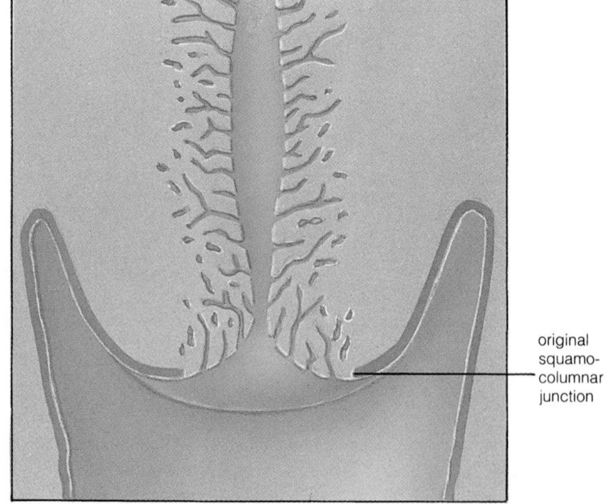

Fig. 1.26 Process of eversion. On completion, endocervical columnar tissue lies on the vaginal surface of the cervix, and is exposed to the vaginal environment.

corresponding to the area of everted endocervical tissue. The term 'erosion' has traditionally been applied to this appearance; at first, this may not seem an inappropriate term, as the tissue shows redness and roughness at naked eye examination, suggesting that it is ulcerated and haemorrhagic.

Redness is due to the more vascular endocervical stroma seen through the thinner 'filter' of endocervical epithelium, and roughness is a consequence of the villous nature of everted endocervical epithelium. Therefore, erosion is a term that is best not used, as it implies an erroneous view of the phenomenon.

A variety of alternative terms have been used, such as 'erythroplakia', 'ectopy' and 'transformation zone'. It is in this zone that physiological transformation to metaplastic squamous epithelium takes place (Fig. 1.27).

More importantly, this is the area where transformation to cervical intraepithelial neoplasia occurs, which may lead to invasive squamous cell carcinoma of the cervix. In fact, this area should not be called a 'transformation zone' until squamous metaplasia has started to develop. The transformation zone is defined as the area of cervix bounded caudally by the original squamocolumnar junction, and cephalically by the highest point that squamous metaplasia reaches.

The transformation zone may be described as normal, either immature or mature, abnormal, or congenital. These concepts will be discussed in separate sections.

Other hormonal effects on the squamocolumnar junction

Apart from adolescence, eversion of the cervix occurs at other times, although it is thought that this period is by far the most significant in the development of cervical malignancy. In the neonatal period, the effect of maternal hormones on the fetus leads to eversion of the cervix. In pregnancy, increased levels of circulating hormones cause the cervix to evert further, beyond the position reached at the end of adolescence. After each pregnancy, the cervix will return to more or less the state that it was in before that pregnancy. The combined oral contraceptive pill has a similar but less marked effect on the degree of eversion.

After the menopause, the levels of sex steroid hormones fall and the eversion reverses (Fig. 1.28) so that the transformation zone passes back into the cervical canal. The original squamocolumnar junction may come to lie further within the canal than it did in childhood. This process of inversion may commence as many as 10 years before the menopause, and for this reason the whole of the transformation zone may be visible at colposcopy in older women.

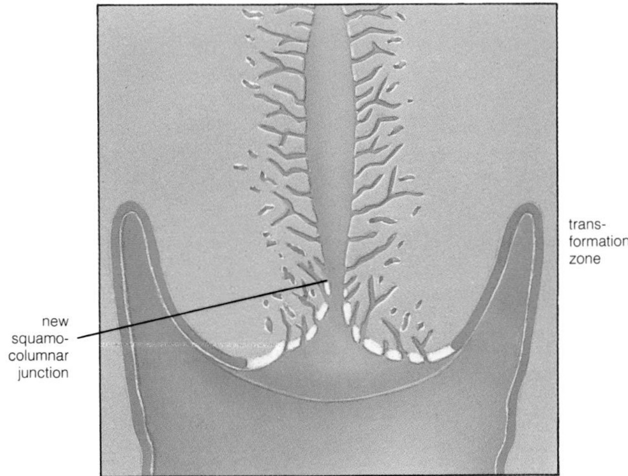

Fig. 1.27 Postadolescent cervix. Acidity of the vaginal environment is one of the factors that encourage squamous metaplastic change, replacing the exposed columnar epithelium with squamous epithelium.

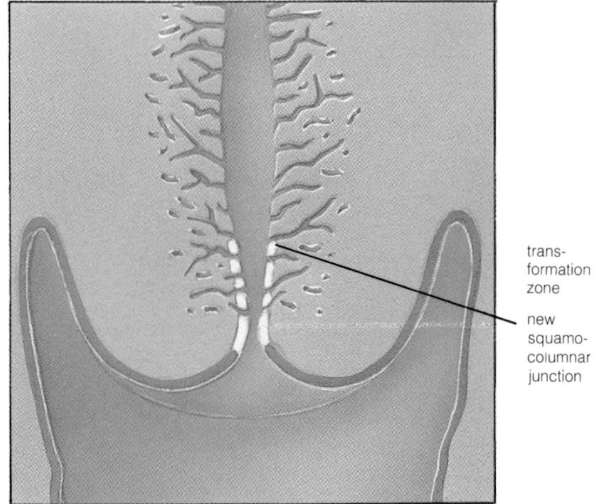

Fig. 1.28 Postmenopausal cervix. At this time, cervical eversion, which was so important in adolescence, reverses; thus, the transformation zone is now drawn into the cervical canal. The original squamocolumnar junction may be situated further within the canal than it was before puberty (see Fig. 1.25), and the new squamocolumnar junction may be out of sight, high inside the canal.

Squamous metaplasia

CONCEPT AND STIMULI

As described above, eversion leaves endocervical epithelium on the vaginal portion of the cervix. This epithelium is highly differentiated and specialized, performing its function most effectively within the cervical canal. The vaginal environment is hostile to this delicate epithelium, as the most important difference between the endocervical and vaginal environments is the much higher acidity in the vagina of a woman of reproductive age, which has been found to be even more marked in pregnancy. This feature is most significant in stimulating the epithelium to undergo squamous metaplasia, whereby an area initially covered by columnar epithelium becomes covered by squamous epithelium.

Mature, fully differentiated epithelial cells cannot change into another type of epithelial cell; the process is one of replacement, in which columnar cells are lost and replaced, not by more columnar cells as would normally happen in the endocervix, but by cells that will eventually differentiate into mature squamous cells.

This process of squamous metaplasia on the cervix is physiological and should be considered a normal event. There is nothing sinister about it, and its relationship with squamous cell carcinoma of the cervix is only that the two conditions share the same early path in the process of their development.

RESERVE CELL HYPERPLASIA

The first sign that the process of squamous metaplasia is beginning in the endocervix is the appearance of reserve cell proliferation. Reserve cells are seen as a single layer of cells beneath and very close to the nuclei of columnar epithelial cells, initially giving the impression that the epithelium has a double line of nuclei.

The origin of reserve cells is not clear; it seems likely that they are normally present in small numbers beneath the endocervical columnar epithelium, and replenish the cells as they are lost.

Alternative, but less probable, origins may be the endocervical stromal cells and blood-borne monocytes. Morphologically, reserve cells have a somewhat similar appearance to the basal cells of the original squamous epithelium, with round nuclei and little cytoplasm. As the metaplastic process continues, reserve cells proliferate and form a layer that is several cells thick. At this stage, the endocervical villi begin to fuse; this development can be appreciated both histologically (Fig. 1.29) and colposcopically (see Chapter 7).

It has also been suggested that the basement membrane of the original columnar epithelium dissolves as reserve cells appear, and is reformed between the proliferative reserve cells and the stroma, as metaplasia continues.

Cytologically, reserve cells appear as small, round cells with a very darkly staining nucleus and coarsely textured chromatin in a small amount of green-

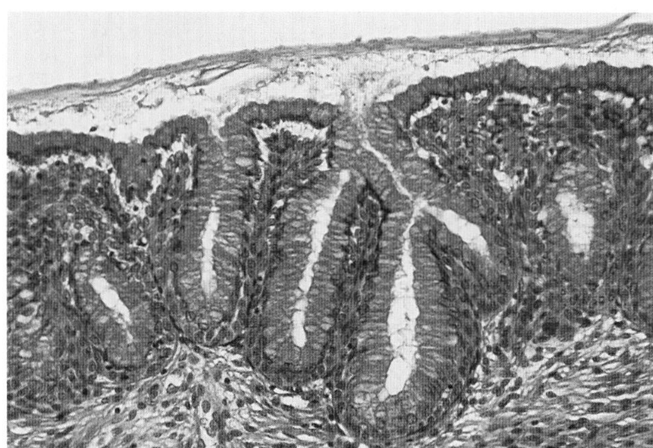

Fig. 1.29 Reserve cell hyperplasia.

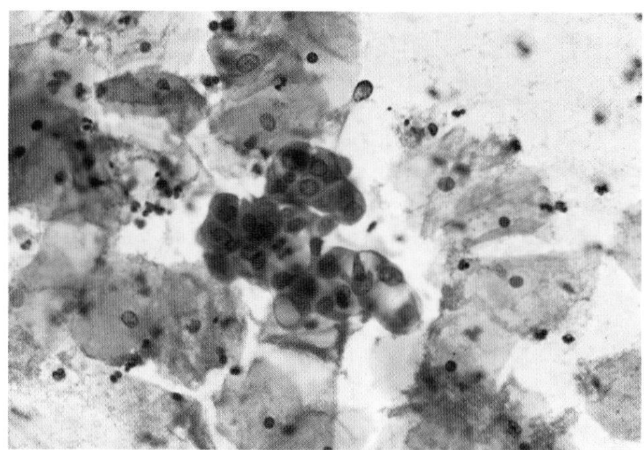

Fig. 1.30 Reserve cell hyperplasia. Small, darkly stained cells with large nuclei and a small rim of cytoplasm are seen.

staining cytoplasm (Fig. 1.30). When they occur discretely they may well be overlooked or be mistaken for lymphocytes or endometrial cells. However, reserve cells are most frequently seen with columnar endocervical cells.

IMMATURE METAPLASIA

As the metaplastic process develops further, reserve cells begin to undergo differentiation and maturation to become initially immature squamous cells. The amount of cytoplasm increases a little, and the nuclei enlarge, often with prominent nucleoli.

Stratification of the epithelium is not apparent at this stage. Residual groups of mucin-containing columnar cells may often be seen both on the surface of immature squamous epithelium and embedded within it (Fig. 1.31); this may be subsequently described as showing immature and incomplete squamous metaplasia. At this stage the epithelium is usually thin, and the junction between epithelium and stroma often presents a 'scalloped' outline, reflecting the fact that endocervical villi have been fused together by the process of immature squamous metaplasia.

For the cytologist, the most important aspect in recognizing metaplastic cells in cervical smears is an appreciation of the spectrum of cell changes that invariably occur, and an awareness that cells of varying degrees of maturation will be seen in any single cervical smear.

In cytology, the term 'immature' is used to describe cells that have a round shape, with a thick, green-staining cytoplasm and a very large, darkly staining nucleus showing a coarse chromatin pattern, sometimes with prominent chromocentres or small nucleoli. Occasionally, the cytoplasm may show some elongation, and the cell tends to take on an oval shape (Fig. 1.32).

MATURE METAPLASIA

As the process of squamous metaplasia continues, the developing squamous cells become more mature. Eventually, the epithelium has fully mature, differentiated squamous cells on its surface, and no residual columnar cells are seen. It is now of almost the same thickness as the original squamous epithelium (Fig. 1.33), and is glycogenated. The purpose of the metaplastic process is fulfilled when the delicate, thin layer of endocervical, columnar cells is replaced by a much thicker, stronger and more protective layer of squamous cells.

As maturation of the metaplastic process progresses, the cytoplasm appears more squamous in nature, staining blue or pink, but not quite achieving the characteristic transparent appearance of the normal, intermediate cell. The cytoplasm gradually becomes more recognizably squamous, taking on a pink hue; the nucleus becomes less dominant, with a less obvious chromatin structure, although it still appears larger in comparison with the nucleus of a normal squamous cell (Fig. 1.34).

In complete maturity, the metaplastic cell is

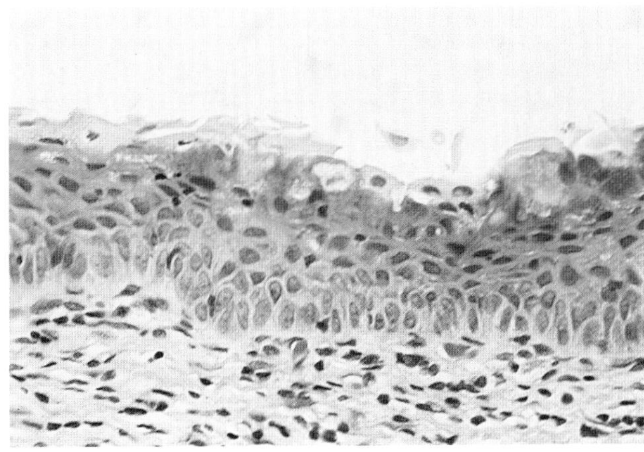

Fig. 1.31 Immature, incomplete squamous metaplasia.

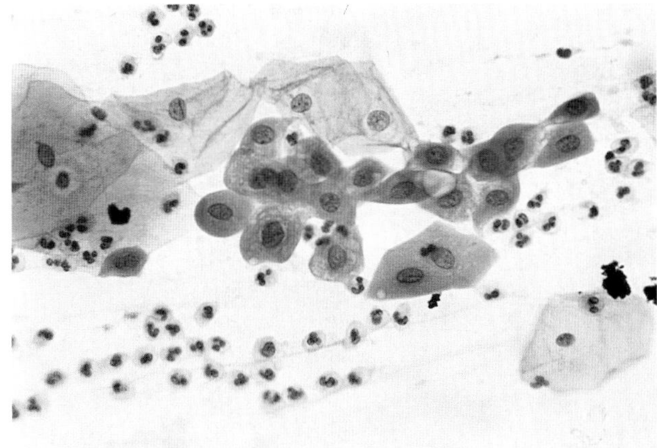

Fig. 1.32 Immature squamous metaplasia. As reserve cells become more mature metaplastic cells, the nucleus is less prominent, although still showing its chromatin structure. The outline of the cell is elongated and resembles more closely that of a squamous cell.

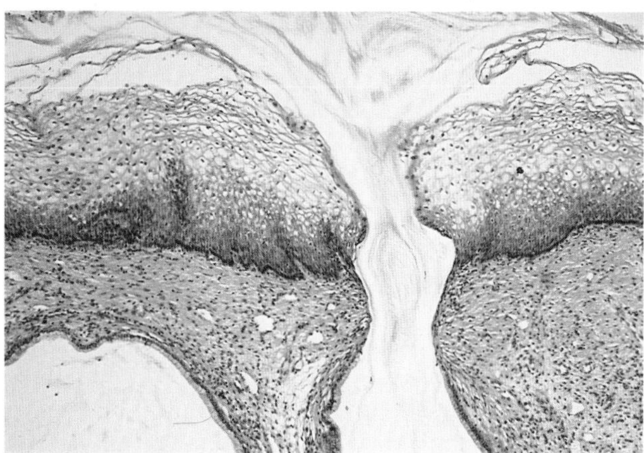

Fig. 1.33 Mature squamous metaplasia. Note the opening of a crypt.

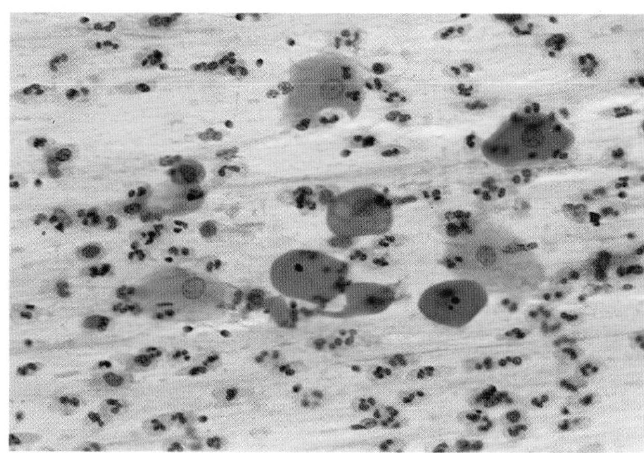

Fig. 1.34 Maturing squamous metaplasia. This shows the features that distinguish a metaplastic cell from a mature squamous cell. The nucleus is now much smaller than that of an immature metaplastic cell, and the cytoplasm closely resembles the shape and texture of a squamous cell.

cytologically indistinguishable from the normal superficial squamous cell that arises from the original squamous epithelium.

METAPLASIA AND CRYPTS

Although squamous metaplasia is most often seen as a process of the surface epithelium, it may involve the crypts of the endocervix, albeit usually only the more superficial ones (Fig. 1.35). The pattern of this involvement can become quite complex, and the inexperienced pathologist must be wary of misinterpreting these appearances as invasive carcinoma.

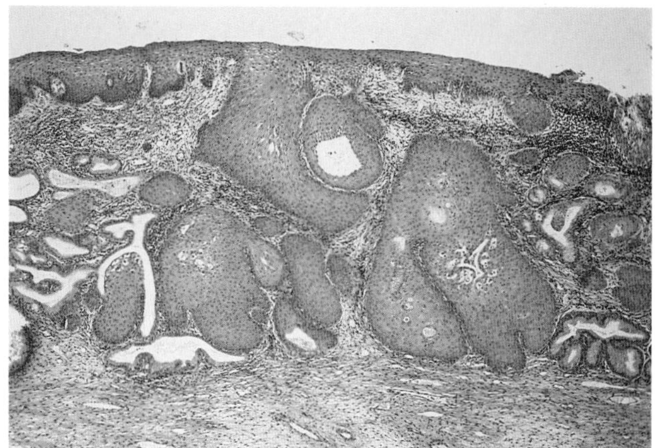

Fig. 1.35 Squamous metaplasia, involving gland crypts.

This misdiagnosis may be avoided by looking at the cell detail of both the overlying epithelium and the apparent invasive islands.

NATURAL HISTORY OF METAPLASIA

In the cervix, squamous metaplasia is an irreversible process: columnar epithelium that has been replaced by squamous epithelium cannot revert to columnar. Thus, when the transformation zone recedes into the cervical canal after the menopause (see Fig. 1.28), the epithelium remains squamous. It also seems likely that once the process of transformation has started, the stimulus must be maintained if the process is to continue and be completed. However, it is not always true that the process of squamous metaplasia, once started, progresses rapidly and inexorably to completion. If the stimulus is withdrawn, for instance by a reversed cervical eversion or reduced acidity of the upper vagina, the metaplastic process may be arrested at any stage. Equally, if the stimulus recurs, progression towards a mature squamous epithelium may recommence.

Furthermore, squamous metaplasia may progress at varying rates in different areas of the same cervix, perhaps reflecting a range of degrees of protection that the cervical mucus offers the epithelium. It is, therefore, very common to observe areas of widely differing maturity in the metaplastic squamous epithelium within the transformation zone.

CONGENITAL TRANSFORMATION ZONE

Histological appearances

The congenital transformation zone (CTZ) is confusing to pathologists as well as to colposcopists. It is poorly understood and not always recognized. The condition is not at all rare, and has been seen in approximately 5% of all women examined at the Colposcopy Clinic of the Samaritan Hospital, London.

The congenital transformation zone is a variant of squamous metaplasia, and has many histological features in common with the latter. Maturation of the squamous epithelium is not fully completed, and typically the congenital transformation zone shows a disorder of maturation that combines excessive maturation on the surface, as exemplified by keratinization, with delayed, incomplete maturation of the deeper layers. These deeper layers show the same features as squamous metaplasia; the nuclei are large but regular, with prominent nucleoli. There is little pleomorphism, and mitotic figures are infrequent. Rapid maturation may occur within the course of the thickness of three or four cells.

Hyperkeratosis or parakeratosis (layers of keratinized cells with retained, although pyknotic, nuclei) is very often present on the epithelial surface. When this layer is thick, it corresponds to leucoplakia which is one of the characteristic colposcopic features of the congenital transformation zone (see Chapter 7).

The most striking histological feature of the congenital transformation zone is the irregularity of the lower margin, the epithelial/stromal junction, which is always dentate, with apparent incursions of squamous epithelium into the stroma (Fig. 1.36). Very often, the tips of these processes appear to be separated from the overlying epithelium, giving the impression of invasive buds. This impression may be further heightened when the centre of the process undergoes differentiation, so that a whorl of keratin is seen in the centre (Fig. 1.37). Careful attention to the cytological details of the section will show that the congenital transformation zone is not an invasive neoplasm.

Cytologically, cells arising from an area of congenital transformation zone will, in general, be indistinguishable from cells arising from the typical transformation zone. However, personal observation (A.R.M.) has led to a belief that, occasionally, cells from an area of immature congenital transformation zone may show exaggerated nuclear features, with very coarsely clumped and densely stained chromatin. Therefore, a differential diagnosis between immature metaplastic cells and cervical intraepithelial neoplasia may be difficult.

HISTOGENESIS

The colposcopic and histological appearance of the congenital transformation zone are the same as some of those seen in diethylstilboestrol exposure *in utero* (see Chapter 20), and it is possible that the mechanism of development of both conditions is similar in some respects.

During embryogenesis, the cuboidal epithelium of the canalized vaginal anlage is replaced by squamous

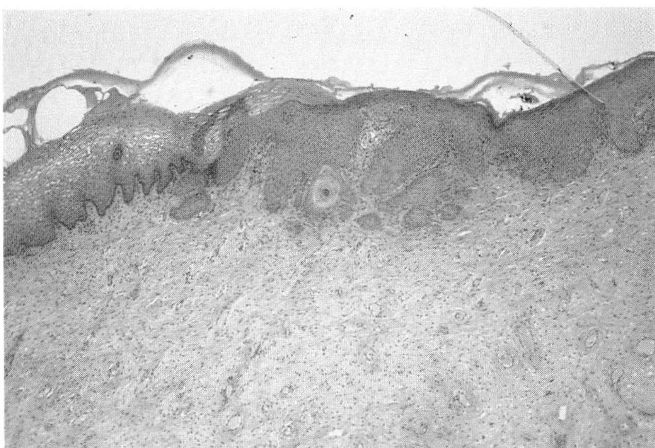

Fig. 1.36 Congenital transformation zone. Normal, original squamous epithelium is present on the left.

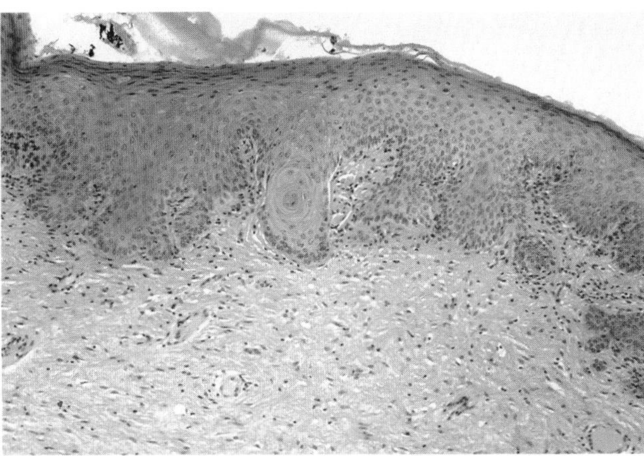

Fig. 1.37 Congenital transformation zone. Keratinization is seen in the centre of one of the 'processes'.

epithelium, a process that is thought to start at the caudal end of the urogenital sinus. This process would normally reach completion, so that the entire length of the vagina and ectocervix becomes covered by squamous epithelium well before the time of birth. If, however, the upward conversion of cuboidal to squamous epithelium happens to be arrested, then some cuboidal epithelium will remain. This epithelium may undergo squamous conversion later in intrauterine life, and perhaps even after birth. The line of demarcation between congenital transformation zone and original squamous epithelium is the point at which normal squamous development stopped, and therefore the congenital transformation zone is believed to be the result of this delayed squamous change.

The difficulty with this theory of histogenesis is that it does not justify the spiky lower margin of the epithelium, which can only be explained as a replacement of superficial gland crypts by metaplastic cells of the congenital transformation zone, but remnants of these gland crypts are not seen. More work is needed to elucidate fully the origin of the congenital transformation zone.

NATURAL HISTORY OF THE CONGENITAL TRANSFORMATION ZONE

The morphological appearances of the congenital transformation zone through the microscope suggest that it is more closely related to squamous metaplasia than to cervical intraepithelial neoplasia, although the colposcopic features have much in common with the latter (see Chapter 7). However, observation of women with areas of untreated congenital transformation zone has shown no propensity to malignant change over several years of follow-up. The finding of a diploid chromosome content by microdensitometry provides further support for the suggestion that the condition has no malignant potential. Gradual maturation of the epithelium is expected over the years, with increased glycogenation.

2. *Cervical intraepithelial neoplasia*

NOMENCLATURE

For many years, the premalignant changes of the cervical epithelium were known as the dysplasias and carcinoma *in situ* (CIS). The definitions of these abnormalities were not precise, and left much to the interpreter. Carcinoma *in situ* was defined as 'a lesion in which all or most of the epithelium shows the cellular features of carcinoma', whereas dysplasia was 'all other disturbances of differentiation of squamous epithelium, of lesser degree than carcinoma *in situ*'.

The chief disadvantage of the dual dysplasia/CIS terminology was that it suggested a distinction between the dysplasias, which were often considered to be benign epithelial changes, and carcinoma *in situ*, the name of which implied significant malignant potential, if not actual malignancy.

These imprecise definitions allowed histopathologists to exercise considerable flexibility in interpreting epithelial changes. For instance, epithelium showing differentiation and stratification (suggesting a diagnosis of dysplasia) may also show a marked degree of nuclear abnormality, leading to its wrong allocation to the category of carcinoma *in situ*.

This looseness of interpretation worsened the imprecision and subjectivity in reporting cervical epithelial abnormalities. When this approach by pathologists was superimposed on a clinical approach whereby carcinoma *in situ* was sometimes overtreated and dysplasia was in some cases inadequately treated, it became apparent that a rather unsatisfactory situation existed which allowed the vague histological concepts of the disease to be compounded by imprecise clinical management protocols.

Over the last three decades, it has become clear that the range of intraepithelial abnormalities of the cervix belongs to one disease process, the components of which vary in degree. 'Cervical intraepithelial neoplasia' (CIN) was suggested as the term appropriate to this spectrum of disease, and it is now being used increasingly. However, practitioners have to be familiar with both systems of nomenclature as occasionally the dysplasia/carcinoma *in situ* terminology is still used.

The concept of cervical intraepithelial neoplasia proposes that all degrees of abnormality should be given the same name, as part of a continuous spectrum of disease, so that the mildest form of cervical intraepithelial neoplasia is equivalent to mild dysplasia, and the most abnormal forms are the same as carcinoma *in situ* (Table 2.1). CIN 3 includes both severe dysplasia and carcinoma *in situ*; this point is important in that it recognizes the lack of actual difference between severe dysplasia and carcinoma *in situ*, which relieves the histopathologist of the problem of distinguishing between them.

Table 2.1 Correlation between cervical intraepithelial neoplasia and dysplasia/carcinoma *in situ*

CIN 1	CIN 2	CIN 3	
Mild dysplasia	Moderate dysplasia	Severe dysplasia	Carcinoma *in situ*

The arguments in favour of the 'cervical intraepithelial neoplasia' terminology are:

1. The unitary terminology is in accord with the modern management approach, whereby cervical intraepithelial neoplasia is regarded as one disease.
2. It is more readily reconcilable with what is known of the nature and natural history of the disease.
3. It recognizes that some of the mildest forms of cervical intraepithelial neoplasia constitute one end of the spectrum which may lead to invasive carcinoma, so that they may be dealt with accordingly.

On the other hand, critics of the 'cervical intraepithelial neoplasia' terminology have claimed that the labelling of very minor, often reversible, and perhaps reactive changes as neoplastic, increases the chances of dealing with them too radically. An understanding of the histopathology of the conditions concerned, together with an appreciation of the guidelines for treatment laid out in this book, should minimize this difficulty.

Approaches to the histological classification of intraepithelial neoplasia that closely parallel the Bethesda cytological classification have been proposed on the basis that subdivision into three categories is artificial. It has been proposed that cervical intraepithelial neoplasia should be split into two categories only: low-grade and high-grade lesions.

Richart (1990) suggests that the conceptual breakpoint should come between those minor lesions that have no evidence of aneuploidy and are associated with a heterogeneous group of human papillomavirus types, and those that have abnormal mitotic figures, indicating aneuploidy, and contain high and intermediate risk human papillomavirus types.

The latter group of lesions (CIN 2 and CIN 3) are considered to be precursors of invasive carcinoma, whereas the former (CIN 1 with human papillomavirus-related changes) has an unpredictable outcome.

This view is a restatement of the long-accepted, pragmatic approach to the subdivision of cervical intraepithelial neoplasia into those lesions that have a high risk of progression to invasion, and those that have an apparently low risk. This can be linked to a sensible approach to treatment.

However, as with cytology, there remains a dividing line between the low-grade and high-grade lesions; therefore, no matter how attractive this concept may seem in theory, practical difficulties will persist in determining the borderline and in allocating lesions that fall near the borderline.

Moreover, the value of an approach that relies, even partly, on the presence and type of human papillomavirus infection is questionable.

HISTOLOGY

Diagnosis

The histopathologist has to make the decision whether or not the epithelium in a cervical biopsy shows cervical intraepithelial neoplasia and, if so, its degree. The histological features used to establish the diagnosis are listed in Table 2.2.

Table 2.2 Histological features of CIN

1 Differentiation, maturation, stratification
- a) Present or absent
- b) Proportion of the thickness of epithelium showing differentiation

2 Nuclear abnormalities
- a) Increased nuclear cytoplasmic ratio
- b) Hyperchromasia
- c) Nuclear pleomorphism
- d) Anisokaryosis

3 Mitotic activity
- a) Number of mitotic figures
- b) Height in epithelium
- c) Abnormal configurations

STRATIFICATION, DIFFERENTIATION AND MATURATION

The meaning of each of these closely related terms has been discussed in Chapter 1. Two aspects are taken into account when assessing a case of cervical intraepithelial neoplasia. First, it should be readily apparent whether or not there is any maturation and stratification. This used to be the main criterion for distinguishing carcinoma *in situ* from severe dysplasia: if no maturation was seen, then the lesion was carcinoma *in situ*, whereas the presence of differentiation indicated a diagnosis of severe dysplasia, a distinction that does not currently seem relevant.

Secondly, the proportion of thickness of epithelium showing maturation and differentiation can be used as a measure of severity in a case of cervical intraepithelial neoplasia. If epithelial cells begin to differentiate, with associated maturation and resultant stratification in the basal quarter of the epithelium, the degree of abnormality is likely to be less severe than where this change is not apparent until the superficial quarter of the epithelium is reached.

In other words, the more severe degrees of cervical intraepithelial neoplasia are likely to have a greater proportion of the thickness of epithelium composed of undifferentiated cells, with only a narrow or non-existent layer of mature, differentiated cells on the surface. However, this is only one of a number of relevant criteria, and should not be taken as the sole criterion, or indeed as the most important one.

NUCLEAR ABNORMALITIES

These are the familiar cytological features that are applied in the diagnosis of dyskaryosis in cervical smears. Increased nuclear cytoplasmic ratio, hyperchromasia, nuclear pleomorphism and variation in nuclear size (anisokaryosis) are all very important features to be taken into account when abnormal epithelium is being assessed.

Enlargement and irregularity of the nuclei are related to the chromosomal abnormalities that have so often been described in cervical intraepithelial neoplasia, although it would seem hazardous to attempt to distinguish between aneuploidy and polyploidy in ordinary histological preparations.

In general terms, there is good correlation between the proportion of epithelium showing maturation and the degree of nuclear abnormality. However, when there is lack of correlation, the degree of nuclear abnormality should be taken as the more reliable criterion in grading.

A comparison of Figs 2.1 and 2.2 illustrates this dilemma: Fig. 2.1 shows an epithelium which is beginning to mature in its middle third, but the nuclei of the basal third show marked abnormalities. Conversely, Fig. 2.2 illustrates an example where maturation is not seen until the top third of the epithelium is reached, but nuclear atypia is quite mild. The former is the more abnormal epithelium, even though the latter has a greater thickness of undifferentiated cells; both have been designated CIN 2.

MITOTIC ACTIVITY

Mitotic figures are present in normal squamous epithelium of the cervix, but they are infrequent and are seen only in the parabasal layers. In cervical intraepithelial neoplasia, the number of mitotic figures increases, and these may be seen not only in the parabasal zone but also higher up in the epithelium. The height in the epithelium at which mitotic figures are found is generally much the same as the level reached by immature cells; the less differentiation in an epithelium, the higher the level at which mitotic figures are likely to be seen.

This is expected, as both mitotic activity and lack of differentiation are expressions of immaturity of cells. At this point, it should be noted that infection with human papillomavirus can produce several morphological changes in the epithelium (see Chapter 12). One of these changes is an increase in the number of mitotic figures, which may result in attributing an erroneously high grade to a cervical intraepithelial neoplasia.

In addition to the number of mitotic figures and their height in the epithelium, note is also taken of abnormal configurations of mitotic figures. The most common aberration is the three-group metaphase (Fig. 2.3), which is seen when most of the chromosomes line up along the equatorial plane of the cell at metaphase, but small collections of chromosomes are left at the poles of the cells. If mitosis is completed, these non-moving elements will confer an uneven distribution of chromatin to the daughter cells. This could be a mechanism by which aneuploidy is perpetuated in an abnormal epithelium. Less common than the three-group metaphase are mitotic figures with more than two spindles, such as the triaster (Fig. 2.4) and quadraster mitotic figures. Other rare forms may also be encountered.

Keratinization

Keratinization may be seen on the surface of cervical intraepithelial neoplasia. It is most frequently found in CIN 3 (Fig. 2.5), but may also sometimes occur with minor forms of cervical intraepithelial neoplasia, the congenital transformation zone and even otherwise normal metaplastic epithelium.

Colposcopically, keratinized epithelium will be

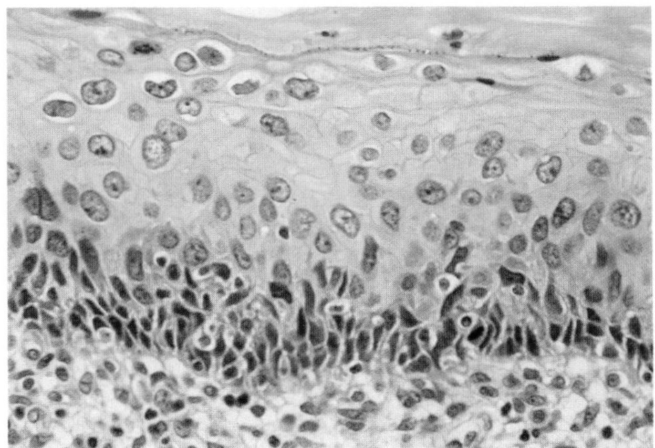

Fig. 2.1 CIN 2. This is an unusual appearance, as the nuclear changes in the basal three or four layers of cells are quite marked. On the other hand, maturation is well developed and less than one-third of the epithelium is showing severe abnormalities. An argument could be made for designating this a CIN 3, on the basis of the abnormalities of the basal layers.

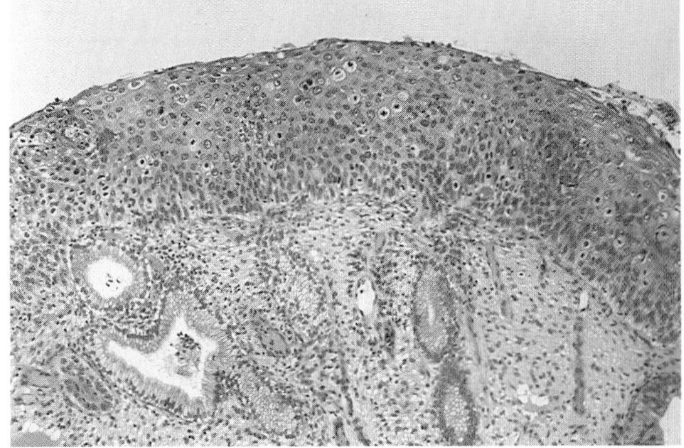

Fig. 2.2 CIN 2. Mitotic figures are quite frequent, and one is seen in the upper half of the epithelium. Nevertheless, the uniformity of nuclei and good maturation justify calling this lesion CIN 2 rather than CIN 3.

seen as leucoplakia; it should be borne in mind that an invasive carcinoma may be hidden under an area of leucoplakia.

GRADING OF CERVICAL INTRAEPITHELIAL NEOPLASIA

Grading may be characterized as follows, taking into account the histological features described above.

CIN 1

There is usually good maturation. Nuclear abnormalities are present, although of minimal degree. These are mainly confined to the deeper layers of the epithelium, but some nuclear abnormalities persist at the surface; if this were not so, cytological recognition of CIN 1 would not be possible. Mitotic figures are present, but not numerous, and do not show abnormal configurations (Fig. 2.6).

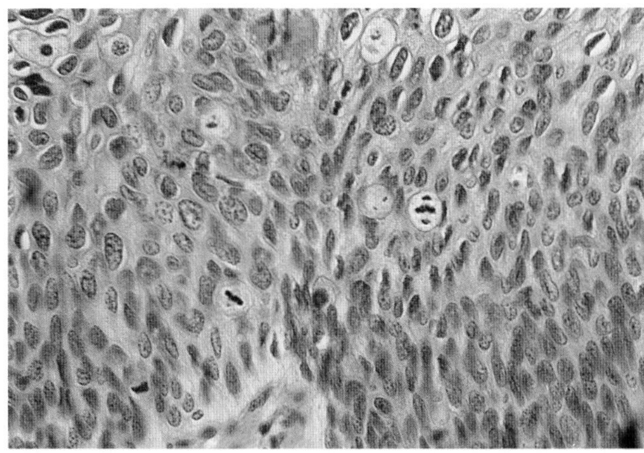

Fig. 2.3 Abnormal mitotic figure; three-group metaphase. The mitotic figure on the left has most of its chromatin at the equatorial plane, but two smaller clumps are present at either end and have not migrated. The mitotic figure on the right is normal.

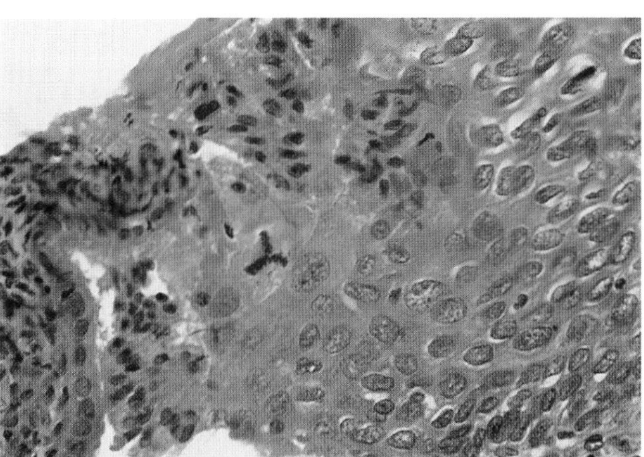

Fig. 2.4 Abnormal tripolar mitotic figure. Three spindles have formed, instead of the normal two.

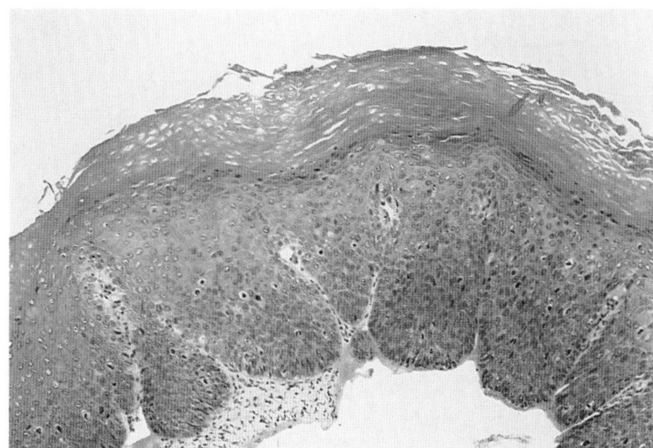

Fig. 2.5 Keratosis on CIN 3. This thick layer of keratin is very obvious colposcopically as leucoplakia. The granular layer is also prominent (see Fig. 8.7, page 93).

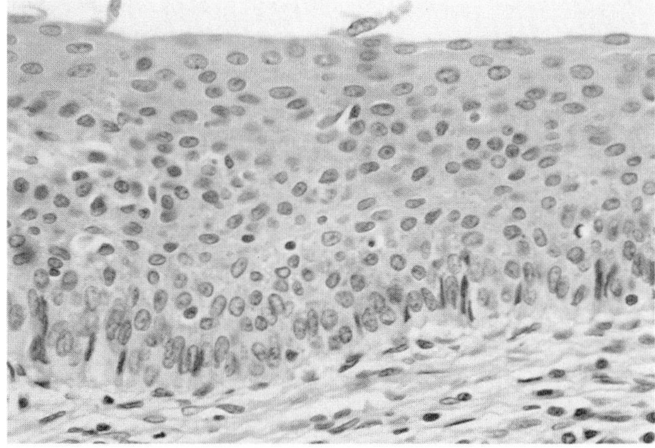

Fig. 2.6 CIN 1. Slight nuclear abnormalities with little pleomorphism and hyperchromasia are seen. Enlarged nuclei persist to the surface, and maturation is obvious.

CIN 2

Maturation is present in the upper half of the epithelium, again with some nuclear atypia persisting at the surface. Nuclear abnormalities are more marked and extend higher in the epithelium than those of CIN 1 (Fig. 2.7). Abnormal mitotic figures may be seen, and these may be present throughout the basal half of the epithelium (Figs 2.8 and 2.9; see also Figs 2.1 and 2.2).

CIN 3

Differentiation and stratification may be completely absent, or present only in the superficial quarter of the epithelium. Nuclear abnormalities may extend through the entire thickness of the epithelium, and are more marked in degree than in CIN 1 and CIN 2 (Fig. 2.10). Mitotic figures may be numerous, and abnormal forms are frequent (Figs 2.11–2.16).

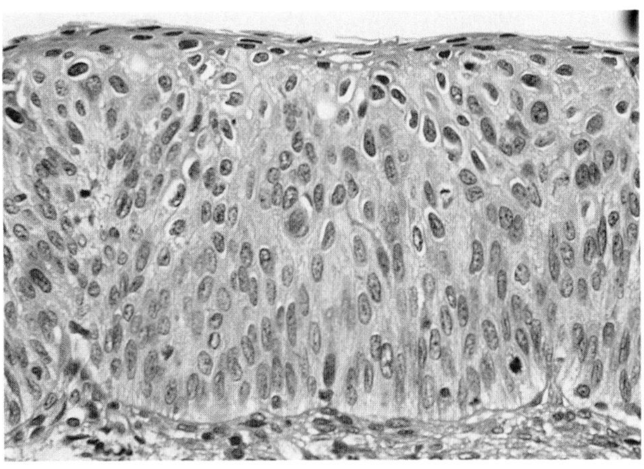

Fig. 2.7 CIN 2. Nuclear crowding is moderate in the basal part of the epithelium. Cytoplasm increases in amount as the surface is reached. A few cells show koilocytic change.

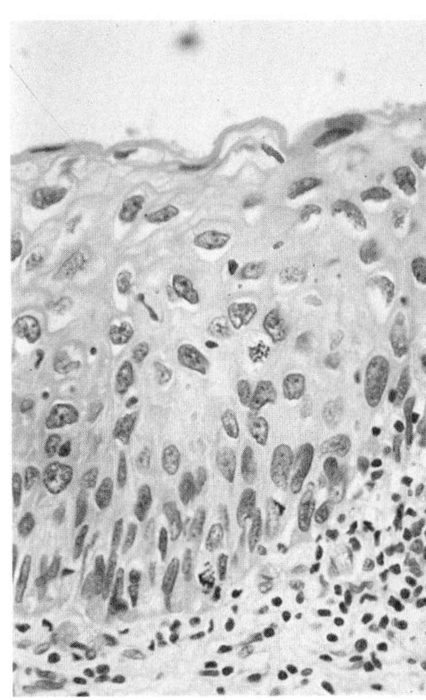

Fig. 2.8 CIN 1–2. Nuclear pleomorphism is apparent, and a mitotic figure is seen halfway up the epithelium. There is abundant cytoplasm in most cells, and maturation is good. As cervical intraepithelial neoplasia is a spectrum, it is quite legitimate to refer to intermediate forms, such as CIN 1–2 or CIN 2–3.

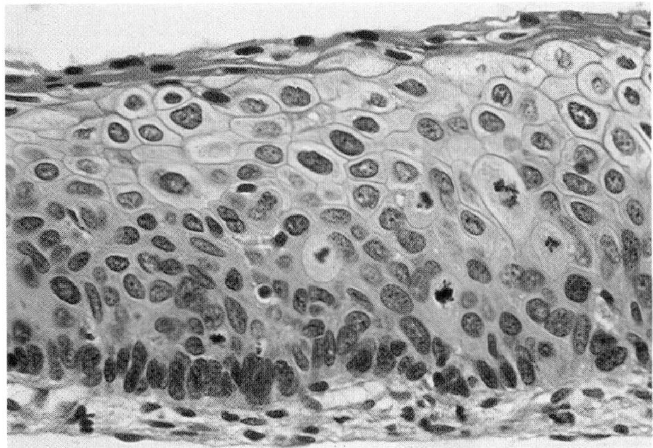

Fig. 2.9 CIN 2–3. Mitotic figures are numerous, two being seen halfway up the epithelium. Very good maturation is present on the surface.

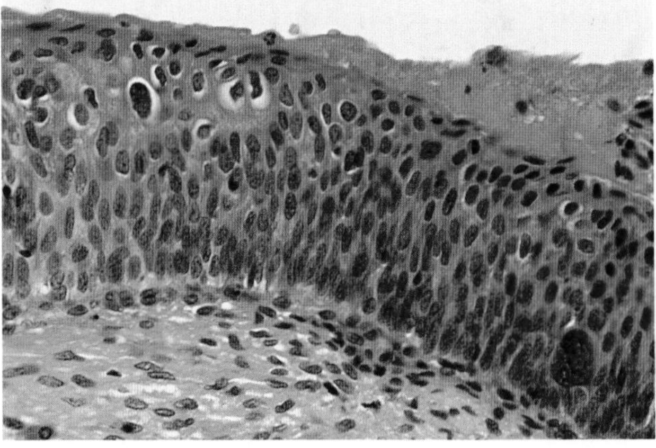

Fig. 2.10 CIN 3. On the right side of the field, there is marked nuclear enlargement with crowding and one giant nucleus. There is some surface maturation. The maturation is better on the left, and some of the more superficial cells show koilocytic change.

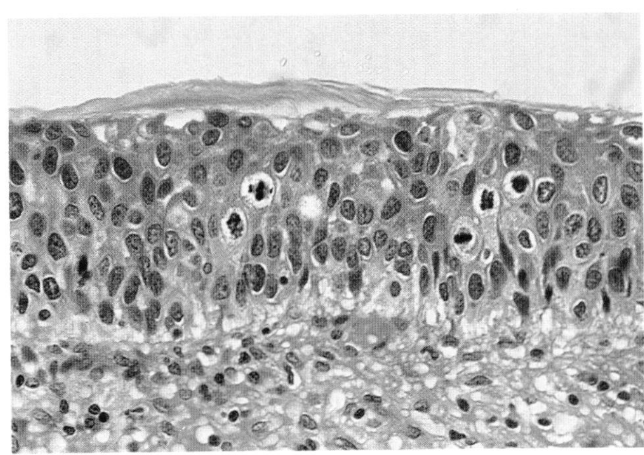

Fig. 2.11 CIN 3. A fairly thin epithelium, showing almost full-thickness loss of differentiation. Mitotic figures are very prominent, several being abnormal. Even so, most cells have a fair amount of cytoplasm.

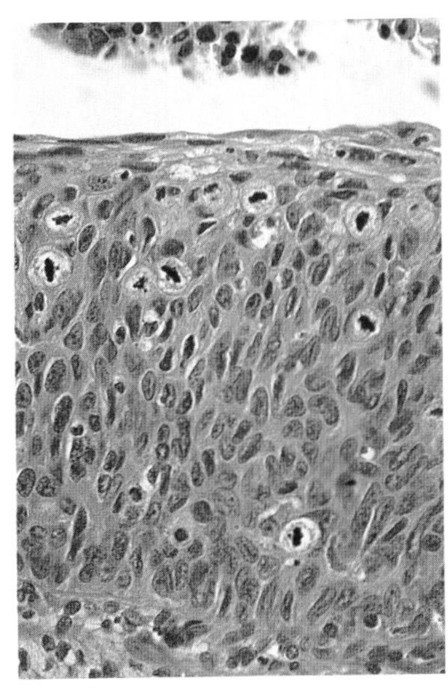

Fig. 2.12 CIN 3. Many mitotic figures are distributed throughout the thickness of the epithelium.

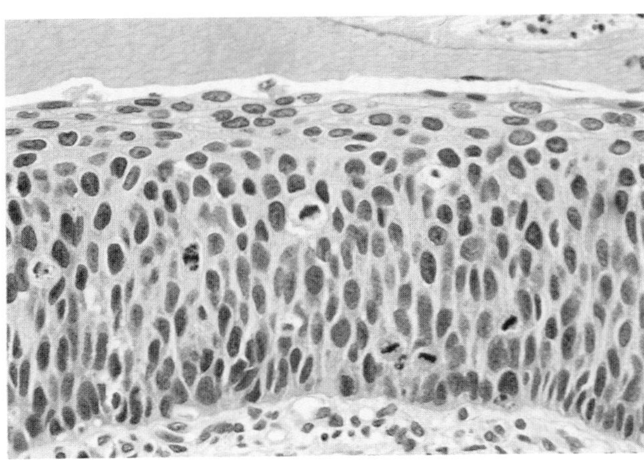

Fig. 2.13 CIN 3. Stratification is seen in one to four or five layers of cells. Nuclear abnormalities are striking.

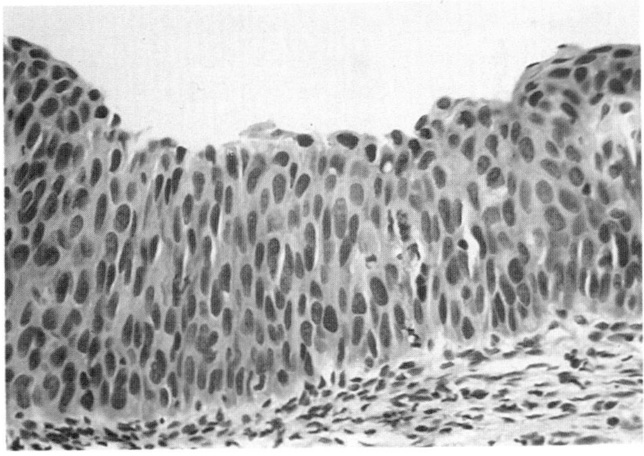

Fig. 2.14 CIN 3. There is virtually no surface maturation or stratification. Mitotic figures are sparse.

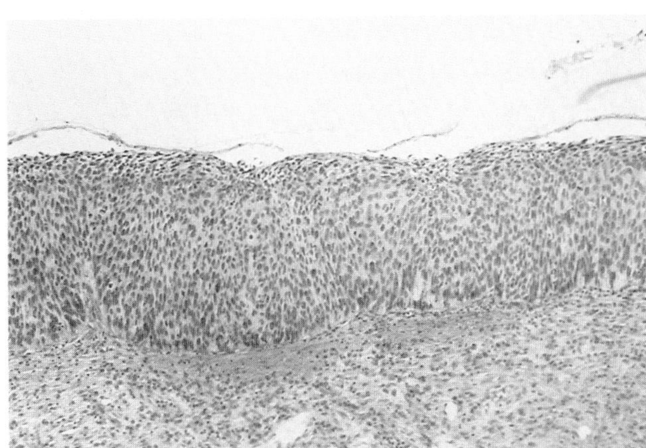

Fig. 2.15 CIN 3. A partially thick example, up to 40 cells thick in places.

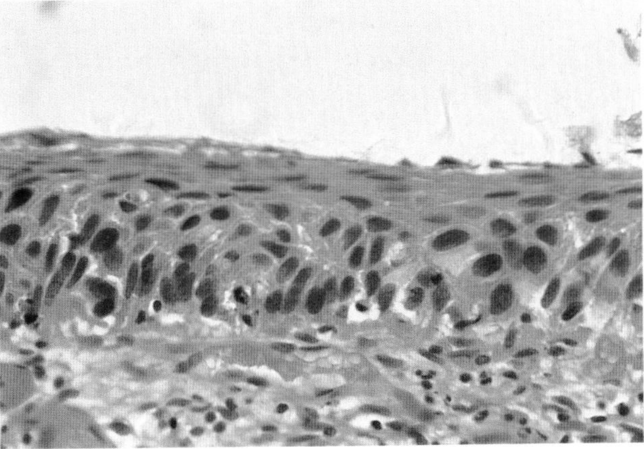

Fig. 2.16 CIN 3. In contrast to Fig. 2.15, this is a remarkably thin epithelium, but the nuclear pleomorphism and hyperchromasia justify the diagnosis of CIN 3.

Subjectivity of diagnosis

The diagnosis and grading of cervical intraepithelial neoplasia are made on a combination of apparently distinct, but often interrelated, morphological criteria. Many of these are features that vary in degree, in quantitative terms, but not in a way that can be precisely measured; their interpretation, therefore, is largely subjective and a matter of opinion.

Furthermore, these criteria have to be applied with different priority to different examples of cervical intraepithelial neoplasia: one example may show numerous mitotic figures, with many abnormal forms but little nuclear abnormality. Another example may show few mitotic figures, but striking nuclear pleomorphism and hyperchromasia. Both are examples of CIN 3, but in each one the morphological criteria have to be applied in slightly different ways.

This introduces further subjectivity into the histological interpretation of cervical intraepithelial neoplasia, so much so that a lesion described by one pathologist as CIN 1 may be diagnosed by another as CIN 3. To make matters worse, it has been demonstrated that even the same pathologist may interpret a slide of cervical intraepithelial neoplasia differently on separate occasions.

These inconsistencies further support the concept of cervical intraepithelial neoplasia as one disease, which is irreconcilable with subdivisions, and the allocation of grades is fraught with exactly the same difficulties that were encountered with the dysplasia/carcinoma *in situ* terminology.

CRYPT INVOLVEMENT

Cervical intraepithelial neoplasia develops in the transformation zone, the field of columnar epithelium that undergoes squamous metaplasia. It follows the contours of the original columnar epithelium, and affects gland crypts as well as the surface.

Gland crypt involvement by cervical intraepithelial neoplasia is often recognizable at colposcopy, and is usually obvious in histological sections (Figs 2.17 and 2.18). In a study of 354 cone biopsies of women with CIN 3, it was found that 88.6% had some degree of crypt involvement. The mean depth of crypt involvement was 1.24 mm, and the mean plus 3 standard deviations (99.7% of the population under study) was 3.8 mm. The latter figure is the depth of tissue that must be consistently and effectively removed for adequate treatment of cervical intraepithelial neoplasia by any method.

Other studies have shown that the depth of crypt involvement increases as cervical intraepithelial neoplasia becomes more severe, as does the size of the area affected by it.

Diagnosis

It is important that crypt involvement is correctly diagnosed and not misinterpreted as invasive carcinoma. Features that help the histopathologist to recognize crypt involvement and distinguish it from invasion are as follows:

1. Crypt involvement occurs in the area where the crypts are found, so that normal or partially

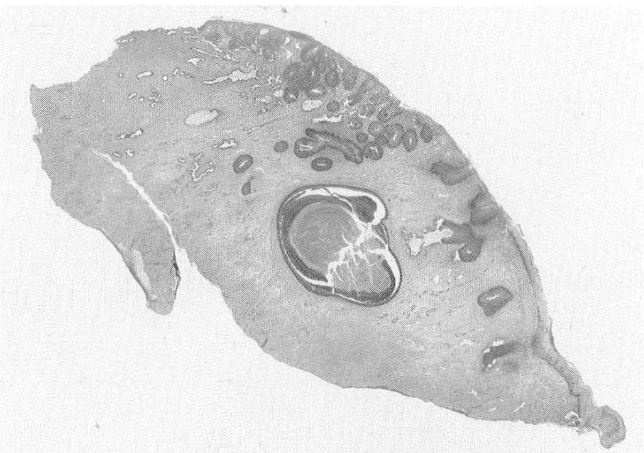

Fig. 2.17 Crypt involvement by cervical intraepithelial neoplasia. This a mounted section from a cone biopsy. Very extensive crypt involvement is present; there is no invasion. The dilated crypt is lined by CIN 3 and, at its deepest point, this cervical intraepithelial neoplasia is just over 6 mm from the surface epithelium in the canal.

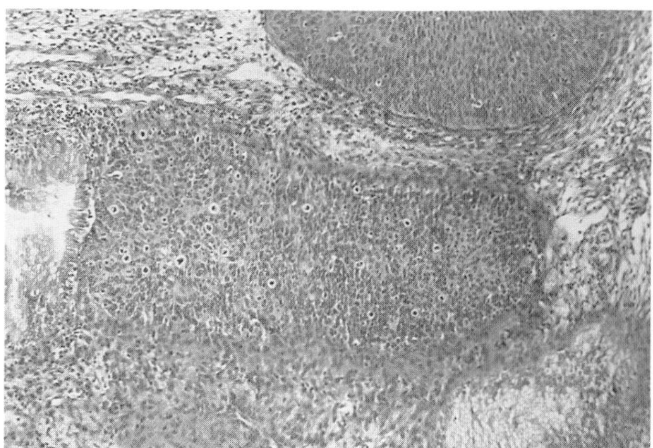

Fig. 2.18 Crypt involvement by cervical intraepithelial neoplasia. The crypt occupying the centre of the field has been cut off-centre, resulting in a non-apparent lumen. Because all the cells are fairly close to the basement membrane, there may be an impression that this epithelial abnormality is more severe than it really is.

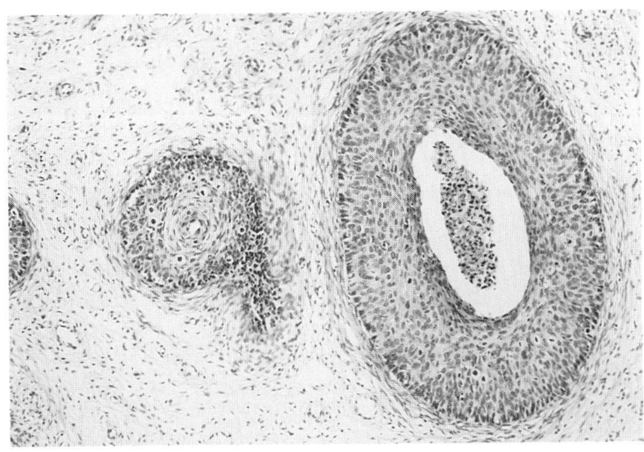

Fig. 2.19 Crypt involvement by cervical intraepithelial neoplasia. The smaller of these two crypts appears to have a spiky projection arising from it, giving the impression of early invasion. However, there is no stromal reaction at this point, and the cells have not changed in morphological appearance. This is an oblique cut of a smaller branch of the crypt.

affected crypts are often seen alongside crypts in which the columnar epithelium is entirely replaced by cervical intraepithelial neoplasia (see Fig. 2.17).

2. Involved crypts have a smooth outline and are surrounded by a basement membrane. Around them, the stroma may show some circumferential thickening of the fibrous tissue.
3. Cells of cervical intraepithelial neoplasia occupying the crypts have the same morphological appearances as cells of the overlying epithelium. This feature may not be obvious if the crypt is cut off-centre, or if the intraepithelial neoplasia completely fills the crypt; in this case, the abnormal epithelium does not have a surface, so maturation appears to be less than that on the surface (see Fig. 2.18). On the other hand, invasive carcinoma, particularly in the early stages, is frequently composed of cells that are better differentiated than those of the intraepithelial neoplasia from which it arises (a finding which is discussed in detail in Chapter 10). Thus, a focus of cells with more abundant eosinophilic cytoplasm is a useful clue to the possibility of invasion.
4. The stroma surrounding a focus of microinvasion often shows a reaction to the infiltrating tumour. There may be an increase in the content of lymphocytes locally, or loosening of the stroma; often, both features are seen together. The stroma around areas of crypt involvement by cervical intraepithelial neoplasia is similar to that under the neoplasia at the surface; if lymphocytes are present, as they very frequently are beneath the neoplasia, then the infiltrate is fairly uniform, and not focused on one or two particular points.

Attention to these points helps to distinguish between crypt involvement by cervical intraepithelial neoplasia and early invasion. However, even to the experienced pathologist this distinction remains a constant problem. Oblique cuts of involved crypts can be very difficult indeed to distinguish from invasion (Fig. 2.19).

Further difficulty is caused by the fact that invasion may sometimes take place by means of rounded islands of infiltrating carcinoma, apparently surrounded by basement membrane.

CYTOLOGY

The confusing and controversial situation concerning the nomenclature of intraepithelial abnormalities, coupled with varying opinions of interpretation among histopathologists, as discussed above, can create difficulties in cytological classification and interpretation.

Cytology is the vital link between clinician and patient; it is the initial indication that all is not well, and that further investigation may be necessary. The clinician therefore relies on the cytologist to give an assessment that is as accurate as possible of the type and degree of abnormality, in a clear and concise report. This will enable the clinician to decide on the course of management, and to advise the patient accordingly. Reassurance and a repeat smear after a specified interval may be all that is necessary, or a more thorough explanation and referral for colposcopy with a view to treatment may be indicated.

Cytological reporting

Various forms of reporting are used, and some of these are shown in Table 2.3.

Most cytologists are aware that a descriptive report using unequivocal terms, together with a recommendation regarding further management, is the type of report most acceptable to clinicians, whether in specialist gynaecological clinics, family planning clinics or general practice. A vague report will convey nothing of real value to the clinician, thus rendering further investigation mandatory, albeit quite unnecessarily in many instances.

Although the 'cervical intraepithelial neoplasia' terminology is used by histopathologists, it is inap-

Table 2.3 Cytological and histological terminology

Histological diagnosis	Normal/benign conditions	BAUS	CIN 1	CIN 2	CIN 3	
	Normal/benign conditions	?Not recognized	Mild dysplasia	Moderate dysplasia	Severe dysplasia	Carcinoma *in situ*
BSCC terminology	Normal/benign conditions including inflammation and repair	Borderline nuclear change	Mild dyskaryosis	Moderate dyskaryosis	Severe dyskaryosis	
Bethesda terminology (cytology)	Normal/benign conditions	ASCUS (includes HPV change)	LSIL	HSIL		
Bethesda terminology (applied to histopathology)	Normal/benign conditions	LSIL (includes HPV change)		HSIL		

BAUS, Basal abnormalities of uncertain significance
CIN, Cervical intraepithelial neoplasia
ASCUS, Atypical squamous cells of undetermined significance
LSIL, Low-grade squamous intraepithelial lesion
HSIL, High-grade squamous intraepithelial lesion
HPV, Human papillomavirus
The divisions indicated by a broken line are poorly defined and do not necessarily correspond from one classification to another

propriate for a cytological approach since cytological criteria must be based on individual cell changes rather than the whole tissue patterns that cervical intraepithelial neoplasia refers to. The term 'dyskaryosis' is, therefore, preferred. For convenience, and to align it as closely as possible with the histological grades, thus facilitating a coherent approach, dyskaryosis is arbitrarily subdivided into mild, moderate and severe degrees. These three grades correlate to the histological grades of CIN 1, CIN 2 and CIN 3 respectively.

The advent of colposcopy, with the resultant availability of histological material from CIN 1 and CIN 2, has enabled the cytologist to compare cytological appearances with histological patterns to an extent that was previously not possible. The cone biopsy was for many years the only treatment for intraepithelial abnormalities, and this procedure was not frequently undertaken until the cellular changes indicated a severe lesion. Although it is often possible for an experienced cytologist to assess a particular degree with accuracy, it would be wrong to suggest that cytology should be used to diagnose the precise degree of cervical intraepithelial neoplasia.

It is important that cytologists exercise some discrimination between the grades of dyskaryosis, because in the UK colposcopy clinics are still expanding to cope with the number of women with abnormal smears who need to be selectively referred, at least initially, for colposcopy.

It is also vital that cytologists understand the nature of an unsatisfactory smear and the importance of reporting it as such, rather than as 'negative' or, worse still, 'showing vague inflammatory change or "irregular" features' (see page 50). These reports do not assist in the management of patients, they erode clinical confidence in the cytologist, and may result in leaving a malignancy unrecognized.

Table 2.4 BSCC terminology guidelines

1 Unsatisfactory for assessment (state reason)	
2 Negative	
3 Nuclear changes bordering on mild dyskaryosis	
4 Dyskaryotic cells:	mild moderate severe
5 Severe dyskaryosis –	some features (specify) suggest the possibility of invasion

The British Society for Clinical Cytology (BSCC) Working Party on Terminology in Gynaecological Cytology addressed these issues in 1986 and recommended a slightly modified approach to terminology (Table 2.4). Some helpful diagnostic features were included with illustrations to assist in categorizing cell change in a consistent way.

Degenerative cell changes associated with inflammation are regarded as insignificant, but, when present, obvious nuclear changes, which may be difficult or impossible to distinguish from dyskaryotic change, are assigned to a 'borderline' category. In many instances the koilocytes associated with human papillomavirus (HPV) infection would fit into the 'nuclear changes bordering on mild dyskaryosis' category, or into dyskaryosis if the nuclear features are consistent with those of dyskaryosis.

Dyskaryosis is separated into mild, moderate and severe. The use of the term 'malignant cells' is not supported because the features associated with invasion are regarded as not sufficiently reliable or readily reproducible, and when an invasive lesion is suspected cytologically it is advised that it should be reported as severe dyskaryosis with some features to suggest that invasion may be present.

Perhaps the most significant feature of the modern terminology is the link with patient management. In 1987 the BSCC published guidelines for linking reports with a recommendation for management, although, of course, the final decision rests with the clinician. This was a courageous and somewhat controversial innovation, but over the years it has been shown to be effective.

All cytology reports should be linked to a recommendation, either for a repeat smear or for colposcopy. The precise protocols for dealing with these recommendations vary and are reviewed from time to time by the National Coordinating Network of the National Health Service Cervical Screening. They help to ensure, for instance, that women who need to be referred for colposcopy are not left for too long, or missed altogether, and that women with minor abnormalities are not unnecessarily referred immediately.

In 1989, the National Cancer Institute also published a statement recommending a new approach to the reporting of cervical and vaginal smears, which has become known as the 'Bethesda classification'. Its development resulted from a perceived need to reclassify the terminology in order to relate it, in a more meaningful way than previously, to patient management.

In addition, it was hoped that a new approach to terminology might improve communication between cytopathologists, as well as between cytopathologists and clinicians. Initial problems resulted in modifications in 1992.

The Bethesda classification discards the Papanicolaou grading system (as does the British Society for Clinical Cytology classification presented above), because it is not related to modern diagnostic cytological practice. It also rejects an association with the CIN terminology, due to its lack of reproducibility between different pathologists, and because it does not offer clear management guidelines.

The Bethesda classification attempts to overcome the shortcomings of other systems of classification, by using a detailed system that may be abbreviated as follows:

1. Within normal limits.
2. Benign cellular change, inflammation and reactive change.
3. Atypical squamous cells of undetermined significance (ASCUS).
4. Low-grade squamous intraepithelial lesion (LSIL).
5. High-grade squamous intraepithelial lesion (HSIL).
6. Glandular cells.
7. Other malignant neoplasms.

Additional comments can be made regarding the presence of human papillomavirus changes (these are put into the low-grade category, even when no features of intraepithelial neoplasia are seen) and the presence or absence of glandular cells, squamous metaplastic cell components.

The main advantage of the original classification in linking the cytological report to a management policy – that lesions reported as being of high grade require colposcopy and treatment, whereas those of low grade may be managed more conservatively – has been lost in the 1992 modification, where the recommendation is not a requirement but is at the discretion of the pathologist.

However, the proposal of this terminology does give the impression of change for its own sake as, whatever system of classification is employed, there will be a need for borderlines to be defined. In this case the breakpoint is between low- and high-grade lesions and little help is given as to how this is identified.

Further criticisms are that the reintroduction of the term 'atypical' seems to be a retrograde step because of its imprecision, and also that the terminology employs what are essentially histological terms; the BSCC believes that cytologists should use cytological terms.

The Bethesda classification has no advantages over the BSCC terminology which has been presented in detail earlier in this chapter. The latter terminology links the cytology report to the management policy for the patient and is more meaningful in practical terms, as well as more flexible in allowing adjustments that may be required to fit in with local considerations.

Furthermore, it fully addresses the dilemmas of persistent minor changes and the unsatisfactory smear. It disregards the inadequate term 'atypical', it uses cytological rather than histological terms, and can be readily adapted to relate to low- and high-risk cellular changes if the point in the spectrum of dyskaryosis at which cellular changes progress from low to high risk can be determined.

CYTOLOGICAL FEATURES

The cytologist relies heavily on individual cell changes for recognizing dyskaryosis and differentiating between degrees of dyskaryosis, in contrast to the histopathologist, who examines the features of the whole tissue and relationships between cells, in addition to cellular detail.

The way that cells are distributed in a cervical smear may bear little relationship to their relative positions *in situ*. However, it is a well-established fact that changes in the cells from the uppermost layers of epithelium do, in the large majority of cases, reflect the overall tissue pattern and degree of cervical intraepithelial neoplasia.

NUCLEAR FEATURES

The nuclear changes in dyskaryosis are summarized in Table 2.5. Nuclear enlargement and chromatin aberration are always present, but not all features are invariably seen.

Table 2.5 Cytological features of dyskaryosis

Nuclear changes
Enlargement
Variation in size and shape
Hyperchromasia
Abnormal appearance and distribution of chromatin
Irregular nuclear outline
Irregular thickening of nuclear membrane
Nucleoli
Mitoses

Cytoplasm
Variable
Indication of degree of dyskaryosis

Nuclear enlargement

This is an essential feature of all dyskaryotic cells. However, not all cells where the nuclear area is much larger than the cytoplasmic area are dyskaryotic; differentiation must be made between dyskaryosis and those cells arising from an area of immature metaplasia (Fig. 2.20) or an atrophic, postmenopausal epithelium (Fig. 2.21).

A postpartum immature pattern can give rise to similar problems of interpretation. However, if due attention is paid to other more diagnostic features misinterpretation should not occur, although immature squamous metaplasia remains the most significant area of cytological misdiagnosis.

Irregular chromatin distribution

This is probably the most important single criterion used in the diagnosis of dyskaryosis (Fig. 2.22). An irregular distribution of chromatin with clumping throughout the nucleus is always present, and very often the nucleus has an irregular shape with indentations and, sometimes, protrusions (Fig. 2.23). Irregular thickening and prominence of the nuclear membrane can also be an important feature (see Fig. 2.23).

Hyperchromasia

Hyperchromasia (increased intensity of staining) is nearly always a prominent feature of dyskaryotic cells. However, it is not an essential feature, and dyskaryotic cells that are not more darkly stained than the normal cells associated with them may be overlooked by the inexperienced and unwary screener.

Mitotic figures

In cytological preparations, mitotic figures are rarely seen, even in CIN 3. This is a finding that lends support to the assumption that only cells from the top layers of epithelium are normally present in most cervical smears. Mitotic figures are, in fact, more frequently seen in association with regenerative changes. It is generally true that the more severe the degree of dyskaryosis, the more pronounced the nuclear features tend to be, although this correlation is not invariable.

Nucleoli

Nucleoli are not an important feature in the identification of dyskaryotic cells, and are virtually never present. Very occasionally small nucleoli may be seen, but these are not a prominent feature of dyskaryosis. Nucleoli are more usually found in regenerative changes.

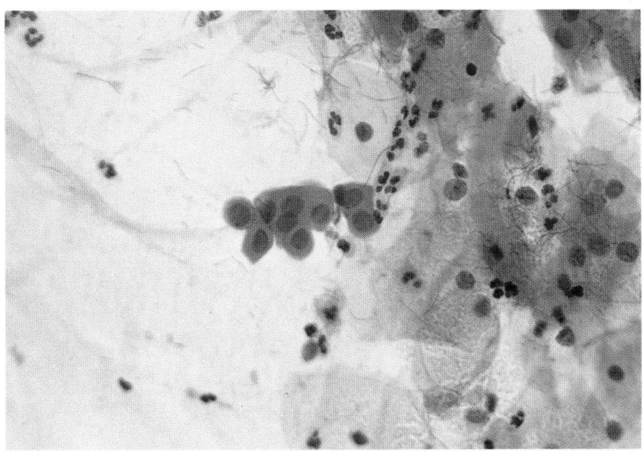

Fig. 2.20 Immature squamous metaplasia. A tight group of cells with enlarged but fairly regular nuclei. Some hyperchromasia is present, but nuclear chromatin is bland and evenly distributed, with regular and even nuclear membranes. The cytoplasm appears thick and homogeneous, with a recognizable squamous shape.

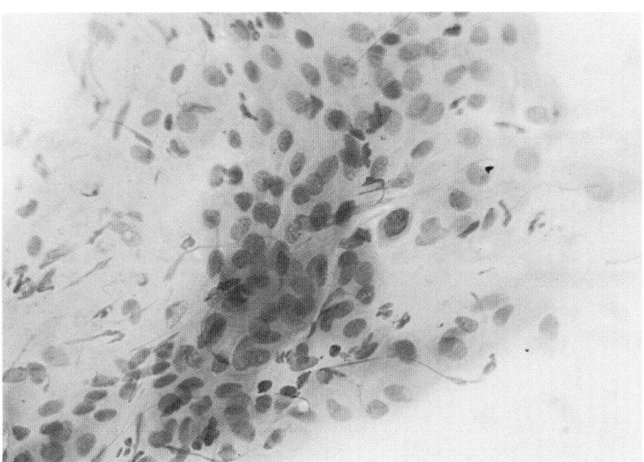

Fig. 2.21 Severe dyskaryosis. A single, severely dyskaryotic cell, although showing hyperchromasia, is easily missed among large numbers of pale-staining, normal parabasal cells in a postmenopausal atrophic pattern.

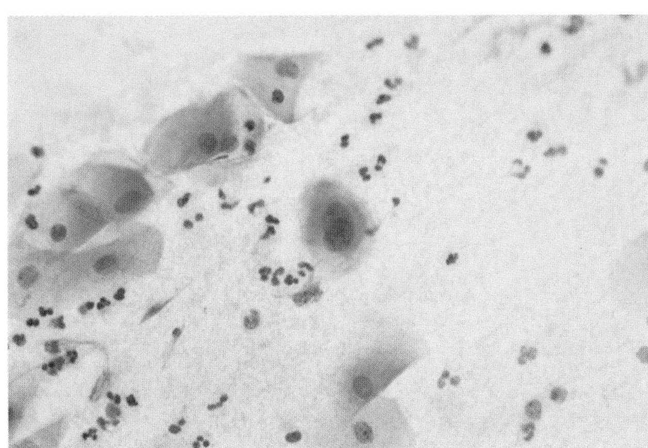

Fig. 2.22 Moderate dyskaryosis. A single binucleate cell, although the nuclei are pale-stained and are not showing hyperchromasia; the chromatin is irregularly distributed, and the nuclei are irregular in shape.

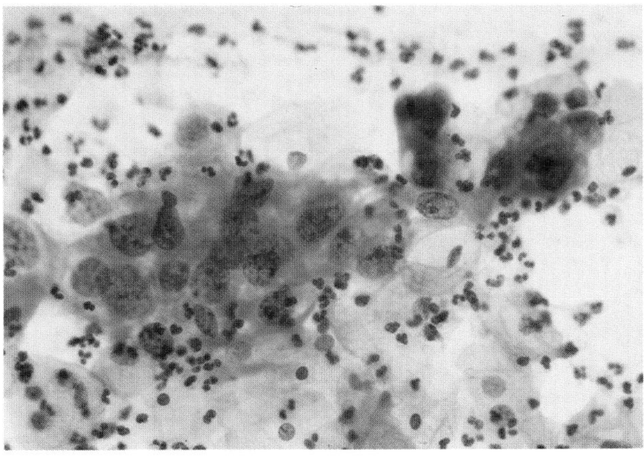

Fig. 2.23 Mild to moderate dyskaryosis. Very large, pale nuclei but irregularly clumped chromatin, variation in size and shape, with irregularly thickened nuclear membranes.

CYTOPLASMIC CHANGES

By themselves, cytoplasmic changes are considerably less important in the identification of dyskaryotic cells than the nuclear changes described above. On the other hand, the amount of cytoplasm in relation to the size of nucleus is one of the most important considerations in assessing the degree of dyskaryosis. The lower the nuclear cytoplasmic ratio, the better differentiated the cell will be, and the milder the degree of dyskaryosis. This implies that individual cell differentiation is suggestive of a better organized and orientated epithelium. On the whole this is true, but there are exceptions.

The staining reaction which results in either acidophilic (pink-staining) or basophilic (blue-staining) cytoplasm may correspond to normal superficial and intermediate cell types, indicating mild or moderate dyskaryosis. However, this should not be regarded as a reliable criterion (Figs 2.24–2.27).

Keratinization

Keratinization of the cytoplasm can be seen in various situations, and cells showing keratinization must be carefully evaluated by close reference to nuclear features. In the context of cervical intraepithelial neoplasia, keratinization can be associated with all degrees of dyskaryosis (Fig 2.28), but it is also an important feature of human papillomavirus infection

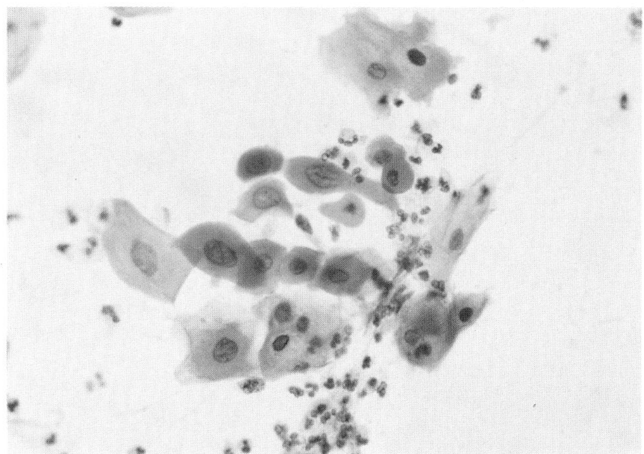

Fig. 2.24 Moderate dyskaryosis. Typical basophilic stained cytoplasm, with enlarged hyperchromatic nuclei showing variation in nuclear size and shape.

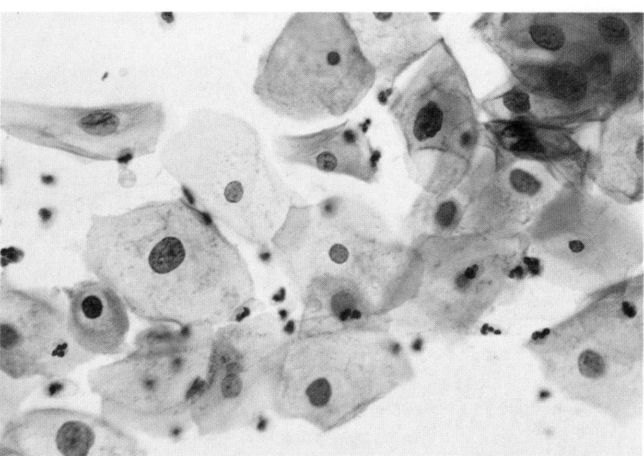

Fig. 2.25 Mild dyskaryosis. Cells are showing typical nuclear features of dyskaryosis, with hyperchromasia and irregular chromatin clumping, enlarged and variously shaped nuclei. The cytoplasm is well defined and ample.

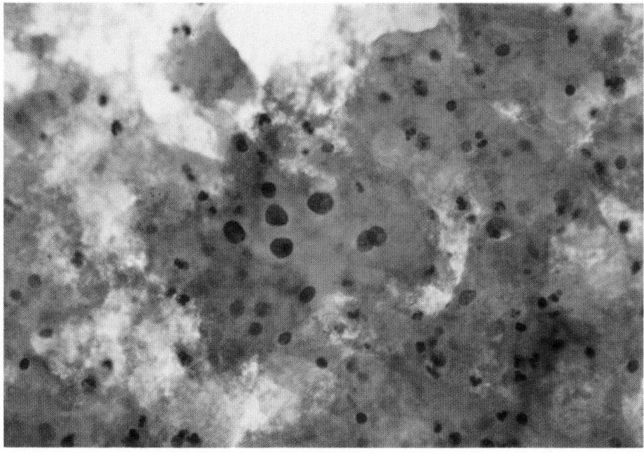

Fig. 2.26 Mild dyskaryosis. Prominent hyperchromatic nuclei, with ill-defined cell borders. The spacing between the nuclei suggests a well-preserved nuclear cytoplasmic ratio consistent with mild dyskaryosis.

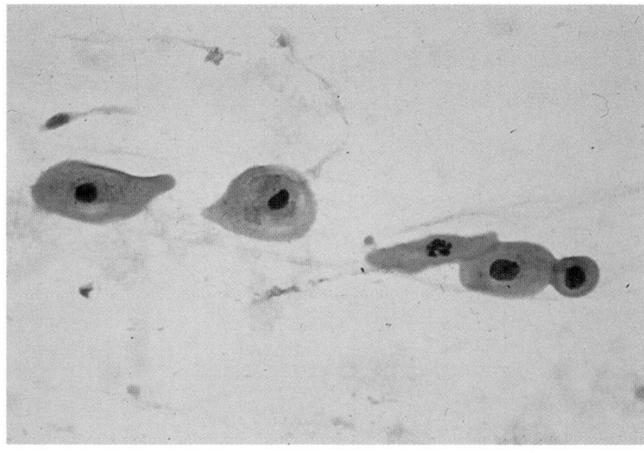

Fig. 2.27 Mild dyskaryosis. Degeneration and karyorrhexis are seen on one cell. The thick, pink-staining cytoplasm suggests maturation, consistent with mild dyskaryosis.

(a) 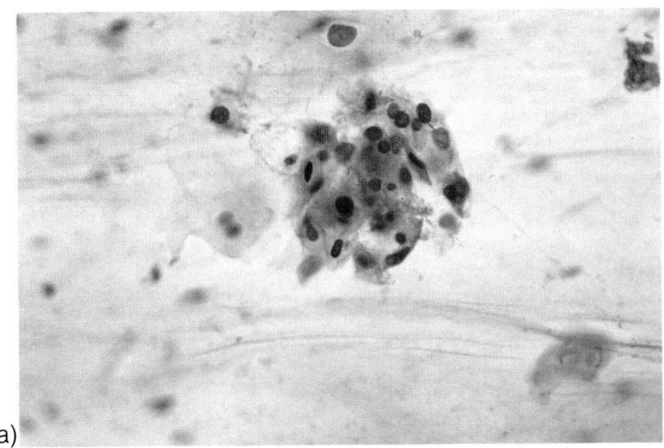

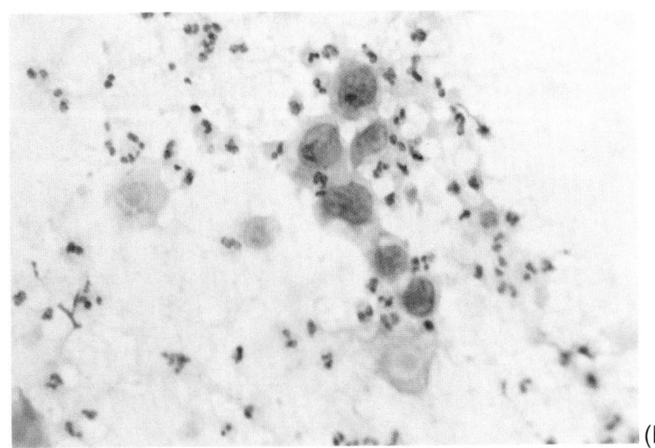 (b)

Fig. 2.28 Severe dyskaryosis with keratinization. (a) Loosely arranged sheets of cells, some with highly keratinized cytoplasm. **(b)** Large, severely dyskaryotic cells, with pale but grossly abnormal nuclei, closely associated with anucleate, keratinized, squamous cells.

which may or may not coexist with all degrees of dyskaryosis. At the other end of the spectrum, atypical keratinization may be found in patients with invasive squamous cell carcinoma; attention to cellular shapes, as well as to the arrangement of plaques and sheets of anucleate keratinized squamous cells, may assist in making a differential diagnosis.

Mixed degrees of dyskaryosis in a smear

Frequently, a cervical smear may contain a mixture of cells showing a variety of degrees of dyskaryosis (Figs 2.29 and 2.30), and a great deal of subjectivity is involved in assessing the overall dyskaryosis of a

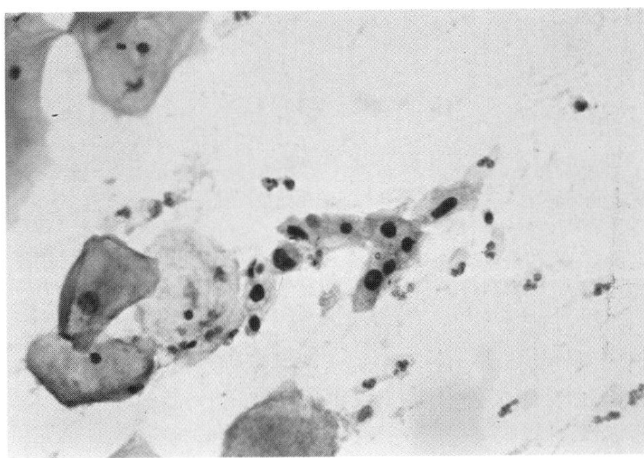

Fig. 2.29 Severe dyskaryosis. The typical, loosely associated sheets of cells are showing severe nuclear features with hyperchromasia, marked variations in size and shape of nuclei, with irregular chromatin pattern and variation in intensity of staining.

(a) 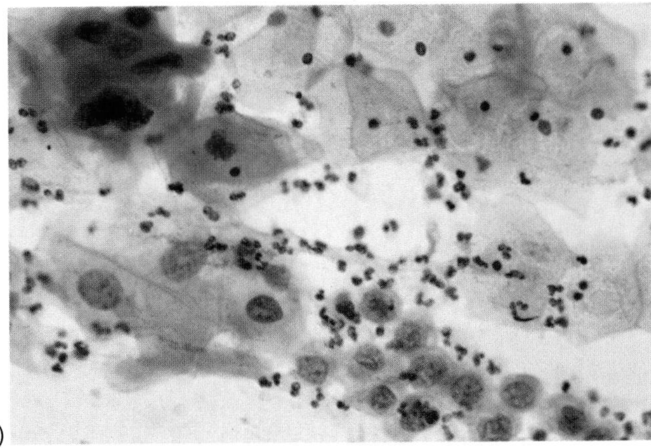

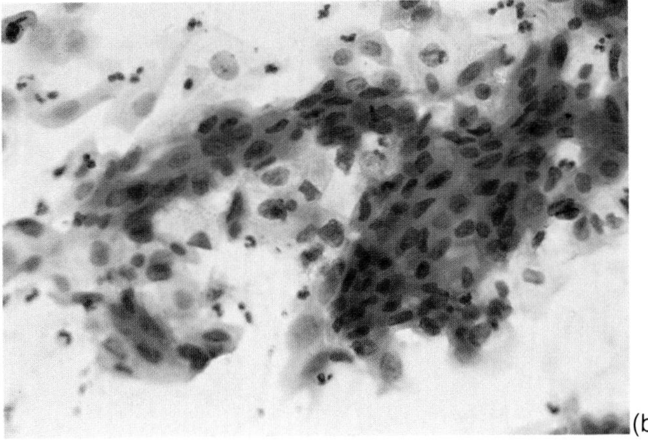 (b)

Fig. 2.30 Moderate and severe dyskaryosis. (a) Note the contrast between the cells at the top left of the field, which show moderate dyskaryosis with hyperchromatic nuclei and darkly stained cytoplasm, and the loose sheet of cells in the bottom right-hand corner, which show severe dyskaryosis with large, pale nuclei but the same degree of pleomorphism. **(b)** Many nuclei appear flattened and elongated, suggesting surface differentiation. Although the nuclei are not round as in most cases, the nuclear features are clearly those of dyskaryosis.

smear. This results in a discrepancy of opinion among cytologists, in the same way that differences of opinion exist among histopathologists.

A smear containing dyskaryotic cells of mainly moderate degree, with only one or two severely dyskaryotic cells, most probably reflects CIN 2. Conversely, if a smear contains the same small number of severely dyskaryotic cells, but none of any other degree of dyskaryosis, it almost certainly reflects CIN 3.

Dyskaryotic cells are often present in loosely associated streaks or small sheets of cells, as well as in large cohesive clumps (Figs 2.31–2.33); the latter appearance is more frequently seen in CIN 3. The quality of the smear in terms of thickness of cell spread, and the presence of physiological or degenerate changes, may also lead to difficulties in interpretation. On occasion, individual dyskaryotic cells may sometimes be seen, and once again it must be emphasized that careful and conscientious screening is of paramount importance if such cells are not to be completely overlooked (see Fig. 2.21; Fig. 2.34).

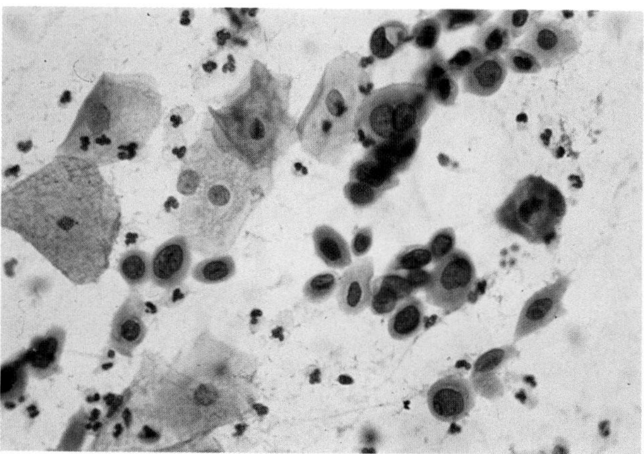

Fig. 2.31 Severe dyskaryosis. The cells are characterized by marked pleomorphism and hyperchromasia.

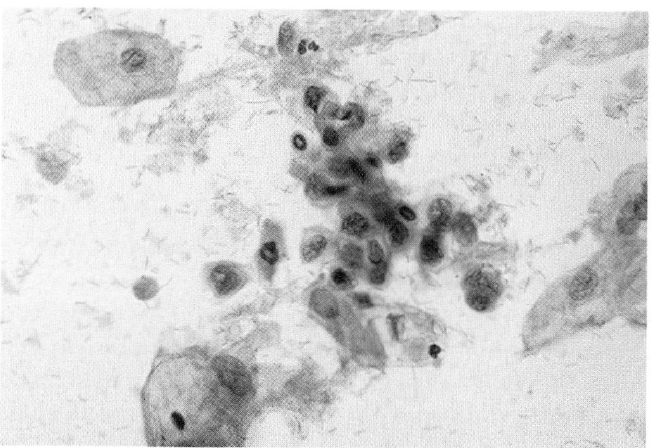

Fig. 2.32 Severe dyskaryosis. Although the dyskaryotic cells can be evaluated and show the features of hyperchromasia and nuclear irregularity, the cytolytic nature of the smear (the result in this case of an exaggerated oral contraceptive effect) makes the background untidy and obscures cellular detail.

(a)

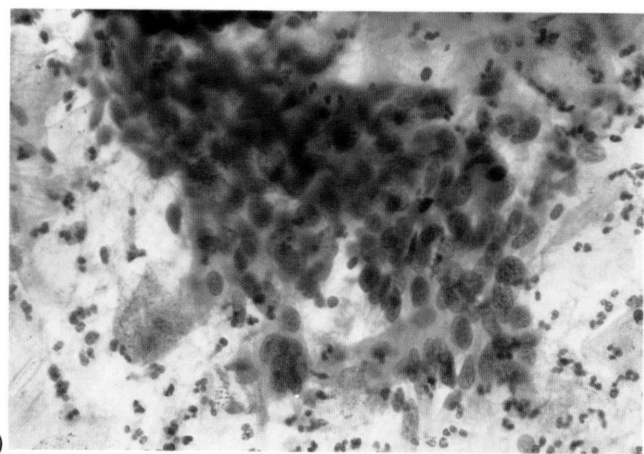

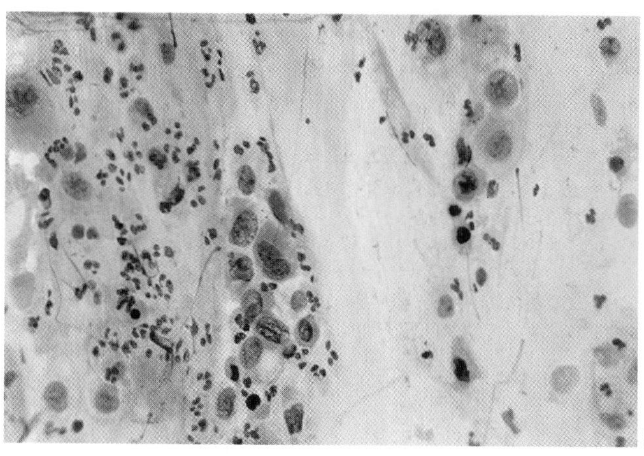

(b)

Fig. 2.33 Severe dyskaryosis. (a) Example of the tight clusters of severely dyskaryotic cells that are sometimes seen. Piling up of the nuclei results in some cells being out of focus. Variation in size and shape is best seen in the cells on the right. **(b)** The severely dyskaryotic cells in some instances show hyperchromasia, but others, particularly the two cells at the top of the string on the right, do not appear hyperchromatic. In addition, degenerative changes, such as pyknosis and karyorrhexis, confuse the pattern.

Experience clearly plays an important role, and close liaison between cytologist, histopathologist and colposcopist can do much to improve expertise in all three disciplines.

With regard to patient management, differentiation between the various degrees of dyskaryosis and cervical intraepithelial neoplasia may not be important. However, in practical terms, it is a good discipline for cytologists to improve their ability to discriminate between various degrees of cellular change. This will enable them to make more critical assessments of the important areas of minimal invasion and glandular abnormalities, where subtle cellular changes are often the only indication of a more significant lesion which may require an alternative method of investigation and therapy.

DIFFERENTIAL DIAGNOSIS OF CERVICAL INTRAEPITHELIAL NEOPLASIA

Although the histological diagnosis of cervical intraepithelial neoplasia is very often unequivocal, there are several conditions that can be confused with it, particularly the less severe degrees. Each of these epithelial states is described in detail in other chapters. Only those features relevant to their distinction from cervical intraepithelial neoplasia will be emphasized here.

Also, in cytological terms, discrimination between intraepithelial neoplasia and other cellular changes is obviously important, and a few areas consistently give rise to difficulty.

Immature squamous metaplasia

HISTOLOGY

By the very nature of its immaturity, this epithelial change has little or no surface differentiation or stratification (Fig. 2.35), and because of this feature it may be confused with cervical intraepithelial neoplasia. Furthermore, the cells of an active metaplasia frequently have an increased nuclear cytoplasmic ratio, with prominent nucleoli.

However, a distinction is usually possible by examining the nuclear detail: the nuclei of metaplastic cells are regular, both in shape and size, and may be hypochromatic rather than hyperchromatic. Mitotic figures may be present, but these are few in number and never show abnormal forms. Squamous metaplasia may involve crypts, but does so less often than cervical intraepithelial neoplasia.

CYTOLOGY

When cells from a maturing area of squamous metaplasia are seen in the smear, few problems are likely to arise, but cells arising from an area of very immature squamous metaplasia may give rise to misinterpretation. The nuclei are always enlarged and frequently have an active and hyperchromatic pattern. However, the chromatin distribution is regular, with a finely granular background matrix. The nuclear membrane is even and finely circumscribed, with no thickening or indentation (see Fig. 2.20).

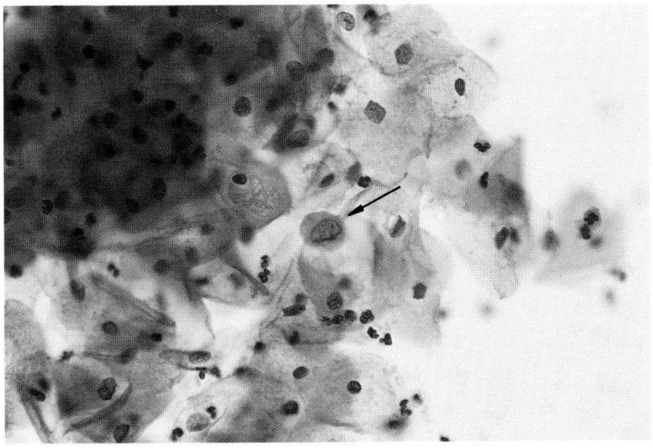

Fig. 2.34 A single severely dyskaryotic cell. This is discretely placed among normal mature squamous cells (arrow).

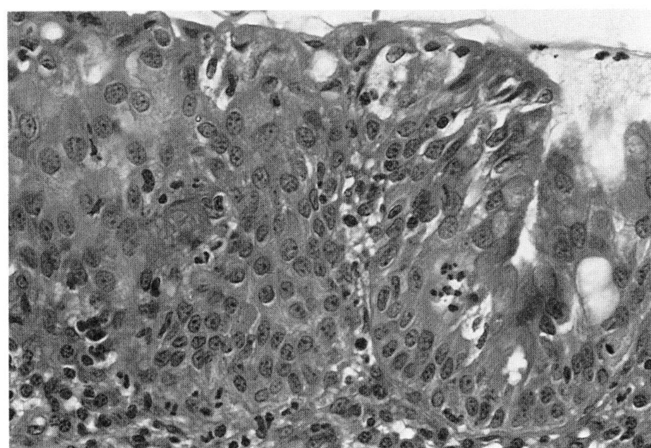

Fig. 2.35 Immature squamous metaplasia. There is significant arrest of maturation, with large nuclei of the basal half of the epithelium. Despite this increased nuclear/cytoplasmic ratio, the nuclei are regular and mitotic figures are very infrequent.

Congenital transformation zone

HISTOLOGY

This is a variant of squamous metaplasia; the epithelium of the congenital transformation zone is composed of maturing metaplastic cells (see pages 83–5 for the colposcopic appearances). There is often a little hyperkeratosis on the surface, but the most alarming feature for the unwary pathologist is the irregular pattern of the basement membrane (Fig. 2.36). This gives the appearance of random, spiky downgrowths of squamous cells into the stroma; to increase the confusion, the centres of these processes may contain whorls of more mature cells. As with squamous metaplasia, the regularity of nuclei and lack of mitotic activity help to distinguish the congenital transformation zone from cervical intraepithelial neoplasia.

Having established that the epithelium does not show the features of intraepithelial neoplasia, irregularity of the epithelial/stromal junction ceases to be alarming.

CYTOLOGY

Cells arising from a congenital transformation zone have no cytological features to distinguish them from any other area of metaplasia.

Healing epithelium

HISTOLOGY

After local destructive treatment for cervical intraepithelial neoplasia, it is common to encounter areas of acetowhite epithelium at colposcopic follow-up. The colposcopist may feel that the appearances are those of residual disease, and will therefore take a biopsy (see Chapter 7).

The histological features of this epithelium are very similar to those of squamous metaplasia, with lack of maturation and large, pale nuclei (Fig. 2.37). It is important that these changes are recognized and not mistaken for cervical intraepithelial neoplasia, although it is equally important not to miss the latter and underdiagnose it as healing epithelium.

In healing epithelium, it is also quite common to find evidence of human papillomavirus infection. With a little experience, distinguishing between this type of epithelium and minor degrees of residual cervical intraepithelial neoplasia becomes easier if attention is paid to the lack of nuclear abnormalities and sparseness of mitotic figures.

CYTOLOGY

Cells arising from areas of regeneration or repair are likely to show active and hyperchromatic nuclei, but

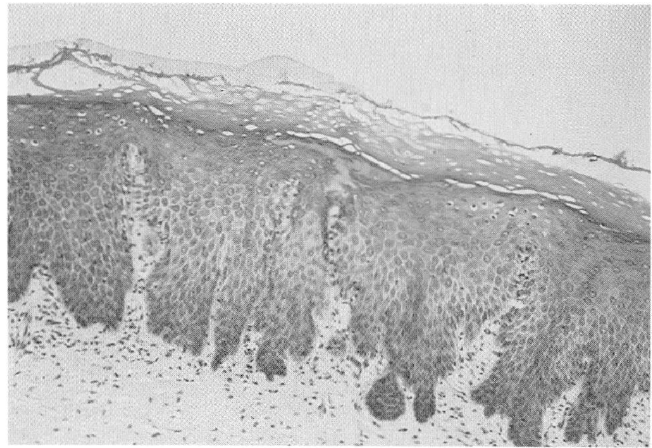

Fig. 2.36 Congenital transformation zone. Keratinization is present on the surface, and the characteristic irregular pattern of the epithelial stromal junction is seen.

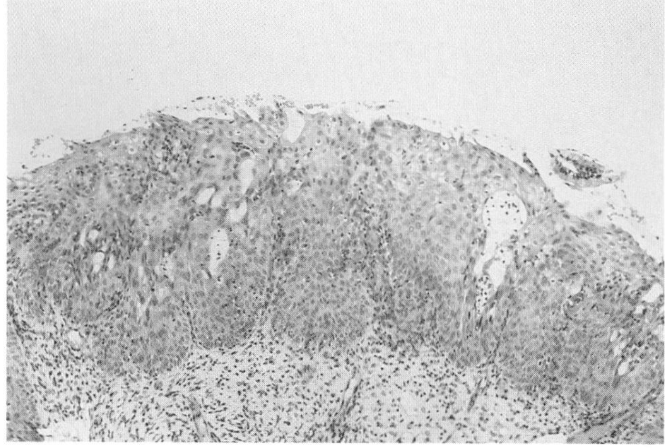

Fig. 2.37 Healing after laser vaporization. The appearances are very similar to those of immature squamous metaplasia. Occasional mitotic figures may be seen, and there is nuclear enlargement.

careful evaluation of chromatin distribution, and the shape and size of nuclei will, in most instances, successfully resolve any difficulties (Fig. 2.38).

Subclinical papillomavirus infection

HISTOLOGY

One of the hallmarks of subclinical papillomavirus infection is koilocytic change in the cell: the nucleus becomes irregular, hyperchromatic and enlarged, surrounded by an exaggerated perinuclear halo. At low magnification, epithelium containing many cells showing koilocytic change gives the impression of widespread nuclear enlargement and irregularity, which may lead to an erroneous diagnosis of cervical intraepithelial neoplasia. In assessing whether or not an epithelium showing subclinical papillomavirus infection also contains cervical intraepithelial neoplasia, the cells not showing koilocytic change must be evaluated. If these show no more than a minimal variation in size and shape, a diagnosis of cervical intraepithelial neoplasia is not justified.

Furthermore, subclinical papillomavirus infection can cause an increase in the number of mitotic figures in the epithelium, therefore the presence of mitotic figures cannot be taken as evidence of cervical intraepithelial neoplasia if the other features of subclinical papillomavirus are also seen.

Very frequently, cervical intraepithelial neoplasia and subclinical papillomavirus infection coexist in the same area of epithelium; in this case, the presence of the latter must not be taken as an explanation for the nuclear changes that may be present as a manifestation of a genuine cervical intraepithelial neoplasia.

CYTOLOGY

The cellular features associated with human papillomavirus infection are discussed in detail in Chapter 12. Here, it is important to stress that whenever the nuclear features of dyskaryosis are present, the cell must be regarded as such and reported accordingly, whether or not the other features of human papillomavirus infection are seen in that particular cell or in associated cells (Fig. 2.39).

Atrophic postmenopausal epithelium

HISTOLOGY

If the oestrogenic stimulus, which encourages the squamous epithelium of the cervix to mature, is withdrawn, the epithelium becomes thin and

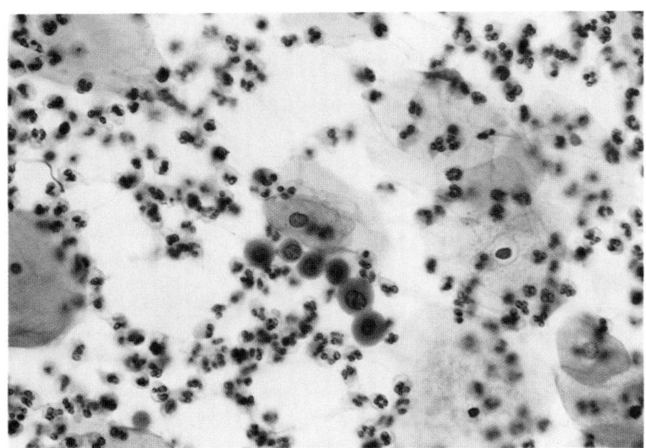

Fig. 2.38 Regeneration and repair. Large hyperchromatic nuclei are granular, but chromatin is regularly distributed throughout the nuclei; nuclear membranes are even and regular.

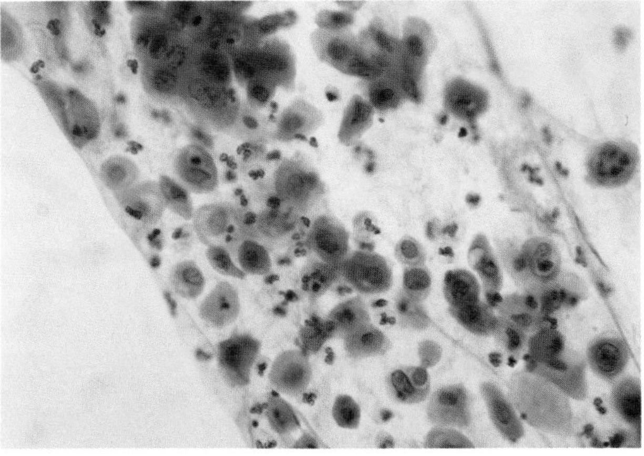

Fig. 2.39 Moderate and severe dyskaryosis with human papillomavirus changes. Quite marked pleomorphism of the nuclei is seen. Also seen are dyskeratosis, with keratinization and occasional koilocytic change, characteristic of papillomavirus infection.

atrophic. It is only a few cells thick, and the nuclear cytoplasmic ratio increases. However, this process is the opposite of that occurring in cervical intraepithelial neoplasia: it is the cytoplasm that is reduced in amount, rather than the nucleus that is increased.

The results of these changes may give an appearance that can be very difficult to distinguish from cervical intraepithelial neoplasia, with large nuclei occupying a significant proportion of the epithelium (Fig. 2.40).

Mitotic figures are not seen in an atrophic epithelium, and an experienced pathologist will recognize that the nuclei are smaller than those found in cervical intraepithelial neoplasia. Nevertheless, an atrophic epithelium can often give rise to difficulties in interpretation, particularly when it is found on a small cervical or vault biopsy.

CYTOLOGY

Cells arising from an atrophic epithelium are easily recognized as the nuclei are often very pale, with a fine chromatin pattern (Fig. 2.41). However, in the

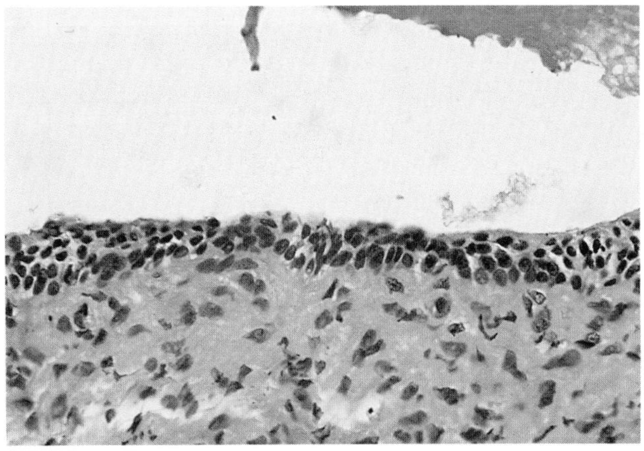

Fig. 2.40 Atrophic postmenopausal epithelium. The nuclei appear large, but this is due to loss of cytoplasm and not an increase in nuclear size. Hyperchromasia is present, but no mitotic activity is seen.

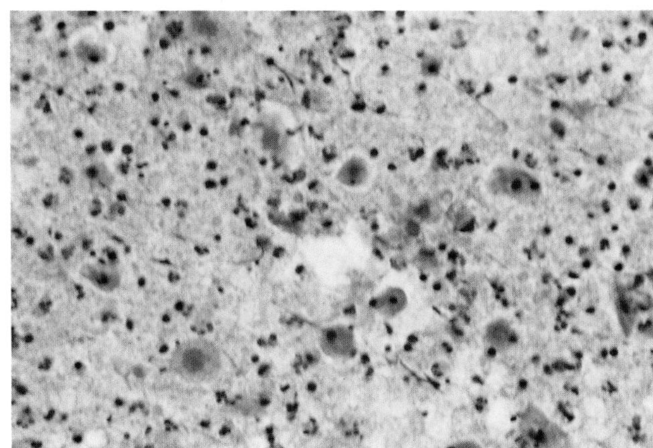

Fig. 2.41 Atrophic postmenopausal pattern. Parabasal cells showing degenerative changes, particularly swelling, bloating and nuclear distortion. Numerous polymorphs, together with pyknosis and karyorrhexis, are frequently seen.

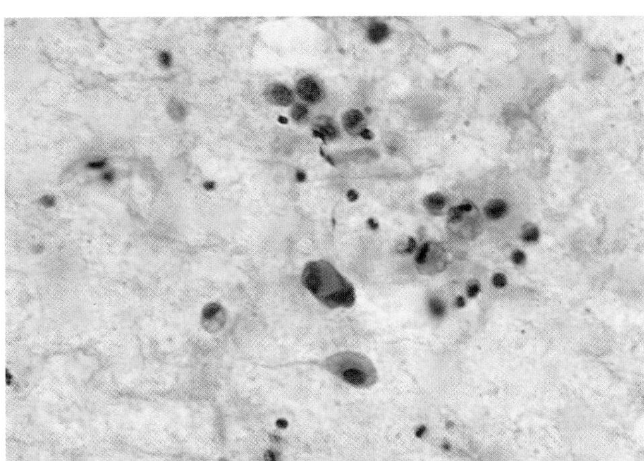

Fig. 2.42 Endometrial cells associated with the use of an intrauterine contraceptive device. Occasional discrete cells show darkly staining nuclei. Although chromatin is clumped, the background matrix is finely granular. These cells are typical endometrial cells of glandular type. Large cells, at the lower centre, are probably stromal and show reactive changes.

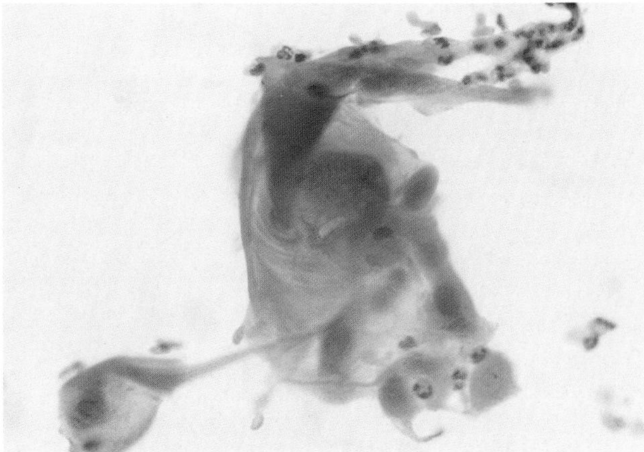

Fig. 2.43 Radiation changes. The cells are showing gross enlargement and variation in shape. The large cells appear bloated, and although the nuclei are enlarged the chromatin has a bland appearance. The cytoplasm is showing vacuolization characteristic of radiation change.

presence of infection the nuclei may appear more active, and such smears remain a source of error leading to a false positive diagnosis.

Equally important is a false negative diagnosis which may result when dyskaryotic cells are mistaken for normal parabasal cells. Postpartum patterns may also give rise to the same problems of differential diagnosis.

Endometrial cells

CYTOLOGY

Endometrial cells may occasionally be mistaken for severely dyskaryotic cells in a smear, particularly when degenerative changes give rise to darkly stained nuclei, or where nuclear changes associated with an intrauterine contraceptive device are seen (Fig. 2.42). In the latter case, the enlarged and active-looking nuclei can be difficult to interpret, but careful attention to other nuclear features and the cytoplasm, as well as the overall smear pattern, will usually resolve the issue.

On rare occasions, it may be impossible to distinguish between cells arising from an area of CIN 3 and endocervical (or endometrial) carcinoma.

Radiation change

CYTOLOGY

Occasionally smears taken from women who have had radiotherapy in the recent past may show changes which can be confused with dyskaryosis or malignancy, especially if this information is not given in the request form. Enlargement of nuclei with bizarre forms is commonly seen, but the nuclei are usually pale-staining with fine chromatin structure and may appear wrinkled (Fig. 2.43.).

3. *Aetiology and natural history of cervical carcinoma*

INTRODUCTION

Squamous cell carcinoma of the cervix and its precursors have been widely investigated, and much has been written about their epidemiology and aetiology. A number of epidemiological factors that appear to contribute to the development of a neoplasm have been identified, but the way in which these factors relate to the causative agent, or agents, is not yet clear.

More importantly, these aetiological agents have not been identified conclusively, although different types of agents have been incriminated from time to time.

Changes in the cervix and interactions of aetiological agents in the development of cervical carcinoma are summarized in Fig. 3.1.

EPIDEMIOLOGY

The results of a large number of epidemiological studies comparing women who have the disease with those who do not, are summarized below. Some studies have looked at invasive cancer as 'the disease', others have considered cervical intraepithelial neoplasia, while a number of them have looked at both invasive cancer and cervical intraepithelial neoplasia.

The results appear to be broadly similar in all three groups. Naturally, these studies do not agree in all respects, but the findings discussed here represent the results of the majority in each case.

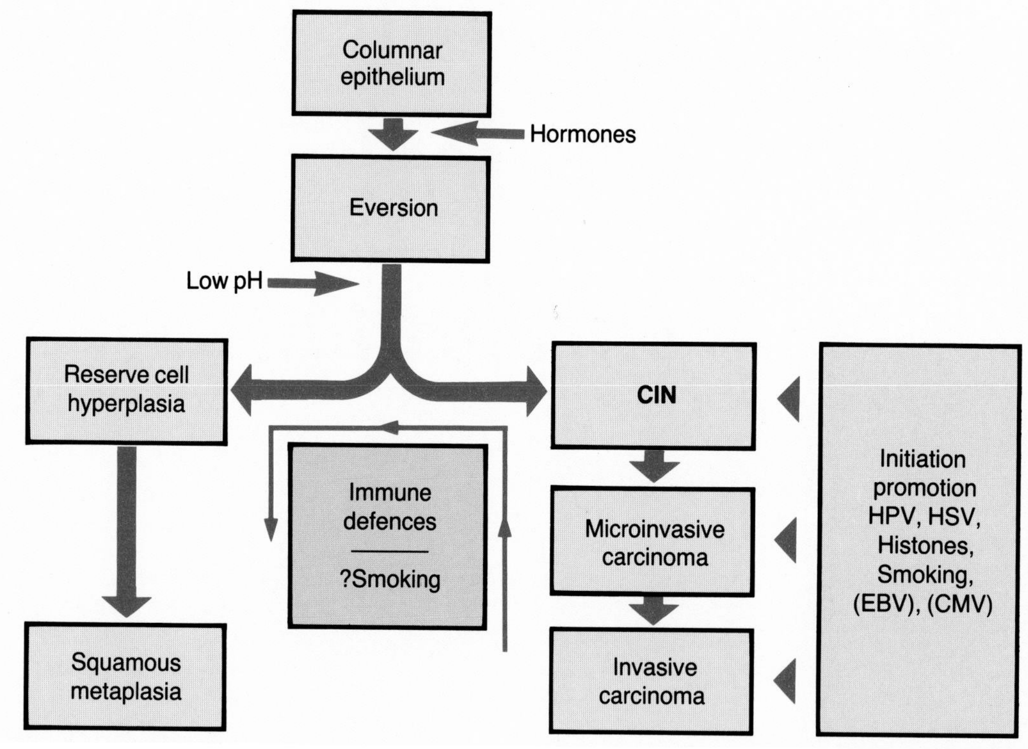

Fig. 3.1 Actions and interactions in the development of cervical carcinoma. Hormonally induced eversion of the cervix and an acidic vaginal environment encourage the development of the transformation zone. In physiological conditions, benign squamous metaplasia is the eventual outcome. In the presence of a sexually transmitted agent, the benign metaplastic process is diverted into a malignant transformation, resulting first in increasingly severe grades of cervical intraepithelial neoplasia and then, in an unknown proportion of women, invasive squamous cell carcinoma. A number of carcinogens are suggested here. Whether the agents act in unison or sequentially as initiators and promoters is also unclear, and it is not known whether continued exposure to the carcinogen (or another agent) is necessary for the progression of cervical intraepithelial neoplasia from mild to severe degrees, or for the estabiishment of an invasive carcinoma. It is likely that local systemic immune defences are important in counteracting the changes generated by the carcinogenic agents, at the stage of development of cervical intraepithelial neoplasia during its progression through the different grades, at the point of beginning invasion and at the time when a microinvasive carcinoma expands to become established as stage Ib carcinoma with metastatic potential.

Coitus

Squamous cell carcinoma of the cervix does not occur in women who have never had sexual intercourse; coitus is the major prerequisite for the development of this tumour.

In the past, extensive investigations of medical records and death certificates of nuns showed how rare cervical cancer of any type was in a group of women who were assumed never to have had sexual intercourse.

Age at first coitus

Several epidemiological studies have shown that women with cervical cancer are more likely to have become sexually active during adolescence than matched controls without the disease.

Age at marriage and age at first pregnancy have also been looked at, and similar results have been observed. These factors obviously reflect the age at first intercourse.

Number of partners

Many investigations have indicated that women with cervical cancer and precancer are more likely to have had extramarital partners than control groups without the disease. In fact, promiscuity in either sex increases the risk of cervical cancer.

Frequency of coitus

There is no evidence that frequency of intercourse is a significant factor, provided that this does not imply a greater number of partners.

Parity

It has been apparent for many years that women with cervical cancer tend to have more children than women without the disease. However, when the obvious correlation between high parity and an early age at marriage is taken into consideration, this association between high parity and carcinoma of the cervix disappears.

It seems that high parity reflects sexual activity starting at an early age; the suggestion that the birth of several children repeatedly traumatizes the cervix, with trauma predisposing to the development of malignancy, is unfounded.

Sexually transmitted diseases

Women with cervical cancer have a high frequency of sexually transmitted diseases (syphilis, gonorrhoea, trichomoniasis, genital herpes, papillomavirus infection and *Chlamydia* infection).

It is possible that all these infections are related to the tumour, but only in the sense that they are a consequence of intercourse, as is cervical cancer, and therefore have a common epidemiological background. However, some of these infections have been incriminated as causative agents, and will be discussed in more detail below.

Male circumcision

There has been a long-standing belief that circumcision of the male protects the female from developing cervical cancer. This belief was established partly because of the low incidence of cervical cancer in Jewish women, and partly as the result of two totally uncontrolled epidemiological studies carried out in the 1940s.

One of these studies demonstrated a lower incidence of cervical cancer among native Fijian women compared with immigrant Hindu women in the same country. The second study compared the incidence of cervical cancer in Hindu and Muslim women in India, finding a higher incidence in the Hindu than in the Muslim population. It was suggested that the differences found in both these investigations were the result of circumcision of Fijian and Muslim men.

A number of subsequent studies have repeated these investigations, using controls for as many other factors as possible, but they give no support to the suggestion that male circumcision protects from cervical cancer.

Racial factors

The interrelationship between racial, cultural and religious factors in the development of cervical cancer is illustrated by reference to cervical cancer in Jewish women, who have repeatedly been shown to have a low incidence of the disease.

However, this apparent partial immunity may be related more to the regulation of sexual life by observing the laws of Niddah, than to circumcision of the male or a hereditary resistance to the disease. Therefore, low incidence is probably due to the fact that orthodox Jews tend not to have intercourse during adolescence and not to have multiple sexual partners. There is some evidence to suggest that the incidence of cervical cancer is higher in Jewish women who adhere less rigidly to this strict sexual code.

Socioeconomic factors

Epidemiological studies in the past have shown that women from lower socioeconomic groups have a higher incidence of cervical cancer than those in the higher-income groups. The reason for this is obscure but, again, it is possible that an early age at first intercourse and marriage may be the most important factor. However, no association has been demonstrated between social class and the risk of developing cervical intraepithelial neoplasia.

Smoking

It has recently become apparent that there is an important correlation between cigarette smoking and the risk of developing cervical intraepithelial neoplasia and cervical carcinoma. This finding was initially explained away by the supposition that young women who smoked were more likely to have intercourse at an early age, and to have multiple partners. Subsequent, carefully controlled, epidemiological studies have indicated that this was a false assumption, and that the risk from cigarette smoking is maintained after controlling for all other factors.

It remains to be shown whether cigarette smoking acts by a local carcinogenic or co-carcinogenic effect, or by suppression of local immune mechanisms in the cervix.

Method of contraception

There have been several major epidemiological studies investigating whether or not there is an association between oral contraceptive use and increased risk of cervical neoplasia, with conflicting results.

The main difficulty with these studies is that a woman's choice of contraceptive method may depend on other factors that influence the possibility of developing cervical cancer. For instance, women who use different methods of contraception are likely to have different attitudes to sexual behaviour.

A small number of well-controlled epidemiological studies have indicated that the risk of developing cervical cancer increases in proportion to the length of oral contraceptive use. Rather than incriminating a direct effect of the contraceptive pill, it could be argued that the rate of cervical precancer has been increasing in parallel with the growing popularity of this form of contraception, and that this increase can be explained by a change in sexual behaviour. Furthermore, progestogens cause eversion of the cervix, which enables endocervical lesions to be more readily diagnosed. Another factor that may bias the results of studies is that women taking oral contraceptives possibly have more frequent cervical smears.

The use of barrier methods of contraception should protect the cervical epithelium from an agent transmitted at intercourse, if it is assumed that cervical cancer is caused by an infective agent. A number of studies have shown that women who consistently use barrier methods of contraception have approximately one-quarter of the risk of cervical neoplasia compared with women who use other methods of contraception.

Male factors

The only satisfactory explanation of the importance of intercourse in the development of cervical cancer is that an agent of some description is transmitted from the male to the female at intercourse. If this agent is carried by some men but not by others, then the woman who is promiscuous is more likely to encounter a man who is a carrier.

If the agent is carried by both sexes and can be transmitted from a female carrier (not necessarily a woman who is developing cervical cancer) to a male, then the chances of a man being a carrier are proportional to the number of his partners. This would mean that a woman who has intercourse with a promiscuous man, although he may be her only sexual partner, is at risk of developing cervical cancer by his promiscuity.

Support for this hypothesis is provided by studies showing that the incidence of the tumour may be related to the occupation of the patient's partner in a way that does not necessarily reflect socioeconomic status but which may be linked with opportunities for promiscuity in the man.

Immunological factors

Cervical intraepithelial neoplasia and invasive cancer are more common in women who are immunosuppressed; a 14-fold increase in the incidence of CIN 3 has been demonstrated in renal transplant recipients. This increased risk may be the result of impaired immunological surveillance, so that malignant cellular changes are not recognized and tumours can develop unchecked.

Alternatively, it is possible that resistance to mutagenic viruses is lowered; this point may be particularly relevant to the cervix in view of the possible role of viruses in the aetiology of cervical cancer.

A third possibility is that immunosuppressive drugs are carcinogenic. Studies on local immune mechanisms within the cervix reveal that an inadequate host response may play a part in allowing progression to cervical intraepithelial neoplasia, after the external mutagen has been encountered.

TRANSMISSIBLE AGENTS

From the above discussions it appears that the development of cervical cancer and its precursors almost certainly depends on the transmission of an agent, or agents, from one individual to another. Therefore, it is now relevant to consider what these agents may be.

Over the years, a large number of substances that could be transmitted from a man to a woman at intercourse have been considered. All of these have, at different times, been put forward as possible causes of cervical cancer. Only a few of them will be discussed here.

Smegma

The question of whether male circumcision protects the woman from cervical cancer has been considered above. The possibility that this factor was linked with a reduced risk of the disease in the female partners of circumcised men rested largely with the assumption that smegma may be a chemical carcinogen. Smegma has also been incriminated as a factor responsible for the higher incidence of this tumour in the lower socioeconomic groups, and in this respect it has been linked to poor cleanliness. However, there is no evidence that human smegma is carcinogenic.

Nevertheless, there seems to be a genuine relationship between absence of circumcision and increased risk of developing penile carcinoma. Furthermore, there is evidence that the wives of men with penile cancer are at greater risk of developing cervical cancer, which suggests a remote but real association.

Spermatozoa

Spermatozoa are packed with deoxyribonucleic acid (DNA), very closely related to the DNA of the metaplastic endocervical cell. Because of this, spermatozoa could be considered a prime suspect for causing mutagenic DNA interactions. Some evidence has shown that endocervical cells are capable of phagocytosing sperm heads, but integration of sperm and endocervical cell DNA has not been demonstrated.

Basic proteins

The possible role of spermatozoa in the aetiology of cervical cancer was further investigated by examining the protein content in sperm rather than its DNA content, and superficial contact with the endocervical cell rather than entry into it. It was suggested that an arginine-rich histone in the sperm head had an effect on DNA filaments originating from the nuclear DNA, which, while remaining connected with the nucleus, protruded through the cell surface. These filaments in the mucoid coat may act as a 'switchgear' which, if suitably stimulated, activates the DNA within the cell, resulting in an increased capacity for protein synthesis and proliferation (both of which are characteristics of cancer cells).

Chlamydia

Chlamydia trachomatis is a common pathogen causing chronic infection of the cervix and fallopian tubes. As with many other sexually transmitted infective agents, it is reasonable to consider that *Chlamydia* may perhaps play a part in cervical carcinogenesis. There is an association between infection with *Chlamydia* and cervical precancer: a higher prevalence of positive cultures and serum antibodies to *Chlamydia* has been shown in women with cervical intraepithelial neoplasia, together with a higher incidence of *Chlamydia*-associated changes in smears, compared with controls. In addition, a higher progression rate to CIN 3 has been seen in women with chlamydial changes in their smears than in a control group of women without such changes. However, these findings may only be due to the fact that both diseases are the consequence of sexual intercourse.

Viruses

HERPES SIMPLEX VIRUS TYPE 2 (HSV-2)

Women with cervical cancer have an increased incidence of HSV-2 antibodies compared with women who have non-malignant gynaecological complaints. Furthermore, HSV-2 is capable of transforming cells in tissue culture. However, HSV-2 DNA has only rarely been found in tumour samples (Fig. 3.2). Further evidence against HSV-2 being related to cervical neoplasia has come from studies demonstrating that the incidence of HSV-2 antibodies is more closely related to sexual behaviour than to the presence of neoplasia.

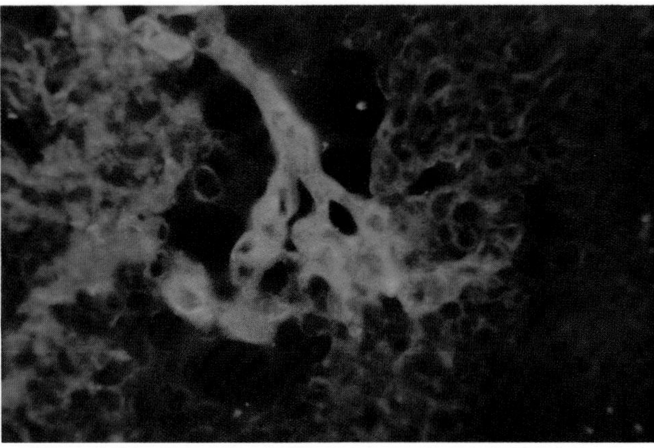

Fig. 3.2 Invasive squamous carcinoma of the cervix. Immunofluorescence using a monoclonal antibody to a herpes simplex virus-specific protein. Cancer cells are positive.

HUMAN PAPILLOMAVIRUS

Since the mid-1970s, human papillomavirus (HPV) infection (Fig. 3.3) has been at the centre of investigations into the aetiology of cervical cancer. Many studies have shown that a high proportion of cervical tumours contain HPV-DNA, in particular HPV-16, HPV-18 and HPV-33. Furthermore, cervical intraepithelial neoplasia is very frequently found in association with morphological features indicative of human papillomavirus infection (see Chapter 12). Studies involving immunocytochemistry (Fig. 3.4) and DNA–DNA hybridization on such specimens have confirmed with sufficient certainty that these appearances, recognized under the light microscope after routine processing and staining, are indeed the result of infection by human papillomavirus.

The inability to culture the virus in the laboratory has led to a system of viral typing based on DNA homology rather than serology, and over 60 different human papillomavirus types have now been reported. Once the cell is infected, the virus persists in the nucleus as circular DNA, referred to as 'episomal', which is distinct from the cellular DNA.

Analysis of the genomes has shown that the viral DNA may be divided into regions, the early and late regions being of most interest. The segment of DNA between the end of late proteins and the start of early proteins contains a number of DNA sequences that are thought to be of importance in controlling viral protein synthesis and replication. In addition, it has been found that the regions encoding the E6 and E7 proteins of HPV-16 and HPV-18 are capable of

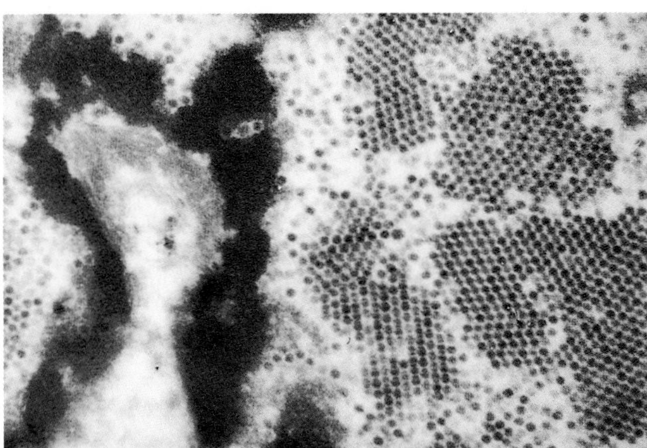

Fig. 3.3 Transmission electron microscopic (TEM) view of koilocyte from a cervical human papillomavirus-induced lesion. Crystalline or 'honeycomb' patterns of human papillomavirus particles are seen (left and right).

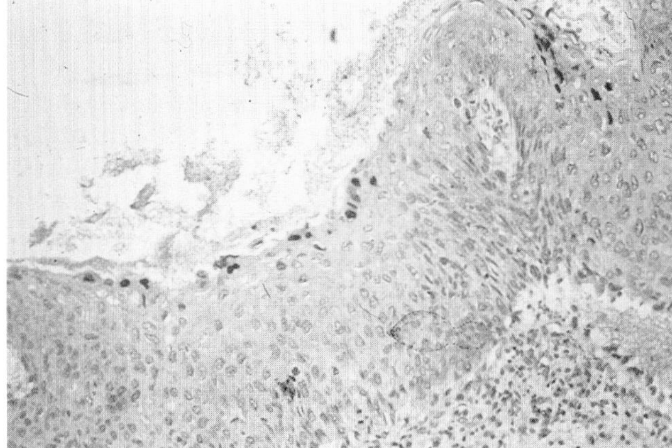

Fig. 3.4 Cervical intraepithelial neoplasia. Immunoperoxidase method for human papillomavirus-associated protein. A positive reaction (brown staining) in the koilocytes is seen near the surface of abnormal epithelium.

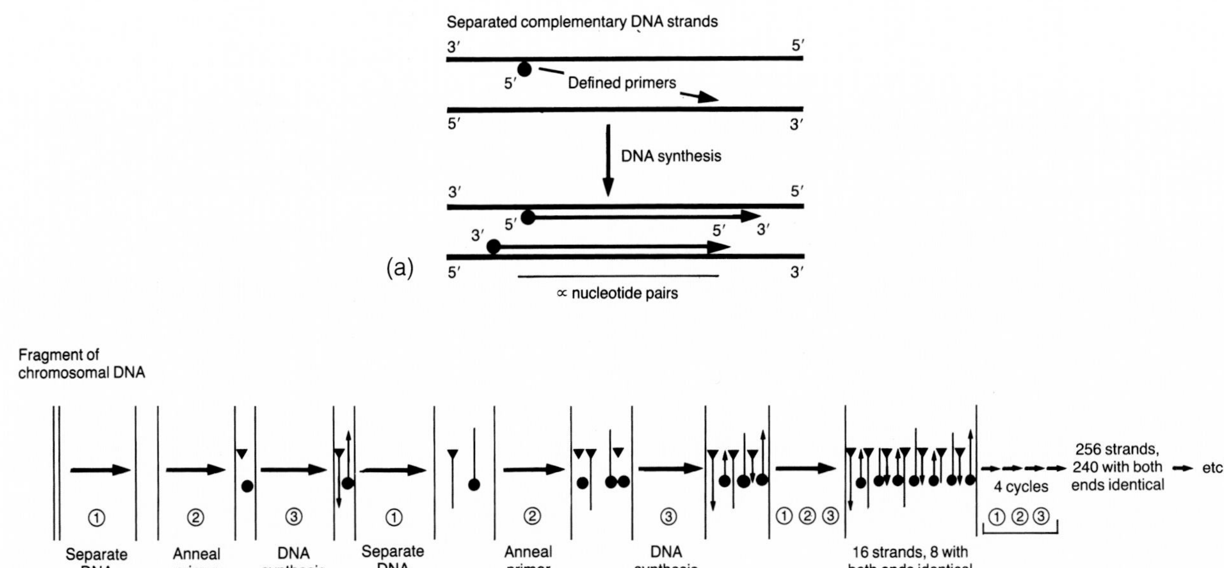

Fig. 3.5 The polymerase chain reaction (PCR) for amplifying specific nucleotide sequences *in vitro*. (a) DNA isolated from cells is heated to separate its complementary strands. These strands are then annealed with an excess of two DNA oligonucleotides (each 15–20 nucleotides long) which have been chemically synthesized to match sequences separated by x nucleotides (where x is generally between 50 and 2000). The two oligonucleotides serve as specific primers for *in vitro* DNA synthesis catalysed by DNA polymerase, which copies the DNA between the sequences corresponding to the two oligonucleotides. **(b)** After multiple cycles of reaction, a large amount of a single DNA fragment, x nucleotides long, is obtained, provided that the original DNA sample contains the DNA sequence that was anticipated when the two oligonucleotides were designed.

immortalizing and transforming tissue cells in culture, and it seems that in HPV-16 the E6 and E7 proteins have the maximum ability to transform cells. There is evidence that this activity is the result of the E7 protein binding with the protein product (RB) of the retinoblastoma gene (*Rb1*) and the E6 protein binding with p53 gene product. These are both tumour suppressor genes and binding with E6 and E7 inhibits their anti-oncogenic, growth-regulating properties, leading to malignant transformation.

Human papillomavirus infection of the cervix may be subdivided into two groups: HPV-6, HPV-11, HPV-31 and HPV-35 are thought to be associated with condylomata acuminata, low-grade intraepithelial neoplasia, and only rarely with invasive tumours. HPV-16, HPV-18 and HPV-33 are associated with subclinical papillomavirus infection, low-grade cervical intraepithelial neoplasia which progresses, high-grade intraepithelial neoplasia and invasive carcinomas. It is this latter group of human papillomavirus types that has the ability to transform cells in culture, and to cooperate with oncogenes in cellular transformation. It has been shown that the majority of cervical tumours contain a proportion of HPV-DNA which, instead of being episomal, is integrated within the host genome.

Prevalence and significance of human papillomavirus infection

The development of the polymerase chain reaction (PCR) has resulted in great advances in the identification of human papillomavirus infection (Fig. 3.5). Hitherto, the detection of HPV-DNA was dependent on a minimum amount of DNA being available, and very small quantities could not be detected. The PCR amplifies DNA dramatically so that very small quantities of DNA may now be identified, and its invention has revolutionized the identification of viral DNA. However, it has brought with it its own problem of such greatly increased sensitivity that the assays were at risk of being invalidated by even the most minute contamination. Now that these problems have been recognized and addressed, epidemiological studies using improved assays are coming up with interesting findings. A number of recent studies has looked at the relationship between HPV infection and the other known risk factors for cervical neoplasia. These show that many of the known risk factors are associated with HPV positivity and these results may be interpreted as meaning that these factors, such as multiple sexual partners and early age at first intercourse, increase the risk of developing cervical carcinoma only because they are indicators of an increased risk of HPV infection, a notion that has been with us since the first suggestion of the concept of the 'high-risk male'.

Case-control studies have shown that most women who have cervical intraepithelial neoplasia also have detectable HPV-DNA compared with a much lower percentage of control women. Relative risks have varied from 10-fold to 40-fold, the latter investigation involving high-grade lesions (CIN 2 and CIN 3) only. The proportion of cases of CIN attributable to HPV infection approaches 90%. It has been stated that relative risks and attributable proportions of this strength and consistency are so rare in cancer epidemiology that the statistical association of HPV and cervical neoplasia is virtually beyond question.

Many prospective cohort studies of cytologically normal women with HPV infection have been under way for some time, but only a few results from long-term studies are as yet available. These show that women with normal cervices infected by HPV have an increased risk of progression to CIN compared with HPV-negative individuals. In one study, the cumulative incidence of cervical intraepithelial neoplasia at two years was 28% among women with a positive test for HPV and 3% among those without detectable HPV-DNA. The risk was highest among those with HPV type 16 or 18 infection. All 24 cases of cervical intraepithelial neoplasia grade 2 or 3 among HPV-positive women were detected within 24 months of the first positive test for HPV. Furthermore, follow-up studies of women with low-grade lesions have demonstrated that the risk of progression is influenced by HPV type.

It is very likely that cervical cancer is caused by a number of factors or agents and has a multistep aetiology which requires initiation by one agent and promotion by another. It is probable that herpes simplex virus, human papillomavirus, smoking, and even other factors not yet considered, all act together or in succession, resulting in the evolution of the disease. It is also possible that different aetiologies may be involved in different women.

NATURAL HISTORY OF CERVICAL CARCINOMA

In order to treat cervical intraepithelial neoplasia most effectively, it is necessary to have an understanding of the relationships between the various grades of cervical intraepithelial neoplasia, and also between cervical intraepithelial neoplasia and invasive carcinoma. A great deal of work has been done in an attempt to establish these relationships, but an accurate knowledge of the natural history of this disease still eludes us.

Progression of cervical intraepithelial neoplasia

There have been several studies of the apparent progression from minor degrees of intraepithelial neoplasia to more severe degrees. Some of these studies have involved examination by colposcopy and cytology, whereas others have added the histology of biopsies.

In general, it has been shown that a mild or moderate degree of cervical intraepithelial neoplasia will either progress to a more severe form, or it will regress. Regression is more likely in the milder forms, and there is evidence that taking biopsies encourages this process, a fact that may invalidate prospective studies in which biopsies are taken at the beginning of or during the study.

It may be reasonable to assume that progression through the grades of cervical intraepithelial neoplasia occurs in a gradual, incremental fashion, but there is no direct evidence for this. Most of the studies that have shown a gradual progression have been sampling the cervix as a whole, either by cytology or by directed biopsies from the most abnormal areas. It is not possible to study a single small area of epithelium by biopsy over a period of time, as the biopsy removes the tissue being studied.

If, as is quite likely, cervical intraepithelial neoplasia represents abnormal clones of cells, a clone with abnormalities of severe degree may develop suddenly within a field of minor abnormality. Furthermore, the same argument can be used to suggest that severely abnormal degrees of intraepithelial neoplasia may develop without necessarily being preceded by minor abnormalities.

Relationship of cervical intraepithelial neoplasia to invasive carcinoma

The success of effective cervical screening programmes that detect cervical intraepithelial neoplasia by cytology and allow its treatment while still in the preinvasive phase, rests largely on two assumptions:

1. A significant proportion of women with cervical intraepithelial neoplasia would eventually develop invasive carcinoma if not treated.
2. Most invasive squamous cell carcinomas are preceded by a demonstrable intraepithelial phase.

However, there is little precise information on the rate of progression from cervical intraepithelial neoplasia to invasive carcinoma, mainly because of the moral and ethical impossibility of observing without intervention women with a known premalignant disease. Even so, some figures are available from a number of studies. In the 1950s, two studies from Scandinavia established progression rates of 65–70% in women with carcinoma *in situ* (CIN 3) who developed invasive carcinoma over the course of up to 12 years. A more recent study from New Zealand found that 36% of women who had persistent abnormal cytology following incomplete treatment for CIN 3 developed invasive carcinoma after 20 years; 18% had developed carcinoma after 10 years.

This figure of 36% of women progressing to invasive carcinoma after 20 years is surprisingly low, but it must be remembered that those patients were partially treated, so that the disease was probably not allowed to run its natural course. This illustrates the other main flaw of this type of study, namely the inability to make a reliable diagnosis without removing tissue, which would interfere with the natural

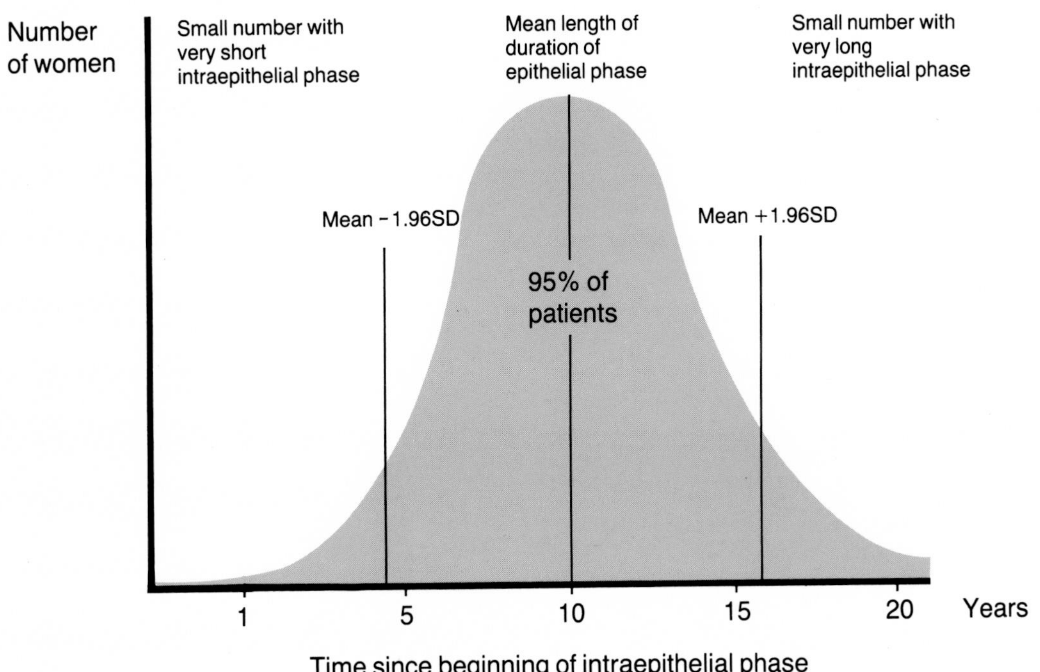

Fig. 3.6 Natural history of cervical intraepithelial neoplasia. The Gaussian curve represents the length of time during which the disease remains intraepithelial before it becomes invasive. It is assumed that duration of the intraepithelial phases in a population of women with cervical intraepithelial neoplasia follows a natural distribution. The mean has been arbitrarily taken to be 10 years; 95% of women will have a length of intraepithelial phase that falls within 1.96 standard deviations on either side of the mean. At the two extreme ends of the curve, there will be women whose intraepithelial phase will be either very long (greater than a lifetime) or very short (weeks or months, rather than years). The curve has been intentionally skewed to lengthen it on the right, to allow for the apparently large number of women who either would not develop invasive disease at all, or would progress to invasive carcinoma only after several years.

progression of the disease. Taken in correlation with the moral barrier to such a study, it seems very unlikely that precise figures for the rate of progression from cervical intraepithelial neoplasia to invasive carcinoma will ever be known.

Duration of the preinvasive phase

It has long been accepted from epidemiological and cytological studies that cervical intraepithelial neoplasia takes at least 10 years to become invasive, although more recent analyses indicate that 3–10 years may be more realistic. The fact that women with CIN 3 are generally some 10–15 years younger than those with invasive carcinoma is taken to support this suggestion.

Nevertheless, there have been worrying reports of young women developing invasive carcinoma of the cervix following recent negative cytology. Some of these smears may have been genuine false negatives, which would have been found to contain malignant cells on review. However, it is impossible to escape the conclusion that, at least in some of these women, there had been a genuine progression from a normal cervix to invasive carcinoma during the short time, reported to be as little as six months, between the initial smear and subsequent diagnosis of carcinoma.

It may be reasonable to suggest that, although the mean time interval for progression through cervical intraepithelial neoplasia to invasive carcinoma may be 10–15 years, a small number of women will fall at the two extremes of the distribution curve of the length of natural history (Fig. 3.6). As a result, some women will have such a long natural history that progression to invasive disease will never occur in the course of a lifetime; these women would be classified as 'non-progressors' . Equally, at the other end of the spectrum there will be some women in whom the natural history of the disease runs a very rapid course, measured in months rather than years; this may be the case described in the above reports. This speculative suggestion reconciles the very diverse progression rates in different women with the belief that one disease process is occurring. These differences in behaviour represent extreme variations in the length of the natural history of the same disease, and it is not necessary to suggest that rapidly progressing cervical cancer is a different disease.

4. *Indications for referral for colposcopy*

APPROACH TO REFERRAL

The decision to refer a woman for colposcopic examination is based on a number of factors, of which by far the most important is the result of the cervical smear. However, consideration must also be given to the facilities available, and to the psychological impact of referral on the women concerned. These factors play a part both in developing a policy at a local or, preferably, a national level for referral of women to a colposcopy clinic, and in determining whether an individual woman should be referred for the examination. Referral of women with very minor abnormalities could overload a clinic with limited resources, thus jeopardizing the prompt treatment of more severe abnormalities, if care is not taken to prioritize referrals.

For many women with minor abnormalities in their smears, the psychological effect of referral for colposcopy, with or without subsequent treatment, may be greater than the risk of serious disease developing from the abnormality that the smear has identified. It is an important requirement of a screening programme that overall it should do more good than harm to the population.

The smear result itself cannot be taken entirely at face value. Although most cytology departments quite rightly claim a good correlation between cytological findings and final histological diagnosis, it cannot always be assumed that a smear report of mild dyskaryosis means that only CIN 1 is present in the cervix. Several studies have shown that, within a group of women with smears reported as showing mild dyskaryosis, there is a proportion, perhaps as many as one-fifth to one-quarter, who are found to have CIN 3 at colposcopy and biopsy.

On the other hand, an even larger proportion of women with mildly dyskaryotic smears have no demonstrable abnormality at colposcopy. Therefore, when deciding whether to refer a woman for colposcopy, it is necessary to bear in mind the possibility of more severe disease being present than the smear suggests, and to assess the probable natural history of the lesion that is predicted by cytology.

While it is accepted that the need to repeat a cervical smear can cause anxiety to women, it has become clear that more anxiety may be caused by the referral for colposcopy and actual colposcopic examination.

The interests of the women concerned are best served by a balanced approach that takes into account not only the most satisfactory clinical management, but also the most effective use of resources in terms of cost and manpower.

It is important that the referral protocol is flexible enough to allow for temporary constraints of whatever nature, and also to tailor management to the needs of individual patients. Furthermore, adjustments need to be made with the changing pattern of understanding and knowledge of cervical intraepithelial neoplasia.

CYTOLOGICAL INDICATIONS

The following model is based on a 'common sense' approach (Table 4.1). All women with cervical smears suggesting moderate or severe dyskaryosis, and those showing any suggestion of invasive disease or adenocarcinoma, should be referred immediately for colposcopy.

In the case of borderline changes, the current approach is to take another smear after six months. If at that time the changes persist, referral for colposcopy should be considered (see page 154).

There is a case for managing mild, and perhaps even moderate, dyskaryosis in the same way as borderline changes, especially if the cytological features of human papillomavirus infection are seen; these can confuse the picture, and lead to either underdiagnosis or overdiagnosis. Repeat smears at intervals may clarify the pattern, and if the abnormality persists on a second or, at most, a third smear, referral is advised.

The case of persistent unsatisfactory smears requires some special discussion (see Table 5.2). Unless some attempt is made to identify and treat the causative agents, there is little point in repeating smears *ad infinitum*. If the cytologist can give an indication that a bacterial infection is present, then microbiological screening would be indicated, with appropriate treatment. Should the smear remain unsatisfactory when repeated on no more than three

Table 4.1 Cytological indications for referral for colposcopy

1 Suggestion of invasive carcinoma
2 Severe dyskaryosis
3 Moderate dyskaryosis
4 Persistent mild dyskaryosis/borderline nuclear changes
5 Persistent unsatisfactory smears
6 Suggestion of glandular lesion
7 Excessive numbers of keratinized cells

occasions over a period (of, say, 6–12 months), then referral for colposcopy is justified.

Women taking the oral contraceptive pill form a special group since some consistently present with a markedly cytolytic smear showing clumping and folding of cells, making interpretation difficult. This pattern must not be confused with that associated with bacterial infection, but if smears are repeatedly unsatisfactory in this group of women, colposcopy may be the only reliable means of excluding cervical intraepithelial neoplasia.

Some areas of real difficulty remain, as in the case of women with smears showing large numbers of keratinized squamous cells and little else. The cells are often anucleate. These appearances suggest extensive leucoplakia; it is impossible to assess any change that may be occurring in the cells beneath the surface and thus to predict the underlying pathology.

One repeat smear after three months may be appropriate, with referral for colposcopy if a similar pattern is seen. However, where the facility exists, immediate referral should be considered.

Atypical glandular changes not sufficiently marked to warrant a diagnosis of adenocarcinoma may be very difficult to manage cytologically. Discussion with the clinician and colposcopist over individual cases is a sensible approach (see Chapter 11).

OTHER REASONS FOR REFERRAL

Reasons for referral other than an abnormal cervical smear should not be overlooked. A woman who has a clinically 'suspicious-looking' cervix to naked eye examination, in spite of whether or not the cervical smear is reported as showing dyskaryotic or malignant cells, should be referred for colposcopy.

It is often claimed that the diagnosis of invasive cancer of the cervix is a clinical one, but, as many general practitioners and clinicians may not see a case of invasive disease in their professional lifetime, early invasive disease can easily be missed. Many women with cervical cancer suffer from intermenstrual and postcoital bleeding, and therefore in such cases colposcopy may be of benefit.

When areas of leucoplakia (hyperkeratinization) can be seen at speculum examination, referral for colposcopy and biopsy ought to be considered as the layers of keratin mask the true nature of the underlying epithelium from the cytologist.

It is clear that women with vulval and vaginal intraepithelial neoplasia, as well as those with vulvovaginal warts, are at increased risk for cervical intraepithelial neoplasia. This group should also have priority in a protocol for referral for colposcopy, even if the cervical smear is negative.

5. *Taking a screening smear*

INTRODUCTION

Some aspects are of special significance with regard to the actual taking of a cervical smear, and these are discussed here. Other considerations relating to the ambience of the clinic, its facilities and the comfort of women undergoing colposcopy, are discussed in detail in Chapter 22.

VISUALIZATION OF THE CERVIX

The first essential prerequisite is that the entire cervix must be fully visualized, and a speculum of suitable size should be chosen. Lubrication should be used sparingly and not be allowed to come into contact with the cervix.

Whether the left lateral or lithotomy position is used is a matter of personal preference, but there should be a source of good illumination and the cervix should be completely and clearly visible.

TYPE OF SPATULA

For many years, the only type of cervical spatula available was the Ayre's design. It has become increasingly clear that no one instrument is ideal in all cases. Currently, there are numerous varieties of cervical sampling devices available; it is recommended that a selection of samplers be available on the clinic trolley, and that some thought is given to selecting the optimal device for various situations (Fig. 5.1).

The Aylesbury spatula is a modified Ayre's spatula in wood with an elongated and thinner prong, and in the vast majority of women it will be the optimal type. Several commercial variants of this design, both in wood and in plastic, are available (Fig. 5.2), but some are relatively expensive. The thinner extended prong allows more effective sampling of the endocervical canal, with a higher yield of endocervical glandular cells at the same time as sampling the ectocervix with the broad part of the blade of the spatula, thus increasing confidence that a truly representative sample has been obtained.

In the case of a large, patulous or multiparous cervix, a broader spread is most suitable, still taking care to sample the endocervical canal. This requires thorough scraping of the ectocervix over the whole area using the broad, flat end of the spatula in a backwards-and-forwards movement that is more akin to painting.

At the other end of the spectrum, a small, tight postmenopausal or postconization os, with no visible transformation zone, demands careful sampling of the canal. On occasions, even the thin prong of an Aylesbury spatula will be too large to sample the target area effectively, and a suitable alternative could be the endocervical brush. It must be emphasized that, apart from the instances where there has been previous colposcopic assessment, the endocervical

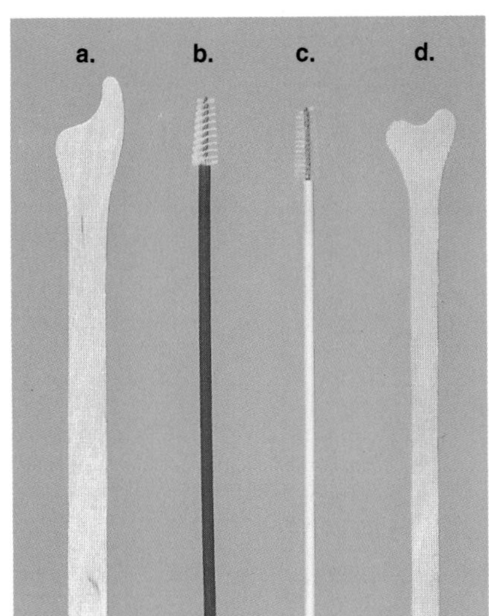

Fig. 5.1 Selection of commercially available sampling devices.
(a) Aylesbury; **(b)** Histolab; **(c)** Medscand; **(d)** Ayre's.

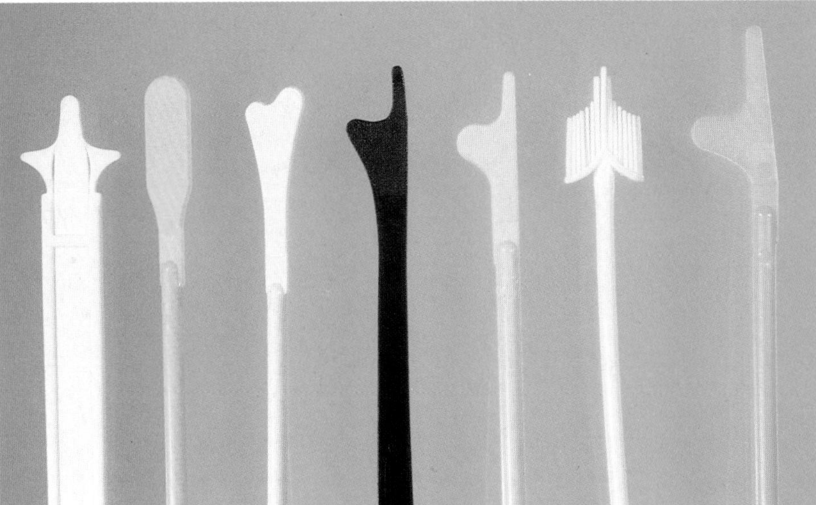

Fig. 5.2 Modifications of Ayre's spatula.

brush should not be used routinely on its own. Problems associated with it include bleeding from the canal, and sometimes damage of epithelium in a visible squamocolumnar junction.

Ideally, the endocervical brush should be used in combination with an Aylesbury or similar type of spatula. The method usually employed is to use each consecutively, inserting the spatula first, smearing it on a slide, taking a specimen with the brush and smearing that on the slide (Fig. 5.3). Speed is important, to prevent the material smeared from the spatula becoming air-dried before the brush material is smeared. The use of two slides would overcome this problem, but would increase the work for the cytology laboratory. Another alternative is to use the spatula and brush together, leaving the brush in the canal while the spatula is being rotated, withdrawing both at the same time and smearing them together on the same slide.

The device used will be a matter of preference based on experience and, to some extent, financial constraints. Perhaps the most difficult concept to grasp is that of variety: learning to tailor the sampling device to suit a particular cervix, as opposed to the established tendency to use one universal sampler for all cervices.

SPREADING THE SMEAR AND FIXATION

The method of spreading the material on to a glass slide also needs to be carried out with care and thought. It is important to spread the material evenly, avoiding thick areas which would result in incomplete penetration of the fixative (Fig. 5.4); the latter would give rise to artefact (Fig. 5.5) or dense staining (Fig. 5.6), making cytological assessment impossible.

The next critical step is fixation. If the sample is allowed to air-dry at all, quality will be seriously impaired in terms of preservation of vital cell detail as well as staining, which may render the smear at best suboptimal and at worst unsatisfactory for a reliable assessment (Fig. 5.7). Once spread evenly, and using all the material obtained on the spatula, the slide must be either completely immersed in 95° alcohol, or flooded with polyethylene glycol fixative (Fig. 5.8). It is important to ensure that the fixative is fresh and not previously used, as cell fragments and debris are frequently lost and quickly contaminate fixative pots and dishes. The slides should be well separated and not touch one another, to allow free circulation and rapid penetration of fixative.

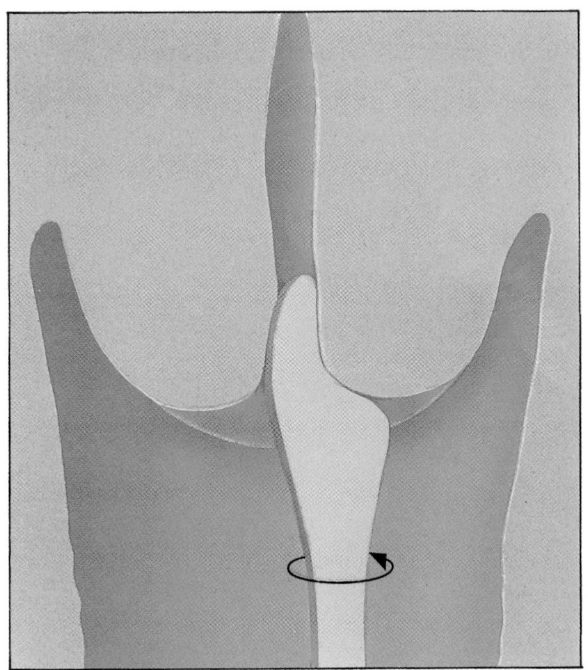

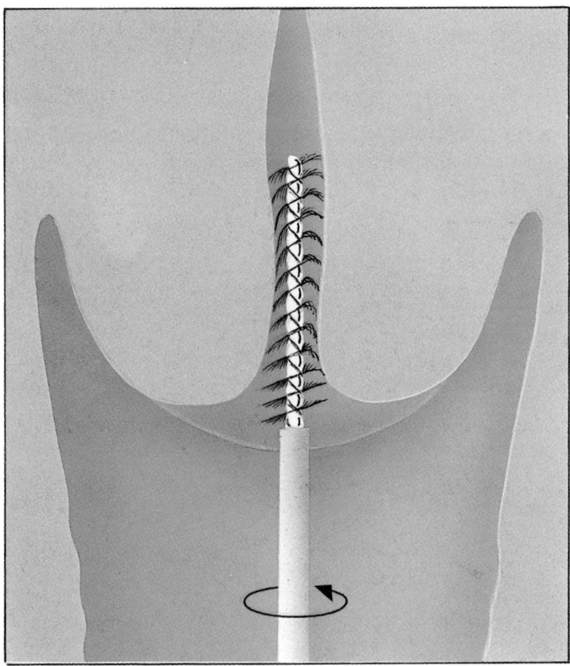

Fig. 5.3 Diagrammatic representation of obtaining a cervical smear, using (a) a spatula and (b) an endocervical brush.

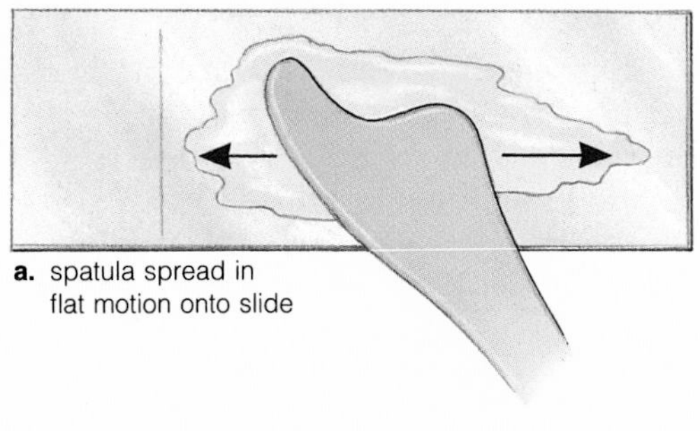

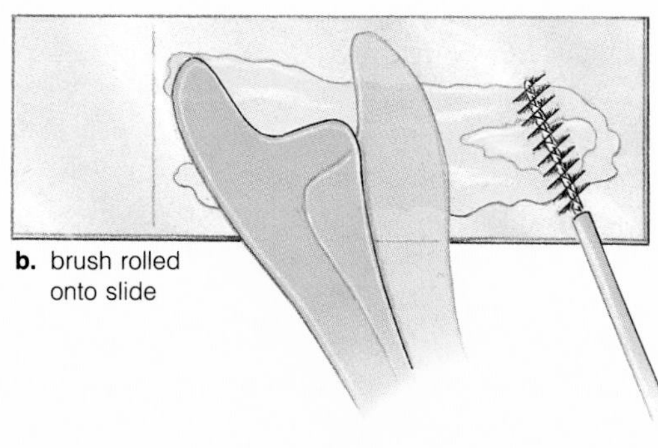

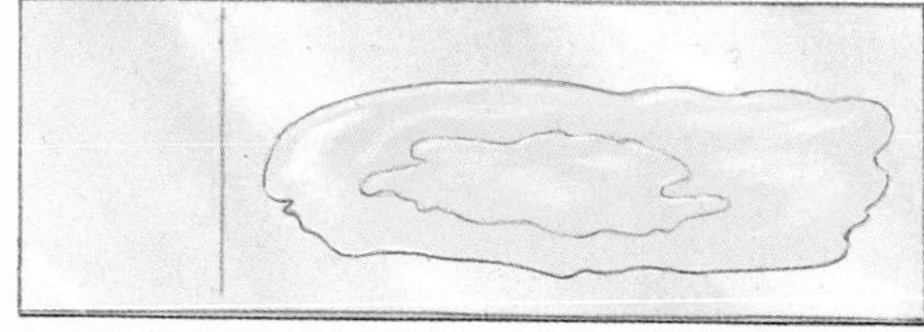

Fig. 5.4 Diagrammatic representation of the optimal method of spreading a cervical smear.

IDENTIFICATION AND LABELLING

Correct labelling of all smears is of prime importance. Frosted end slides should be used. On each slide there should be the surname of the woman, together with forename for more common surnames, clinic number or name, date, and type of specimen, for example cervical or vaginal. A lead pencil should be used, since most inks are soluble in alcohol fixative. It is important that this information is written on the slide before the smear is taken, as vital seconds can be lost and the smear rendered unsatisfactory if it is added after the smear has been spread.

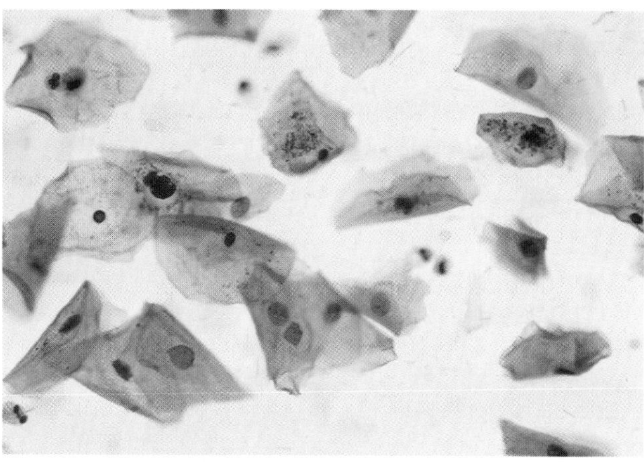

Fig. 5.5 Unsatisfactory smear: fixation artefact. Numerous cells show a brown precipitate over the nuclei, which is the result of delayed fixation in this case. A similar appearance can be due to poor staining or mounting in the laboratory.

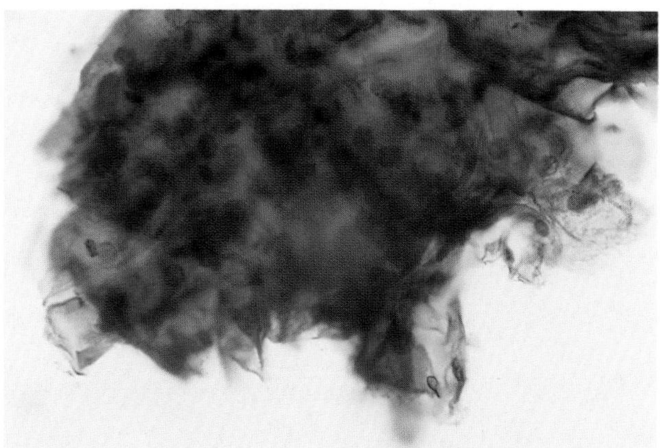

Fig. 5.6 Unsatisfactory smear: too thickly spread. The nuclear detail is quite impossible to assess in this thick clump of cells, and there is evidence of incomplete penetration of fixative and stain in the central area.

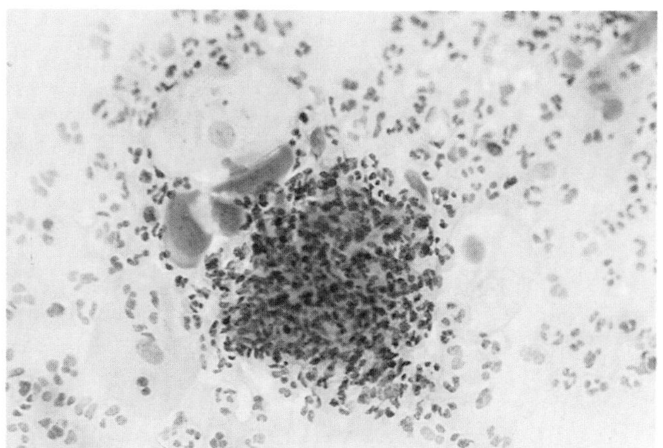

Fig. 5.7 Unsatisfactory smear: air-drying. Delay before fixation has resulted in a bloated appearance to the cells, so that chromatin detail is lost, making interpretation difficult. The larger cells at the upper left edge of the central group are almost certainly dyskaryotic.

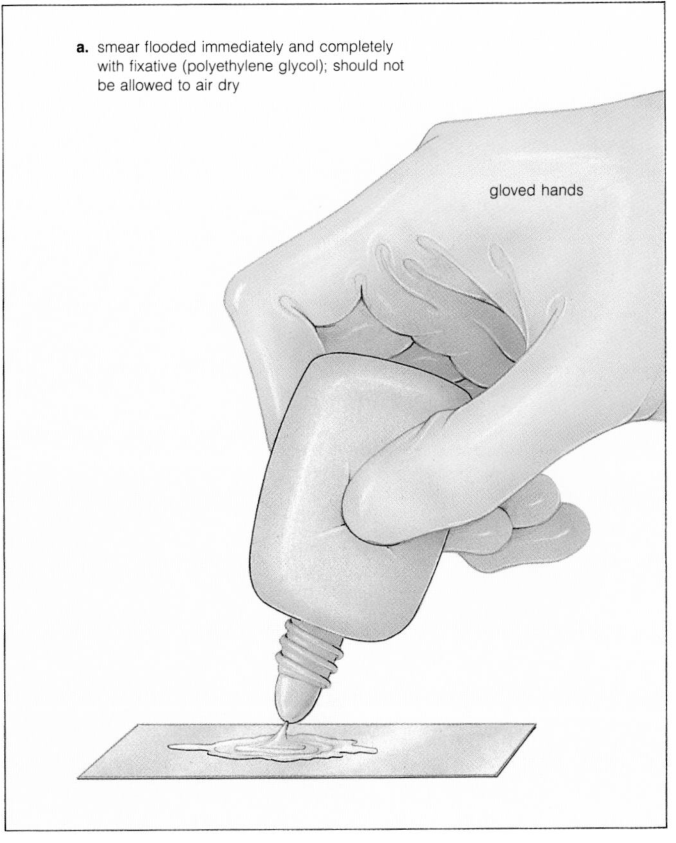

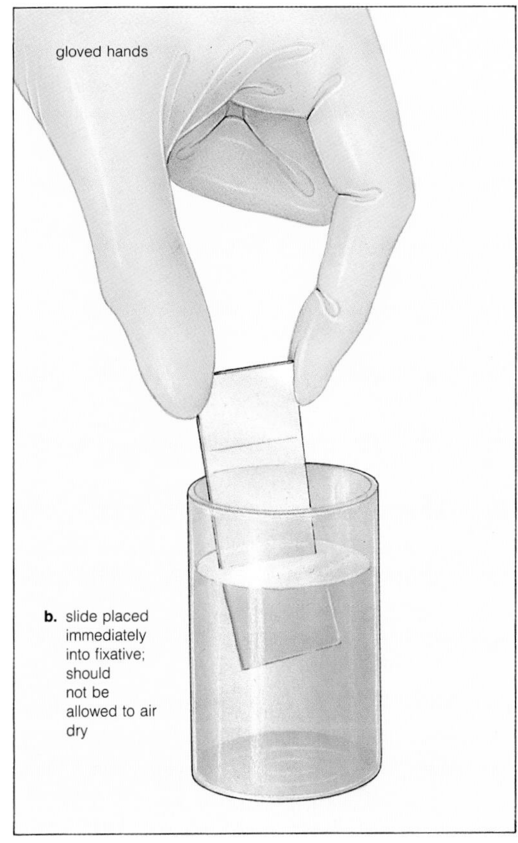

Fig. 5.8 Diagrammatic representation of fixing a cervical smear. The slide is immersed in 95% alcohol, or flooded with polyethylene glycol.

Every smear should be accompanied by a completed request form, clearly filled in in block capital letters to minimize incorrect interpretation (Table 5.1). Surname, forename, date of birth and relevant clinical data should be included, particularly if there is a history of intermenstrual or postcoital bleeding (see page 68). It is helpful to know if there is a history of a previous abnormal smear or whether any treatment has been given, as follow-up and recommendations may be dependent on the type and time of such treatment. A menstrual history, with the date of the last menstrual period, is important in all cases.

The cytologist should also be informed of any use of hormones, including oral contraception, if a proper assessment is to be achieved. It is necessary that information regarding the type of specimen is included, since cellular constituents will vary from one site to another; cell types may be quite acceptable in a cervical smear, but are of special significance in a vaginal smear. Recommendations for referral or follow-up may be inappropriate if misleading information is given. It is now mandatory for a woman as well as her physician to be informed of the result of any cervical smear, and therefore the full postal addresses of both are necessary.

UNSATISFACTORY SMEARS

Table 5.2 summarizes the reasons for unsatisfactory smears. Those relating to faulty clinical technique have already been discussed, and can be improved by proper training (see above). Similarly, the cytological decisions regarding the suitability of smears for a reliable assessment can be improved by an awareness of the areas of difficulty and application of quality assurance, both within the laboratory and

Table 5.1 Information required on cytology request forms

Patient identification
- Surname
- Forename
- Date of birth
- Full postal address
- Full postal address of family doctor

Clinical details
- Type and source of smear (cervix, vulva, endocervical brush)
- Relevant symptoms (e.g. intermenstrual bleeding, profuse discharge)
- Details of any hormonal treatment or other medication
- Date of last menstrual period
- Previous history of abnormal smear with details of any treatment

Clinic details
- Name of clinic or ward
- Clinic or hospital registration number
- Name of consultant
- Name of taker of smear

All information should be clearly written, preferably in block capitals, in order to avoid misinterpretation. Additional information may be required for local reasons or as the result of national policies.

Table 5.2 Reasons for unsatisfactory smears

1 Faulty clinical procedures
- Too scanty
- Too thickly spread
- Inadequate fixation
- Incomplete visualization of cervix

2 Hormonal status
- Menstrual
- Excessive progesterone effect
- Late secretory
- Oral contraceptive

3 Cytological appearances
- Red blood cells
- White blood cells
- Bacteria
- Unrepresentative sample

by involvement in external systems. A balance has to be kept between smears that need to be repeated, and those that are satisfactory.

Unsatisfactory smears due to physiological reasons can be minimized by screening, as far as possible, between the tenth and the sixteenth day of the menstrual cycle. This should definitely be arranged for women having cervical smears as part of the call/recall programme. For diagnostic purposes, arrangements cannot always be convenient in this respect.

While a menstrual smear, or a smear taken in the late secretory phase, is not inevitably unsuitable, it should not be a surprise if the report is classified as 'unsatisfactory'; it must be accepted that a proportion of smears will be justifiably reported as such, and a repeat smear will be required.

The question of absence of endocervical glandular cells in cervical smears is hotly debated, and opinions differ. In the USA, the view of the National Institutes of Health is that a cervical smear without endocervical glandular cells should be regarded at least as suboptimal. Some authorities are suggesting that such a smear should be reported as unsatisfactory.

However, the British Society for Clinical Cytology, together with the British Society for Colposcopy and Cervical Pathology, have issued a statement suggesting a more reasoned approach. This does not overemphasize the absence of endocervical glandular cells in a cervical smear as a sufficient reason in itself to render a smear unsatisfactory. Other factors should also be taken into account, including the age and hormonal status of the woman.

With practice, the procedure for obtaining an optimal cervical smear can be carried out with ease and in a few minutes. However, it is important not to become overconfident; a less than fastidious technique can compromise a woman being screened and undermine confidence in cytology. Furthermore, it could unfairly diminish the confidence of the cytologist.

6. *Introduction to colposcopy and documentation*

THE COLPOSCOPE

Introduction and historical background

The colposcope is a microscope designed to allow examination of the cervix with magnifications ranging between six- and 40-fold. It was invented by Hinselmann, and was first described by him in 1925. Hinselmann, like others in his time, felt the need to diagnose cancer of the cervix in its earliest possible form, and thought that if the cervix could be magnified with the use of an optical instrument, cancer would become visible at its earliest stage, as either a small ulcer or a small exophytic lesion. Hinselmann soon realized that his suppositions were incorrect, but nevertheless found it possible to see changes in the cervical epithelium that fell outside the limits of normality.

In the early days, the technique of colposcopy was confined to German-speaking countries, and it was not until the 1960s that the English-speaking nations began to take an interest in it. Although its lack of popularity outside Germany was, to some extent, due to the fact that the original work was published in German, it was further hampered by an impression that its only value was as a research instrument. While accepting the value of the colposcope in research, its main function is, undoubtedly, purely clinical.

When Hinselmann first came across cervical cytology, his reaction was that this method would mean the end of colposcopy. However, after seeing and assessing cytology, he realized that the two techniques were complementary, and stated that 'the man who thinks that cytology is better than colposcopy, or that colposcopy is better than cytology, is a fool who knows nothing of either'.

At this point, the place of histology should be stressed: while it is important that the colposcopist is aware of the terminology used by the cytologist, it is even more important that the colposcopist has a working knowledge of the histology of the normal and abnormal cervix, and is fully familiar with the terminology used by the histopathologist.

Types of colposcope

Several types of colposcope have been produced, but all are based on the principles of magnification, usually ranging between six- and 40-fold, and adequate illumination in order to visualize the cervix. Modern light sources usually rely either on a tungsten or halogen lamp, or on a fibreoptic cable.

The colposcope is usually mounted on a freely movable stand. Alternatively, it can be fixed to the side of an examination table, or be attached to a wall or the ceiling of the colposcopy room (Fig. 6.1).

The focal length of the colposcope usually ranges between 200 and 250 mm, which is a comfortable working distance for most practitioners. However, some colposcopists, like Kolstad, use an objective lens of 125 mm, while others use lenses of up to 400 mm. The longer working distance may be preferable when operative procedures are being carried out under colposcopic direction. There are varying magnifications for eyepiece lenses, ranging between six- and 12-fold, and drum changers for large magnifications.

Most colposcopes have various accessories, such as:

1. A monocular teaching arm.
2. A still or video camera (the latter has largely superseded 1).

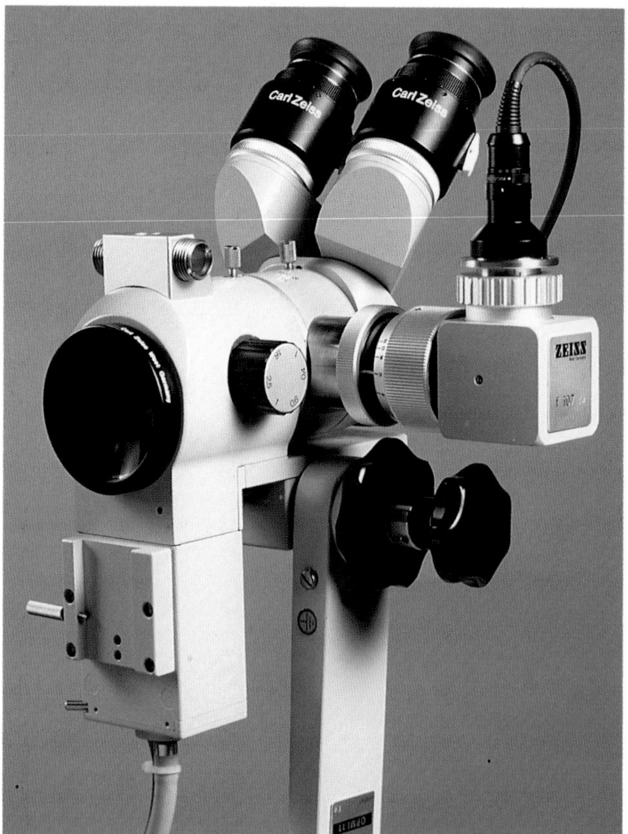

Fig. 6.1 Modern video documentation. A tiny, unobtrusive, colour video camera (actual size: 2 × 2 × 2 inches) is attached via a beamsplitter between the colposcope body and eyepiece section. Courtesy of Carl Zeiss, Germany.

3. A green filter which is interposed between the light source and the objective lens of the colposcope. The green filter absorbs red light, so that red blood vessels become much darker and appear black. The green filter is a particularly important accessory if the saline technique is being practised for colposcopy.

TECHNIQUE OF COLPOSCOPIC EXAMINATION

Instrumentation

THE EXAMINATION TABLE

Any form of examination table that allows the patient to be placed in a modified lithotomy position is suitable for colposcopic examination. The patient's feet can be placed either in heel rests or in knee crutches (Fig. 6.2). It is not essential to have a chair

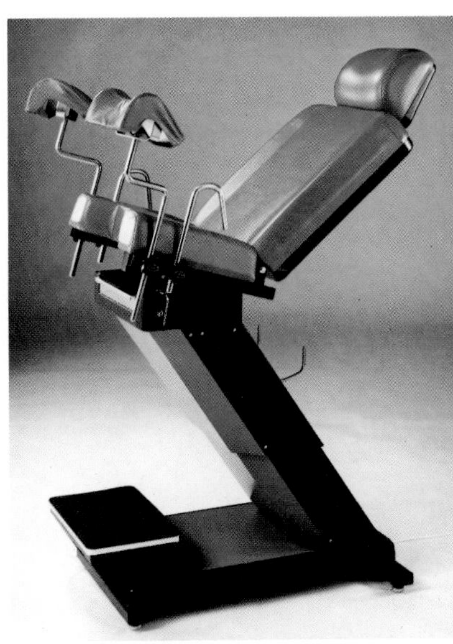

Fig. 6.2 Colposcopy couch with knee rests. This can be moved up and down, and will tilt. Courtesy of Rocket of London.

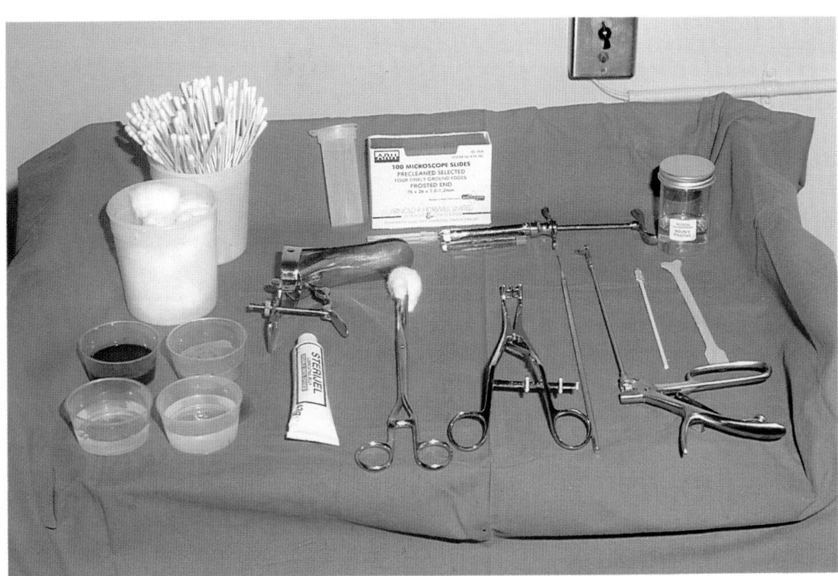

Fig. 6.3 Colposcopy instrument trolley.

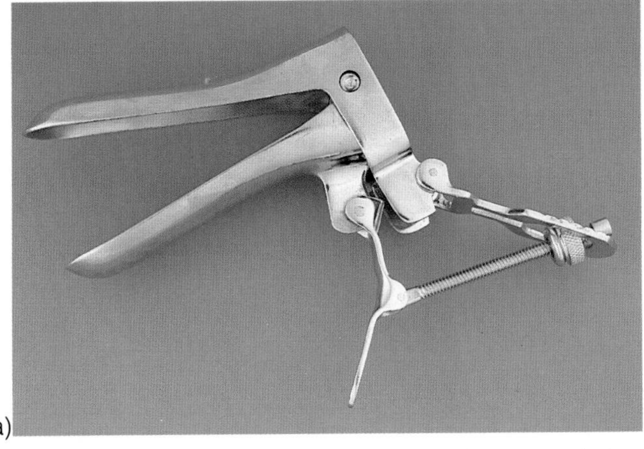

(a)

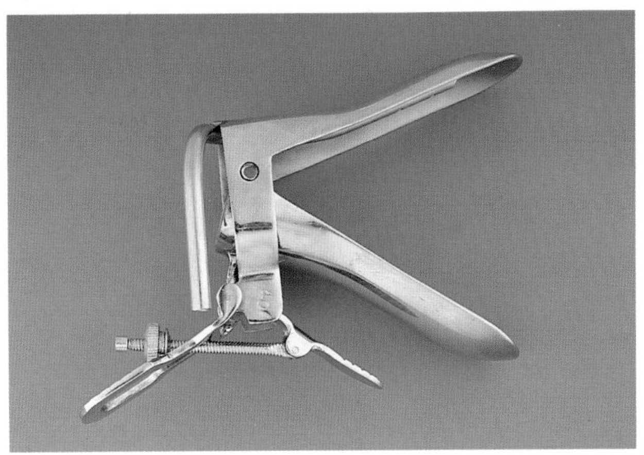

(b)

Fig. 6.4 Cusco speculum. (a) Bivalve. **(b)** With smoke extractor attachment: this is necessary for laser and diathermy treatment.

that can be moved up or down (see Fig. 6.2), although this has an advantage, particularly where operative procedures are being carried out under colposcopic direction.

A typical range of instruments is shown in Fig. 6.3. These are placed on the trolley situated alongside the colposcopist. The following instruments are essential:

1. Bivalve speculum (Fig. 6.4). Varying widths of specula should be available, and the colposcopist should be encouraged to use the widest size that can most comfortably be inserted into the vagina. Routine use of a narrow speculum is to be discouraged, as visualization of the cervix will often be restricted by lax vaginal walls.
2. Cotton wool balls.
3. Sponge-holding forceps, to hold the cotton wool balls.
4. Cotton swabs or orange sticks with a tip covered in cotton wool.
5. Endocervical speculum, useful for examining the endocervical canal (Figs 6.5 and 6.6).
6. Hooks. Fine two- or three-pronged hooks can be inserted into the cervical or vaginal epithelium with minimal or no discomfort, thereby allowing manipulation of the cervix or vagina under direct vision (Fig. 6.7). The hook is usually detachable, and the length of the handle can be adjusted to suit individual needs. Alternatively, a skin hook may be used, which has a larger hook than the iris type.
7. Biopsy forceps (Fig. 6.8), several types of which are available. A number of them are purpose-

(a)
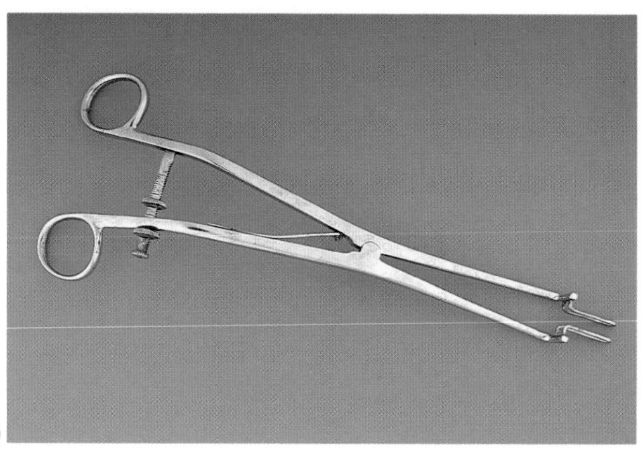

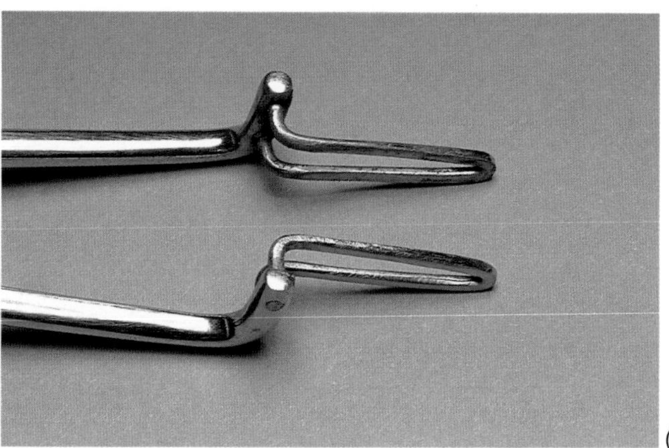
(b)

Fig. 6.5 (a) Kogan's endocervical speculum. (b) Magnified view of the distal end.

(a)
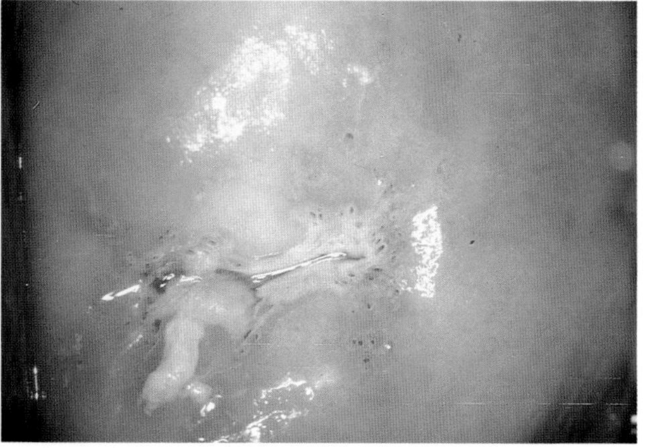

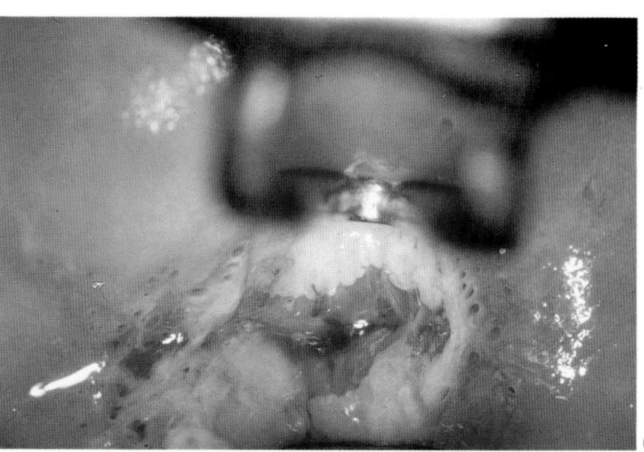
(b)

Fig. 6.6 Visualization following insertion of endocervical speculum. (a) Acetowhite epithelium is seen extending into the endocervical canal. **(b)** The endocervical speculum allows the upper limit of the lesion to be very clearly seen.

made, but some colposcopists use bronchoscopy or sigmoidoscopy biopsy forceps.

8. Four small containers. These hold normal saline solution, acetic acid (3% or 5%), Schiller's iodine (iodine 2 g, potassium iodide 4 g and distilled water 300 ml) and Monsel's solution.
9. Endocervical curette.

Examination procedures

The patient is placed in a modified lithotomy position, and the cervix is exposed using a bivalve speculum. If bimanual palpation of the pelvic organs is part of the clinic routine then it should be performed and recorded at this stage. Keep lubricant to a minimum so as not to affect the quality of the subsequent cervical cytology specimen. There are two basic schools of colposcopy: that which practises 'classical or extended' colposcopy, and that which uses the 'saline technique'.

CLASSICAL OR EXTENDED COLPOSCOPY

This is the method most widely used. The cervix and upper vagina are first examined at six- to 16-fold magnifications. If a cervical smear is thought necessary, it should be obtained at this stage, taking care not to scrape the cervix too vigorously, otherwise bleeding may occur, causing difficulties in interpreting the subsequent colposcopic picture.

Following this, excess mucus is gently removed from the cervix with a dry or saline-soaked cotton wool swab. Again, the cervix is inspected. Routine smear taking at the first visit is not always necessary, as usually the colposcopist will already know that the cytology is abnormal.

Acetic acid test

Acetic acid (3% or 5%) is gently applied with a cotton wool swab. Acetic acid is left *in situ* for approximately five seconds; it is then relatively easy to remove most of any remaining mucus. The acetic acid causes the tissue to swell, especially columnar and abnormal epithelium; the latter appears as white epithelium (acetowhite), which is usually quite easily distinguishable from normal epithelium because of a sharp line of demarcation between the two. Normal squamous epithelium appears pink as colposcopic illumination picks up the redness of the subepithelial capillary pattern.

As the effect of acetic acid depends on the amount of nuclear protein or specific cytokeratins present, it follows that abnormal epithelium, because of its higher nuclear density and consequent higher concentration of protein, will undergo maximal coagulation and prevent light from passing through the epithelium. As a result, the subepithelial vessel pattern is less easy to see, and therefore the epithelium appears white. The higher the concentration of protein, the more intense the white appearance will be following application of acetic acid. The acetic acid effect wears off after approximately 30–40 seconds, but reappears if application is repeated. Following application of acetic acid, Schiller's iodine may be used.

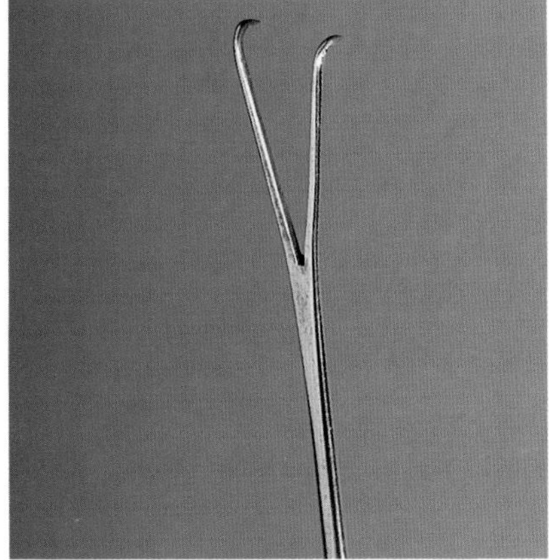

Fig. 6.7 A double-pronged skin hook.

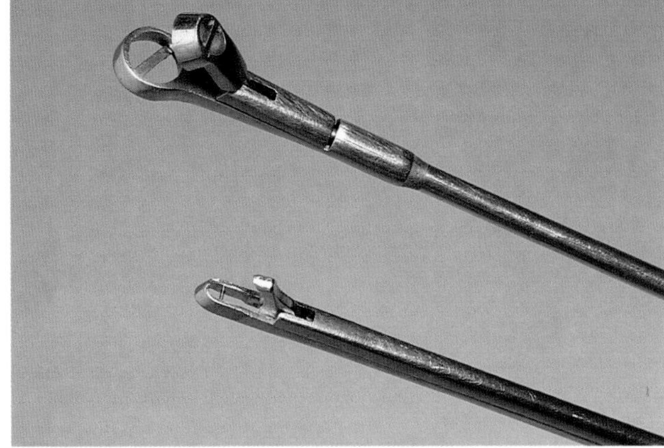

Fig. 6.8 Tips of two commonly used cervical punch biopsy forceps.

Schiller's iodine test

The rationale behind this test is that normal, mature, squamous epithelium is characterized by an abundance of glycogen, whereas abnormal epithelium contains relatively little or no glycogen. Therefore, application of Schiller's solution to normal squamous epithelial cells will produce a dark brown, almost black, stain, whereas columnar and abnormal epithelial cells, both of which contain little or no glycogen, remain relatively unstained.

Most experienced colposcopists do not routinely use this test, although it is essential that beginner colposcopists use it as occasionally minor degrees of abnormality that would otherwise remain undetected will be recognized.

Colposcopists should also remember that false positive Schiller's tests are relatively common. In particular, immature metaplasia and a congenital transformation zone will be non-staining. Sometimes, these conditions cover large areas of the cervix and may even extend on to the vagina; since they do not require treatment, it is important that they are recognized for what they are – variations of normal epithelium.

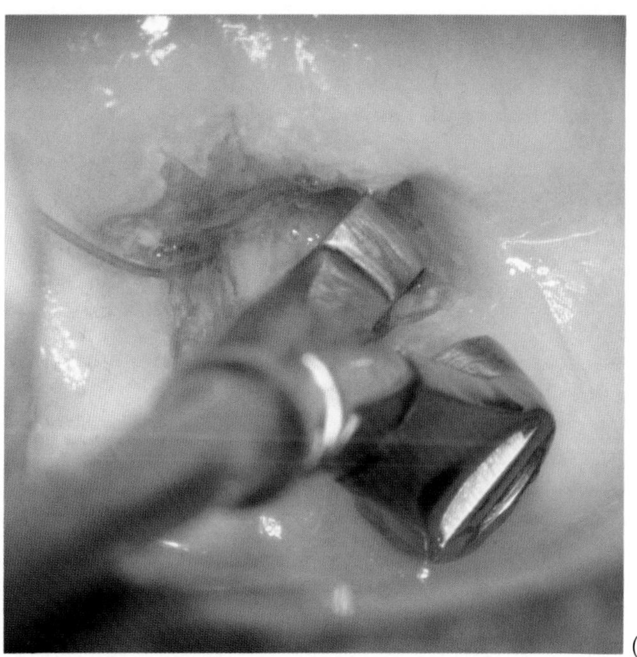

(a)

Fig. 6.9 (a) A cervical punch biopsy. (b) Immediately after punch biopsy. **(c)** After application of Monsel's solution for haemostasis.

SALINE TECHNIQUE

The use of acetic acid or Schiller's iodine makes a study of the angioarchitecture of the cervix difficult. For this reason, the saline technique was devised by Koller and developed by Kolstad, both from the Norwegian Radium Hospital in Oslo.

After the cervix is exposed, mucus is gently removed with a cotton wool swab and the cervix moistened with physiological saline; this allows the subepithelial angioarchitecture to be studied in great detail. In order to see capillaries most clearly, it is advisable to use a green filter at high magnification; the red capillaries will appear darker and stand out more clearly. This method depends entirely on the visualization of various vessel patterns, and although it is a more difficult technique to master, it allows the colposcopist to predict the underlying histological pattern with greater accuracy than does the acetic acid method.

COLPOSCOPIC BIOPSY

If the colposcopist contemplates treatment of cervical intraepithelial neoplasia by destruction (cryocautery, cold coagulation, deep radical diathermy or laser), it is imperative that a colposcopically directed biopsy is taken and assessed by an expert pathologist before such treatment is undertaken (Fig. 6.9).

However, if the patient is to be treated by cone biopsy, there is little point in taking an out-patient biopsy unless there is suspicion of invasion. Several forceps are available, all of the punch biopsy type. The biopsy site must be chosen with care, and should be that part of the cervix which shows the greatest degree of abnormality. If necessary, several biopsies should be taken. Occasionally, the biopsy forceps may slip off the ectocervix, in which case the epithelium can be raised by using an iris hook or, alternatively, a single-toothed tenaculum. Bleeding can be arrested quite simply with a silver nitrate stick or Monsel's solution (Table 6.1 and Fig. 6.9(c)).

For best haemostatic results, Monsel's solution should be used as a paste. This is produced by leaving a small amount (10–20 ml) of the solution in a small, open container for 24–72 hours. If the paste solidifies through being exposed for a longer time, a little of the original solution may be added and stirred until the paste-like consistency is restored. The paste is applied directly to the biopsy site using a small cotton wool-tipped stick.

Cartier first described the method of taking cervical biopsies using a diathermy loop. This technique is now widely used to allow removal of the entire transformation zone in the out-patient department, if desired, using a large diathermy loop (see Chapter 13, pages 167-8).

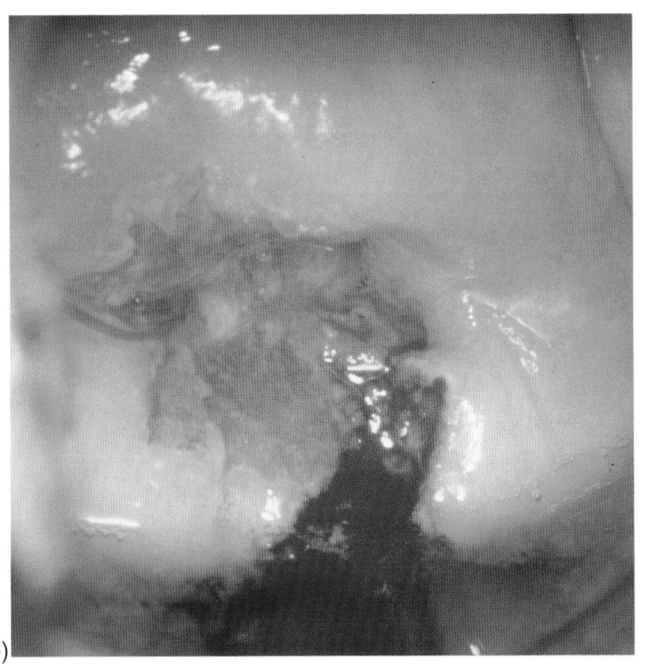
(b)

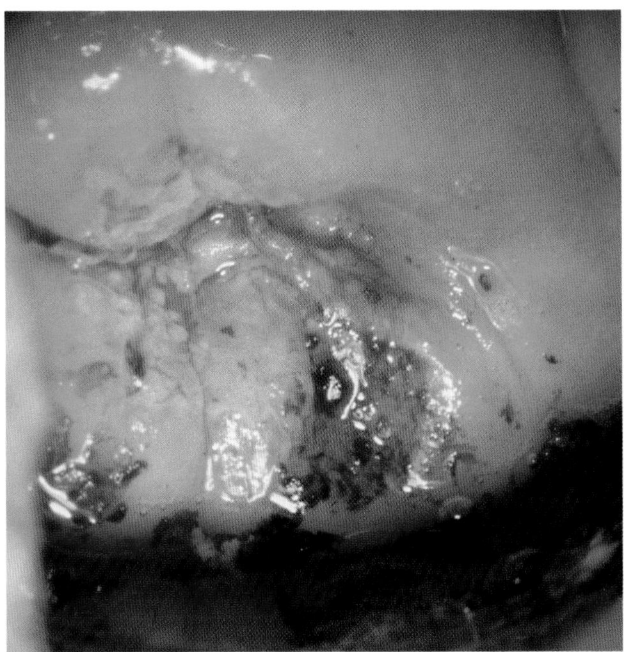
(c)

A biopsy from the endocervical canal may be obtained with an endocervical curette. This technique is performed routinely in most North American centres; the aim is to detect unsuspected abnormality in the endocervical canal above the squamocolumnar junction.

A routine endocervical curettage may be helpful in preventing litigation if the colposcopist admits to being relatively inexperienced. However, most experienced colposcopists reserve endocervical curettage for patients who have been treated by destruction or conization, and in whom the squamocolumnar junction is not visible; a sample is taken from the endocervical canal, to confirm that treatment has removed the entire epithelial abnormality. Alternatively, an endocervical brush may be used for obtaining a cytological sample from the canal.

PSYCHOLOGICAL EFFECTS OF COLPOSCOPIC EXAMINATION

To be told that a cervical smear is abnormal and that colposcopy, and probably treatment, is required, may be a devastating experience for a woman. The utmost care must be taken to deal with the patient in a sensitive and understanding manner, with full awareness of her distress and fear. The patient should be carefully counselled when first told of her abnormal smear, and again before and after the colposcopic assessment; time for this should be available during her visit to the clinic. As the cervical smear is usually thought of as a 'cancer test', many women with abnormal results will believe that they have cancer unless it is explained to them that they do not. During the examination, it needs to be made clear to the patient that she is the most important person in the colposcopy room. This is difficult to achieve in a teaching and research environment, but it is essential that observers are kept to a minimum. It is a good rule to allow only one observer, in addition to the colposcopist and nurse, with the patient's consent. Some clinics use suitable background music to good effect. A colposcopic examination can be an unpleasant experience for a woman, but with sufficient thought and care by the clinic staff the psychological effects can be minimized.

DOCUMENTATION

History of the patient

Documentation of the patient's history may be performed using some modification of a standard gynaecological record layout, a specifically designed colposcopy page for insertion in the standard case records, a punchcard layout, or a specially designed software run on a microcomputer. Obviously, personal preferences and financial considerations tend to dictate the choice, together with the caseload of the doctor or clinic. Also, the need to undertake intermittent clinical, research or other audit would influence the choice of a simple punchcard system, or, if it can be afforded, a computerized colposcopy patient record and management system.

Table 6.1 Monsel's solution (ferric subsulphate solution) (20 × 100 ml)

Ferrous sulphate BP	–2100 g
Nitric acid BP	–150 ml
Sulphuric acid BP	–110 ml
Freshly distilled water	–up to 2 litres
Nitric acid BP	–qs (sufficient amount)

- This product is to be prepared in the NSM fume cupboard as toxic fumes are given off (nitrogen dioxide). Fume cupboard fan to be on **maximum** and doors to weighing room kept ajar (to maximize ventilation).
- The operator must wear protective gloves, face mask and apron.
- Concentrated acids must be handled with extreme care and the equipment cleaned with care.

Method

Do not allow volume to go below 2250 ml. Stir constantly with magnetic stirrer.

1 Place 500 ml distilled water in a 5-litre beaker (previously tared to 2 litres).
2 Measure out sulphuric acid. Have checked. Add it to the beaker.
3 Place the beaker on a hot-plate/stirrer and heat to almost boiling.
4 Measure out 150 ml nitric acid. Have checked. Add it to solution in the flask.
5 Turn hot-plate down to a low heat. Weigh out ferrous sulphate and have it checked. Gradually add it to the acid mixture with constant stirring: wait until it has dissolved and the effervescence has stopped before adding more. (Do not allow a sediment to form on the bottom.) Make up to 2250 ml approx. Bring to the boil.
6 Keep simmering gently on a medium heat. Gradually add approximately 40 ml nitric acid, then add dropwise until the red-brown fumes stop evolving and the solution is a deep red colour. This usually needs about 70 ml. Watch for the red colour developing, using a glass pipette to view the drops. Keep the volume between 2250 ml and 2500 ml.
7 Ask **Quality Control** to check that the solution is free from nitrate and ferrous ions. If not free of nitrates then boil it until it is. If ferrous ions are present not enough nitric acid has been added – repeat steps 6 to 8.
8 Aim to get the volume of solution to 2250 ml then allow it to cool.
9 Check the volume of the solution at room temperature in a measuring flask – make up to the volume with distilled water if below 2 litres.
10 Store in 100 ml brown glass bottles, and label. 30 ml are required for **Quality Control.**

Specimen label

NOT TO BE TAKEN 100 ml

FERRIC SUBSULPHATE SOLUTION

(Monsel's solution)

DO NOT STORE BELOW 22°C

If exposed to low temperatures crystals may form which will redissolve on warming and shaking vigorously. Loosen cap before exposing bottle to heat.

KEEP OUT OF REACH OF CHILDREN

USE BEFORE: ....

REFERRAL VISIT

COLPOSCOPY CLINIC EIM 62

Visit no. ____
Date ____
Seen by ____
LMP ____

Pat. No. ____
Name ____
DoB ____
Consultant ____

Reason for Referral:-
1. Abnormal smears de novo
2. Abnormal smears after previous treatment of CIN
3. Abnormal smears after previous treatment of Ca
4. Clinically suspicious cervix
5. DES exposure
6. Routine after treatment elsewhere
7. After colposcopy elsewhere
8. Cervical warts
9. Vulval warts
10. Transplant recipient
11. Breast cancer
12. Other Immunosuppression
13. Lymphoma
14. HIV+
15. Clinically suspicious vulva
99. Other (specify):-

Cytology at referral:-
0. Inadequate specimen
1. Negative
2. Pattern suggests borderline changes
3. Pattern suggests CIN 1
4. Pattern suggests CIN 2
5. Pattern suggests CIN 3
6. Pattern suggests CIN 3 / Invasive
7. Pattern suggests glandular abnormality
8. Pattern suggests adenocarcinoma
9. Inflammatory
10. Not known
11. Not done
99. Pattern suggests other abnormality

Duration of Abnormality (mnths)____
Approx. no. of abnormal smears____
Date of last normal smear____

Coitarche____ Number____

Previous history CIN / Carcinoma:-
1. None
2. Cone
3. Laser
4. Cold Coagulator
5. Cryocautery
6. Diathermy Loop
7. Diathermy cautery
8. Hysterectomy
9. Wertheim
10. Radiotherapy
99. Other (specify):-

Other gynae history:-
1. None
2. D & C for menstrual problems
3. PID
4. Cautery (not CIN)
5. T.Hyst. (not CIN)
6. Subtotal hyst
7. Amputn cervix (PFR)
8. Tubal / ovarian surgery
9. Infertility
10. Vulval / Vaginal warts
11. Laparoscopy
99. Other (specify):-

No. of Births......... Spon. abortions.......... Induced abortions........

Current contraception:-
1. Comb. Pill
2. Prog. only
3. Condom
4. Diaphragm
5. IUCD
6. Female sterilisation
7. Male sterilisation
8. None
9. Depo Provera
99. Other (specify):-

Duration < 1 year 1-5 years > 5 years

Ever used:-	Duration		
Comb. Pill Yes / No	< 1 year	1-5 years	> 5 years
Prog only Pill Yes / No	< 1 year	1-5 years	> 5 years
IUCD Yes / No	< 1 year	1-5 years	> 5 years

Current gynae symptoms:-
1. None
2. Abnormal discharge
3. IMB
4. PCB
5. PMB
6. Pregnant
7. Infertile
8. Vulval / Vaginal warts
9. Dyspareunia
10. Amenorrhoea
11. PID
12. Menorrhagia
13. Pain
99. Other (specify):-

Menstrual cycle (e.g.Reg K = $^{5}/_{26\text{-}28}$):-
1. None
2. Regular
3. Irregular
4. Post menopausal

Menstrual flow:-
1. None
2. Not heavy
3. Heavy

Dysmenorrhoea:-
1. None / slight
2. Moderate
3. Severe

Serious medical disease:-
1. None
2. Renal transplant recipient
3. Other Transplant recipient
4. Other immunosuppression
5. Diabetes
6. Lymphoma
7. HIV+
99. Other (specify):-

Drugs:-
1. None
2. Steroids
3. Imuran
4. Cyclosporin
5. Other immuno-suppressive drugs
99. Other (specify):-

Drug Allergies:-

Smoking in the past 12 mnths? Yes / No
Approx. no. per day____
Past history of regular smoking? Yes / No

Any other information?

Fig. 6.10 Specifically designed colposcopy referral visit record page, for history details of patients.
Courtesy of Dr G Smart, Edinburgh.

STANDARD GYNAECOLOGICAL PAGE

This is the usual initial choice for the newcomer to colposcopy, involving no start-up expense and allowing total personalization of the history record. However, there are clear disadvantages in assessing clinical and other outcomes, especially if the caseload becomes substantial.

Furthermore, this approach lacks the advantages of *aide mémoire*, offered by other methods as a consequence of their systematized approach to direct questions in a patient's history.

SPECIFICALLY DESIGNED COLPOSCOPY PAGE

In addition to standard questions relating to the general gynaecological and obstetric history, this page would include a number of systematized questions pertinent to the range of disorders met in diagnostic colposcopy (Fig. 6.10).

If such an individualized sheet is to be redesigned and printed, it would be worth adding to the artwork diagrammatic representations of the cervical, vaginal and vulval outlines, with the anal region included, in the form of 'blanks' for drawing in in longhand the colposcopic findings (see below).

PUNCHCARD SYSTEM

This is similar to the above page, but printed on a punchcard format (Fig. 6.11). Each individual element of a patient's history occupies one allocated closed perforation and, if present in a given case, it is converted to an open perforation using a special punching device.

Other perforations are attributed to elements of colposcopic findings, biopsies taken, histopathological diagnosis, cytological results, treatment employed with appropriate details, and any information required for research purposes.

The example in Fig. 6.11 also allows for longhand graphic recording of the topography and nature of any atypia within the transformation zone.

This method of documentation, by the use of a long needle-like device passed through the unpunched perforations in a uniform stack of cards, allows simple sorting of the group into sets and subsets, and subsequent counting by hand. This facilitates clinical and research audit, and is of value provided that patient numbers do not become too great.

Beyond a certain critical mass, the punchcard method becomes laborious, and has a further disadvantage in that these cards have to be kept separate from the case folder, which may not be acceptable to a hospital records officer. Wasteful duplication of documentation may result.

COMPUTERIZED RECORDS AND MANAGEMENT SYSTEMS

Suitable software is available for integrating computerized records and management of colposcopy patients. Such programs should offer a complete record of all aspects of a case (Fig. 6.12), including full personal details of patients, indications for referral, history, general clinical findings, specific colposcopic findings, biopsy sites, cytological and histopathological reports, and reports of other tests carried out during a visit (for example, bacteriological, virological). Details of decisions in relation to management should be recordable, and treatment detailed.

Subsequent follow-up observations must be catered for, and the ultimate fate of the patient on discharge documented. Computer-generated, standard letters to referring doctors and others with an interest in the case should be possible, with secretarial efficiency in mind. These should be user-definable. Preferably, the system should be capable of interfacing with the local 'well woman' cervical cytology call and recall computer, the cytopathology and histopathology reports computer system, and the hospital patient administration system. The software must be user-friendly and attractive to clinicians. It is an advantage if the system can print out a visit summary for inclusion in the case records as hard copy, signed by the clinician for legal purposes.

With this type of documentation comes the problem of confidentiality, and therefore appropriate data protection and access codes are essential. Furthermore, in a large and busy clinic it is important to avoid unnecessary duplication of effort and material.

Findings

On completion of a diagnostic colposcopic examination, it is essential to document the findings in the interests of good practice, for research purposes, and also for medicolegal reasons.

Documentation options include a simple longhand drawing, one of the variants of colpophotography, recording of a video image, and possibly the use of a microcomputer system with a sophisticated graphics element in the software.

(a)

HISTOLOGY LAB No.
OTHER
VIN
VAIN
KOILOCYTOSIS
ADENOCA
GIN
SQ CA
MICROINVASIVE
CIN 3
CIN 2
CIN 1
NORMAL

MANAGEMENT: FOLLOW-UP, COLD COAG., LLETZ, HYSTERECTOMY, CRYOTHERAPY, DIATHERMY, LASER, KNIFE CONE, RADIOTHERAPY, OTHER, DISCHARGED

AGE

PARITY: LIVE BIRTHS:, SPONTANEOUS MISCARRIAGES:, T.O.P.s, ECTOPICS

CIGARETTE: YES, NEVER, STOPPED

MARITAL STATUS: SINGLE, MARRIED, WIDOWED, DIVORCED, SEPARATED

CURRENT CONTRACEPTION: NONE, PILL, IUCD, INJECTION, CONDOM, CAP, CHEMICAL, STERILISED, PARTNER STERILISED

PREVIOUS CERVICAL SURGERY: NONE, COLD COAGULATION, CAUTERY, CRYOTHERAPY, LASER, PUNCH BIOPSY, KNIFE CONE, LASER CONE, LLETZ, REPAIR, HYSTERECTOMY

PRESENT SYMPTOMS: NONE, I.M.B., P.C.B., P.M.B., DISCHARGE, OTHER

SYMBOLS:

ADDRESSOGRAPH:

MAIDEN NAME:
OCCUPATION:
HUSBAND's OCCUPATION:
LMP/MENOPAUSE
DATE OF FIRST COLPOSCOPY APPOINTMENT OFFERED:
DATE COLPOSCOPY PERFORMED:
? PREGNANT:

THB(MR)165

PELVIC FINDINGS:
Examined by:

PREVIOUS CYTOLOGY: NONE, ALL NORMAL, ABNORMAL, UNSATISFACTORY, INFLAMMATORY, NOT KNOWN

Referring Cytology Lab. No.: NONE, NORMAL, BORDERLINE, MILD DYSKARYOSIS, MOD. DYSKARYOSIS, SEVERE DYSKARYOSIS, CIN 3? INVASION, GLANDULAR ABNORMALITY, ADENOCARCINOMA, OTHER, NOT KNOWN

? SMEAR TAKEN AT FIRST COLPOSCOPY

COLPOSCOPIC ASSESSMENT

NORMAL

ABNORMAL:
FAINT A.W.E.: FLAT, Micropapillary Microconvoluted
DENSE A.W.E.: FLAT, Micropapillary Microconvoluted
FINE PUNCTATION
COARSE PUNCTATION
FINE MOSAIC
COARSE MOSAIC
THIN LEUKOPLAKIA
THICK LEUKOPLAKIA
IODINE NEGATIVE
ATYPICAL VESSELS
SUSPECT MICROINVASION
SUSPECT INVASION

Unsatisfactory: S.C.J. NOT VISIBLE, SEVERE INFLAMMATION, SEVERE ATROPHY, CERVIX NOT VISIBLE

MISCELLANEOUS: NON ACETOWHITE MICROPAPILLARY, EXOPHYTIC CONDYLOMA, INFLAMMATION, ATROPHY, ULCER, OTHER

(b)

FOLLOW UP VISITS

DATE	L.M.P.	P.M.P.	
CONTRACEPTION	I.M.B.	P.C.B.	
DISPOSITION SMEAR BIOPSY TREATMENT MEDS.		REVIEW	SEEN BY
DATE	L.M.P.	P.M.P.	
CONTRACEPTION	I.M.B.	P.C.B.	
DISPOSITION SMEAR BIOPSY TREATMENT MEDS.		REVIEW	SEEN BY
DATE	L.M.P.	P.M.P.	
CONTRACEPTION	I.M.B.	P.C.B.	
DISPOSITION SMEAR BIOPSY TREATMENT MEDS.		REVIEW	SEEN BY
DATE	L.M.P.	P.M.P.	
CONTRACEPTION	I.M.B.	P.C.B.	
DISPOSITION SMEAR BIOPSY TREATMENT MEDS.		REVIEW	SEEN BY
DATE	L.M.P.	P.M.P.	
CONTRACEPTION	I.M.B.	P.C.B.	
DISPOSITION SMEAR BIOPSY TREATMENT MEDS.		REVIEW	SEEN BY
DATE	L.M.P.	P.M.P.	
CONTRACEPTION	I.M.B.	P.C.B.	
DISPOSITION SMEAR BIOPSY TREATMENT MEDS.		REVIEW	SEEN BY

Fig. 6.11 Specifically designed punchcard for documentation of colposcopy history and findings. (a) Obverse. **(b)** Reverse. Courtesy of Dr I D Duncan, Dundee.

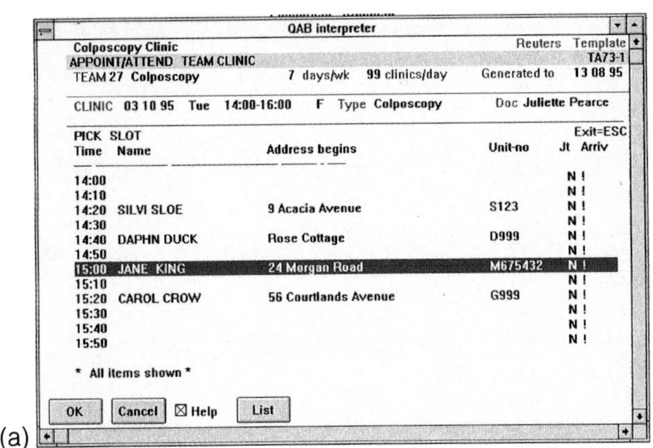

(a)

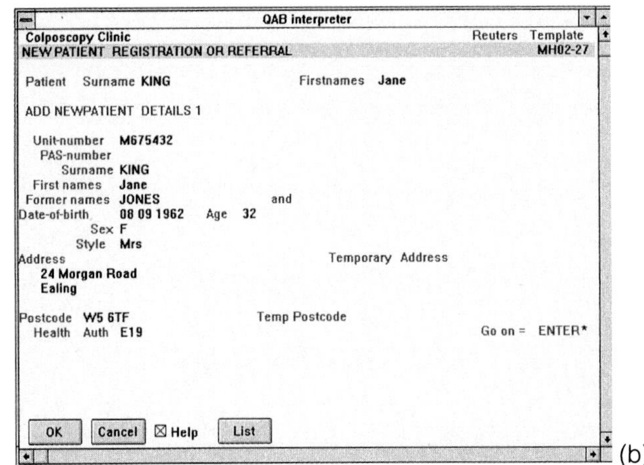

(b)

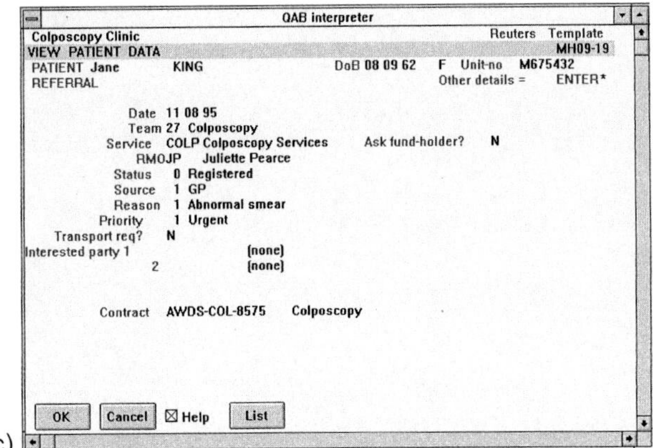

(c)

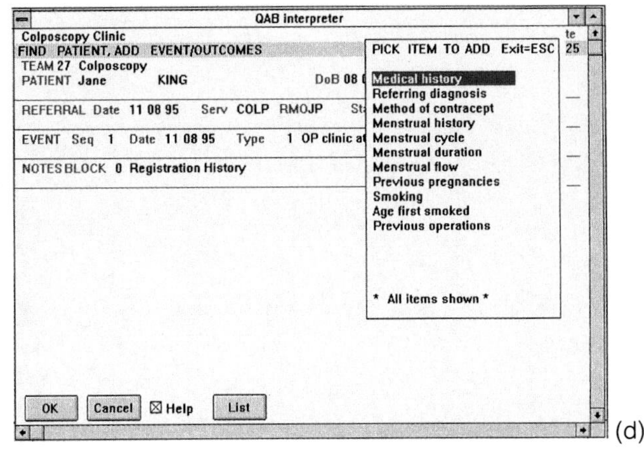

(d)

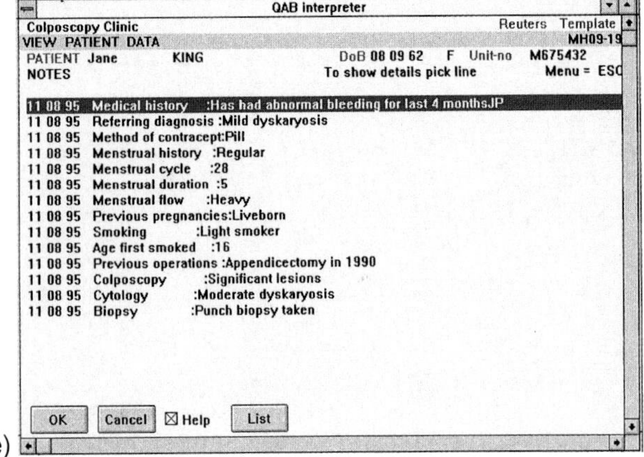

(e)

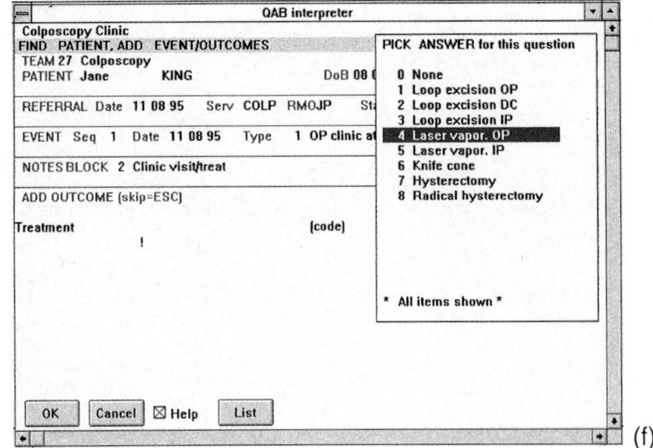

(f)

Fig. 6.12 Computerized colposcopy patient records and management system: examples of screens and documentation. (a) Colposcopy Clinic appointments screen. **(b)** New patient registration data. **(c)** New patient referral data. **(d)** New patient clinical data selection screen with drop down menu. **(e)** New patient clinical data completed from previous drop down menu. **(f)** Patient events/outcomes data. Courtesy of Gilbert Plant and Reuters, London.

COLPOSCOPIC ASSESSMENT

COLPOSCOPY CLINIC

EIM 63

Visit No. ____________________

Date ____________________

Seen by ____________________

LMP ____________________

Pat. No. ____________________

Name ____________________

DoB ____________________

Consultant ____________________

Reason for examination:-
1. First Visit
2. Routine
3. Abnormal cytology post treatment
4. Post Partum
5. First colposcopy unsatisfactory
6. Bleeding following treatment
7. Recalled because of default
99. Other (specify):-

Appearance of vulva:-
1. Normal
2. Atrophic
3. Warts
4. Dystrophic
5. Tumour
6. Bartholins cyst
99. Other

Appearance of vagina:-
1. Normal
2. Inflammation
3. Adenosis
4. Warts
5. Tumour
99. Other

Cervix:-
1. Present 2. Absent

Initial colposcopic appearance:-
1. Normal
2. Polyp
3. Warts
4. Leukoplakia
5. Adenosis
6. Inflamed
7. Atrophic
8. Malignant
9. Cx Stenosis
99. Other

Endocervical curettage:-
1. Not done
2. No curettings
3. Tissue obtained

Appearance with acetic acid
1. Normal
2. Acetowhite
3. Fine punctation
4. Coarse punctation
5. Fine mosaic
6. Coarse mosaic
7. Micro-invasive
8. Invasive
9. Unsatisfactory

Upper limit of TZ
1. Seen
2. Not seen
3. Equivocal

Extent of TZ
1. < 25%
2. 25 < 50%
3. > 50%
4. → Vagina
5. Not seen
6. Not evaluated

Diameter of TZ (cms) ____________________

Extent of abnormal epithelium with acetic acid:-
1. < 25%
2. 25 < 50%
3. > 50%
4. -> vagina
5. None seen
6. Not evaluated

Extent of non staining with Lugol's iodine
(corresponds with acetic acid YES / NO

1. < 25%
2. 25 < 50%
3. > 50%
4. → vagina
5. None seen
6. Not evaluated

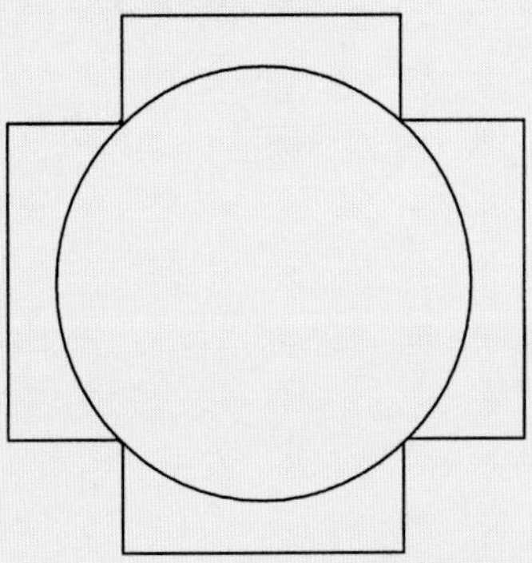

Biopsy taken:-
1. Frozen Section only
2. Frozen and Paraffin section
3. Paraffin section
4. Not done

Bx (o'C)

Histology

Smear taken YES NO

Photograph taken YES NO

PV findings:-
1. Normal
2. Significant uterine enlargement
3. Clinical cervical carcinoma
4. Cervical excitation pain
5. Adnexal mass(es)
6. Pregnant
7. Not done
8. Cx bled on contact
99. Other

Any other information

Fig. 6.13 Specifically designed and printed colposcopy record page, with a facility to document findings for the cervix and upper vagina. Courtesy of Dr G Smart, Edinburgh.

LONGHAND DRAWING

This is the simplest method of documenting colposcopic findings. Diagrams may be drawn on printed outlines of the cervix, vagina and vulva, as discussed above (Fig. 6.13), but if these are not available they must be drawn as part of the representation (Fig. 6.14). For the cervix it is imperative that, as a minimum, some indication is given of the limits of the transformation zone. In addition, the position of the anatomical external os is indicated. If the new squamocolumnar junction lies out of sight within the canal, this should be shown. The colposcopist carefully draws in areas of abnormality, using a devised system of shading, cross-hatching, annotation, etc.

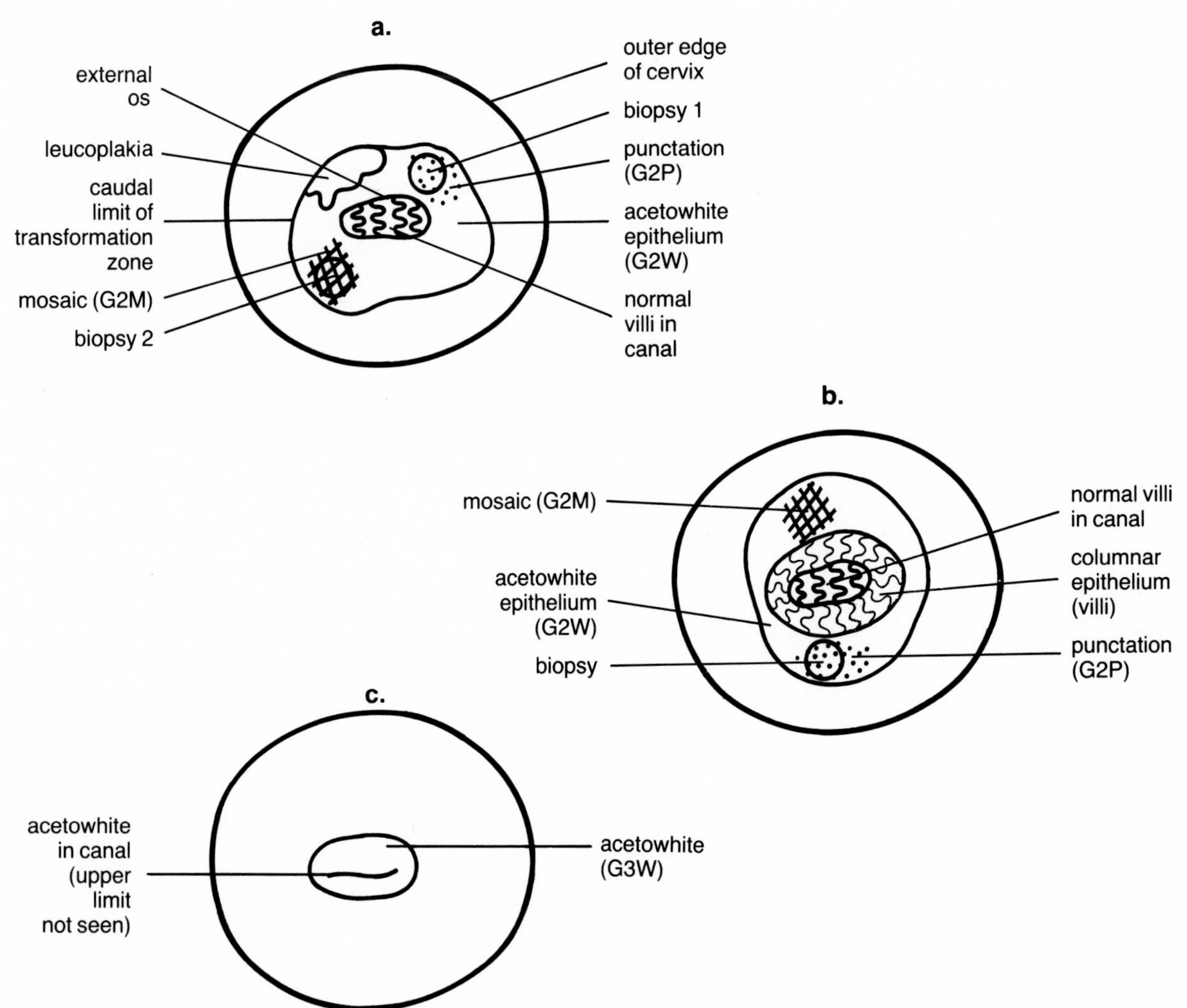

Fig. 6.14 Longhand drawing of the cervix. (a) This example represents a common distribution of abnormality. The transformation zone is totally ectocervical and composed mainly of acetowhite epithelium, with areas of punctation and mosaic. It is good practice to indicate the grade of abnormality on the labels of the diagram. An area of leucoplakia is also present. Normal, villous columnar epithelium in the canal is represented by parallel wavy lines, with confirmation in writing. The positions of the biopsy sites are shown by red circles. **(b)** In this example, normal endocervical tissue is present on the ectocervix and is represented by parallel wavy lines. Crescentic areas of acetowhite epithelium, showing mosaic anteriorly and punctation posteriorly, are present; biopsy is recorded from the posterior lip. **(c)** A small area of acetowhite epithelium is present on the ectocervix and passes into the canal; this is shown by an absence of the pattern that indicates columnar epithelium, with confirmation in the written label.

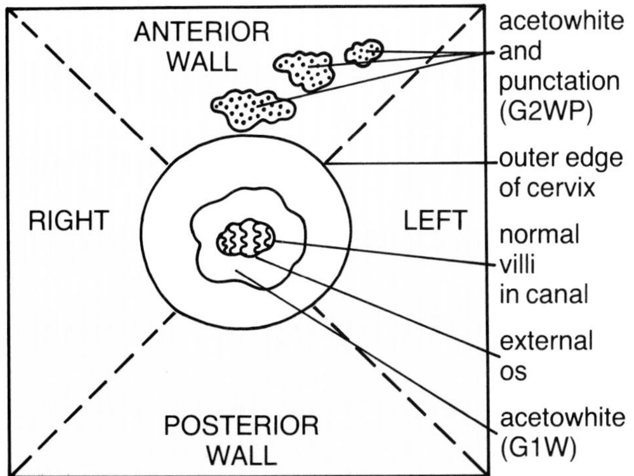

Fig. 6.15 Longhand drawing of the vagina. If the cervix is still present, it can be represented in the central part of the diagram. The anterior, posterior, left and right segments of the vaginal wall are identified diagrammatically, so that the location of the lesions can be recorded.

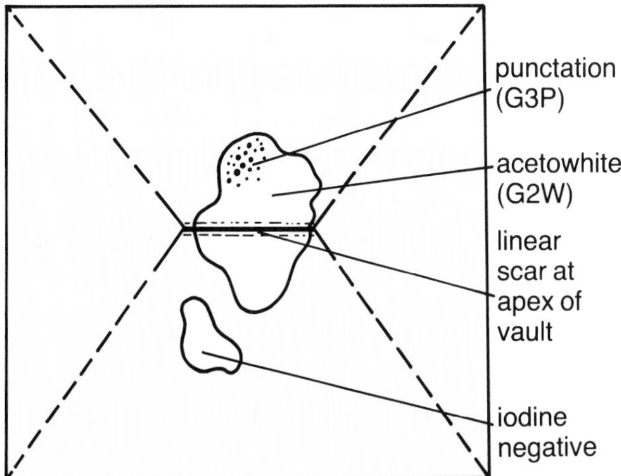

Fig. 6.16 Longhand drawing of the vagina posthysterectomy. In the absence of the cervix, the linear scars at the apex of the vault act as the central landmark. In other respects, the diagrammatic representation is similar to that shown in Fig. 6.15.

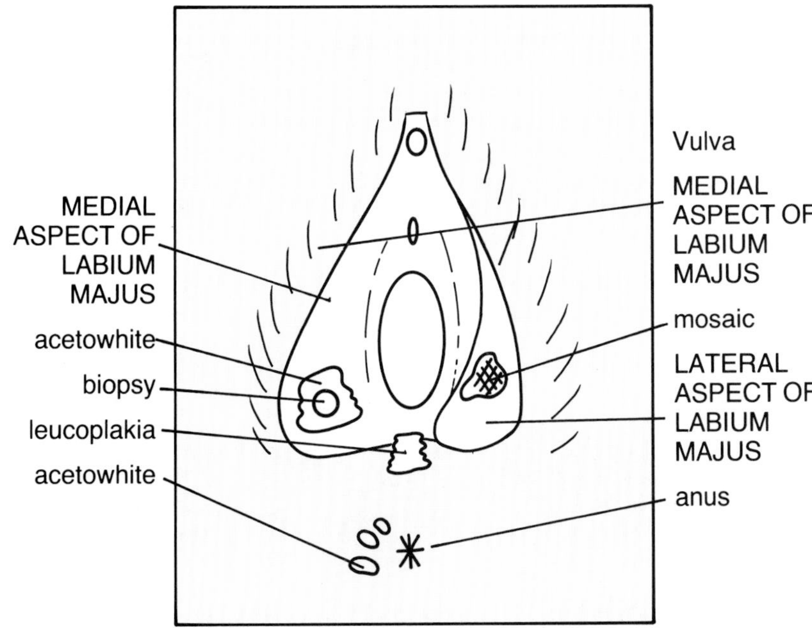

Fig. 6.17 Longhand drawing of the vulva. This should identify the exact position of the lesions so that the labia majora, both surfaces of the labia minora, vestibule, fourchette and perianal region are represented.

The system should cover glandular mucosa and gland openings, leucoplakia and acetowhite change, mosaic, punctation and atypical vascular patterns. Inflammatory vascular patterns, raised or uneven surface and macropapillary change should also be indicated.

For cervicovaginal lesions, the findings may be represented as in Figs 6.15 and 6.16, and for the vulva as in Fig. 6.17. Also, in the vulval diagram, hair-bearing skin should be shown, especially if this is a site of suspected intraepithelial neoplasia.

Some indication should be given of the correlation of findings following Schiller's test and those on colposcopy, particularly after application of acetic acid. Finally, the diagram should highlight the sites of any punch or other biopsies taken.

Colpophotography

The use of colour photography offers the ultimate in accuracy of representation, but it may be considered excessive for routine documentation. Regardless, it is essential as teaching material, and an important research tool.

Photographs are probably the most accurate way of comparing colposcopic images at intervals of time. This may be of some importance in circumstances where a given lesion is kept under surveillance over a period without treatment.

With colour, it is usual to employ a 35 mm format, which can also be used as lecture or teaching material. Polaroid colour cameras (Fig. 6.18) are also available and offer the advantage of an instant image, ensuring that the intended field and exposure have been obtained. The instant print can also be annotated immediately and affixed to the patient's records.

Several special attachments are required to mount the camera on to the colposcope: a beamsplitter, which is inserted between the main colposcope body and binocular eyepiece; an adapter to connect the beamsplitter to the camera body (Fig. 6.19); and a flash unit (Fig. 6.20) attached near or around the objective lens of the colposcope.

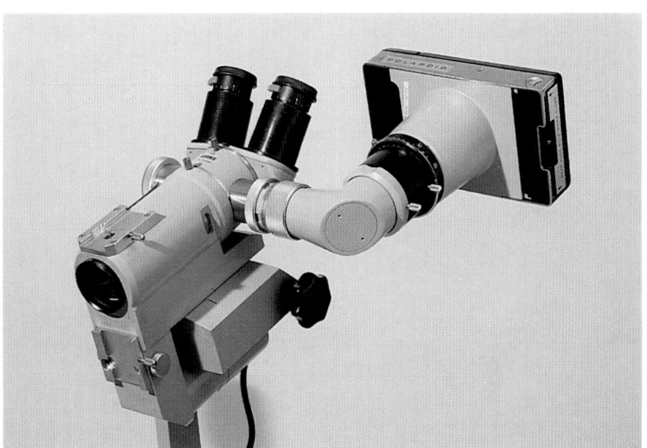

Fig. 6.18 Polaroid camera attached to colposcope via a beamsplitter and adapter.

Closed-circuit television

Using a similar arrangement, with a beamsplitter and a special C-mount adapter, a colour video camera may be attached to record part of or the entire colposcopic examination (Fig. 6.21). This is used as a 'real-time' display, or as archives for teaching purposes. Video could be used in routine documentation, although this is uncommon. In the future, the video medium may find a place if video laser disk technology for documentation becomes available. At present, it should be noted that apparatus is available that allows a virtually instant colour print to be produced from an image 'frozen' in a video frame. This process is less expensive per print than Polaroid.

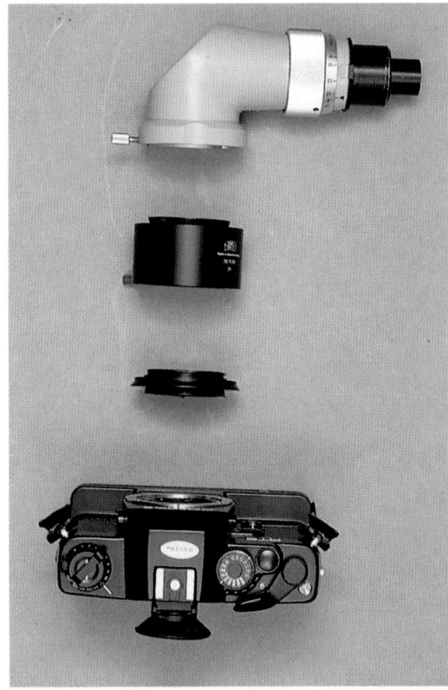

Fig. 6.19 Special attachments of 35 mm colpophotography (beamsplitter and adapters).

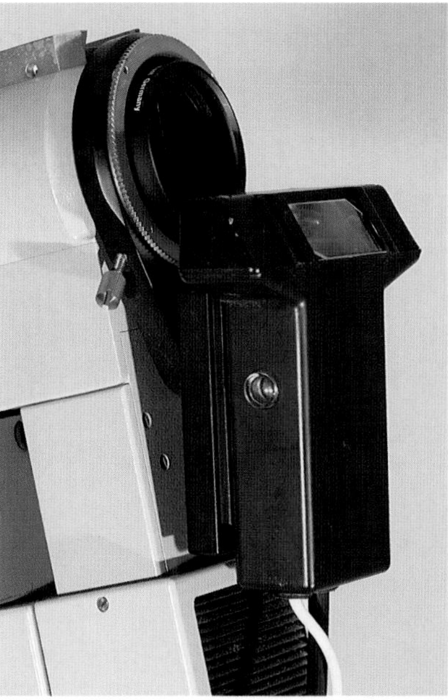

Fig. 6.20 Flash unit, attached below objective lens on a colposcope body.

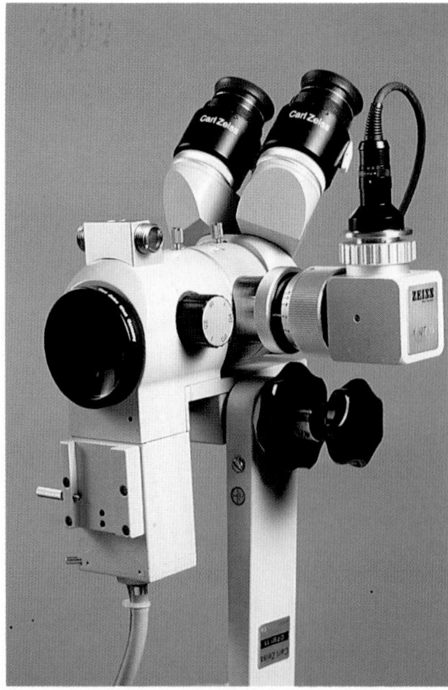

Fig. 6.21 Video camera attached to colposcope via a beamsplitter and C-mount adapter.

7. *Colposcopic appearances of the normal cervix*

INTRODUCTION

There is a great deal more to colposcopy than simply the recognition of acetowhite epithelium, or epithelium that is non-staining after application of Schiller's iodine. The colposcopist must be aware of the following easily observable characteristic features of normal and abnormal cervical epithelium, as described by Kolstad:

1. Vascular pattern.
2. Intercapillary distance.
3. Colour tone relative to the junction of normal and abnormal tissue.
4. Surface contour.
5. Sharp line of demarcation between different types of epithelium.

ORIGINAL SQUAMOUS EPITHELIUM

The original squamous epithelium is easy to recognize, and with care four types of capillaries can be identified. These were first described in detail by Koller and Kolstad.

Hairpin capillaries

Terminal vessels of this type are characterized by one ascending and one descending branch of very fine calibre, forming a small loop. If the surface epithelium is not thick, it might be possible to observe the whole loop by colposcopy; generally, only the tip of the loop is visible, so that these hairpin capillaries are usually seen as regularly and densely arranged small dots (Fig. 7.1).

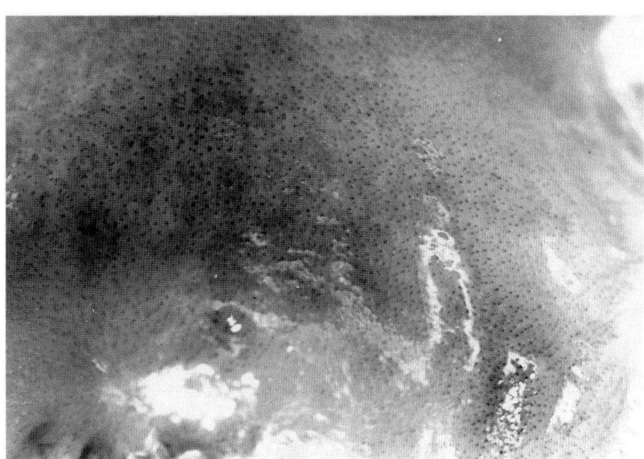

Fig. 7.1 Fine hairpin capillaries. The intercapillary distance varies between 50 and 200 μm.

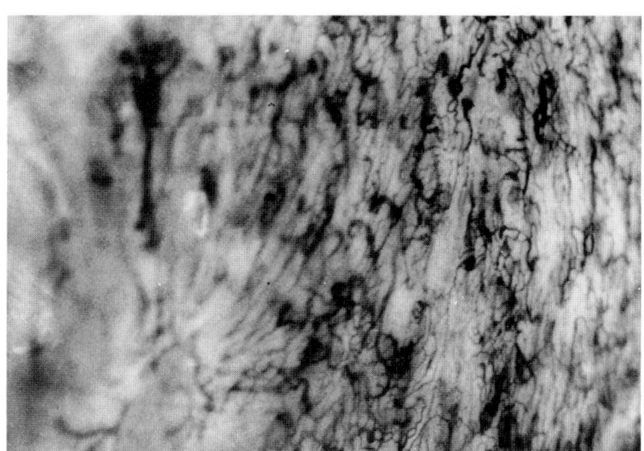

Fig. 7.2 Fine network capillaries.

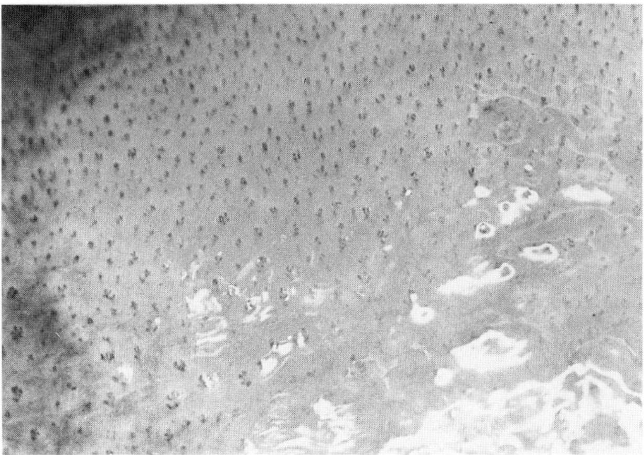

Fig. 7.3 Double hairpin capillaries, due to *Trichomonas vaginalis*.

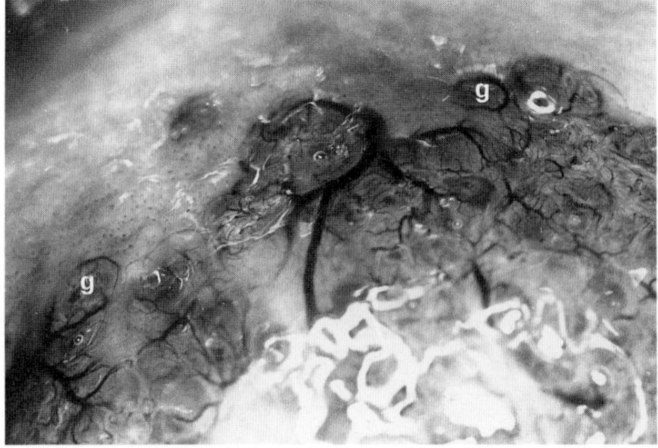

Fig. 7.4 Branching vessels, seen in a normal transformation zone. Some are arranged around a gland opening (g)

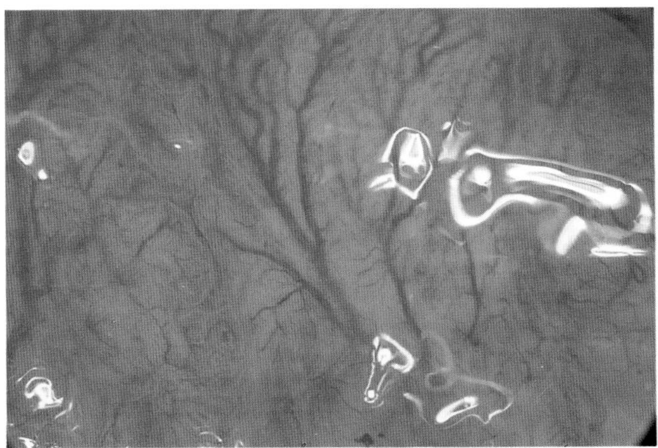

Fig. 7.5 Branching vessels in a normal transformation zone.

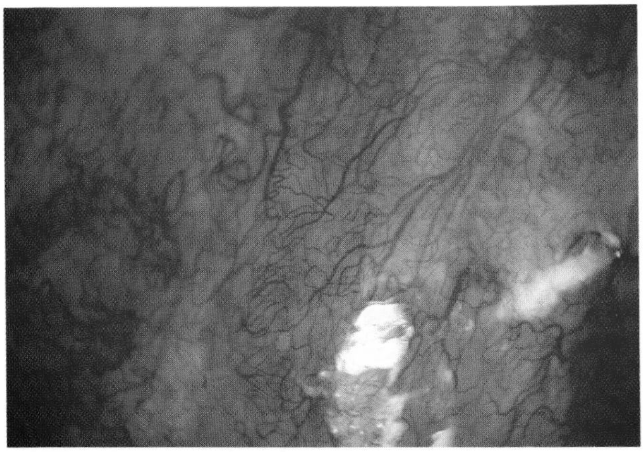

Fig. 7.6 Branching vessels in a normal transformation zone.

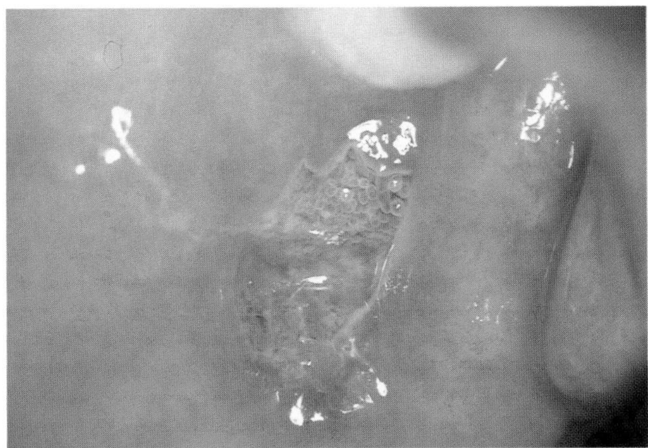

Fig. 7.7 Normal pink squamous epithelium. The entrance to the endocervical canal is seen surrounded by columnar epithelium (centre). The junction of squamous and columnar epithelium is the squamocolumnar junction.

Network capillaries

Occasionally, the terminal vessels of normal squamous epithelium are seen to form a dense, fairly irregular meshwork of very fine capillaries, referred to as network capillaries (Fig. 7.2).

Double capillaries

This term is applied to terminal capillaries of the hairpin type showing two or more crests at the top of the loop. Their shape may be described as resembling a fork, antler or clover leaf.

These latter loops are typically found in the presence of *Trichomonas vaginalis*, but can occasionally be seen within areas of cervical intraepithelial neoplasia (Fig. 7.3).

Branching vessels

These are larger, terminal vessels showing irregular branching patterns. The branches decrease stepwise in diameter, to terminate in a fine-meshed capillary network. These vessels are confined to the transformation zone. They are particularly visible in the walls of retention cysts (Nabothian follicles), and around gland or cleft openings (Figs 7.4–7.6).

The inexperienced colposcopist may confuse these vessels with those of invasive carcinoma, but even with a little experience the two can easily be distinguished.

Original squamous epithelium is characterized by its typical, smooth, pink appearance (Fig. 7.7). If the surface is cleaned and moistened with saline, the typical hairpin-like capillaries will be recognized. Following application of acetic acid, the epithelium will still be pink, but the subepithelial capillaries will be more difficult to see. Whichever technique is used, there should be little difficulty in recognizing this epithelium.

COLUMNAR EPITHELIUM

Normal columnar epithelium is easily recognized by its characteristic grape-like or villous appearance. Before application of acetic acid, the colposcopist will see that each columnar epithelial villus contains a fine capillary (Fig. 7.8). As the villus is covered by no more than a single layer of columnar cells, the blood in the capillary gives columnar epithelium its typically red appearance (Figs 7.9–7.12).

Following application of acetic acid, the villi often appear white and are more easily recognizable.

SQUAMOUS METAPLASIA

The transformation zone is the part of the cervix which is covered by mature normal squamous metaplasia, but which, at some point in the patient's life cycle, was covered by columnar epithelium. The new epithelium results from transformation of columnar to squamous epithelium, through the process of squamous metaplasia.

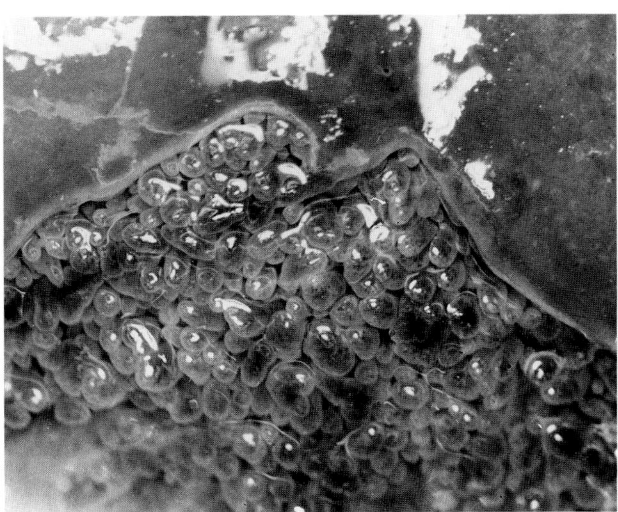

Fig. 7.8 Normal columnar epithelium. This shows capillaries in the villi; normal squamous epithelium; and the squamocolumnar junction.

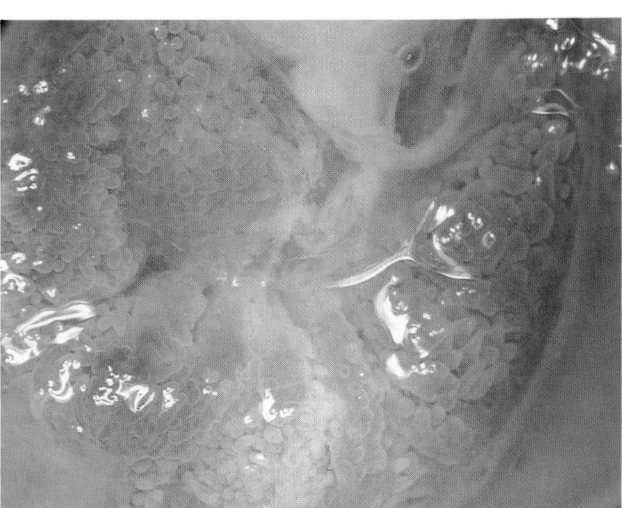

Fig. 7.9 Columnar epithelium.

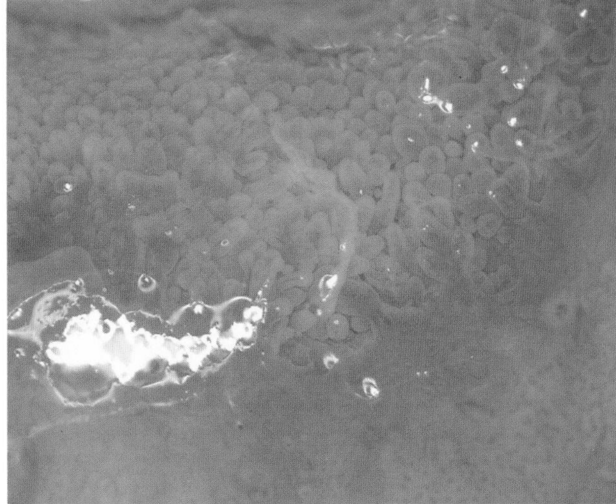

Fig. 7.10 Columnar epithelium.

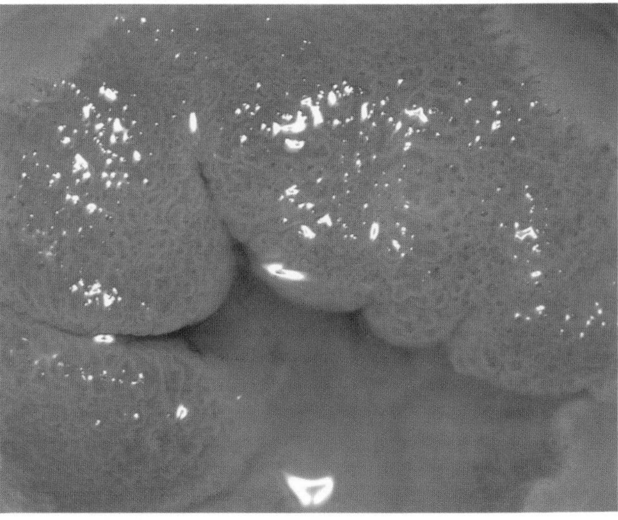

Fig. 7.11 Cervix of a neonate. This shows normal columnar and squamous epithelium.

Mature metaplasia

Fully mature squamous epithelium is characterized by the presence of gland openings and typical branching vessels, as described above (see Figs 7.4, 7.5 and 7.12). Nabothian follicles or retention cysts are also characteristic (Figs 7.13–7.15).

Immature metaplasia

Recognition of immature or active metaplasia, i.e. epithelium that is in the process of being transformed from columnar to squamous, is more difficult at this stage in the metaplastic process: the epithelium is acetowhite and can be very easily confused with abnormal epithelium. This situation may be further complicated, because a cytological smear taken from immature metaplasia may not be reported as normal. Indeed, it is often difficult to differentiate between immature metaplasia and cervical intraepithelial neoplasia (Figs 7.16 and 7.17).

Coppleson and Reid (1986) described as follows the three stages of metaplasia that may be colposcopically recognizable (Fig. 7.18).

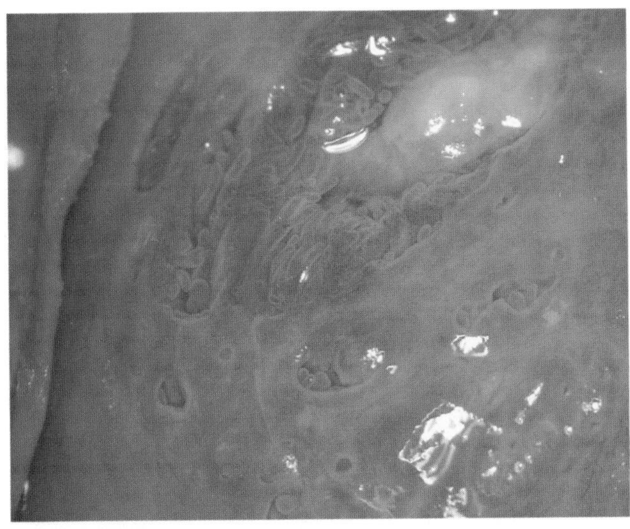

Fig. 7.12 Normal transformation zone. This shows gland openings.

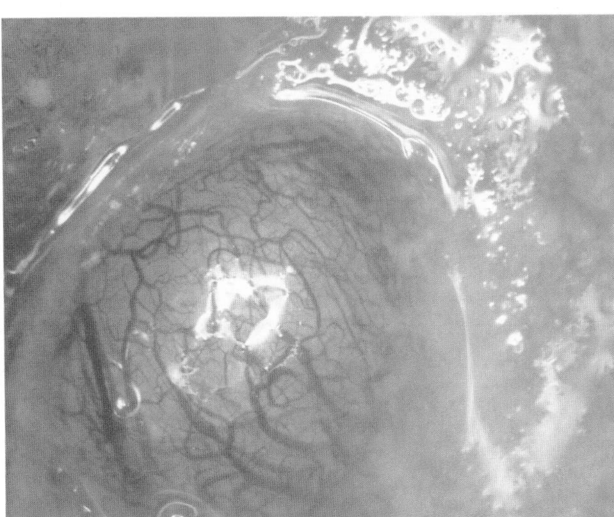

Fig. 7.13 Nabothian follicle.

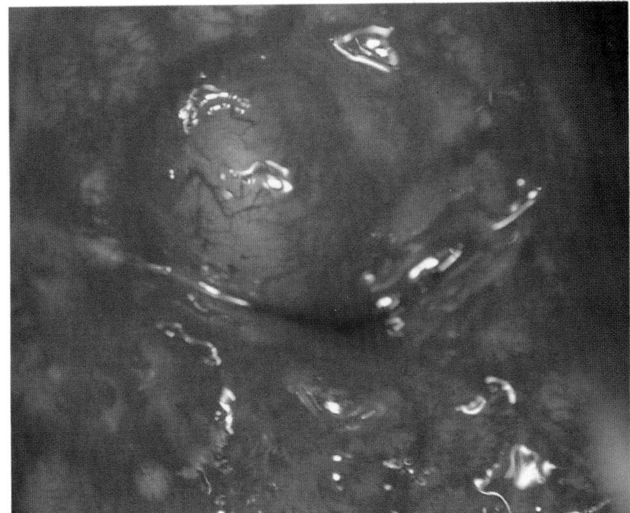

Fig. 7.14 Multiple Nabothian follicles.

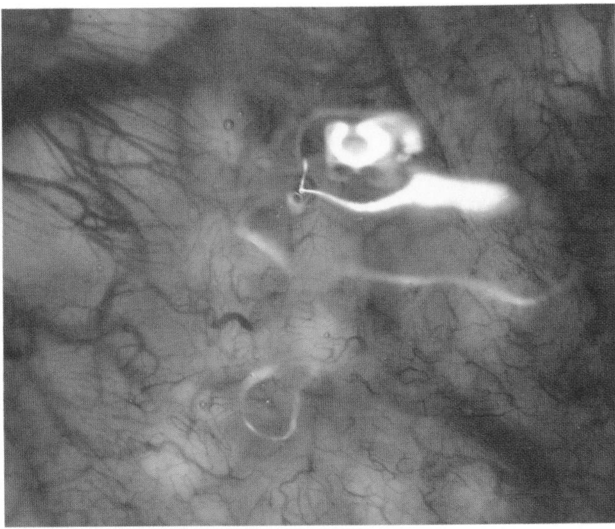

Fig. 7.15 Multiple Nabothian follicles.

STAGE I

There is loss of translucency of the columnar epithelial villi, with each individual villus assuming a ground-glass appearance.

STAGE II

The grape-like configuration disappears as successive villi are fused and their intervening spaces filled in.

STAGE III

The villous configuration is lost, and the new surface takes on the appearance of a decreasingly translucent vascular area. Following fusion of the villi, the end result is normal squamous epithelium.

Scanning electron microscopy of metaplasia

The first stage of metaplasia is observed at the tips

(a) 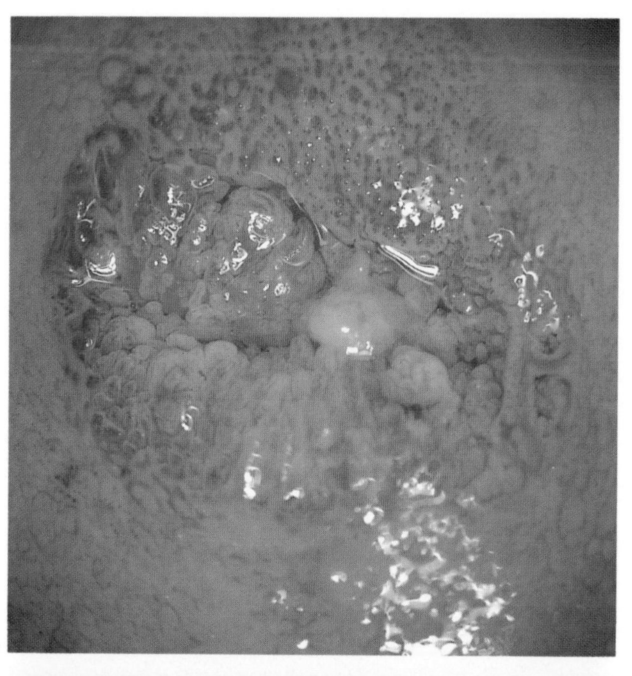

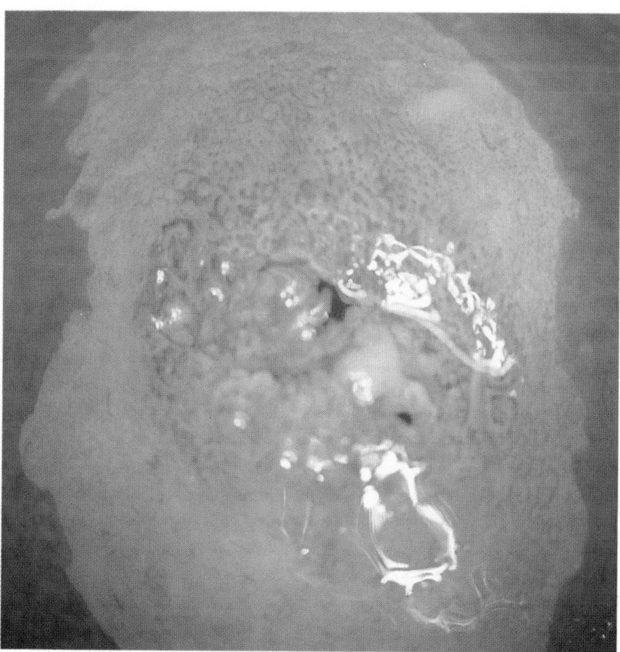 (b)

(c) 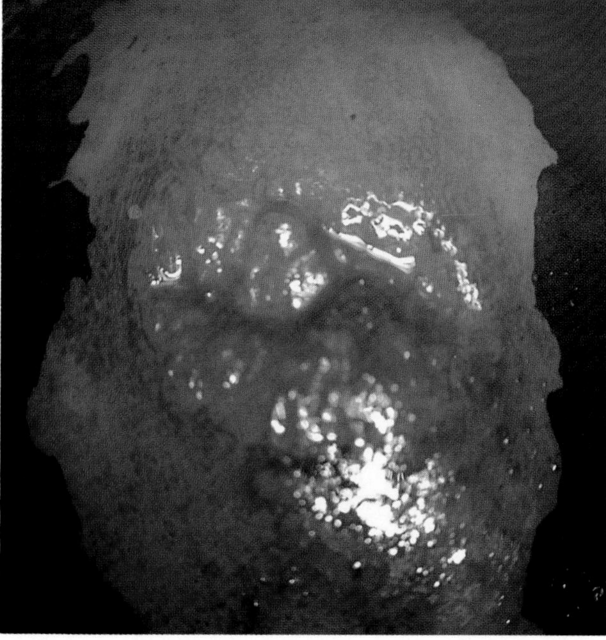

Fig. 7.16 Immature metaplasia. (a) This 18-year-old woman presented with abnormal cervical cytology. **(b)** Colposcopy following application of acetic acid, showing acetowhite changes, punctation and mosaic capillary patterns. **(c)** Following application of Schiller's iodine, the epithelium is seen to be partially glycogenated. Histology confirmed immature metaplasia, with no cervical intraepithelial neoplasia. The woman was on combined oestrogen/progestagen contraceptive pills; the columnar epithelium in (b) shows enlargement and irregularity of the villi.

of columnar villi, where islands of larger metaplastic cells can be seen surrounded by normal columnar epithelium (Figs 7.19 and 7.20). In the second stage, fusion of the columnar epithelial villi (Fig. 7.21) can be seen with islands of flattened, irregular polygonal cells surrounded by easily recognizable, smaller columnar cells.

In the first two stages of metaplasia, cells are covered with short microvilli, and there are no terminal bars between them. In the third stage of metaplasia, terminal bars can be observed, similar to those seen between mature squamous epithelial cells, but the surface of these cells is still largely covered by short microvilli (Fig. 7.22)

When large areas of squamous metaplasia are examined at low magnification, its multifocal nature can be clearly seen. Cervical columnar epithelium often presents in a configuration of a series of ridges and clefts; if this is the case, it is the epithelium along the surface of the ridges that undergoes metaplasia first (Fig. 7.23).

(a) 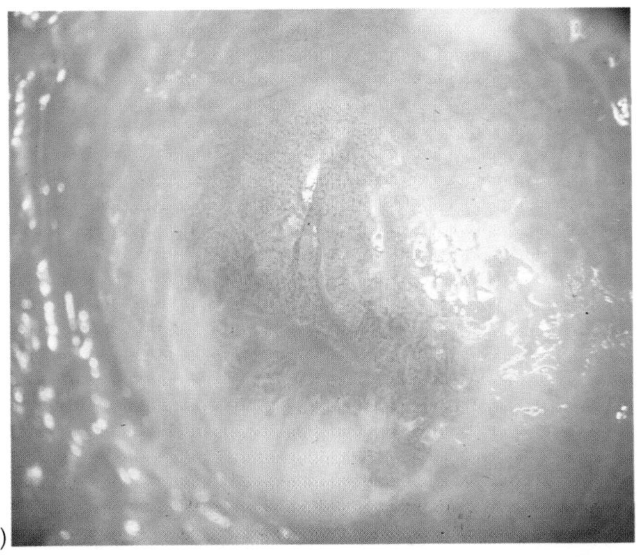

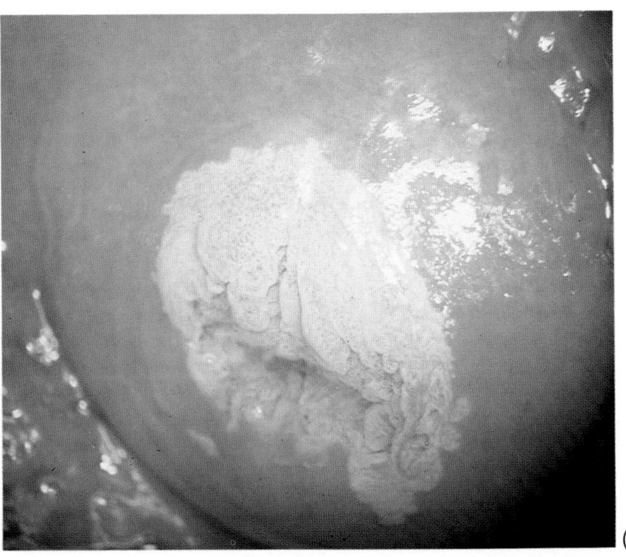 (b)

Fig. 7.17 Immature metaplasia. This 17-year-old woman presented with abnormal cervical cytology. The cervix is seen before **(a)** and after **(b)** application of acetic acid. The acetowhite epithelium was immature metaplasia.

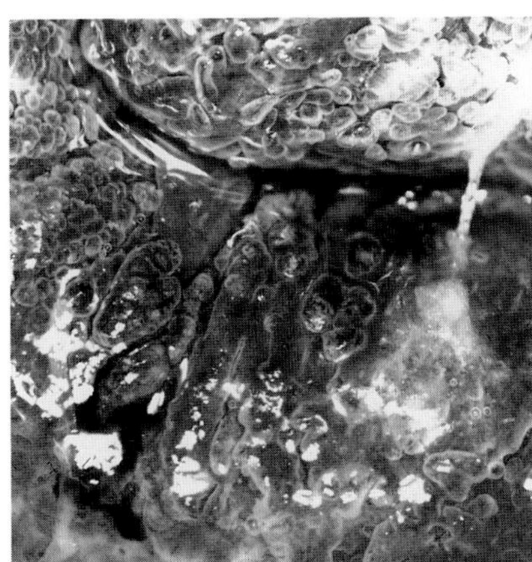

Fig. 7.18 The three stages of metaplasia. See text for explanation.

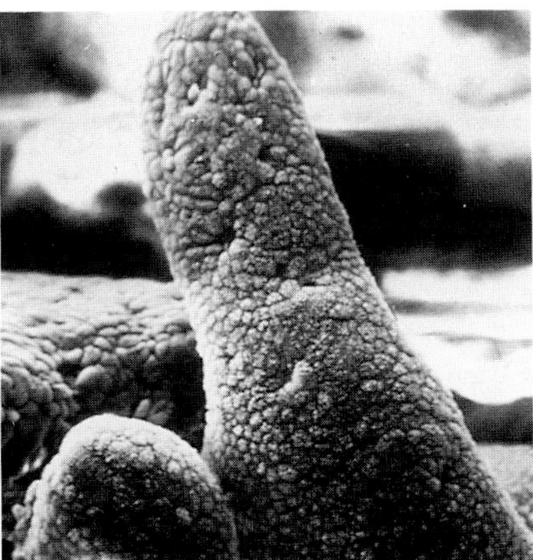

Fig. 7.19 SEM of a columnar epithelial villus. Each villus is covered by columnar cells.

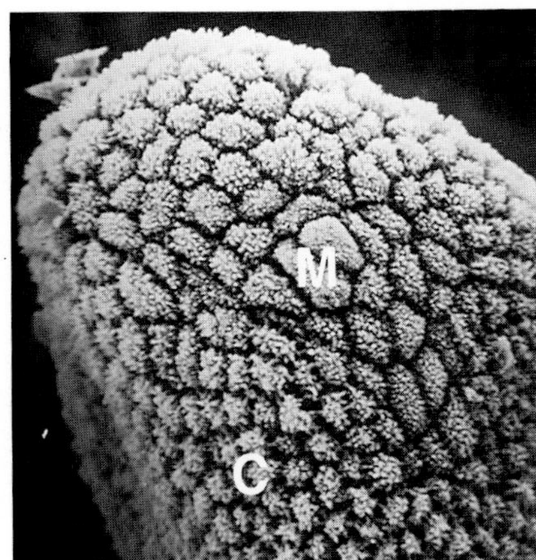

Fig. 7.20 Metaplasia, Stage I. Scanning electron microscopy (SEM) of the tips of a villus showing columnar (c) and metaplastic cells (m).

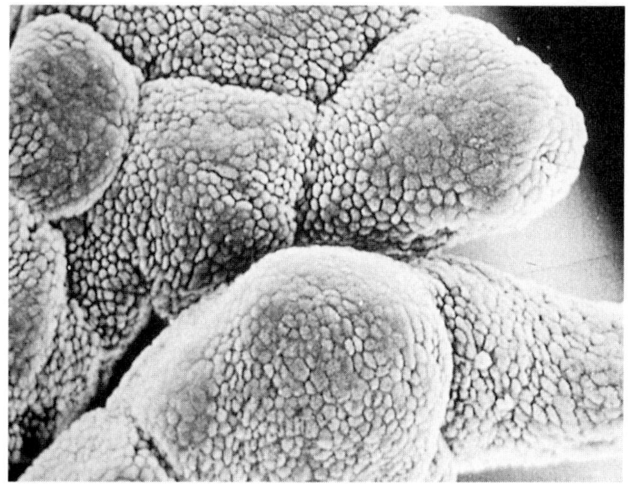

Fig. 7.21 Metaplasia, Stage II. SEM of fusing villi.

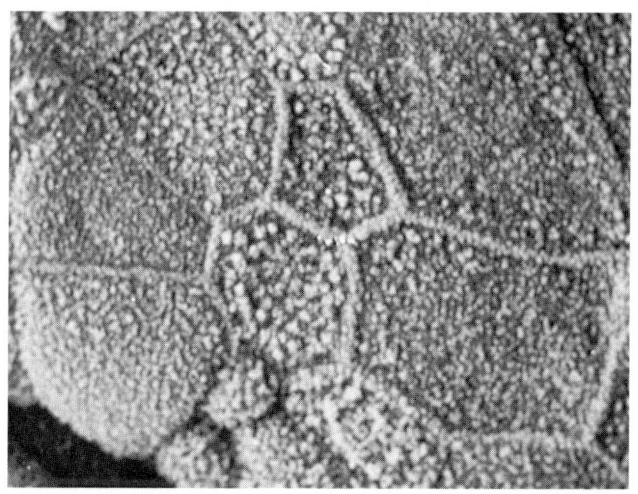

Fig. 7.22 Metaplasia, Stage III. SEM showing flat, almost mature, squamous cells.

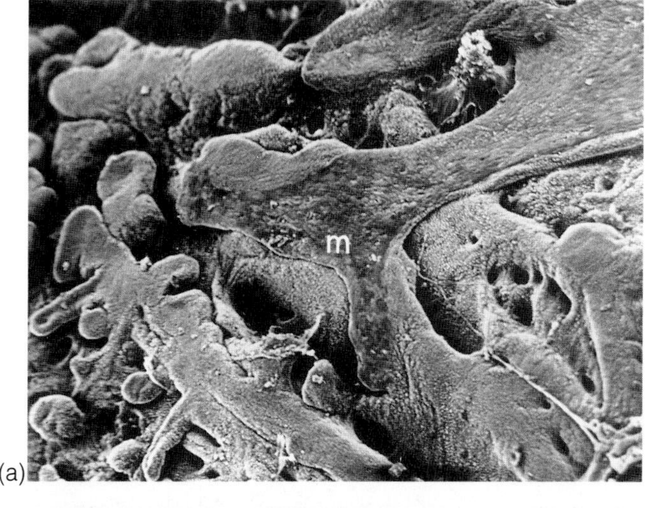

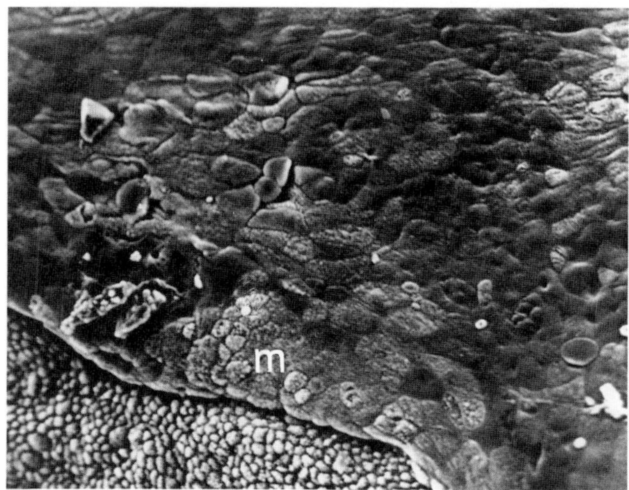

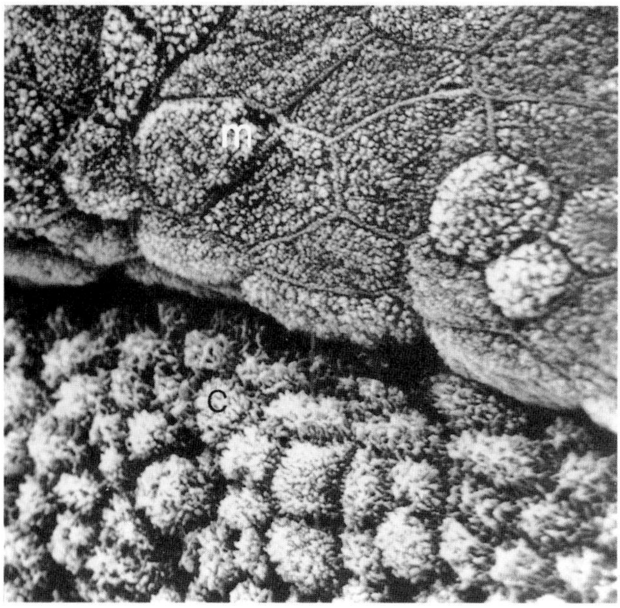

Fig. 7.23 Metaplasia. (a) Low-power view of metaplasia (m) forming along the ridges, with columnar epithelium still present in the clefts. **(b)** Same area (m) showing the new squamocolumnar junction. **(c)** High-power view of the same area, showing details of individual metaplastic (m) and columnar (c) cells.

CONGENITAL TRANSFORMATION ZONE

While most areas of columnar epithelium undergoing squamous metaplasia reach full maturation into glycogenated squamous epithelium, showing the features described above, in a small number of patients metaplastic change results in a persistently acetowhite epithelium which is non-glycogenated. These changes are primarily confined to the cervix, but in approximately 4% of women this type of epithelium will extend from the cervix to involve the vagina, usually anteriorly and posteriorly (Figs 7.24–7.26).

This type of transformation zone may develop during intrauterine life, or before sexual activity, and is at no increased risk of neoplastic change. Its colposcopic significance is related to the following features: the epithelium is acetowhite, has a fine mosaic pattern (cf. cervical intraepithelial neoplasia), and is either non-glycogenated or partially glycogenated.

With histological confirmation of its benign nature no further treatment is required. However, the biopsy material is at risk of being misinterpreted, and the pathologist should be familiar with the typical histological appearances of this benign condition (Fig. 7.27). Therefore, if in the colposcopist's opinion such areas, which are usually very extensive, represent nothing more than a congenital transformation zone, the pathologist should be informed accordingly.

POSTMENOPAUSAL CERVIX

Following the cessation of oestrogen production, the squamous epithelium becomes atrophic with significantly fewer layers of cells. Because of this, one would expect the subepithelial capillaries to show through the thin epithelium, thereby giving the cervix a very red appearance. However, the underlying connective tissue is also changed, becoming less vascular; as a result the squamous epithelium looks pale and is hardly affected by application of acetic acid (Figs 7.28–7.30).

Columnar epithelium becomes atrophic; the villi, characteristic of premenopausal columnar epithelium, become significantly smaller and in many instances disappear.

Application of Schiller's iodine also tends to stain the cervix and vagina a characteristic pale yellow. This is because there is lack of maturation of the squamous epithelium, which contains relatively little glycogen for staining with iodine. The endocervical mucus, characteristic of the premenopausal cervix, is now scanty and thick.

As the epithelium is very thin, insertion of a bivalve speculum may traumatize the small capillaries close to the surface, thereby producing subepithelial petechiae.

The postmenopausal cervix is often difficult for the inexperienced colposcopist to assess, particularly when the patient presents with an abnormal smear; often the squamocolumnar junction cannot be seen

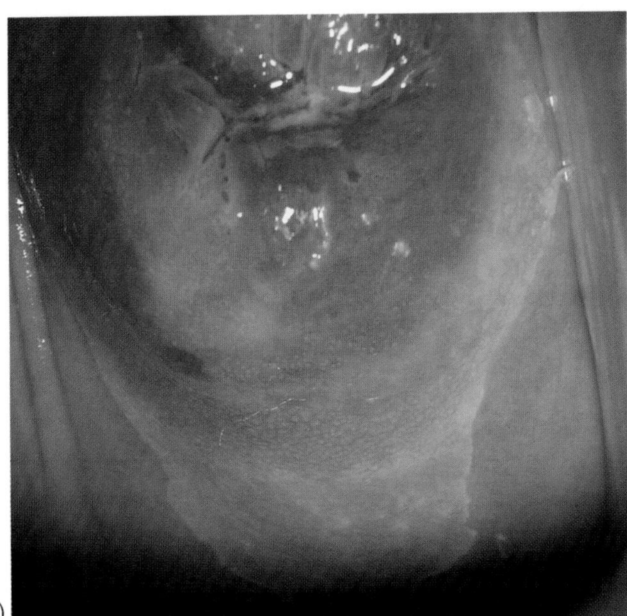
(a)

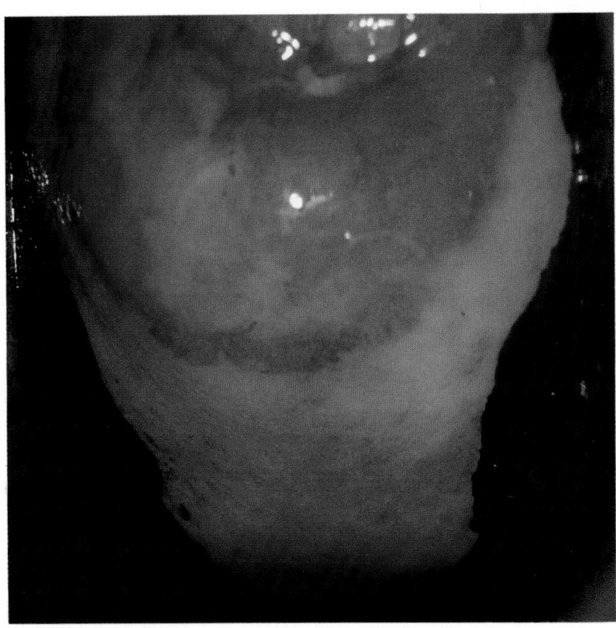
(b)

Fig. 7.24 Congenital transformation zone, extending to the posterior vaginal wall. (a) Following application of acetic acid. **(b)** Following application of Schiller's iodine.

if it lies in the endocervical canal, which is a common postmenopausal feature. Under these circumstances, a short course of oestrogen will be very helpful; glycogenation increases, the mucus becomes clear, the cervix generally becomes softer, and an endocervical speculum can often be inserted to allow visualization of the squamocolumnar junction. Oestrogen may be administered as a cream or, alternatively, as an oral or transdermal preparation.

CERVICAL POLYPS

Cervical polyps almost invariably arise from endocervical columnar epithelium, and usually begin with the enlargement of a single epithelial villus. Their histological appearance is described in Chapter 1 (see page 7).

At its onset, the polyp is covered by columnar epithelium and may only be discovered during colposcopic assessment of the endocervical canal. As

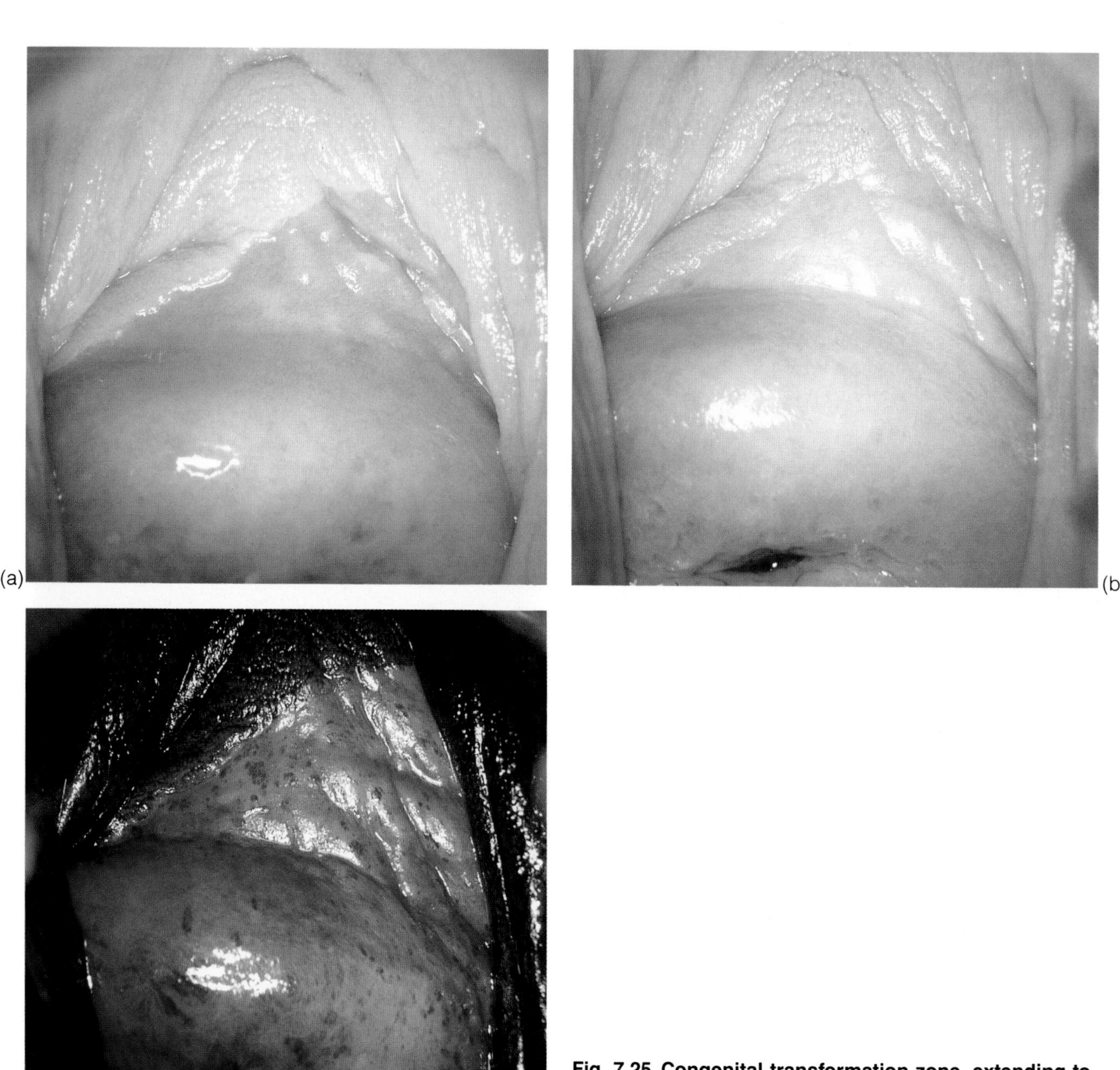

Fig. 7.25 Congenital transformation zone, extending to the anterior vaginal wall. (a) Before application of acetic acid. **(b)** Following application of acetic acid. **(c)** Following application of Schiller's iodine.

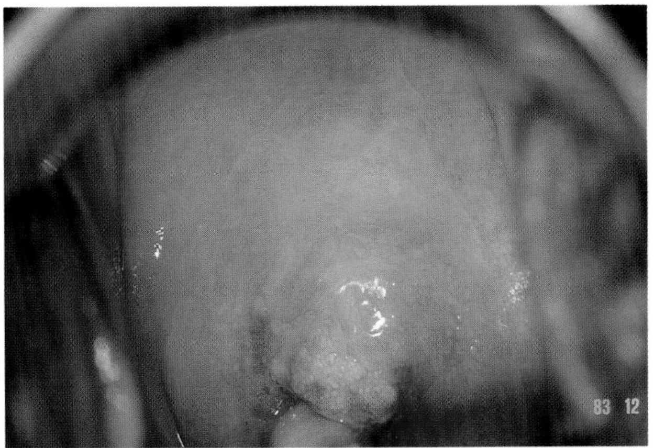

Fig. 7.26 Congenital transformation zone, associated with cervical intraepithelial neoplasia. This extends on to the anterior vaginal wall. Centrally, around the cervical os, there is an area of cervical intraepithelial neoplasia. In this case, provided the colposcopist can distinguish this from the congenital transformation zone, only the cervical intraepithelial neoplasia will require treatment.

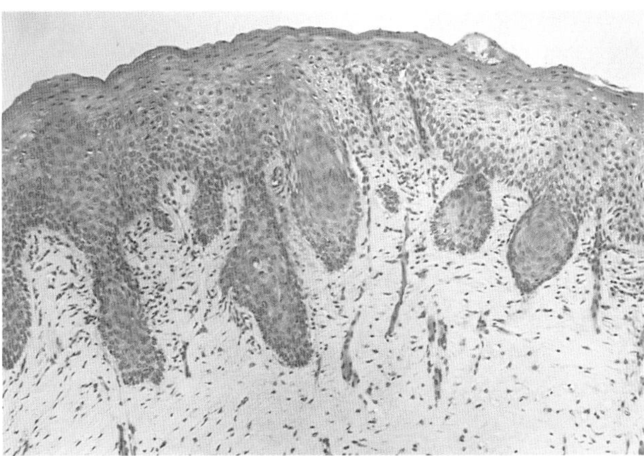

Fig. 7.27 Congenital transformation zone; histology.

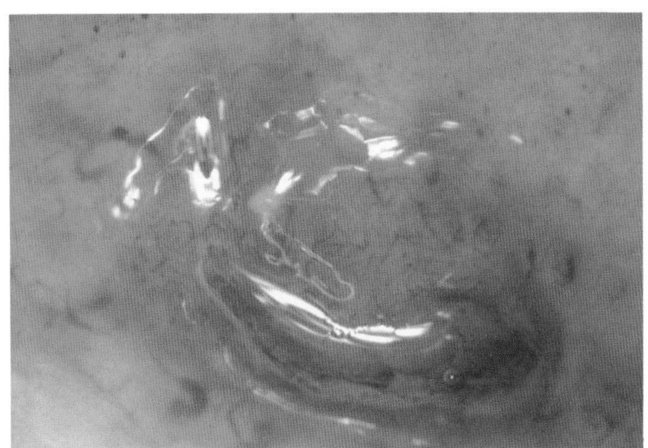

Fig. 7.28 Postmenopausal cervix. The epithelium is pale and atrophic, and subepithelial vessels can be seen. In some areas there are subepithelial haemorrhages caused by taking a cervical smear with a wooden spatula.

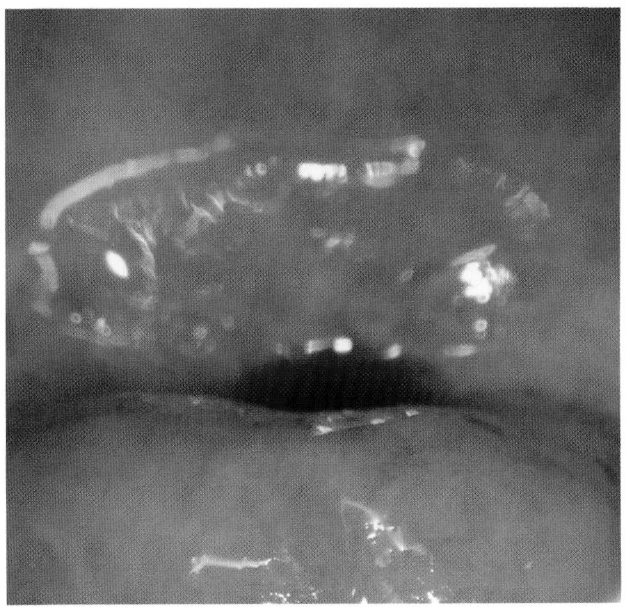

Fig. 7.29 Postmenopausal cervix. The transformation zone has retreated into the canal. Thin covering of epithelium. Squamocolumnar junction not seen.

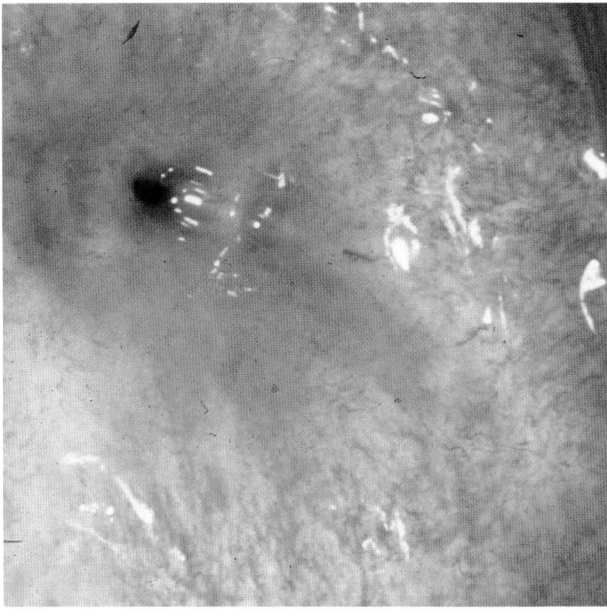

Fig. 7.30 Postmenopausal cervix. Pinpoint os. Thin epithelium exaggerates underlying normal vessel pattern.

the polyp continues to grow, it will protrude beyond the external os. At this stage, metaplasia occurs: the tip of the polyp is covered first by immature and later by mature squamous epithelium, while the stalk, which usually remains in the endocervical canal, is covered by columnar epithelium (Figs 7.31 and 7.32).

The origin of the polyp, i.e. the point at which the stalk begins, must be determined, as removal of the tip but not the stalk will simply result in regrowth (Fig. 7.33). In order to identify the base of the stalk, the colposcopist must be aware that the polyp may not in fact arise from the endocervical canal; occasionally, endometrial polyps will present at the external os.

Less commonly, a submucous fibroid will develop a stalk and protrude through the endocervical canal, frequently causing irregular bleeding and appearing necrotic. Sometimes a necrotic polyp may lead to a false diagnosis of cervical carcinoma. The number of polyps should also be determined, as often more than one will be found. Malignancy in a cervical polyp is very uncommon but should always be considered.

Unless the base of the polyp is clearly visible and accessible, the endocervical canal should be assessed under general anaesthesia. The polyp and its stalk are removed, and the base of the stalk is treated by diathermy to prevent recurrence. Hysteroscopy will prove helpful where the base of the polyp is still not visible after dilatation of the cervix.

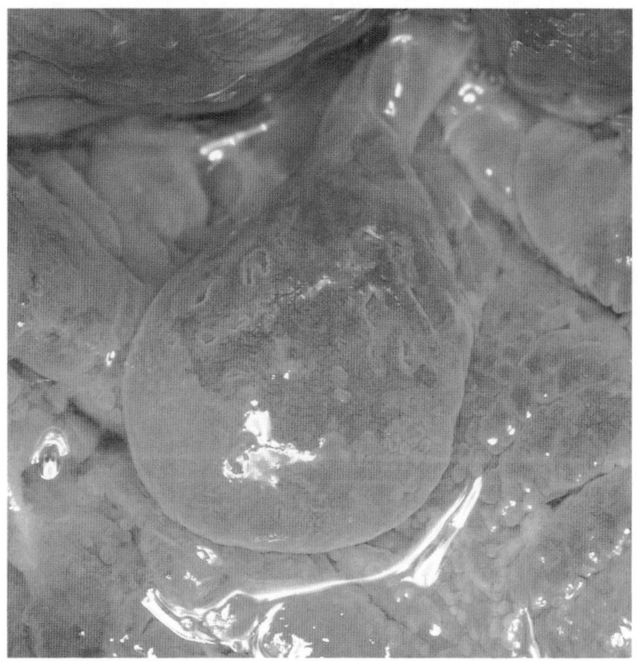

Fig. 7.31 Endocervical polyp. The stalk and base of the polyp are covered by columnar epithelium, while the tip is covered by squamous epithelium.

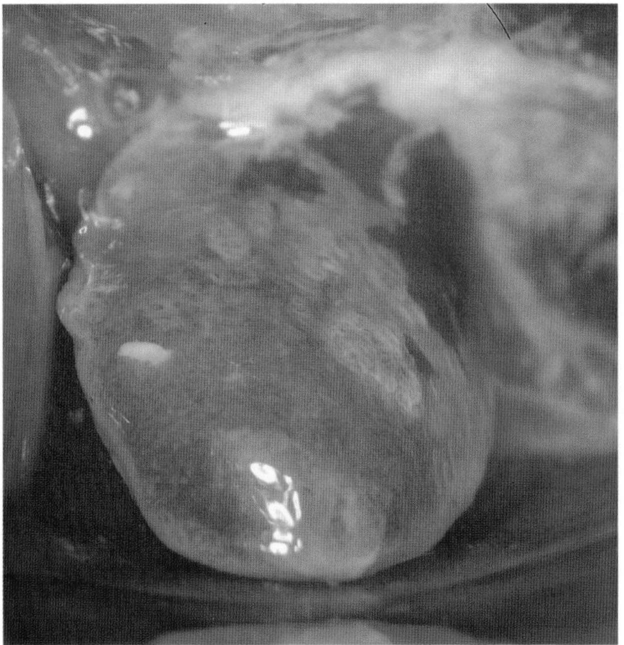

Fig. 7.32 Endocervical polyp. This is showing columnar and immature metaplastic epithelium.

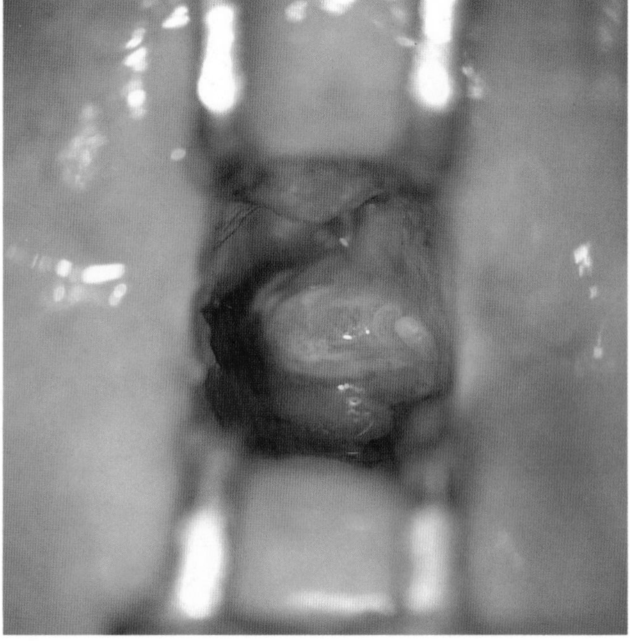

Fig. 7.33 An endocervical polyp arising in the endocervical canal. This is seen with the aid of an endocervical speculum.

8. *Colposcopic appearances of cervical intraepithelial neoplasia*

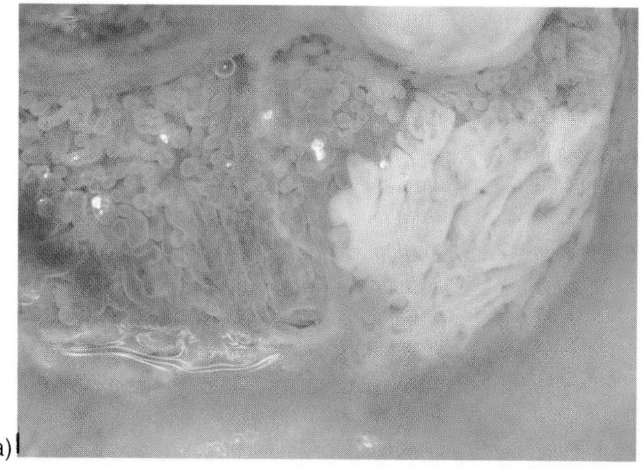

(a)

INTRODUCTION

With the saline technique, cervical intraepithelial neoplasia can be recognized: the abnormal epithelium is dark, there is a sharp line of demarcation between normal and abnormal epithelium, and the capillaries are readily visible, having a punctation or mosaic pattern or showing the presence of atypical vessels.

With the acetic acid technique, the abnormal epithelium appears white. There is a sharp line of demarcation between normal and abnormal epithelium, and the vessels, although less readily visible than with the saline technique, are much more

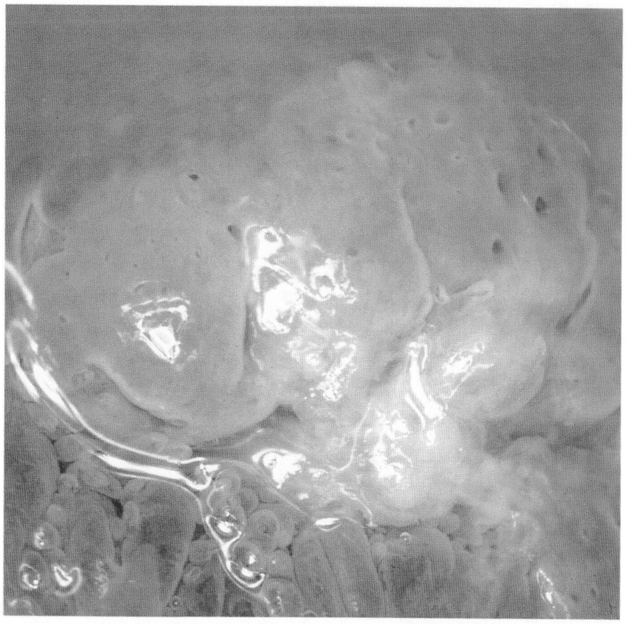

(b)

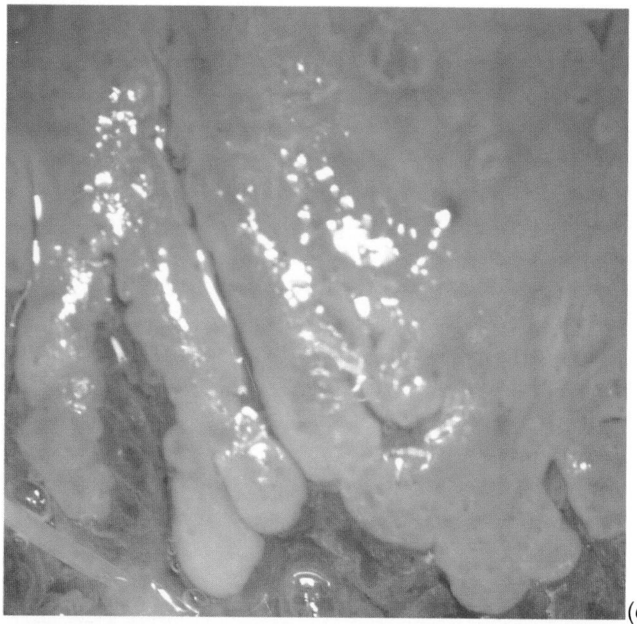

(c)

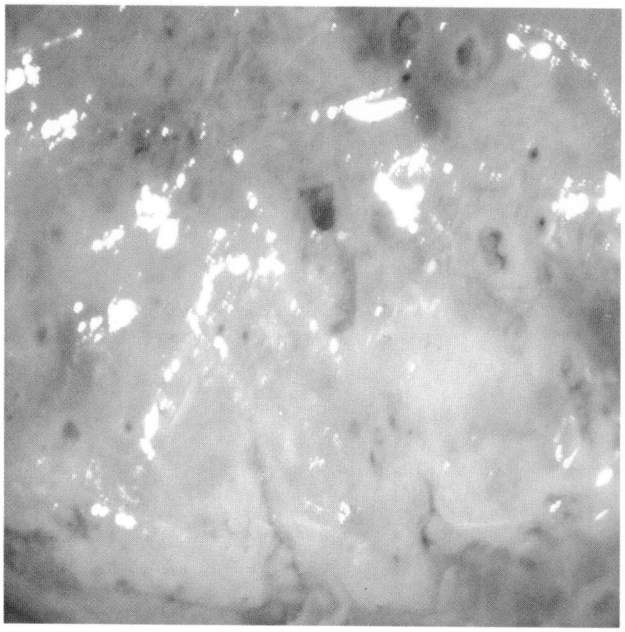

(f)

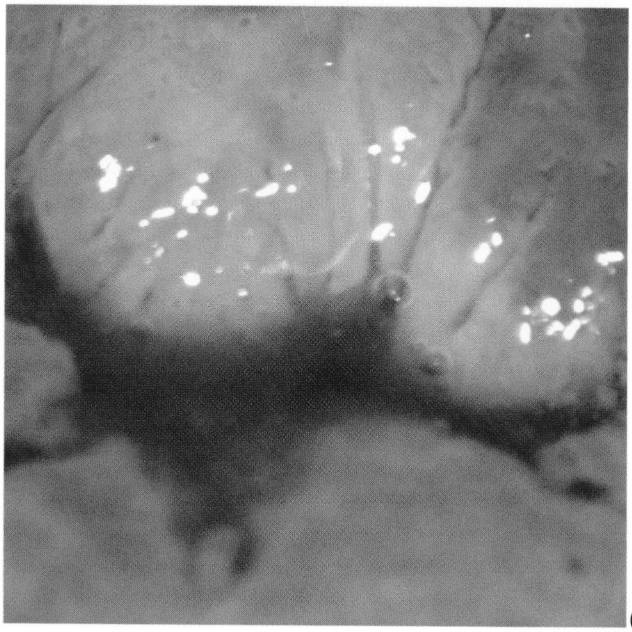

(g)

Fig. 8.1 Acetowhite change within the transformation zone. (a) No abnormal vascular pattern. **(b)** Similar, with gland openings and squamocolumnar junction clearly visible. **(c)** Same as (b), with more pronounced acetowhite change. **(d)** Very marked acetowhite change. CIN 3 was confirmed on biopsy. **(e)** White gland openings in CIN. Field of acetowhite epithelium, containing white gland openings with 'doughnut ring' appearance, implying gland involvement. **(f)** High-grade CIN. The acetowhite lesion occupies the anterior transformation zone. (Note gland openings.) Visible villi and squamocolumnar junction. **(g)** Acetowhite change. Note clefts and gland openings indicating the transformation zone. **(h)** Atypical transformation zone, extending widely posteriorly. Note chevron-like clefts. (i) Epithelial 'stripping' in high-grade CIN. The area denuded of epithelium is obvious within a field of (fading) acetowhite change with punctation. This easily traumatized epithelium raises suspicion of microinvasion.

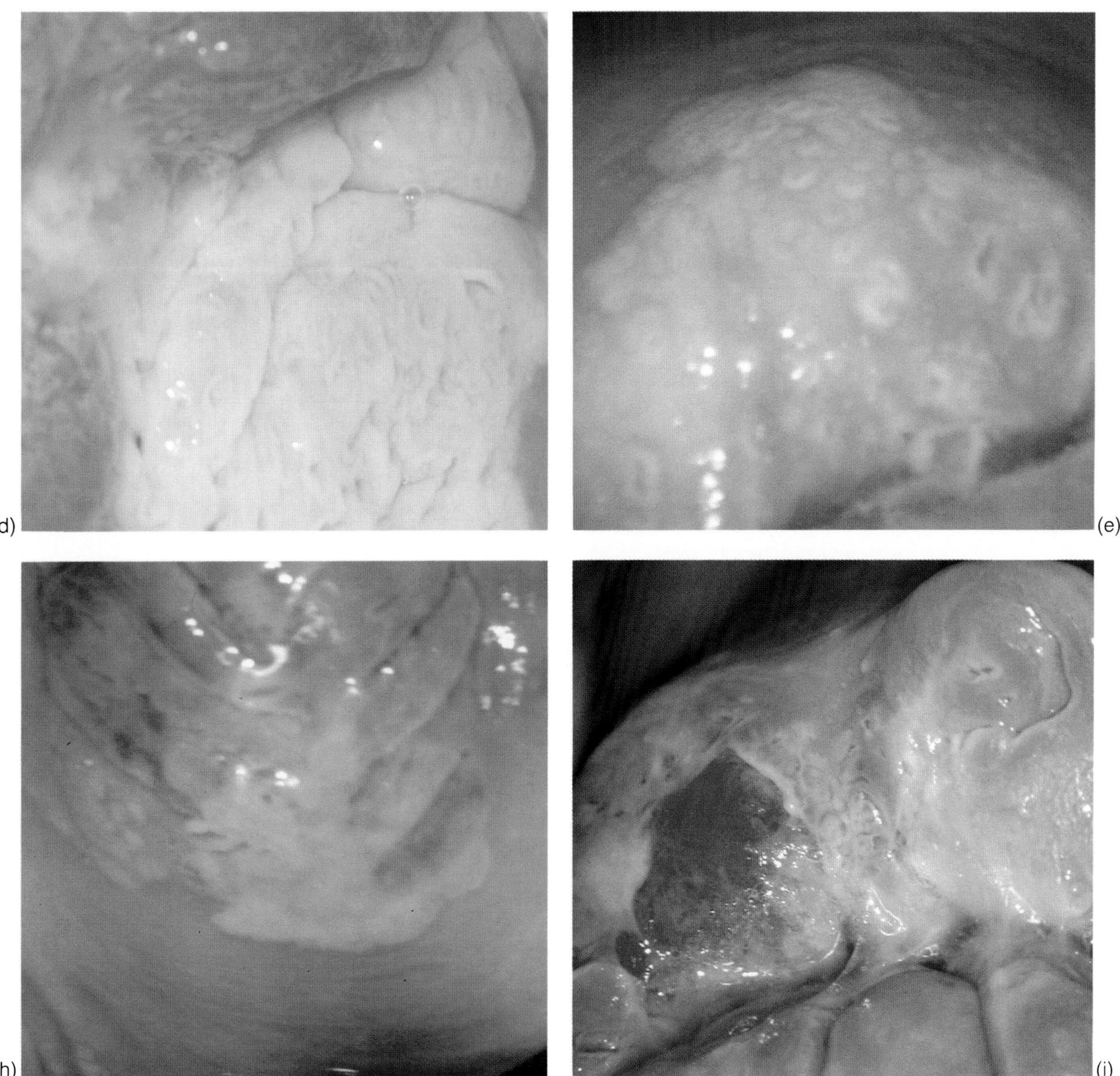

visible than in normal epithelium. Occasionally, in minor degrees of cervical intraepithelial neoplasia there is no vessel pattern to be seen following the application of acetic acid – the abnormal epithelium simply appears white (Fig. 8.1).

Acetowhite change

Acetowhite change is the most important of all colposcopic features (see Fig. 8.1). All examples of cervical intraepithelial neoplasia, unless covered by keratin, will show some degree of acetowhiteness.

Table 8.1 Epithelial changes that may be acetowhite

Cervical intraepithelial neoplasia
Human papillomavirus infection
Combined CIN and HPV
Immature squamous metaplasia*
Healing/regenerating epithelium*
Congenital transformation zone
Inflammation*
Adenocarcinoma CGIN*
Invasive squamous cell carcinoma*

*These conditions are often, but not invariably, acetowhite

Unfortunately, epithelial changes other than cervical intraepithelial neoplasia may also become white with acetic acid (Table 8.1), and it is important that these physiological and minor changes are recognized. Distinction by colposcopy alone is not always possible, and all abnormal areas should be biopsied.

Vascular pattern of abnormal epithelium

The vascular patterns associated with abnormal epithelium are as follows:

PUNCTATION

This pattern is easily recognized, being characterized by dilated, elongated, often twisted and irregularly terminating vessels of the hairpin type, arranged in a prominent punctate configuration (Fig. 8.2). This is usually a well-defined area so that there is a sharp line of demarcation between the normal and abnormal epithelium (Fig. 8.3). The dilated hairpin capillaries seen in inflammatory states (Fig. 8.4) should not be confused with punctation: when the capillaries are dilated and recognizable because of inflammation, the pattern is very diffuse, the capillaries are close together, and there is no sharp line of demarcation as would be seen between normal and abnormal epithelium.

(a) 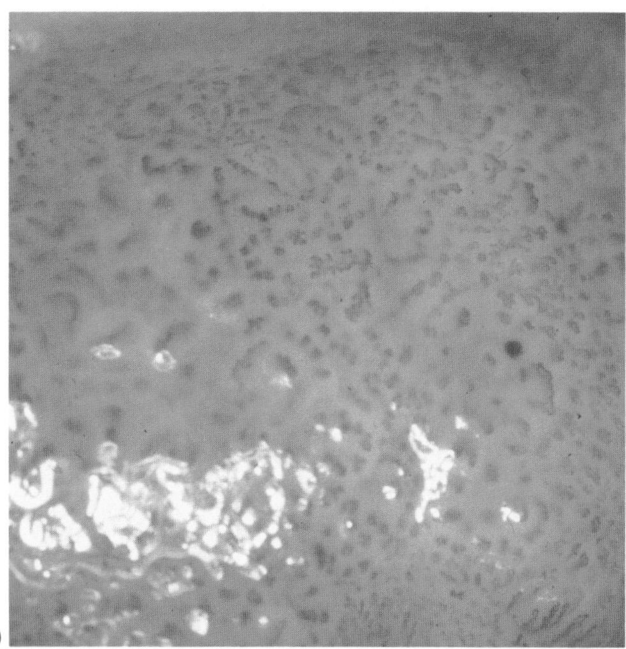

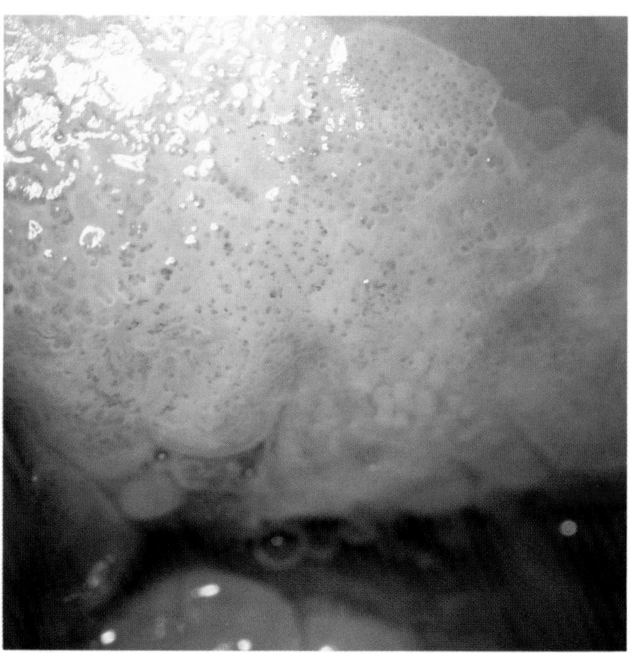 (b)

Fig. 8.2 Punctation. (a) Saline technique, before application of acetic acid. **(b)** After application of acetic acid. Note that the vascular pattern is now less pronounced.

Punctation vessels are more widely spaced than the hairpin capillaries seen in normal squamous epithelium, and because they extend closer to the surface they are more readily seen. Their shape may be hairpin-like, but occasionally they will resemble double capillaries, or the capillary loops may appear like a little ball.

MOSAIC

The capillaries are arranged parallel to the surface in a characteristic mosaic or 'crazy paving' pattern (Fig. 8.5). Therefore, vessels enclose a vascular field which may be small, large, round, regular or irregular in shape. Mosaic vessels may be fine and smoothly curved, coarse and irregularly curved, or they may consist of intertwining strands of dilating capillaries. However, whatever the fine structure, the overall pattern is characteristically mosaic and easily recognized.

ATYPICAL VESSELS

These are terminal vessels which are easily seen by the colposcopist (Fig. 8.6). Typically, they are irregular in size, shape, course and arrangement, and the intercapillary distance is significantly greater than that which is found in normal epithelium. There is no particular pattern, the vessels being arranged in a totally haphazard way.

Intercapillary distance

This is the distance between vessels or space encompassed by the mosaic vessels. In normal squamous epithelium, the maximal intercapillary distance of the hairpin and network capillaries varies, but is approximately 50–200 μm with an average of 100 μm. On the other hand, the maximal intercapillary distance increases as the lesion becomes more severe, i.e. in CIN 1 the average intercapillary distance may be 200 μm, whereas in CIN 3 the greatest intercapillary distance is often 450–500 μm (see Figs 8.3 and 8.5(b)).

It is not necessary to measure the vessels, as in time the colposcopist will be able to tell immediately whether these are close together or widely spaced. If comparison is needed, then the vessels in a lesion should be compared with vessels in the adjacent normal squamous epithelium.

Colour tone

Following application of saline, abnormal epithelium appears much darker than normal epithelium (see Figs 8.3 and 8.5(a)), whereas after application of acetic acid the abnormal epithelium appears very white (acetowhite epithelium; see Fig. 8.5(b)). In both cases, and particularly with acetic acid, an easily recognizable, sharp line of demarcation between normal and abnormal epithelium can be observed.

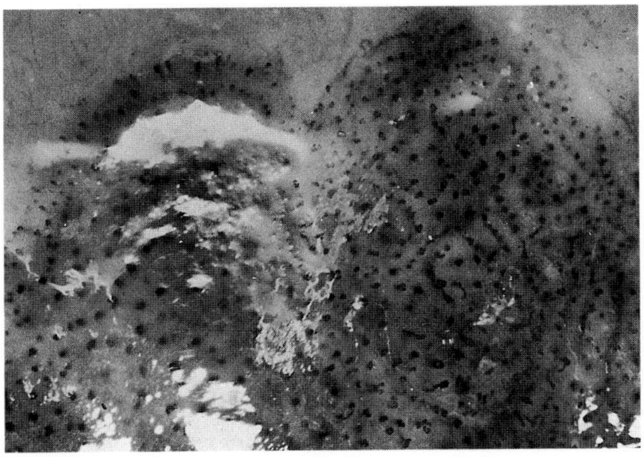

Fig. 8.3 Punctation within a field of cervical intraepithelial neoplasia. The saline technique has been used. The abnormal epithelium appears dark, and punctation vessels can be clearly seen. There is a sharp line of demarcation between the normal (light) and abnormal (dark) epithelium. The capillaries on the left are more spaced, which is indicative of a higher degree of cervical intraepithelial neoplasia compared with the epithelium on the right.

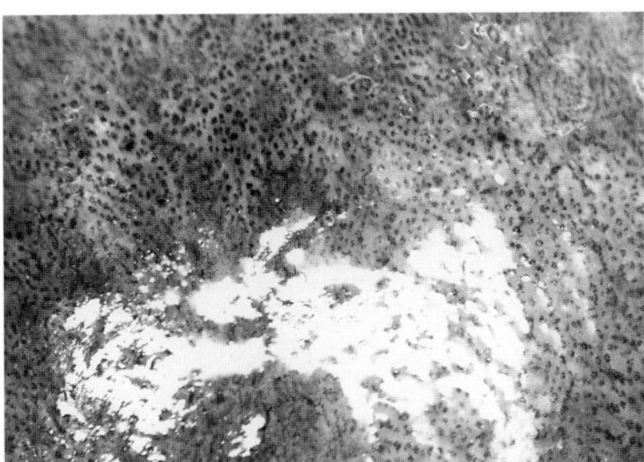

Fig. 8.4 Inflamed cervix. Widespread, uniform pattern of hairpin dilated capillaries. Compare this with Fig. 8.3.

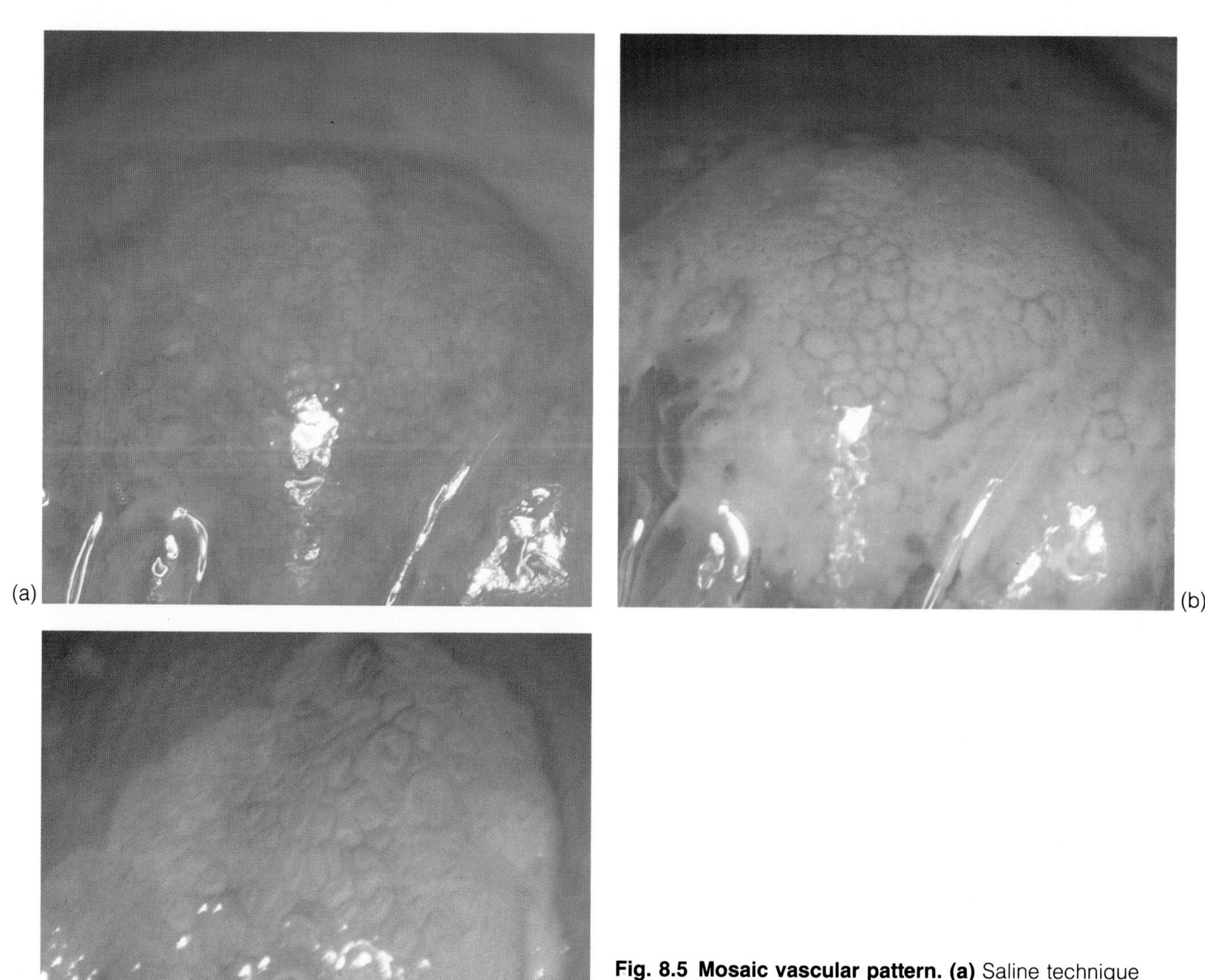

Fig. 8.5 Mosaic vascular pattern. (a) Saline technique before application of acetic acid. Note the dusky colour tone. **(b)** Same as (a), following application of acetic acid. Note also the increased intercapillary distance and the line of demarcation from normal epithelium. **(c)** Coarse mosaic with saline technique. **(d)** Coarse mosaic within a wide field of acetowhite change. Note the gland clefts and white gland openings. **(e)** Field of acetowhite change with associated coarse mosaic vessel pattern.

Surface contour

The surface of a lesion can be described as smooth and even, or irregular. For example, normal squamous epithelium has a smooth surface, while columnar epithelium is easily recognized by its typical grape-like or villous appearance. At the other extreme, invasive cancer is characterized by an uneven or often exophytic growth pattern (see Fig. 10.29, page 117).

Line of demarcation

The borderline or line of demarcation between normal and abnormal squamous epithelium is usually sharp, due to the change in colour that is present in the abnormal epithelium. In contrast, the line of demarcation between normal squamous epithelium and inflammatory lesions is more diffuse. Also, almost always a sharp line of demarcation will be seen between normal squamous and normal

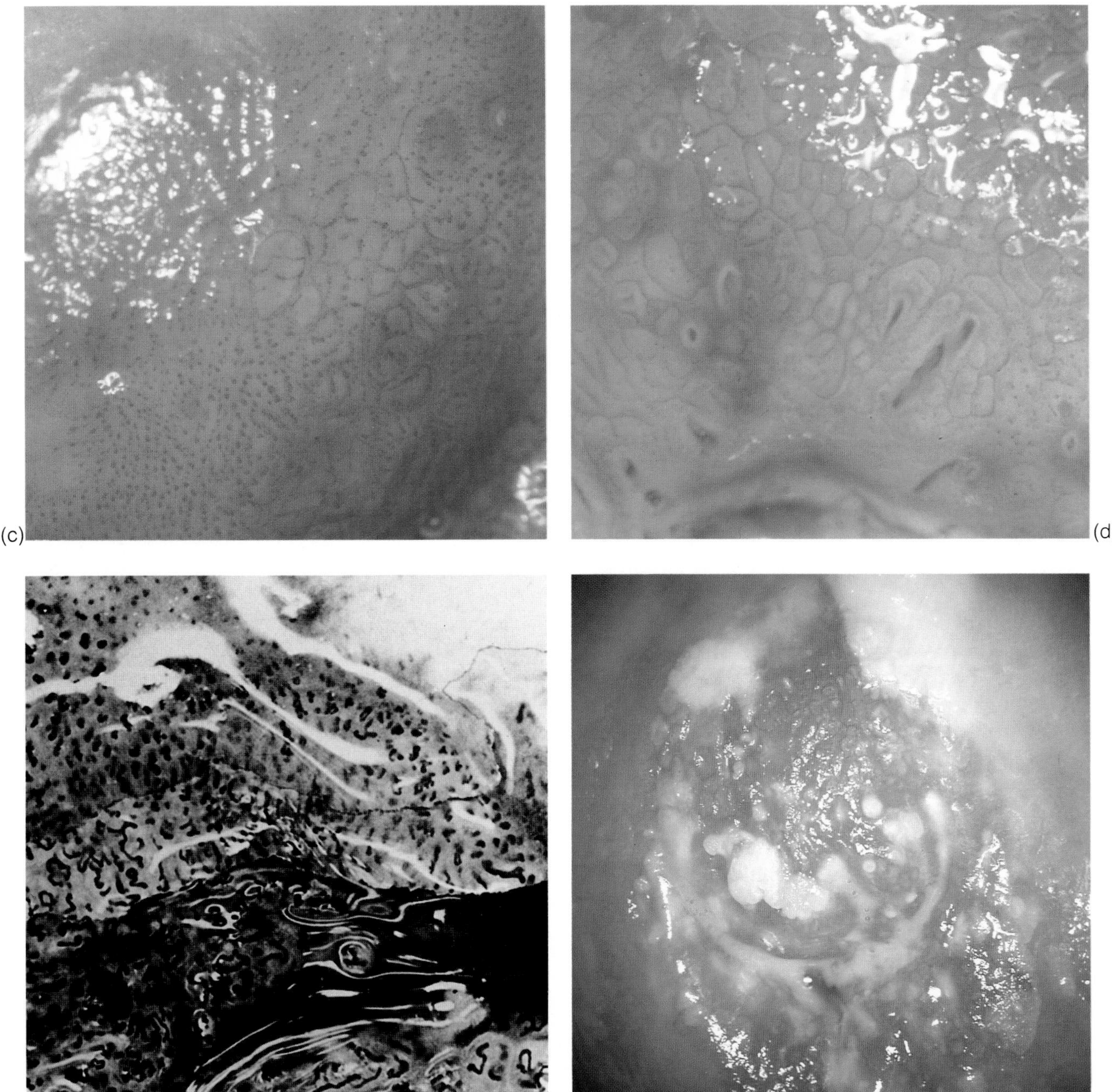

Fig. 8.6 Highly atypical vessels within a small focal lesion in the transformation zone. Note the corkscrew- and comma-shaped vessels, and other bizarre forms.

Fig. 8.7 Multifocal waxy leucoplakia, seen within the transformation zone. No application of acetic acid.

columnar epithelium (squamocolumnar junction), particularly after application of acetic acid.

Leucoplakia

Leucoplakia is seen less commonly on the cervix than acetowhite epithelium, and the vascular abnormalities are detailed above. Normal original or mature metaplastic squamous epithelium of the cervix does not have a layer of keratin on the surface, but in some circumstances keratosis occurs and leucoplakia is seen at colposcopy.

An area of leucoplakia is white before acetic acid is applied (Fig. 8.7), and does not change in colour after application. It is usually seen as one or more raised plaques which may coalesce as the area becomes larger (Fig. 8.8). The outline of the area is usually irregular. When keratosis is only slight, such as in the congenital transformation zone, all that may be observed is a waxy, non-wettable surface which is slightly white before acetic acid is applied but may become a little whiter after application.

Leucoplakia presents problems to the colposcopist when assessing the cervix because its presence hides the diagnostic changes of the underlying epithelium (Fig. 8.9). Although fully developed leucoplakia on the cervix is usually associated with cervical intraepithelial neoplasia, it may be seen overlying otherwise completely normal epithelium, often outside the transformation zone, or an early invasive carcinoma. For this reason, the presence of more than a very small area of leucoplakia within the transformation zone must be an indication for considering excision of the zone.

GRADING OF COLPOSCOPIC FINDINGS

It has already been pointed out that, in mosaic and punctation patterns, the intercapillary distance increases as the degree of histological abnormality in the epithelium becomes greater. Punctation and mosaic may be additionally graded on the basis of coarseness of vessels and regularity of their pattern: the more severe the underlying lesion, the coarser the vessels are likely to be and the more irregular the pattern, the extreme being the atypical vessels of early invasive disease.

Acetowhite epithelium may also be graded, primarily according to the degree of acetowhiteness that is reached at the maximum whiteness. Of secondary importance are the rapidity with which the lesion reaches its maximum degree of whiteness, the length of time that whiteness is retained, and the sharpness of the line of demarcation. Not only do severe abnormalities become whiter than minor lesions, but they tend to become white more quickly and retain their whiteness longer than the mild changes, the latter also usually having a less distinct outline. These features are summarized in Table 8.2.

Two further points need to be made about grading colposcopic abnormalities. First, there is difficulty in comparing different areas of the same cervix if mosaic and punctation as well as acetowhiteness are present. It is not always easy to determine whether a particular area of punctation represents a more severe abnormality than an adjacent area of acetowhite epithelium. This dilemma may be important in deciding from which area to take a directed biopsy. If in doubt, both areas should be sampled.

(a) 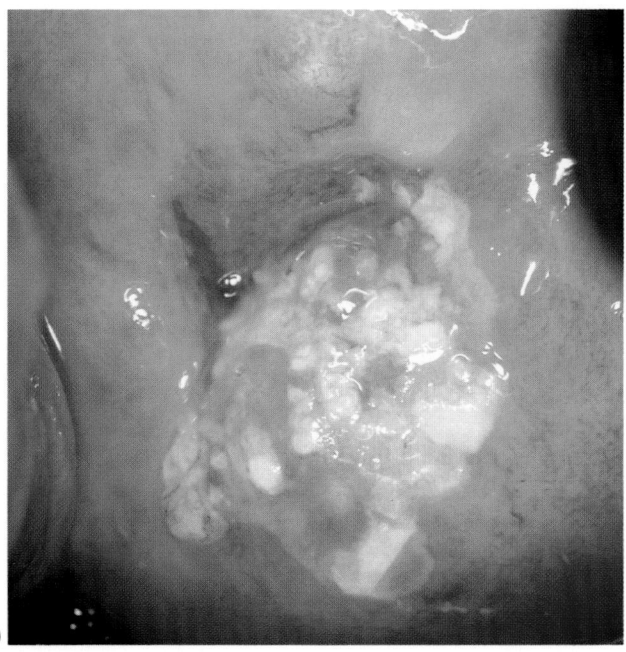

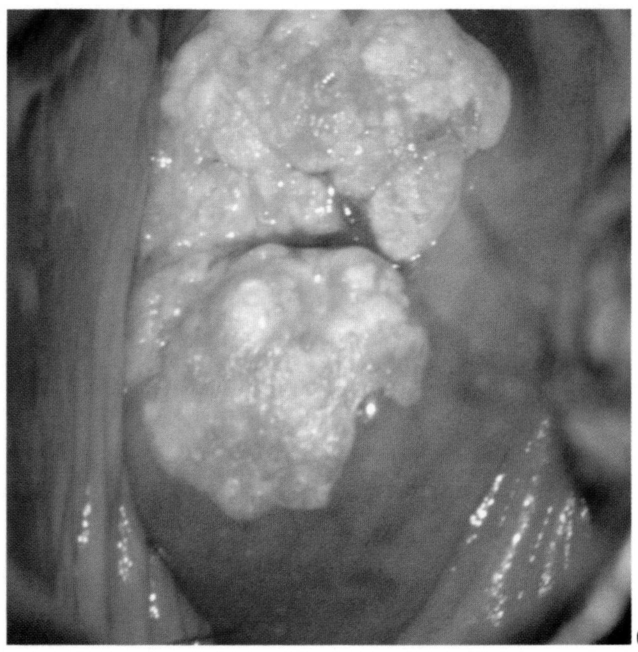 (b)

Fig. 8.8 (a) Coalescent leucoplakia on the cervix. (b) Leucoplakia. The whole area of the transformation zone is the seat of dense, white, waxy change before the application of acetic acid.

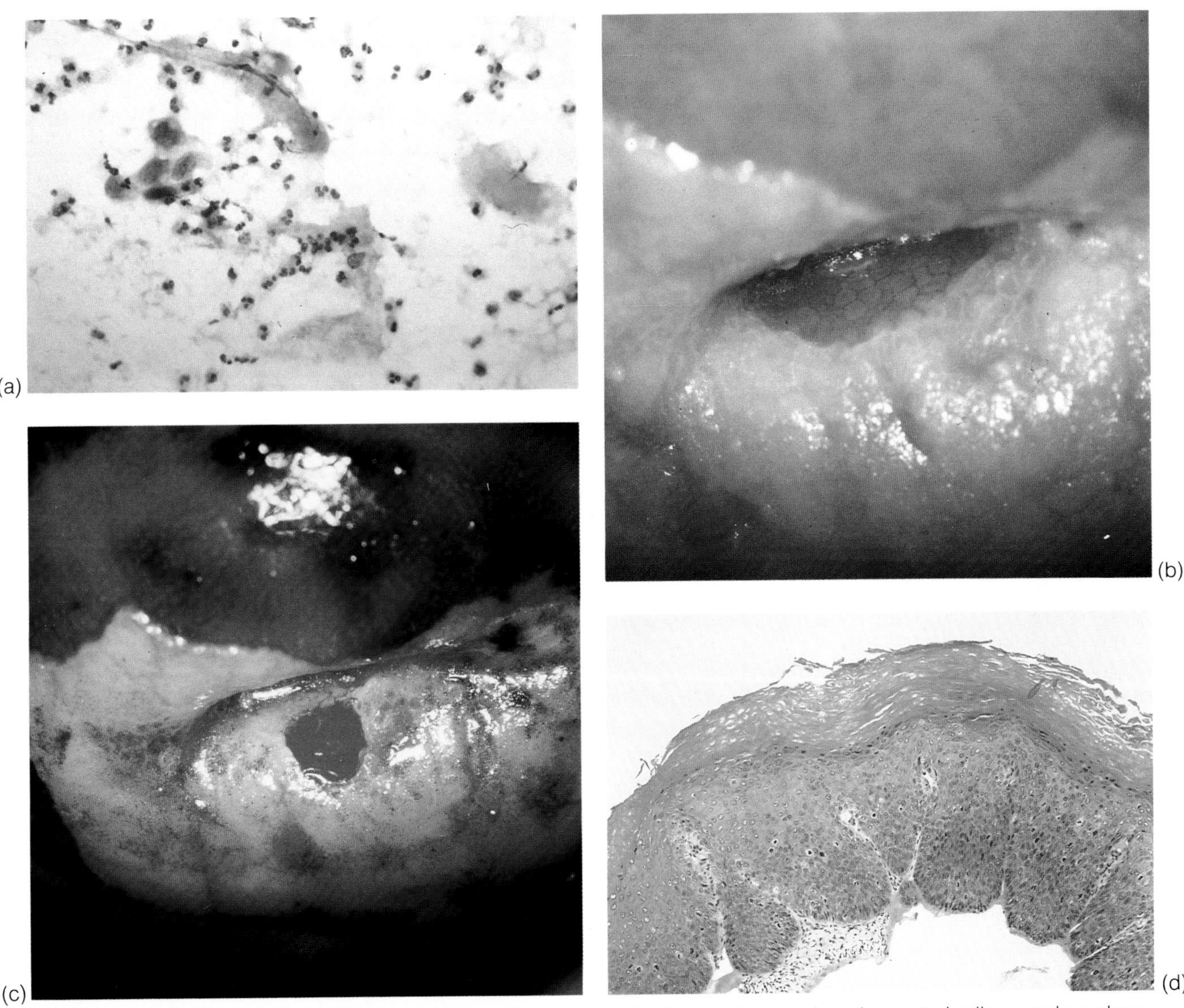

Fig. 8.9 (a) Cervical smear, showing a cluster of moderately dyskaryotic cells above and to the left. Note the smudgy, pink, anucleate, squamous cells. **(b)** Same cervix, showing extensive, dense, waxy leucoplakia. Careful inspection of the small area of visible underlying epithelium in the canal on the posterior lip reveals a clear mosaic pattern. **(c)** Appearance after Schiller's test. Note the biopsy site at the '6 o'clock' position. **(d)** Histopathology of the biopsy reveals cervical intraepithelial neoplasia, with dense, overlying hyperkeratosis.

Second, it has to be emphasized that colposcopic grading is just that: a grading of the colposcopic features; it is not an assessment of the histological grade of the underlying lesion. With experience, it may often be possible for the colposcopist to predict with accuracy the degree of cervical intraepithelial neoplasia present; indeed, trying to guess the degree of abnormality is a useful exercise, as it increases the care with which the examination is carried out.

However, colposcopy is not sufficiently sensitive to discriminate consistently and with certainty between the grades of cervical intraepithelial neoplasia, especially when comparing one woman with another. This is particularly true in the case of acetowhite epithelium, where features other than the degree of epithelial abnormality contribute to the acetowhiteness. For example, an area of CIN 3 in a woman of 60 years is usually quite thin, thinner than an area of CIN 1 in a woman of 25 years. Despite the fact that CIN 3 in the older woman is more nuclear-rich, CIN 1 in the younger woman may be more acetowhite because of its greater thickness.

Table 8.2 Features assessed in colposcopic grading

Acetowhite epithelium
Maximum whiteness reached
Rapidity of development of maximum whiteness
Length of retention of whiteness
Sharpness of outline
Mosaic and punctation
Intercapillary distance
Coarseness of vessels
Regularity of pattern

Table 8.3 Colposcopic features suggestive of invasion

Atypical vessels
Irregular, raised nodular surface
Large, complex lesion
Wide intercapillary distance
Severe changes with canal involvement

First and foremost, colposcopy defines the distribution of lesions; hopefully, early invasive lesions may also be identified (Table 8.3; see Chapter 10). In most cases, high-grade lesions can be determined from minor lesions, and many examples of herpes papillomavirus infection, squamous metaplasia and congenital transformation zone can be correctly identified. However, the capabilities of the technique do not extend to a precise histological grading of cervical intraepithelial neoplasia, or a confident distinction between intraepithelial neoplasia and other causes of acetowhiteness.

A colposcopic report should identify the distribution of the abnormal areas with their colposcopic features and colposcopic grading. The grade of cervical intraepithelial neoplasia can only be added to the report when the histology of the biopsy is known.

Congenital transformation zone

The congenital transformation zone is confusing in terms of acetic acid application (see Figs 7.24–7.27), as it becomes acetowhite slowly but usually retains its whiteness for a long time. Thus, as the whiteness of a central area of cervical intraepithelial neoplasia is fading, it may still be increasing in a surrounding area of congenital transformation zone. Eventually, the congenital transformation zone may be considerably whiter in appearance than the significant cervical intraepithelial neoplasia adjacent to it, which could mislead the inexperienced colposcopist into biopsying the wrong area.

9. *Handling biopsy specimens*

INTRODUCTION

A number of different tissue specimen types originate in the colposcopy clinic. It is therefore useful for the colposcopist to be aware of the way biopsy specimens obtained in the clinic or operating theatre are dealt with in the laboratory, as this has a direct bearing on the handling of material at the time of taking a biopsy.

It is important that those engaged in colposcopy and the histological assessment of biopsy material are familiar with its proper handling. The specimens involved are: (i) punch biopsies (from the cervix, vagina and vulva); (ii) wedge biopsies; (iii) cone biopsies; and (iv) endocervical curettage specimens.

As a total hysterectomy may sometimes be carried out on women with cervical intraepithelial neoplasia and glandular abnormalities, it is also relevant to consider the examination of a hysterectomy specimen. However, details of handling a radical hysterectomy specimen are beyond the scope of this book.

FIXATION

On removal, all specimens are placed in a container with fixative, the purpose of which is to inactivate the cellular enzymes so that autodigestion of the tissue does not take place; furthermore, the tissue is preserved in the state that it was in at the time of fixation. A wide variety of agents are available as fixatives.

Formalin

The most widely used fixative is formalin (formol saline), a solution of formaldehyde in water, buffered so that it is isotonic with tissue. Formalin has a number of advantages as a general-purpose fixative: it is easily available and inexpensive, and has probably the least toxicity when compared with other fixatives. Furthermore, histopathologists are familiar with the appearances of formalin-fixed tissues. However, for cervical histology, formalin is not ideal.

Bouin's fluid

This contains formalin, acetic acid and picric acid, and is preferred because of the greatly enhanced preservation of nuclear detail it gives compared with that of formalin.

The disadvantages of Bouin's fluid are that it is relatively expensive, picric acid is explosive if allowed to dry out, and its vapour is even more irritating than that of formalin. Furthermore, it has deleterious effects on the stainless steel that is now commonplace in laboratory cut-up and processing areas. However, these disadvantages are outweighed by the superior quality of the final stained section. Virtually all histological material illustrated in this book has been fixed in Bouin's fluid.

Formol sublimate

This contains mercuric chloride, and also results in excellent histological fixation. However, because of the health risks associated with mercury-containing compounds, formol sublimate has been banned from most histology laboratories.

FIXATION TIME

Fixation time is finite, and the size of a biopsy specimen determines the length of time necessary for penetration of the fixative. A small punch biopsy will fix in Bouin's fluid in one or two hours, but even a fairly small cone biopsy should not be further processed until it has been left in fixative for at least six hours. Prolonged immersion in Bouin's fluid results in increasing hardening of tissue, which is another of its drawbacks.

PUNCH BIOPSY

Specimens obtained from the cervix, vagina or vulva, using any of the several types of punch biopsy forceps available, are handled in the same way. It is very important that these specimens are correctly dealt with so that the maximum information can be obtained from them. The biopsy, if taken properly, will consist of an ellipse of epithelium approximately 5 mm in length, and in the cervical biopsy the underlying stroma will have a depth of 3–5 mm (Fig. 9.1(a)). Vaginal and vulval biopsies tend to have less underlying lamina propria and dermis because of the different consistency of these elements.

Biopsies are immediately placed in Bouin's fluid. In addition to the other advantages over formalin, small specimens are easier to handle after fixation in Bouin's fluid, due to the yellow staining. Fixation results in curling of the specimen, so that epithelium is on the outer, convex surface and the stroma on the inside (Fig. 9.1(b)). This facilitates correct orientation.

The use of filter paper, glass coverslips or even cucumber squares has been advocated, but none of these aids is necessary for proper orientation of a specimen.

The fixed, curled biopsy is transversely bisected, producing two approximately pyramid-shaped pieces (Fig. 9.1(c)). These are then embedded in wax with the flat, cut surface downwards (Fig. 9.1(d)), so that this surface is cut by the microtome. Each piece is cut at three levels, and thus a total of six levels are examined through the biopsy.

This number of sections should be adequate for most purposes, and therefore step–serial sectioning is not necessary. Routine staining is by haematoxylin and eosin; mucin stains are sometimes used when glandular abnormalities are suspected or found.

Biopsies smaller than the ideal size can be handled in the same way. Although the absence of underlying stroma can make orientation difficult, the combination of tissue curling in Bouin's fluid and sectioning at several levels nearly always means that at least one out of the six sections cuts the epithelium at right-angles, enabling a diagnosis of the epithelial abnormality to be made.

Histopathological reporting

The histopathologist reporting on a colposcopic biopsy should, of course, indicate what degree of epithelial abnormality is present, and whether invasion is seen or not. It is good practice always to make a definite statement on whether there is evidence of invasion or not, as absence of evidence of invasion is a requirement that must be met before local destructive treatment of cervical intraepithelial neoplasia can be carried out. If there is no stroma, no comment can be made about invasion.

As the definition of microinvasive carcinoma requires that a cone biopsy or a larger specimen is examined, microinvasive carcinoma cannot be diagnosed on a punch biopsy; more precisely, it cannot be distinguished from stage Ib invasive carcinoma. A statement such as 'stromal invasion is present' should be used, usually without further qualification. This indicates that a further diagnostic procedure, normally a cone biopsy, is required. Nevertheless, it is sometimes possible to make a definitive diagnosis of stage Ib invasive carcinoma on a colposcopic biopsy where the whole of a large biopsy is virtually replaced by invasive carcinoma.

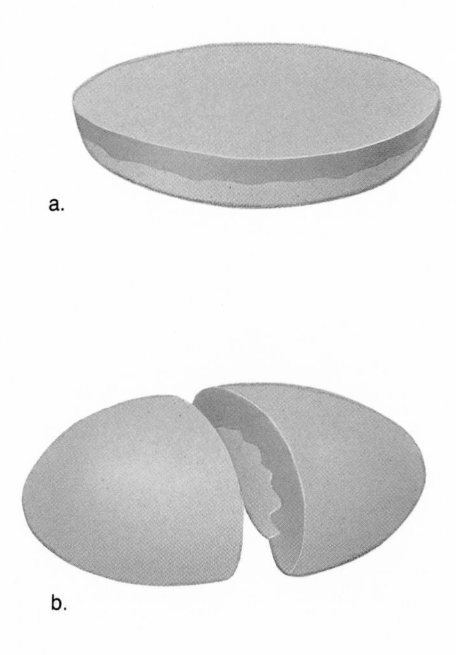

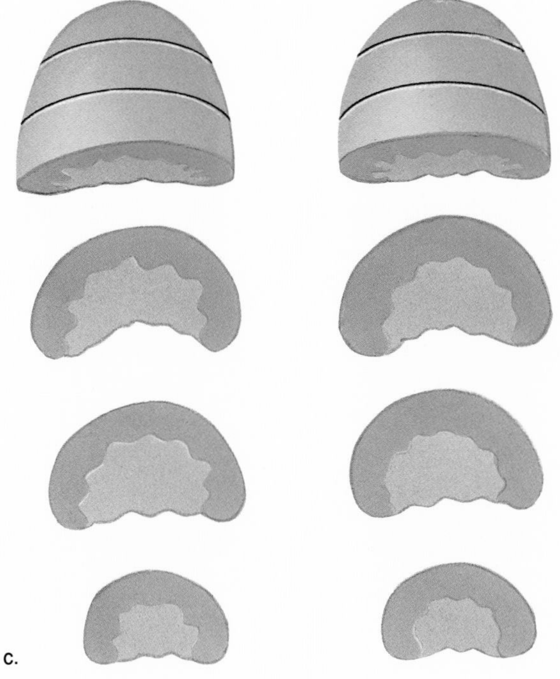

Fig. 9.1 Handling a punch biopsy specimen. (a) When freshly taken, the biopsy has a fairly flat layer of epithelium on the surface and stroma underneath. After fixation in Bouin's fluid, the biopsy curls and the epithelium forms a rounded, convex surface. **(b)** The biopsy is bisected transversely. **(c)** Both halves are embedded in wax, with the cut surface facing down, and cut at three levels.

WEDGE BIOPSIES

Wedge biopsies are not usually taken in the colposcopy clinic, and are required when invasive carcinoma is strongly suspected. These specimens are best fixed in Bouin's fluid and, if possible, orientated so that sectioning perpendicular to the surface is carried out.

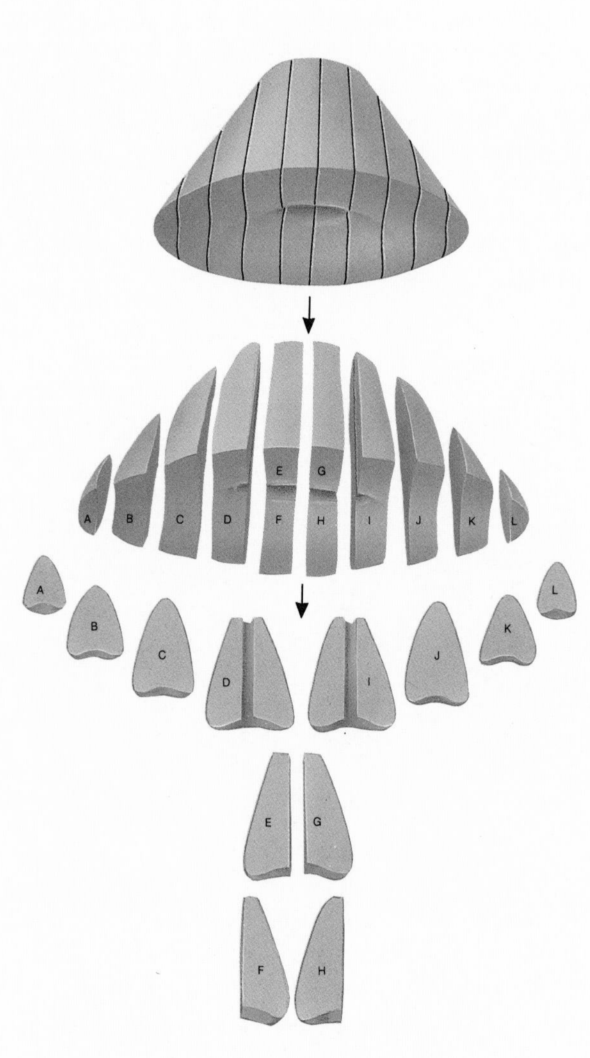

Fig. 9.2 Taking blocks from a cone biopsy. After thorough fixation in Bouin's fluid, the unopened specimen is divided into individual blocks of 2–2.5 mm thickness, each of which is initially sectioned at one level.

CONE BIOPSY

The term 'cone biopsy' describes the procedure of excising the transformation zone and producing a specimen suitable for histological examination. Excision may be carried out using a scalpel, laser (laser excision cone), or low-voltage diathermy loop. The advantages and disadvantages of each of these methods are discussed in Chapter 13.

The specimens produced by all these methods are roughly similar and traditionally cone-shaped, the base being the ectocervical surface and the apex the endocervical extreme. The current view is that the excised tissue should be cylindrical in shape, rather than conical, to avoid incomplete excision of the deeply involved endocervical crypts high in the canal. Because of the different emphasis in the indications allowing these procedures to be carried out in the out-patients department, laser excision cone specimens and low-voltage loop diathermy specimens often tend to be shallower than knife cone biopsies. Therefore, it has been traditional for the surgeon to attach a stitch at one point of the circumference of the cone, to enable orientation. With the application of alternative methods, this practice seems generally to have been abandoned, and it is questionable whether knowledge of the exact position of the lesion in a biopsy is of any help in establishing future management. However, this knowledge is useful in correlating colposcopic findings with histological outcome.

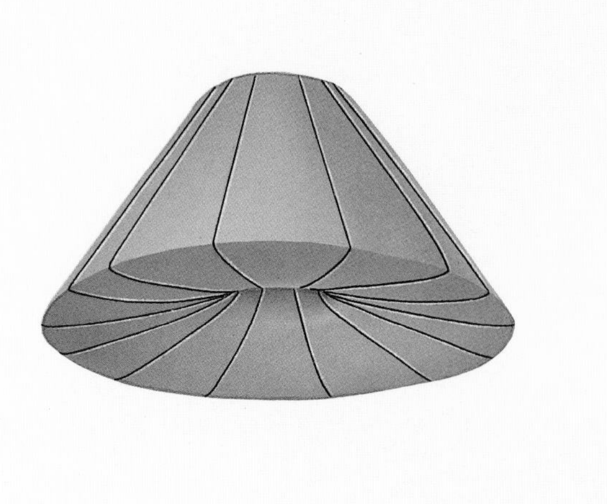

Fig. 9.3 Method of block-taking when the cone has a wide-open os.

Examination of cone biopsy specimens

A number of techniques have been proposed for the examination of cone biopsy specimens. To a certain extent, the method applied depends on the configuration of a specimen. Immediately upon removal, the specimen should be immersed intact into Bouin's fluid. It is common practice for the specimen to be opened, either by the gynaecologist or the pathologist; the cone is then pinned open and fixed. However, before fixation this will damage the fragile abnormal epithelium, and it is likely that the resultant stretching of the delicate endocervical epithelium significantly contributes to epithelial loss in the final sections. Opening of the cone biopsy specimen in no way facilitates examination of resection margins.

After fixation, most cone biopsy specimens can be dealt with in the same way (Fig. 9.2), by taking parallel cuts throughout the tissue. This must be done with a very sharp knife (such as a dermatome) at 2–2.5 mm intervals, taking care to keep the cuts straight and parallel (this is more easily achieved after fixation in Bouin's fluid than in formalin because of the greater firmness of Bouin-fixed material). The corresponding surface of each block is sectioned (see Fig. 9.2), so that sampling is as even and thorough as possible. Oblique cuts are unlikely to be a problem with this technique.

Longitudinal sections are examined, and both ectocervical and endocervical edges of the specimen can be easily assessed.

It is unusual for the os to be circular and open. When it is, it may be necessary to take radial blocks (Fig. 9.3); this technique has the disadvantage that blocks end up being wedge-shaped, possibly causing a problem with embedding and sectioning. This approach is very rarely needed.

If the cone biopsy is long, an alternative approach can be used to good effect (Fig. 9.4). The endocervical part of the specimen is cut transversely, to obtain several circular blocks; if necessary, the block from the tip of the cone may be cut at levels, to assess the endocervical extreme. The ectocervical part of the specimen is handled in the same way as the more usual cone biopsy. This method avoids the problem of unmanageably long blocks.

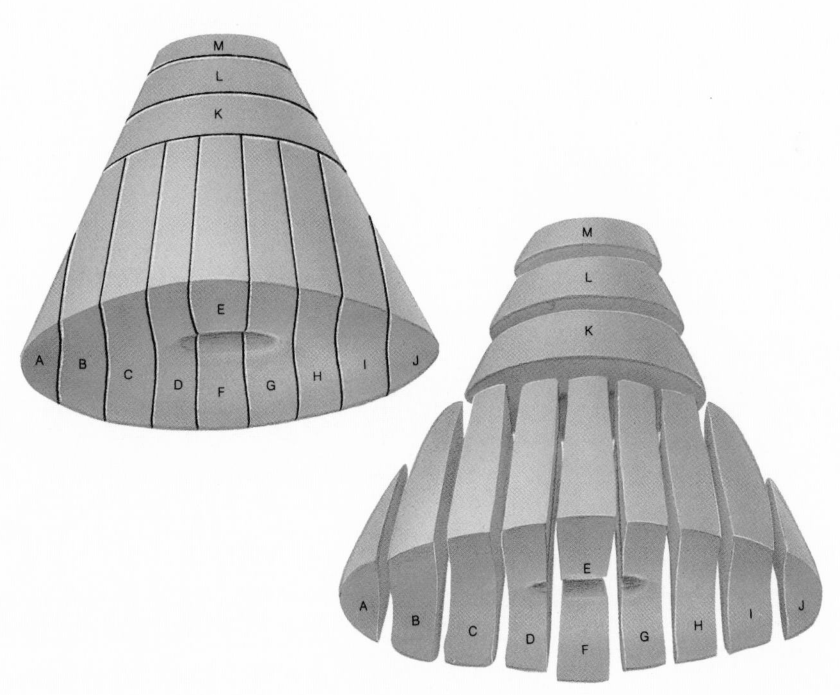

Fig. 9.4 Method of block-taking for a long cone biopsy. A transverse cut is made approximately 1.5 cm from the ectocervical edge, and serial transverse blocks are taken up to the endocervical end. The ectocervical part of the specimen is handled in the same way as the more usual cone biopsy. This method avoids the problem of unmanageably long blocks.

cone biopsy is handled in the manner that has already been described, taking parallel anteroposterior cuts (see Fig. 9.4).

The cone biopsy specimen is sometimes not perfect and, perhaps as a result of distortion of the cervix, it may be open at one side. It is usually possible to handle this using a modification of the above methods.

The techniques described above will generate approximately 6–25 sections, depending on the size of the cone biopsy. It is standard practice to examine, initially, just one good section from each block taken in this manner. If this first block shows anything suspicious, such as a focus of better differentiation within a gland crypt or an isolated focus of lymphocytic infiltration, both of which may indicate an adjacent area of invasion, deeper levels or step–serial sections are cut on that block, and usually also on adjacent blocks.

On the other hand, some centres advocate routine step–serial sectioning, resulting in perhaps 250 slides from the whole specimen. The policy of examining only one section from each block may be supported by the suggestion that, if an area of invasion is too small to be identified in sections taken at intervals of 2–2.5 mm, even if it was found by more meticulous sectioning it is also too small to necessitate any change in the management of the patient.

THE CONE BIOPSY REPORT

The pathologist's report on a cone biopsy must give the following information:

1. The degree of cervical intraepithelial neoplasia, if any is present. It should also record whether crypts are involved or not, although this does not affect subsequent management. It will be helpful to the colposcopist if the distribution of the lesion (if the specimen can be orientated) and number of blocks involved by cervical intraepithelial neoplasia are indicated.
2. Whether invasion is present or not. The majority of specimens will not show invasion, but it is essential that a statement is included in the report making it clear to the gynaecologist that invasion has been looked for and not found. If invasion is present, the report must include the measurements of maximum depth of invasion and maximum width of the invasive tumour. It should also stipulate whether lymphatic channels are involved or not, whether the growth pattern is confluent or not, and whether the invasive lesion passes to the edge of the specimen.
3. Whether or not the intraepithelial lesion has been completely excised, at both endocervical or ectocervical extremes. Stripping of epithelium at the edges of the specimen should also be stated, as this would make it impossible to comment on the completeness of excision.
4. A point should be made if no abnormality is found but extensive epithelial loss is present; it is important to distinguish between a negative biopsy and one that is inadequate because of epithelial loss.
5. Other incidental findings, such as papillomavirus infection, congenital transformation zone, squamous metaplasia, microglandular hyperplasia and inflammation should be recorded.

ENDOCERVICAL CURETTAGE

This procedure usually produces multiple tiny fragments of tissue, often with abundant blood and mucus. Fixation should be in Bouin's fluid, and meticulous care must be exercised to ensure that all the material is processed. Step–serial sections are advisable.

TOTAL HYSTERECTOMY

If, perhaps for reasons of coexistent benign gynaecological disease, the patient with cervical intraepithelial neoplasia is treated by hysterectomy rather than more conservatively, the cervix is amputated to produce a piece of tissue approximately 2 cm thick; then, after fixation, this is serially blocked in the same way as a cone biopsy (Fig. 9.5). Also, transverse serial blocking of the adjacent upper segment of the cervix should be carried out.

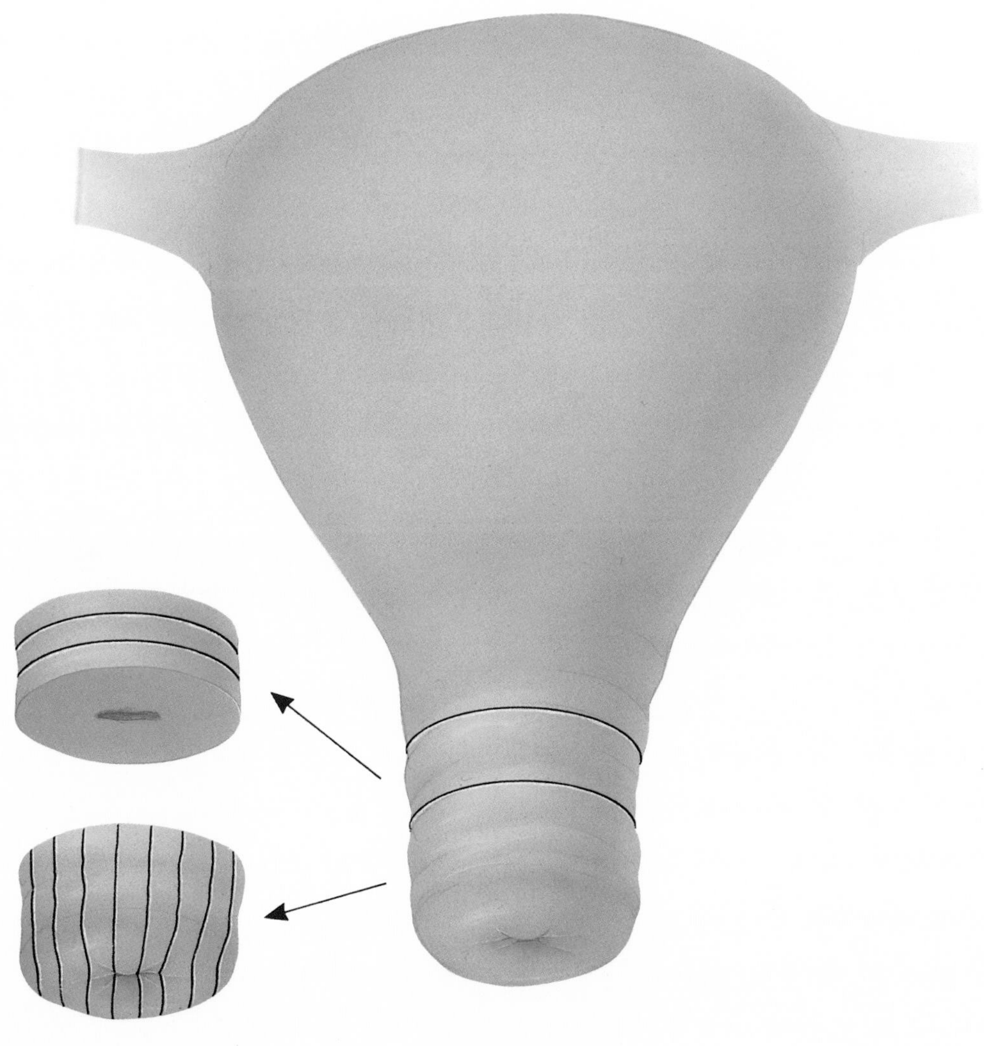

Fig. 9.5 Method of block-taking when hysterectomy is performed for cervical intraepithelial neoplasia (or glandular abnormalities). The cervix is amputated in the fresh state, and the adjacent 1.5–2 cm area is removed separately; both specimens are fixed in Bouin's fluid. Serial blocks are taken from the caudal piece in the same way as in a cone biopsy. The cylinder of tissue, through which the canal runs, is serially blocked transversely. The body of the uterus may be blocked in the usual way.

10. *Invasive squamous disease*

STAGING

The complete FIGO staging system for cervical carcinoma is given in Table 10.1. A simplified, diagrammatic representation of the relationships between the subdivisions within stage I is shown in Fig. 10.1. The colposcopist is almost entirely concerned with the preclinical stages of the disease; clinical carcinoma will only be covered in brief.

Table 10.1 1995 modification of FIGO staging of carcinoma of the cervix uteri

Stage		Description
Stage 0		Preinvasive carcinoma (CIN 3, carcinoma *in situ*).
Stage I		Carcinoma strictly confined to the cervix (extension to the corpus should be disregarded).
	Ia	Measured stromal invasion with maximum depth of 5.0 mm and no wider than 7.0 mm.
	Ia1	Measured invasion of stroma up to 3.0 mm in depth and no wider than 7.0 mm.
	Ia2	Measured invasion of stroma of 3.0–5.0 mm and no wider than 7.0 mm.
	Ib	Clinical lesions confined to the cervix or preclinical lesions greater than stage Ia.
	Ib1	Clinical lesions no greater than 4.0 cm in size.
	Ib2	Clinical lesions greater than 4.0 cm in size.
Stage II		Invasive carcinoma that extends beyond the cervix but has not reached either lateral pelvic wall; involvement of the vagina is limited to the upper two-thirds.
Stage III		Invasive carcinoma that extends to either lateral pelvic wall and/or the lower one-third of the vagina.
Stage IV		Invasive carcinoma that involves urinary bladder and/or rectum or extends beyond the true pelvis.

PRECLINICAL INVASIVE SQUAMOUS CELL CARCINOMA

Preclinical invasive carcinomas may be either stage Ia or stage Ib (see Fig. 10.1). The majority of stage Ib carcinomas are clinically obvious, but preclinical stage Ib invasive carcinoma (formerly referred to as stage Ib [occult]) is an important group to recognize because of different treatment implications compared with stage Ia carcinoma. Stage Ia invasive squamous cell carcinoma of the cervix is usually referred to as 'microinvasive carcinoma'.

Microinvasive carcinoma

The concept of microinvasive carcinoma was introduced by Mestwerdt in 1947, and it referred to lesions which invaded no more than 5 mm into the cervical stroma, in the belief that these had a better prognosis than the other stage I lesions. Currently, this difference in prognosis and, by implication, treatment of microinvasive carcinomas, as opposed to stage Ib carcinomas, is crucial to our perception of preclinical tumours; can very early invasive carcinoma be treated in a relatively conservative way, and if so, is it possible to define by histology the stage in the growth of the tumour at which radical treatment becomes necessary? This is the question underlying the histological definitions of stage Ia and stage Ib invasive carcinoma of the cervix, which will be discussed after a histological description.

HISTOLOGICAL FEATURES

The earliest stage at which invasion can be recognized is shown in Fig. 10.2. A tiny bud of invasive cells is seen to penetrate the basement membrane and push into the underlying stroma. These cells are similar in morphological appearance to CIN 3 from which they arise.

As invasion becomes more advanced, the cells frequently become better differentiated than the overlying cervical intraepithelial neoplasia (Fig. 10.3). There may be a stromal reaction to the infiltrating tumour, characterized by a localized lymphocytic reaction or loosening of the stroma, or both (Figs 10.4 and 10.5).

As invasion progresses even further, other histological features need to be taken into account. These are tumour dimension, lymphatic channel involvement and pattern of growth (Table 10.2).

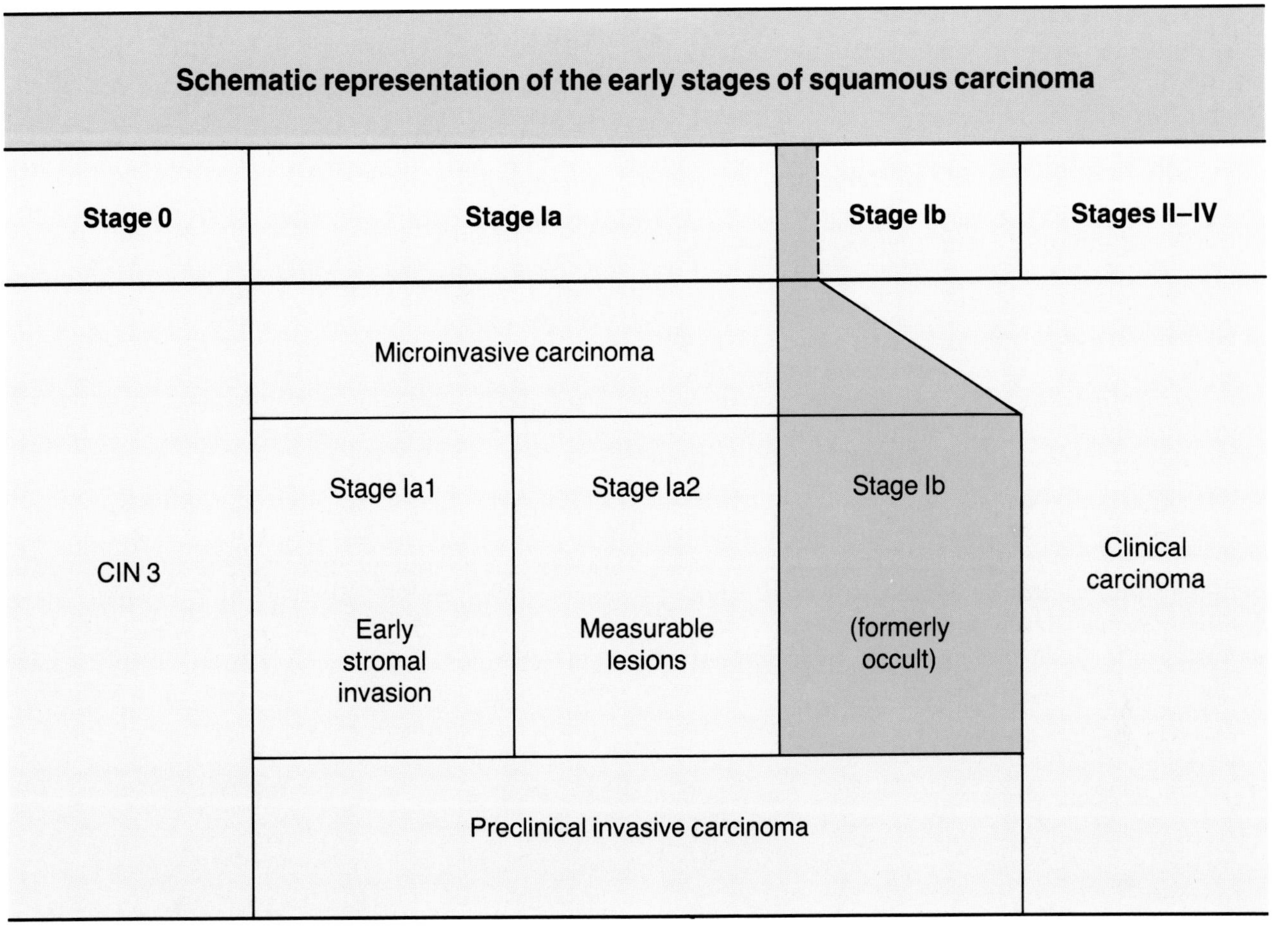

Schematic representation of the early stages of squamous carcinoma

Stage 0	Stage Ia		Stage Ib	Stages II–IV
CIN 3	Microinvasive carcinoma			Clinical carcinoma
	Stage Ia1 Early stromal invasion	Stage Ia2 Measurable lesions	Stage Ib (formerly occult)	
	Preclinical invasive carcinoma			

Fig. 10.1 Staging of squamous cell carcinoma of the cervix. Schematic representation.

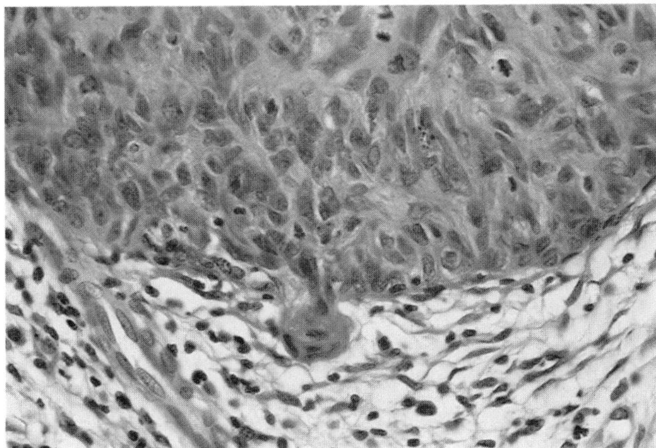

Fig. 10.2 Early stromal invasion. This is the earliest stage of invasion that can be recognized. A small group of cells have breached the smooth contour of the epithelial/stromal junction and invade into the stroma.

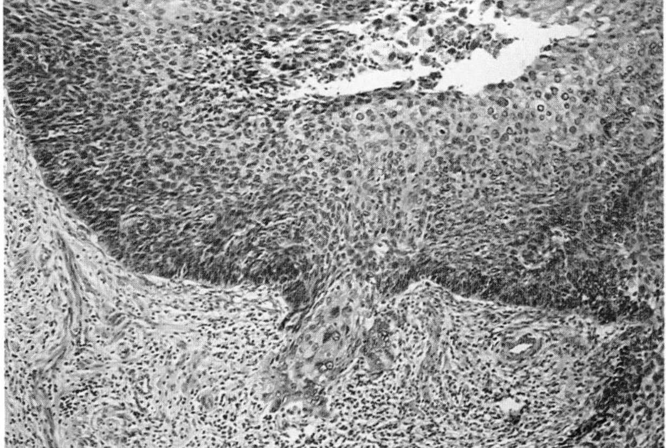

Fig. 10.3 Early stromal invasion. This example is showing very early invasion which is barely measurable. However, the disruption of the contour of the epithelium is clearly seen, and the invasive cells show better differentiation than the matrix cervical intraepithelial neoplasia. This better differentiation is also shown by cells maturing upwards, towards the surface of the epithelium.

TUMOUR DIMENSION

It is generally accepted that as the invasion of a preclinical carcinoma in the cervix advances, the prognosis worsens and the need for radical treatment becomes greater. It has been customary to measure invasion only by its depth, but Burghardt has suggester that the tumour volume gives a more reliable indication of prognosis than measurements in only one or even two dimensions. This volumetric assessment necessitates examination of step–serial sections; when the distance between the sections is known, the third dimension can be calculated, in addition to the two dimensions of depth and width in the section which shows the greatest extent of invasion.

It has been demonstrated that there is no risk of metastatic spread up to 500 mm^3 of tumour size, provided that no vascular invasion is seen. In most laboratories this form of assessment is considered too time consuming, but it is recommended that a two-dimensional (depth and width) measurement of tumour size is given, rather than a measurement of the depth alone (Fig. 10.6).

Table 10.2 Histological features taken into account in the assessment of early invasive tumours

Tumour dimensions (measured in two or three dimensions)
Capillary-like space involvement
Growth pattern (finger-like, spray or confluent)

LYMPHATIC CHANNEL INVOLVEMENT

This can be identified in some preclinical invasive squamous cell carcinomas (Fig. 10.7). It would seem reasonable to argue that a tumour which has lymphatic channel involvement is more likely to have lymph node metastases than one in which such

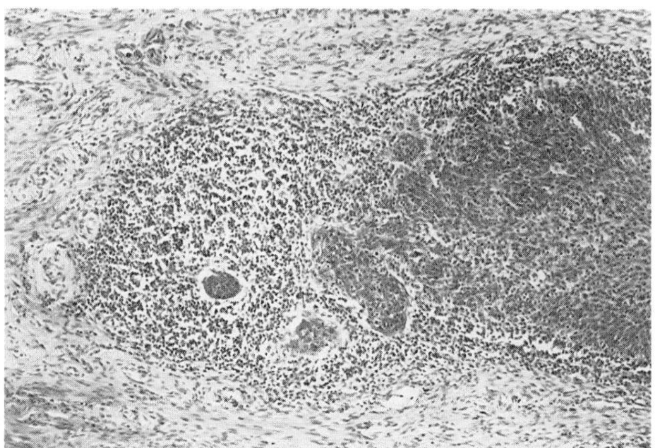

Fig. 10.4 Early stromal invasion. Islands of invasive cells, less than 1 mm from their epithelial origins, are surrounded by a dense infiltrate of lymphocytes.

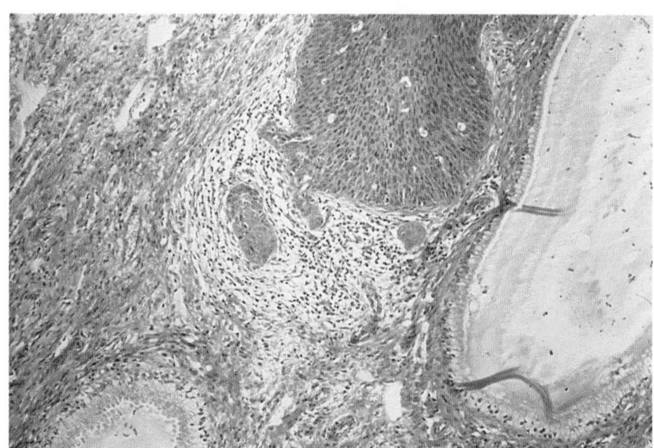

Fig. 10.5 Early stromal invasion. There is striking loosening of the stroma surrounding the invasive islands, with a slight increase in the number of lymphocytes.

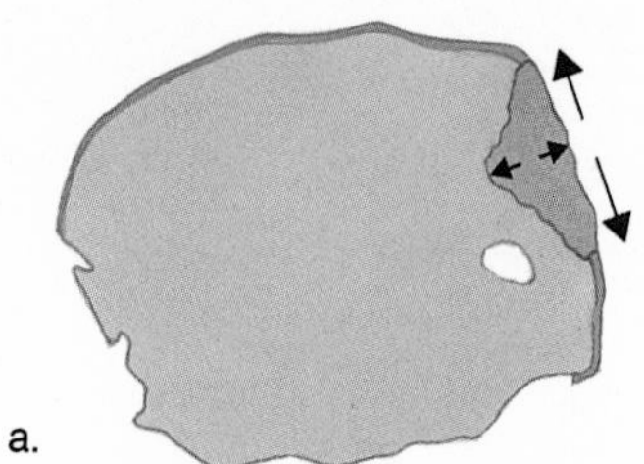

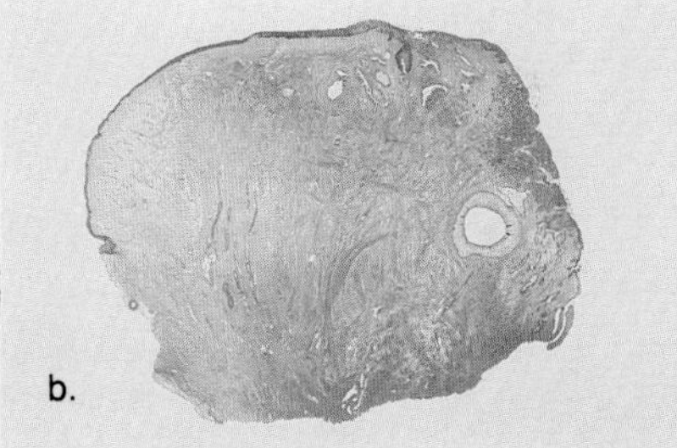

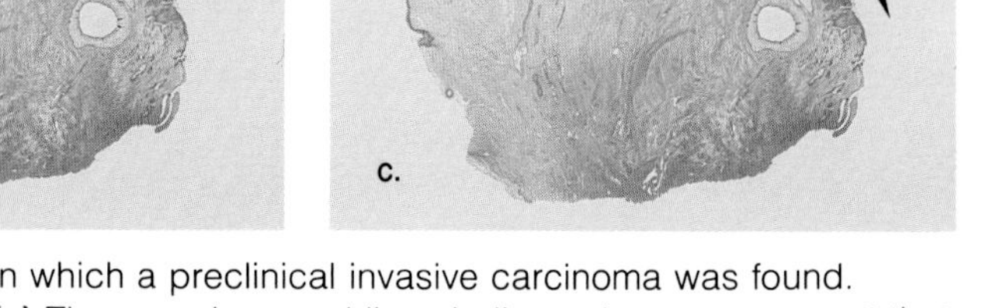

Fig. 10.6 Microinvasive carcinoma. (a) Diagrammatic representation, showing the tumour measurements that need to be taken. **(b)** Measurement of microinvasive carcinoma: this is a section from a hysterectomy specimen in which a preclinical invasive carcinoma was found. **(c)** The superimposed lines indicate the measurement that should be recorded.

involvement is not seen, implying a worse prognosis and the need for a more radical treatment.

Unfortunately, information on this point is conflicting and hampered by the diversity of lesions that have been accepted as microinvasive. In one often-quoted study, Roche and Norris took step–serial sections from 30 cervices which had been diagnosed as containing microinvasive carcinoma, with invasion of 2–5 mm from the surface epithelium; 57% of the patients had 'capillary-like space' involvement. These women had all been treated by radical hysterectomy with pelvic lymphadenectomy, but no metastatic deposits were found in any lymph nodes.

From this study, the authors concluded that the presence of tumour in lymphatic spaces was of no value in predicting which patients were likely to have secondary involvement of lymph nodes.

Nevertheless, subsequent studies have suggested that the presence of lymphatic channel involvement in early invasive carcinoma of the cervix is, indeed, an indication of increased risk of metastases, and this risk becomes greater as the tumour increases in size. The results of these studies indicate that lymphatic channel involvement does not predict an increased risk of pelvic lymph node involvement if invasion is less than 3 mm, but its presence should be taken into account when planning treatment of patients with invasion of 3–5 mm. However, there are individual cases where invasion may be only as much as 2 mm, but with lymphatic channel involvement and pelvic node metastases.

Sometimes the pathologist finds it difficult to decide whether lymphatic channel involvement is present or not; confusion may be caused by tissue shrinkage around invasive buds, leaving a clear space which can be readily mistaken for a lymphatic channel. Only if the nuclei of endothelial cells can be identified should the diagnosis of lymphatic channel involvement be made.

GROWTH PATTERN

The earliest 'finger-like' pattern of growth is illustrated in Figs 10.2–10.5. As the tumour becomes more advanced, this often changes to produce a confluent growth pattern (Fig. 10.8). It has been suggested that the latter is more likely to be associated with metastatic spread, but as this pattern is likely to be seen in more advanced tumours, it may simply be a factor of depth of invasion. Occasionally, multiple finger-like processes of invasion are seen over a wide area, creating a 'spray-like' configuration which is distinct from a confluent pattern (Fig. 10.9).

CYTOLOGICAL FEATURES

The cytological diagnosis of microinvasive carcinoma of the cervix is controversial. Some cytologists believe that a distinction between CIN 3 and the earliest stages of invasive disease cannot be made with cytology. This view is partly supported by the corresponding problems of histological interpretation.

However, there is evidence that, in a significant proportion of cases, it is possible to recognize

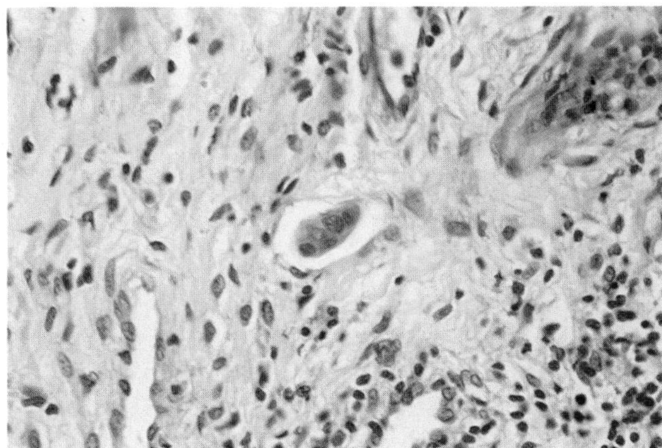

Fig. 10.7 Lymphatic channel involvement. A clump of tumour cells is present within a preformed space. The nuclei of the endothelial cells are easily recognized.

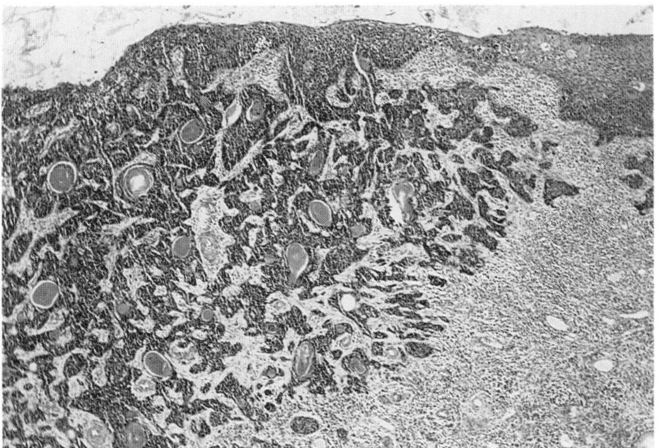

Fig. 10.8 Preclinical invasive carcinoma with a confluent growth pattern. This is the same case as in Fig. 10.7. The tumour is invading as a confluent mass of irregular islands, in contrast to the pattern shown in Figs 10.3–10.5.

cytological features that strongly suggest the beginning of invasiveness of a lesion, or at least the point at which the lesion is no longer intraepithelial. The application of cytology in this area is difficult; diligence and experience are required in order to recognize the subtle changes and interpret them in a meaningful way (Table 10.3).

A striking histological feature of minimal invasion is cytoplasmic differentiation, and this can be recognized with cytology. The cell borders are less well defined than in severe dyskaryosis. The cytoplasm appears more finely granular, frequently staining a pinkish hue (Fig. 10.10), although blue- or green-staining cytoplasm is also seen. The cytoplasmic differentiation must be distinguished from that associated with human papillomavirus infection; the absence of keratinization and dyskeratosis will allow this distinction on most occasions.

Occasionally the cells assume an elongated or elliptical shape. Odd-shaped cells with tails and rounded projections are sometimes observed. Unlike cervical intraepithelial neoplasia, where the cells tend to be seen in lines or small groups, in microinvasion the cells tend to appear loosely associated in sheets (Fig. 10.11). The nuclei may show marked pleomorphism and hyperchromasia (Fig. 10.12), but the chromatin may appear less coarsely clumped than in intraepithelial neoplasia, frequently with more obvious nuclear clearing. Variation in intensity of staining between one nucleus and another may also be seen.

As colposcopic recognition of minimal invasive disease is also difficult, it is important that the cytology is carefully reviewed; where cellular features suggest that the lesion is no longer typical of cervical intraepithelial neoplasia, the colposcopist should be alerted to the possibility of invasion by the appropriate wording of the report.

However, it is equally important not to overdiagnose early invasive disease cytologically, as this would lead to difficulties in managing the patients, and would also undermine the confidence of clinicians and colposcopists in the cytological opinion.

It is not possible to make a confident distinction between stage Ia and stage Ib invasive carcinoma with cytology.

Table 10.3 Cytological features associated with microinvasive carcinoma

1 Tendency to form large sheets of cells rather than strings
2 Smaller, paler-staining nuclei/cells
3 Cytoplasmic differentiation
4 Small tails and rounded projections to cytoplasm/sometimes keratinized
5 Increased pleomorphism
6 More obvious nuclear 'clearing'
7 Loss of round appearances to cells

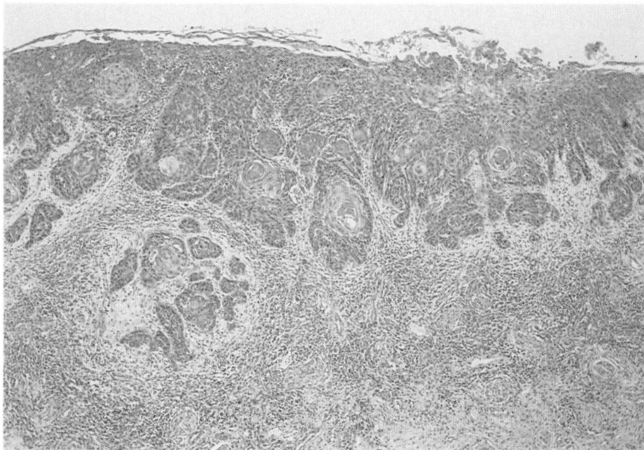

Fig. 10.9 Preclinical invasive carcinoma with a confluent growth pattern. Although in this example the maximum depth of invasion is under 2 mm, it is taking place over a broad field with a confluent, 'spray-like' growth pattern.

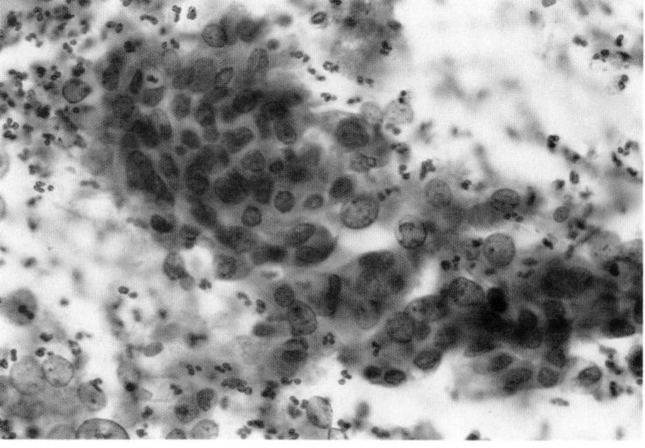

Fig. 10.10 Microinvasive carcinoma. Loosely associated sheets of cells, showing cytoplasmic differentiation staining a pinkish hue.

DEFINITIONS

The search for a definition of microinvasive carcinoma is the quest for the histological features that allow a reliable identification of the maximum disease which can be safely treated in a conservative manner; this ideal definition is not yet available, although the most recent recommendations for the staging of cervical carcinoma by FIGO appear to come close to it (Table 10.1).

Stage Ia lesions are defined as having a depth of invasion of no greater than 5 mm and a lateral width of not more than 7 mm. Stage Ia lesions are further subdivided into stage Ia1, where invasion is no deeper than 3 mm, and stage Ia2, with invasion between 3 mm and 5 mm. Examples of small stage Ia1 lesions are illustrated in Figs 10.2–10.5. These tumours, with invasion of less than 1 mm, have no metastatic potential, and radical treatment is not indicated. Most tumours falling into the FIGO (1995) stage Ia1, particularly if there is no evidence of vascular space involvement, probably also have very little metastatic potential and may be treated conservatively. The dilemma remains over the more advanced cases that fall into stage Ia2, most of which probably merit radical treatment. However, in both categories, each case must be handled individually and all factors taken into consideration.

Stage Ib lesions are of greater dimensions than stage Ia2, irrespective of whether they are clinically apparent or not.

INVASIVE SQUAMOUS CELL CARCINOMA

Gross features

With colposcopy, an early invasive carcinoma of the cervix may appear striking. However, to the unaided eye diagnosis is not always easy to make, as the features are not characteristic. The surface may be slightly raised, and the tumour may present as a rough, red, granular area, bleeding to the touch. There is often little to distinguish an early invasive carcinoma from an ectopy, where vascular endocervical tissue is present on the vaginal part of the cervix.

Many invasive squamous cell carcinomas, by the time they become clinically apparent, are visible on speculum examination and involve the external os. However, some remain entirely within the canal, and although of squamous origin they are clinically classified as endocervical carcinomas. The growth pattern may be either predominantly exophytic, with polypoid or papillary excrescences, or ulcerating with necrosis. Frequently, a combination of these two patterns is seen.

Histological features

Squamous cell carcinomas are conventionally subdivided into large-cell keratinizing carcinoma,

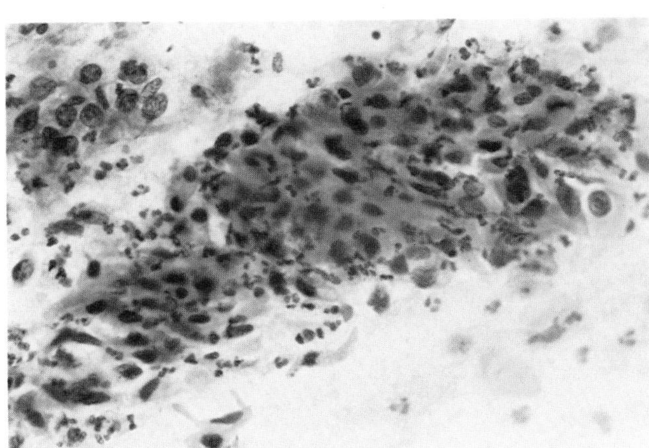

Fig. 10.11 Microinvasive carcinoma. Loosely associated sheets of cells, with marked pleomorphism and some cytoplasmic tails.

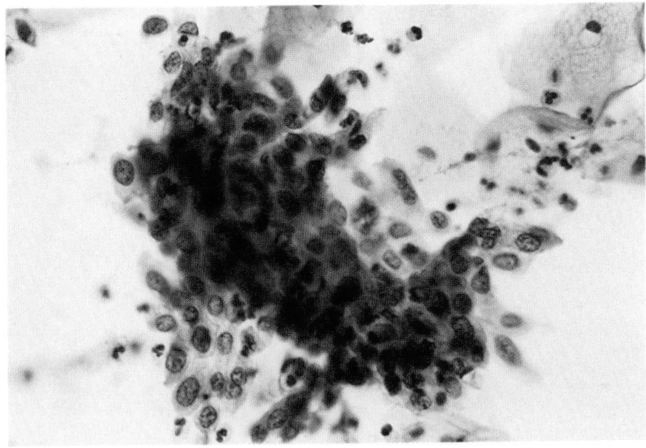

Fig. 10.12 Microinvasive carcinoma. Cells are showing hyperchromatic nuclei with clearing. The cytoplasm in some cells has rounded projections.

large-cell non-keratinizing carcinoma, and small-cell non-keratinizing carcinoma (Table 10.4). Although, in general terms, the small-cell carcinomas are poorly differentiated and the keratinizing carcinomas are well differentiated, the classification given in Table 10.4 describes the cell type rather than the grade; the nuclear grade should also be assessed in this cell type. Some keratinizing carcinomas (Fig. 10.13) may show areas of high nuclear grade.

LARGE-CELL KERATINIZING CARCINOMA

This consists of typical epidermoid cells, with characteristic central whorls of cells containing central nests of keratin ('keratin pearls'). Intercellular bridges are seen, along with keratohyaline granules and cytoplasmic keratinization (see Fig. 10.13).

LARGE-CELL NON-KERATINIZING CARCINOMA

This is composed of cells which are usually recognizable as being squamous because of their polygonal shape. There may be a little individual cell keratinization, but keratin pearls are absent (Fig. 10.14). These tumours are often, but not necessarily, of a worse nuclear grade than the keratinizing tumours.

SMALL-CELL NON-KERATINIZING CARCINOMA

This consists of small, round cells with fairly uniform, dark nuclei. There is often little to characterize these tumours as squamous, although on rare occasions keratinizing examples are seen (Fig. 10.15). Some tumours, classified as small-cell non-keratinizing squamous cell carcinomas, contain argyrophil cells with a pattern resembling the small-cell anaplastic ('oat cell') carcinoma of the bronchus (Fig. 10.16). These tumours are associated with a particularly poor prognosis.

Table 10.4 Classification of squamous cell carcinomas of the cervix

Cell type	
	Large-cell, keratinizing
	Large-cell, non-keratinizing
	Small-cell, non-keratinizing
Grade	
	Grade 1 – well differentiated
	Grade 2 – moderately differentiated
	Grade 3 – poorly differentiated

Cytological features

The cytological appearances associated with invasive squamous carcinoma have been well described (Table 10.5). However, the reliability of cervical smears in the identification of squamous cell carcinoma of the cervix has been questioned. To some extent this may be related to the experience of the individual cytologist, and also to the mistaken expectation that

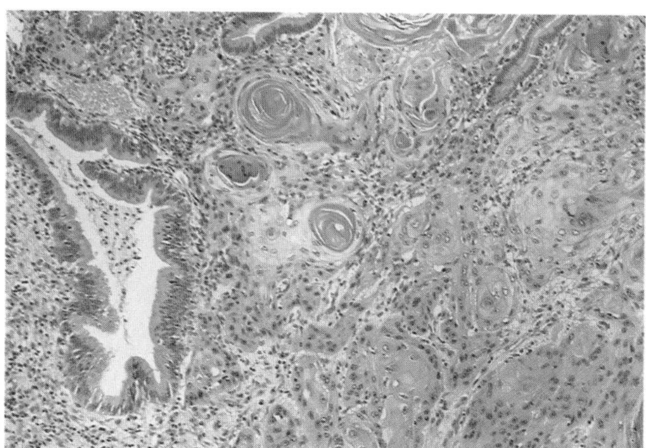

Fig. 10.13 Invasive squamous cell carcinoma; large-cell keratinizing type. The characteristic keratin pearls are prominent.

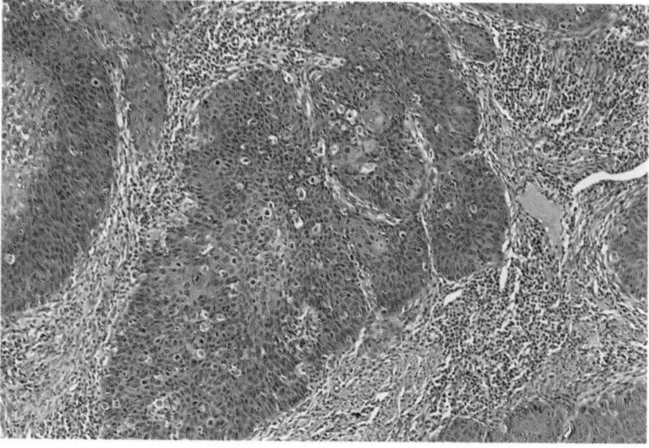

Fig. 10.14 Invasive squamous cell carcinoma; large-cell non-keratinizing type. A moderately lymphocytic infiltrate is present in the stroma.

all invasive disease will present with a large number of bizarre and keratinized malignant cells.

It is certainly true that, in the case of large-cell keratinizing carcinoma, the malignant cells are sometimes grossly enlarged, with obvious pleomorphism, and associated with bizarre tadpole or spindle forms which may show excessive keratinization (Fig. 10.17). In the large-cell non-keratinizing type, either no evidence of keratinization is seen, or only occasional small keratinized cells are present (Figs 10.18–10.20). However, in a case of squamous cell carcinoma, the cervical smear will quite frequently contain very few malignant cells. Consequently, smears must be care-

Table 10.5 Cytological features associated with invasive squamous carcinoma

1 Nuclear pleomorphism
2 Marked anisocytosis and anisonucleosis
3 Occasionally bizarre 'tadpole' and 'spindle' forms
4 Highly keratinized cytoplasm (in some cases)
5 Much associated cell necrosis and debris, frequently with red blood cells

(a) 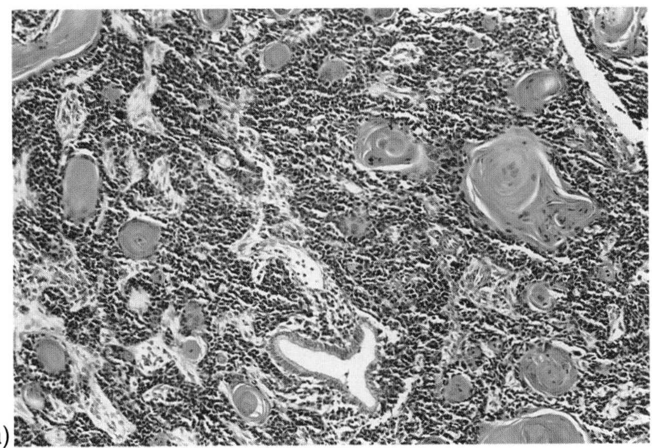

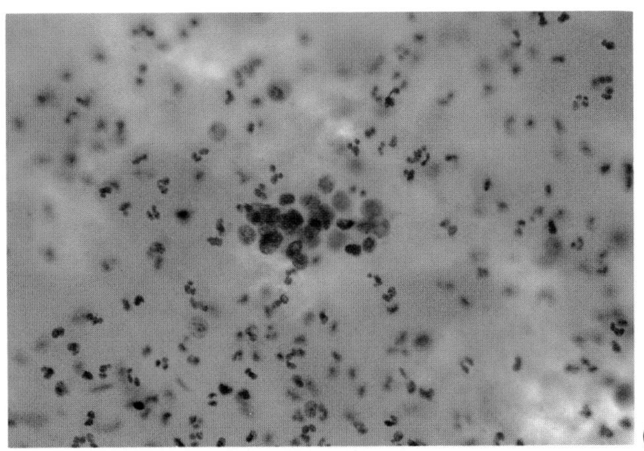 (b)

Fig. 10.15 Invasive squamous cell carcinoma; small-cell keratinizing type. (a) This is an unusual variant of squamous cell carcinoma, and is the same example as shown in Figs 10.6(b) and 10.10. Keratin pearls are prominent. **(b)** The cells appear as a loosely associated group in a blood-stained background. Although the nuclei are small, they are notably pleomorphic.

(a) 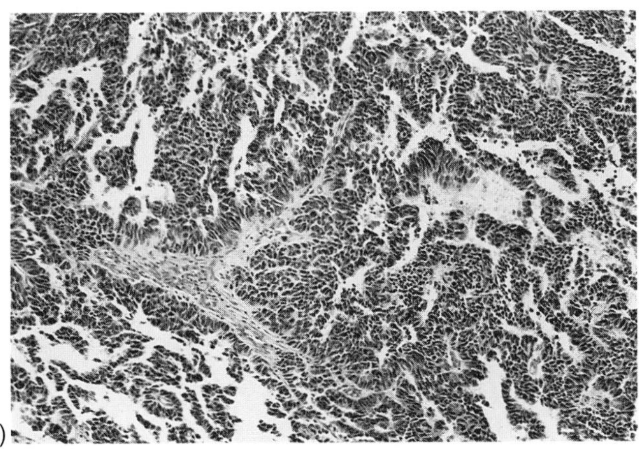

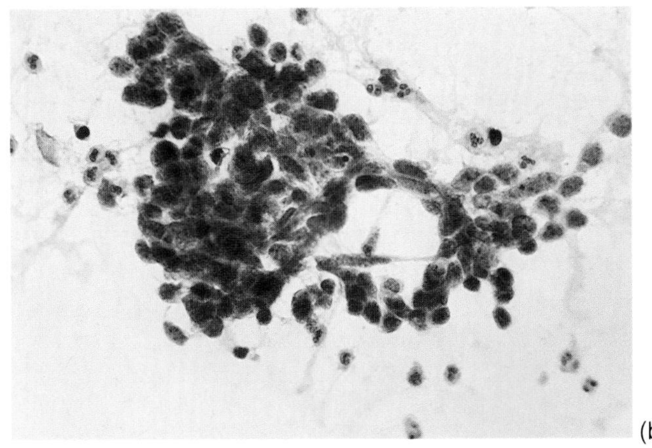 (b)

Fig. 10.16 Invasive carcinoma; small-cell anaplastic type. (a) There are no features to suggest a squamous origin of this tumour, the appearances of which are similar to the small cell anaplastic 'oat cell' carcinoma of the bronchus. **(b)** The nuclei show hyperchromasia and pleomorphism with a homogeneous appearance of chromatin; there is obvious moulding.

fully screened to pick out the few malignant cells among the red blood cells and necrotic debris (Fig. 10.21).

At the other end of the spectrum, cells from a well-differentiated lesion may not show bizarre and keratinized forms but only minimal nuclear change with abundant cytoplasm, and these may closely resemble cells of squamous metaplasia (Fig. 10.22). Cells arising from a small-cell anaplastic carcinoma (oat cell type) show moulding of the nuclei (see Fig. 10.16(b); Fig. 10.23) very similar to the characteristic appearances of oat cell carcinoma in sputum.

The absence of striking cytoplasmic change may add to the difficulty of recognition. The ability to discriminate between necrotic change associated with inflammation and that associated with invasive cancer is only improved by careful evaluation both of individual cell changes and overall smear pattern.

Differentiation from human papillomavirus infection depends on identifying the other features seen with that infection. The background and other cell types seen, as well as the distribution of keratinized cells together with dyskeratosis and dyskaryosis, all need to be considered in arriving at a final diagnosis.

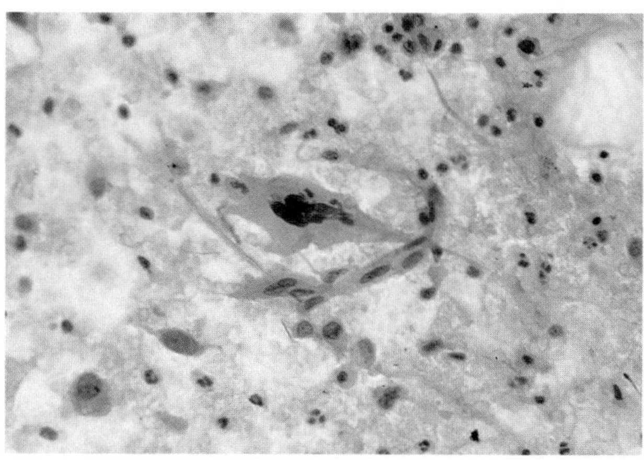

Fig. 10.17 Invasive squamous cell carcinoma; large-cell keratinizing type. A bizarre, keratinized, multinucleated cell is present in the centre, surrounded by necrotic debris.

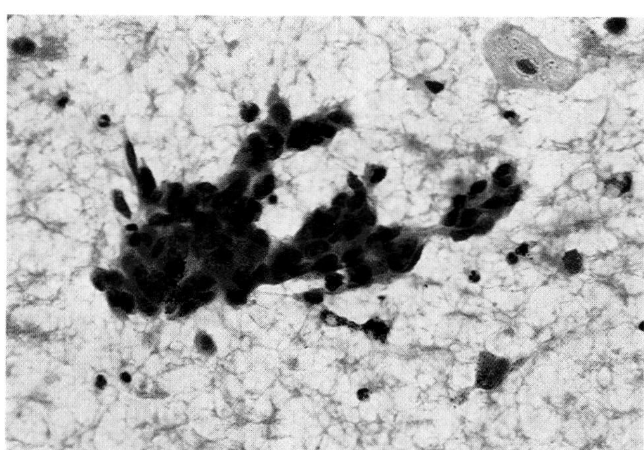

Fig. 10.18 Invasive squamous cell carcinoma, large-cell non-keratinizing type. An irregular sheet of pleomorphic cells with hyperchromatic nuclei and sparse cytoplasm is seen, characteristic of this type of tumour.

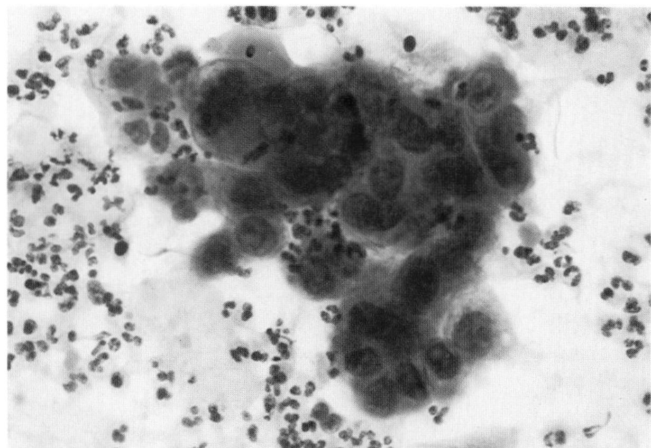

Fig. 10.19 Invasive squamous cell carcinoma, large-cell non-keratinizing type. This group of grossly pleomorphic cells demonstrate a greatly increased nuclear/cytoplasmic ratio.

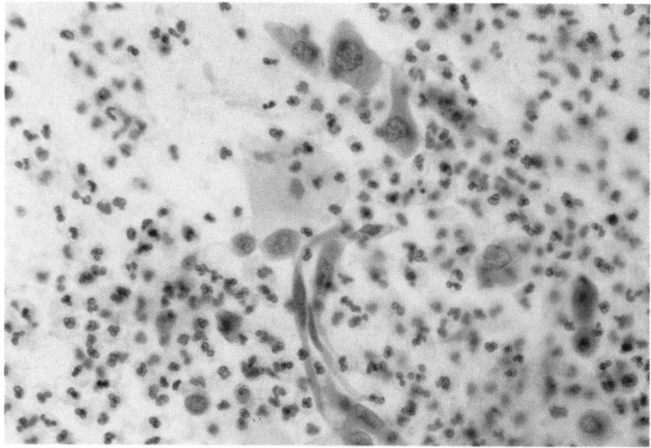

Fig. 10.20 Invasive carcinoma. One elongated keratinizing 'spindle' form is present, together with discrete, pale-staining but pleomorphic cells.

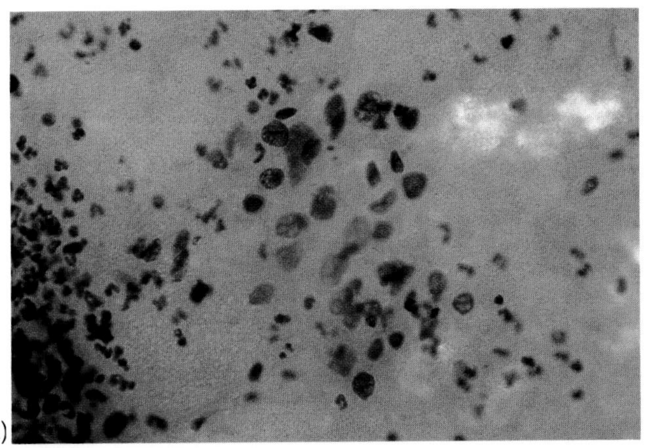

(a)

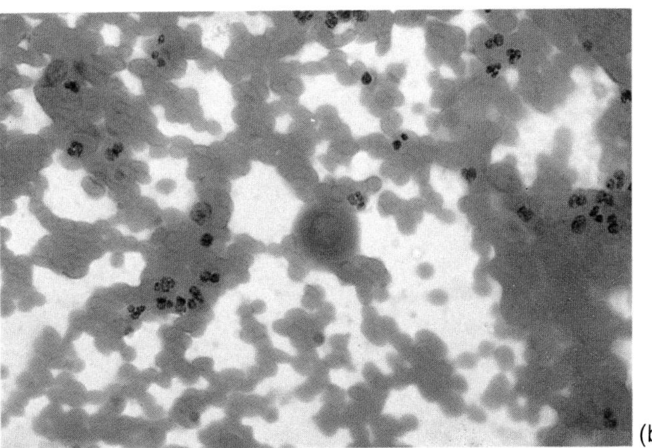

(b)

Fig. 10.21 Invasive carcinoma. (a) Discrete, poorly displayed malignant cells are seen in a sea of blood-stained debris and polymorphonuclear leucocytes. **(b)** One large, pale, necrotic cell in a sea of blood. The nucleus is poorly displayed but is greatly enlarged, with an irregular shape and chromatin pattern.

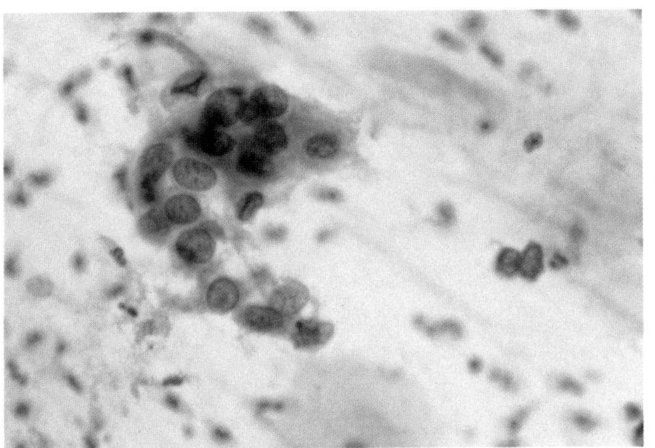

Fig. 10.22 Invasive carcinoma. This small group of cells has well-defined, blue–green cytoplasm and enlarged nuclei which do not show bizarre changes. Careful evaluation is required to recognize the more subtle features suggestive of invasion.

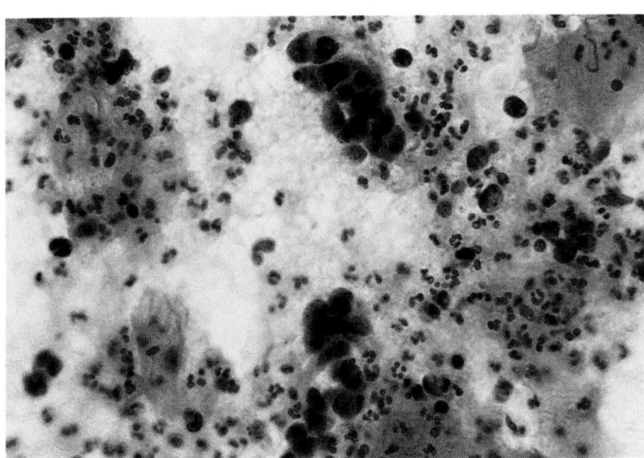

Fig. 10.23 Small-cell anaplastic carcinoma. The two groups of small, densely stained cells show clear evidence of moulding reminiscent of bronchial 'oat cell' carcinoma.

COLPOSCOPIC FEATURES

Invasive carcinoma is generally thought of as an area of ulceration or gross and irregular hypertrophy. However, in many instances, the disease will be clinically unsuspected and will be recognized for the first time when the patient is referred for colposcopy following an abnormal cervical smear.

Colposcopically, atypical vessels are often thought to be the hallmark of an invasive carcinoma. These are focal colposcopic appearances in which the blood vessel pattern shows not as punctation, mosaic or delicately branching vessels, but as irregular vessels with abruptly changing courses, with 'comma', 'corkscrew' or 'spaghetti-like' forms. Atypical vessels are coarser than normal vessels, and are irregular in width, shape and course. They have a horizontal component, and may appear and disappear abruptly.

Even where the cervix is macroscopically normal, wide intercapillary distance, the presence of atypical vessels, and an irregular surface, often with ulceration, will alert the colposcopist to the possibility of invasive disease (Figs 10.24–10.31). Nevertheless, many early invasive lesions have no atypical vessels. In a series of 180 patients with preclinical invasive

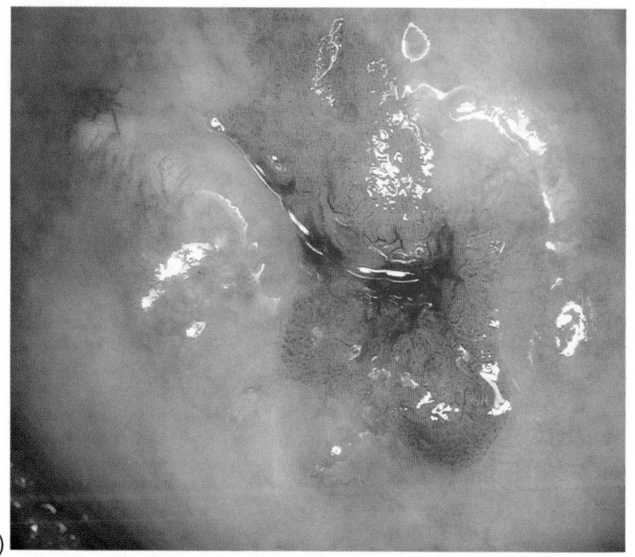
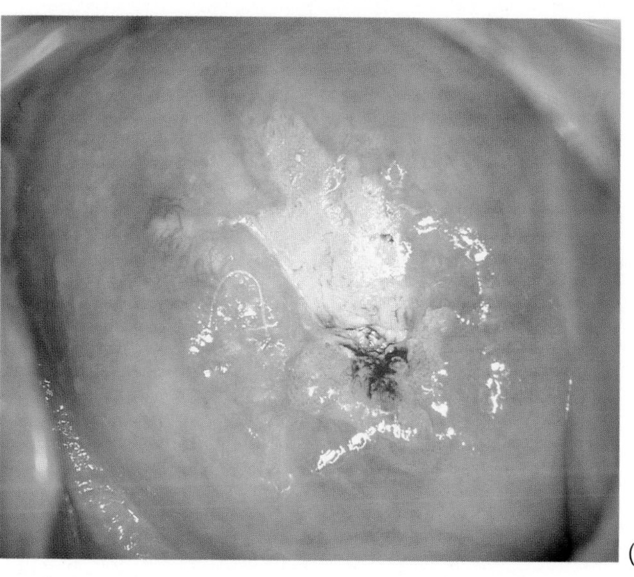

Fig. 10.24 Microinvasive carcinoma. (a) Before and **(b)** after application of acetic acid. The possibility of microinvasion was raised by the irregular, friable epithelium at the '6 o'clock' position. Such lesions require an excisional cone biopsy.

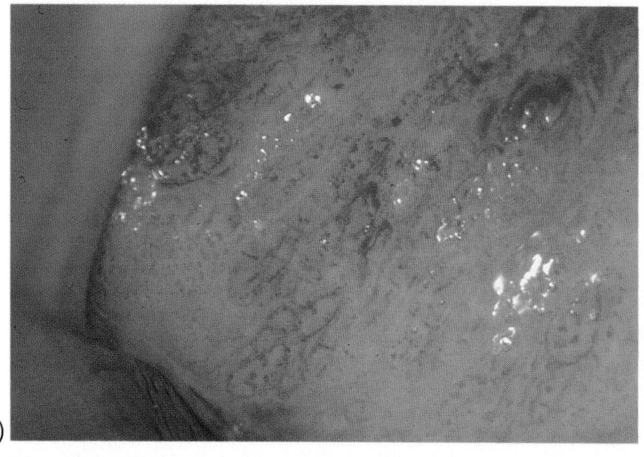
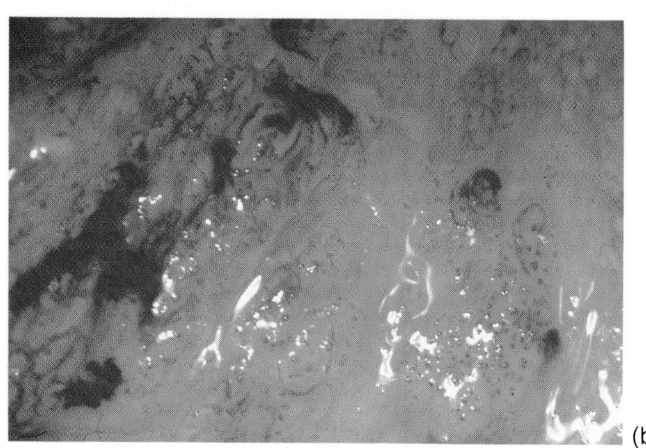

Fig. 10.25 Microinvasive carcinoma. (a) Before and **(b)** after application of acetic acid. The lesion demonstrates atypical vessel and a surface that is irregular and friable.

disease (stage Ia and Ib), Benedet, Anderson and Boyes (1985) reported that no markedly atypical vessels were found at colposcopy. The main features associated with invasion were large lesions with complex patterns (i.e. combination of acetowhite, mosaic and punctation), a raised, irregular surface and CIN 3 with cervical canal extensions.

If the lesion is ulcerated, surface epithelium is lost and there may be a few or even no vessels to be seen in the ulcer cavity. On the other hand, if the lesion is hypertrophic, there is proliferation of epithelial tissue, and the vessels in this instance are usually very prominent. Even in the presence of obvious invasive disease, the cervix and upper vagina should be examined by colposcopy to assess the limits of abnormality. Frequently, unsuspected premalignant disease is found to extend beyond the borders of invasion; it is therefore important that any treatment regimen takes the extent of both malignant and premalignant disease into consideration.

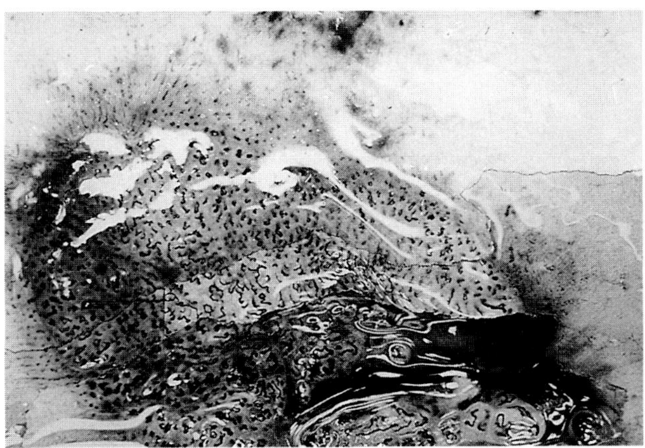

Fig. 10.26 Microinvasive carcinoma and CIN 3. Using the saline technique and a green filter, the vessels are clearly seen. The anterior part of the lesion is showing the coarse punctation pattern of CIN 3. The part of the lesion around the external os displays atypical vessels and an irregular surface. The lesion extends into the canal, and requires an excisional biopsy.

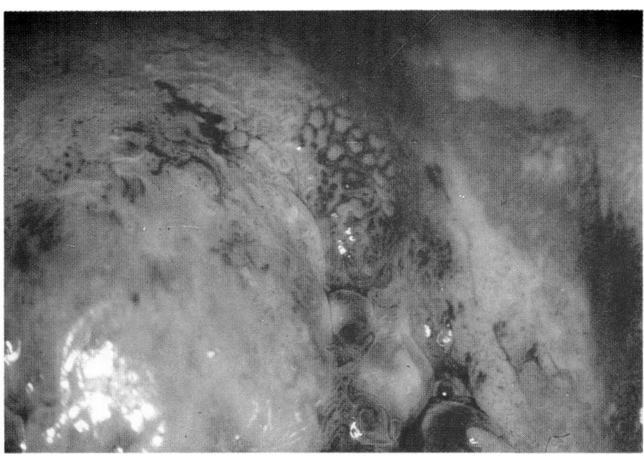

Fig. 10.27 Microinvasive carcinoma. Atypical vessels are seen after application of acetic acid.

(a)

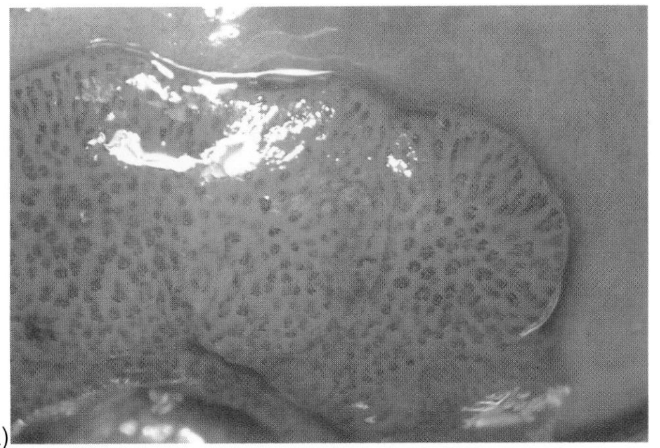

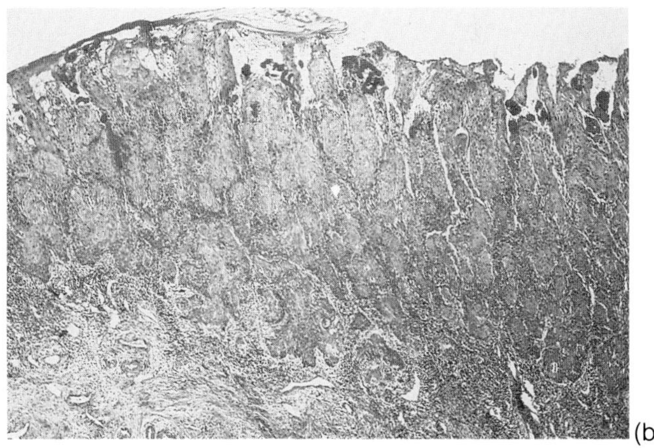

(b)

Fig. 10.28 (a) Microinvasive carcinoma. This was suspected because of the very prominent, coarse punctation, atypical vessels and a surface that is raised above the adjacent normal squamous epithelium. **(b)** Histology of the same lesion.

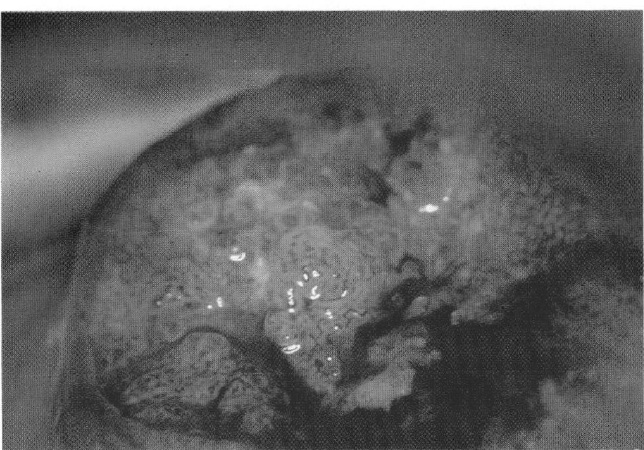

Fig. 10.29 Invasive carcinoma. Even without application of acetic acid, the lesion is raised, irregular, friable and contains atypical vessels.

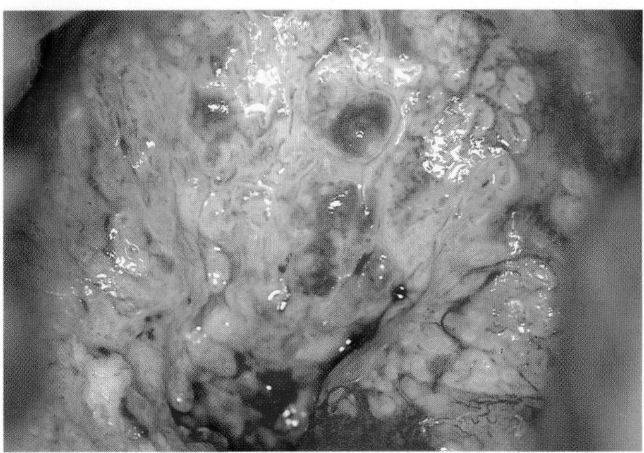

Fig. 10.30 Invasive carcinoma after application of acetic acid.

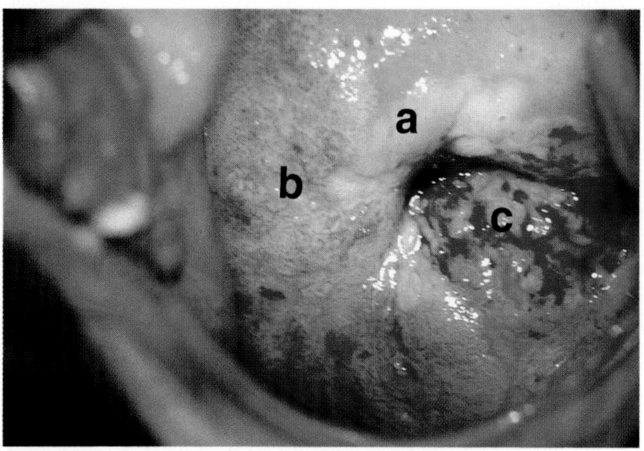

Fig. 10.31 Full range of cervical neoplasia. (a) Acetowhite area at '12 o'clock' on the anatomical os – CIN 3. **(b)** Right half of cervix (left of figure) covered by atypical vessels – microinvasive carcinoma. **(c)** Left posterior quadrant (lower right of figure) and disappearing into the canal, irregularly raised, bleeding surface – frank invasive carcinoma.

11. *Glandular lesions*

HISTOPATHOLOGICAL CLASSIFICATION

Malignant and premalignant changes of the glandular epithelium of the cervix make up a small but important group of diseases. The proportion of patients with adenocarcinoma, reported in various series of cervical carcinoma, ranges between 4.5% and 34%.

More recently, there has been an apparent increase in the proportion of adenocarcinomas. This may be due to a reduction in the number of squamous cell carcinomas, perhaps as a result of screening and treatment at the preinvasive stage, rather than an increase of adenocarcinomas. However, there is some evidence of an absolute increase of cases of adenocarcinoma.

Table 11.1 Classification of adenocarcinoma of the cervix

Cervical cell adenocarcinoma
Mucinous adenocarcinoma
Endometrioid adenocarcinoma
Clear cell carcinoma
Minimal deviation adenocarcinoma
Serous papillary carcinoma
Adenosquamous (mixed) carcinoma
Mucoepidermoid carcinoma
Glassy cell carcinoma

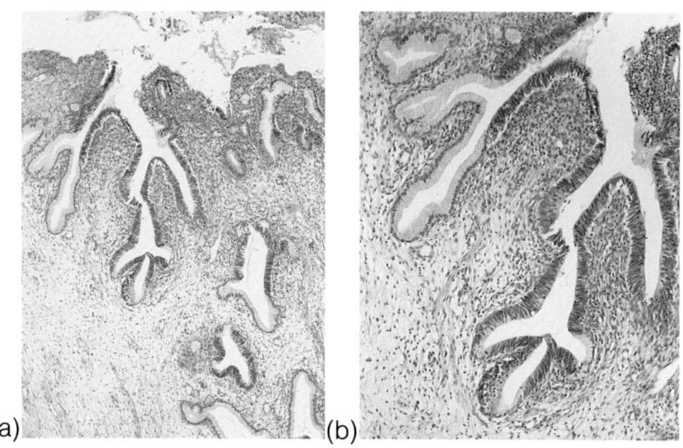

Fig. 11.1 High-grade cervical glandular intraepithelial neoplasia (CGIN). (a) At low magnification, the architectural pattern of the endocervical crypts is seen to be undisturbed. **(b)** The highly abnormal epithelium follows exactly the same contours as the normal epithelium, sharing the same basement membrane.

Some three decades ago, the observed proportion of adenocarcinomas within the total number of cervical carcinomas encountered was typically in the region of 4–5%. By comparison, in one recent large study using routine data from a British regional cancer registry, adenocarcinomas represented approximately one in six of all cervical invasive malignancies reported, which is a clear and worrying increase. Moreover, almost 8% of those lesions occurred in single women, compared with just over 4% for squamous lesions in the same group.

In another large study of the incidence of adenocarcinoma, using recent data from three British cancer registries and covering a span of 15 years, the number of cases per million in women between 20 and 34 years of age almost tripled (from 2.4 to 6.6 cases per million), an alarming increase in this young and potentially fertile group. Little change was observed in women aged 35 years and over.

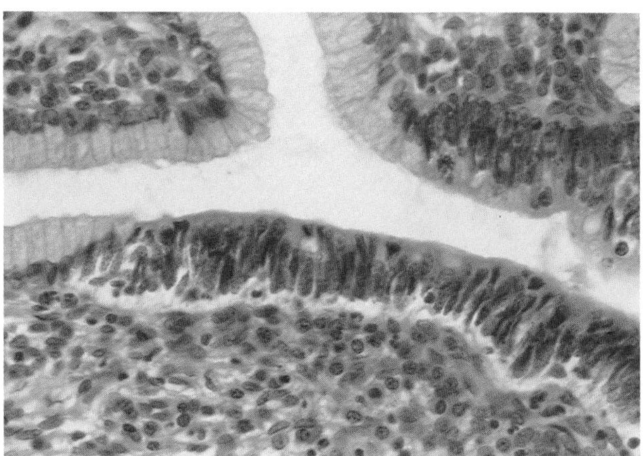

Fig. 11.2 High-grade CGIN. The contrast between normal and abnormal epithelium is clearly demonstrated. The area of high-grade CGIN demonstrates all the features listed in Table 11.1.

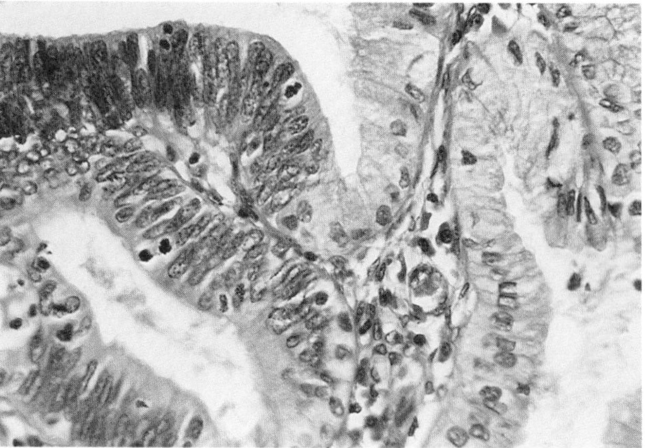

Fig. 11.3 High-grade CGIN. There are numerous mitotic figures.

Table 11.2 Classification of glandular intraepithelial abnormalities of the cervix

Low-grade CGIN	=	Glandular atypia or glandular dysplasia
High-grade CGIN	=	Adenocarcinoma *in situ*

CGIN, cervical glandular intraepithelial neoplasia

Glandular abnormalities of the cervix may be invasive or intraepithelial; a classification of invasive adenocarcinoma is given in Table 11.1. As the colposcopist is mainly concerned with preclinical disease, invasive intraepithelial adenocarcinoma will be covered in brief.

Similar to intraepithelial squamous neoplasia, glandular intraepithelial neoplasia appears to form a spectrum of disease, ranging from very mild to severe forms. Various classifications have been suggested; the most widely used is shown in Table 11.2. The most severe abnormalities are classified as high-grade CGIN, and lesser degrees of change are referred to as low-grade CGIN.

Table 11.3 Histological features of cervical glandular intraepithelial neoplasia

Architectural features

Often retains normal architectural pattern
Slight crowding is accepted
Slight variation in size and shape of glands is accepted

(If architectural changes are marked, even in the absence of striking cellular changes, or if atypical crypts are found outside the normal crypt field, a diagnosis of invasive carcinoma must be considered)

Cellular changes

Increased nuclear/cytoplasmic ratio
Variation in nuclear size and shape
Mitotic activity
Loss of polarity
Stratification
Reduced mucin production

CERVICAL GLANDULAR INTRAEPITHELIAL NEOPLASIA

Cervical glandular intraepithelial neoplasia (CGIN) of high grade has been recognized for over 30 years and is also known as adenocarcinoma *in situ* (AIS). However, it has been reported most frequently in recent years, often in association with squamous cervical intraepithelial neoplasia, or adjacent to an invasive adenocarcinoma.

Microscopically (Table 11.3), CGIN maintains the architectural pattern of normal endocervical crypts, and often involves only the superficial crypts (Fig. 11.1). The abnormal epithelium of high-grade CGIN shows loss of polarity, increased nuclear size, nuclear pleomorphism and anisokaryosis, mitotic activity,

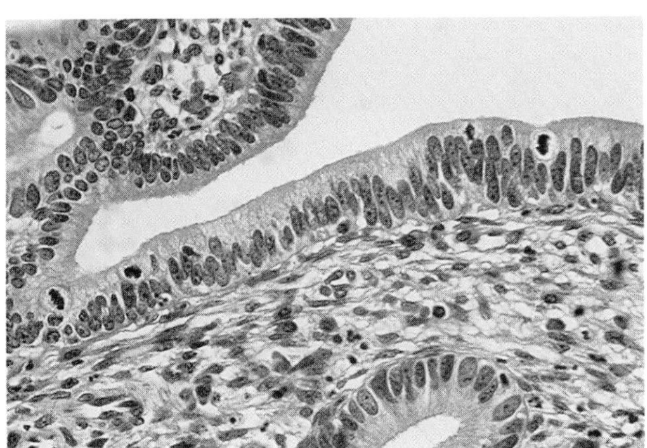

Fig. 11.4 Low-grade CGIN. Mitotic figures are seen, and there is an increase in nuclear size with some nuclear pleomorphism. However, polarity is largely maintained, and mucin-containing cytoplasm is apparent.

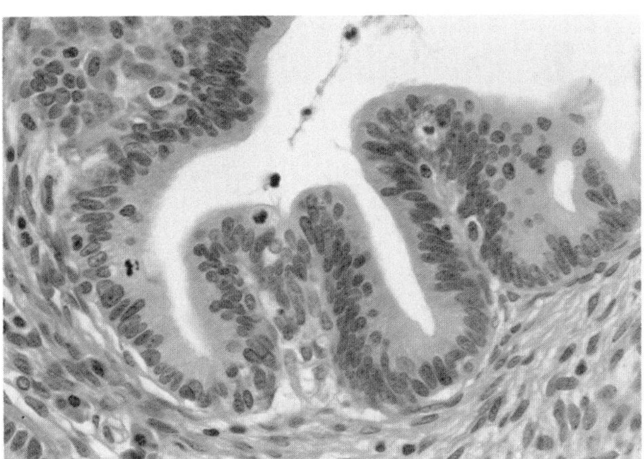

Fig. 11.5 Low-grade CGIN. This example shows rather less abnormality than that in Fig. 11.4.

reduction in cytoplasmic mucin and, frequently, stratification (Figs 11.2 and 11.3).

The low-grade lesions show the same changes, but to a less marked degree (Figs 11.4 and 11.5). For example, a low-grade lesion will show fewer mitotic figures, more preservation of polarity, less stratification and more mucin production than a high-grade CGIN (compare Figs 11.2 and 11.4). However, as in squamous CIN, a distinction between the grades of glandular intraepithelial neoplasia is artificial and arbitrary.

Strictly speaking, the term 'glandular intraepithelial neoplasia should be used only when the crypt architecture is not appreciably altered (see Fig. 11.1).

Even so, some authors show examples of CGIN in which there is reduplication and budding of the crypts (Fig. 11.6), sometimes with a 'back-to-back' pattern of the glands (Fig. 11.7). It is very difficult to recognize the beginning of invasion in an adenocarcinoma, as it invades by newly formed glands pushing into the stroma (Fig. 11.8) rather than by cells invading individually or in groups, which is the case with squamous cell carcinoma. This difficulty is compounded by the application of the term 'microinvasive adenocarcinoma', the criteria for which are equivocal; in our present state of knowledge, there seems little value in using this term.

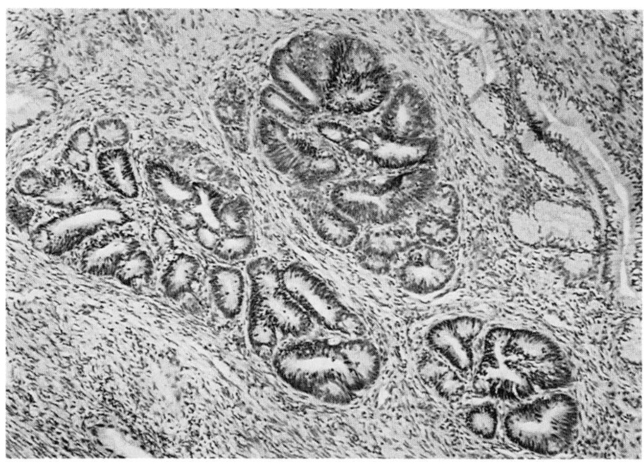

Fig. 11.6 High-grade CGIN. The architectural pattern is disturbed, with glandular reduplication and formation of 'tunnel clusters'.

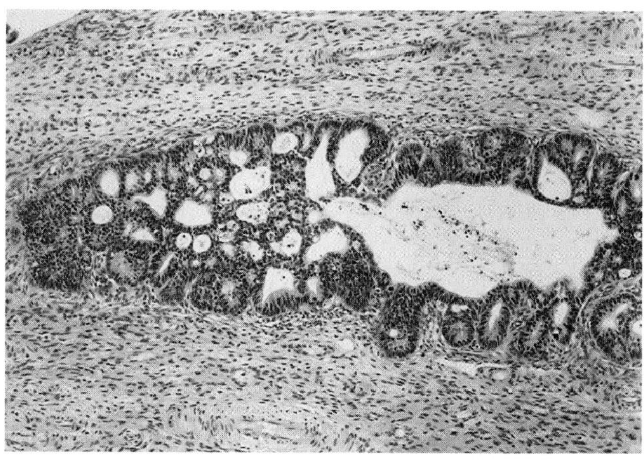

Fig. 11.7 As the complexity of the reduplicating glandular structures increases, a 'back-to-back' cribriform pattern develops. It is questionable whether this should be regarded as CGIN or as invasive adenocarcinoma.

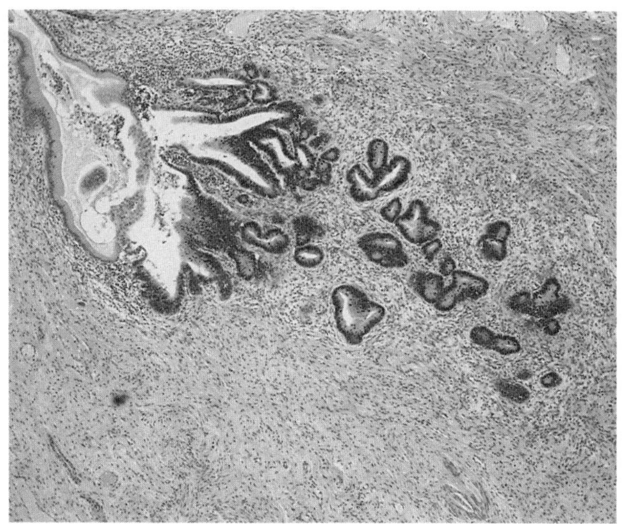

Fig. 11.8 High-grade CGIN, with early invasion. Although a management-related category or microinvasive cervical adenocarcinoma is not recognized, very early stromal invasion is seen. There is little disturbance of the architectural pattern, but a stromal response, with some clearing and an increase in lymphocytes, can be seen. This example illustrates that a well-differentiated adenocarcinoma invades by producing well-formed, new glandular structures.

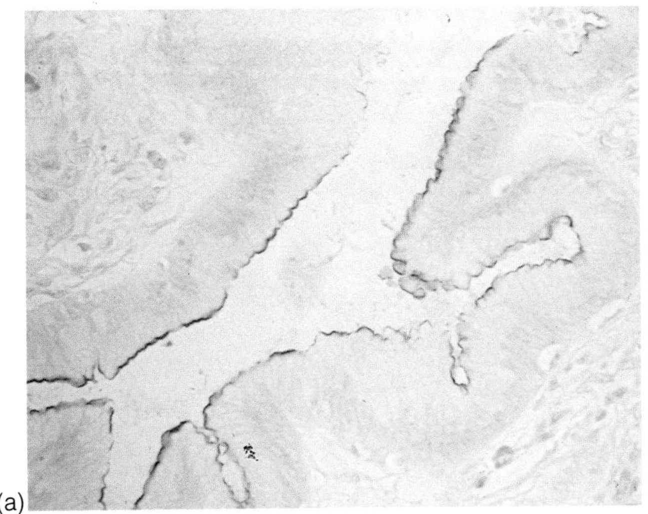
(a)

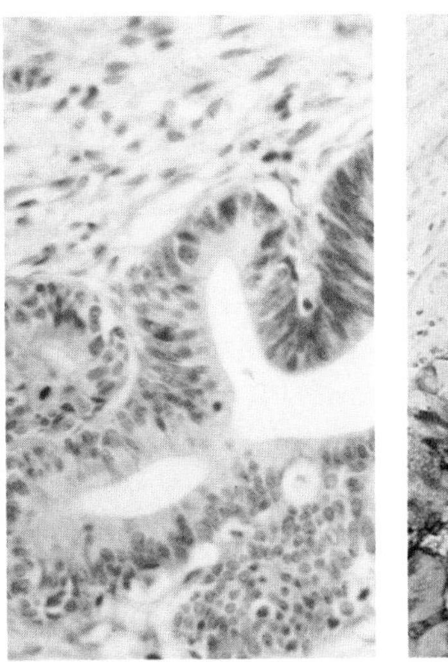
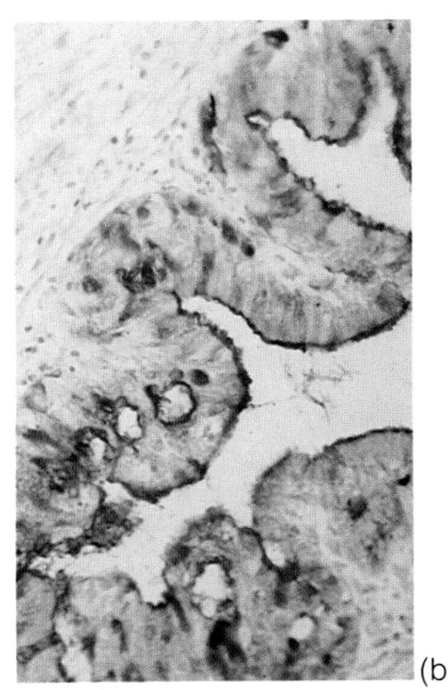
(b)

Fig. 11.9 HMFG1 expression. (a) Normal cervical columnar epithelium (cuticular expression only). **(b)** Low-grade CGIN (cuticular and cytoplasmic expression) on the right, with H&E section for morphology on the left Immunoperoxidase staining; reaction product is brown. Courtesy of Professor Michael Wells, Leeds.

Distribution of glandular intraepithelial neoplasia

In theory, glandular abnormalities may affect any part or all of the endocervical glandular field of the cervix. However, in practice, most examples of CGIN are found adjacent to the squamocolumnar junction, affecting both the surface epithelium and the superficial gland crypts. Very few examples have been described in which only deep crypts are involved; their rarity may, of course, be due to the fact that they cannot be recognized until a clinical carcinoma develops. Skip lesions are only rarely found.

Glandular and squamous intraepithelial abnormalities: association

As many as 50% of reported cases of high-grade CGIN have been associated with coexistent squamous cervical intraepithelial neoplasia, which raises interesting questions regarding the aetiology and histogenesis of both conditions. However, practical considerations are also posed by this association. Most importantly, a woman may harbour squamous CIN together with CGIN, but there is a chance that only the squamous abnormality will be recognized by cytology and colposcopy.

Failure to diagnose a glandular abnormality may possibly affect the eventual outcome if conservative treatment is designed solely for the intraepithelial neoplasia. With an increase in the cases of CGIN being diagnosed, this is a strong argument for using excisional rather than destructive procedures in treating cervical intraepithelial neoplasia.

In situ and invasive adenocarcinomas: relationship

The way in which CGIN is regarded depends upon whether it is genuinely a premalignant state. Cases of progression of an adenocarcinoma from *in situ* to invasive have been described. The shortest progression time documented lies in the region of three to seven years, but a period as long as 14 years has been reported. Another less strongly supportive observation is that the average age at diagnosis is around 15–18 years, lower than the average for adenocarcinoma.

There is one small study of women with adenocarcinoma where antecedent cervical cytology smears were available for further scrutiny. In six out of 13 cases, atypical glandular cells were evidently being exfoliated over an interval of two to eight years before the adenocarcinoma became obvious. It seems unlikely that a covert adenocarcinoma would have remained asymptomatic for so long, which implies that it was preceded by a non-invasive precursor yielding the atypical cells. Strong evidence supporting a progression from *in situ* to invasive adenocarcinoma is the finding of the former at the periphery of an invasive adenocarcinoma, and also the earlier stage of a field of predominantly *in situ* adenocarcinoma with unjustifiable invasion.

Finally, in support of CGIN being a precursor of adenocarcinoma, there are some recent studies of human milk fat globulin (HMFG1; Fig. 11.9) and *c-myc* oncogene expression and amplification (Fig. 11.10) in the cancer and putative precursors. The presence and pattern of expression were similar, suggesting a relationship.

INVASIVE ADENOCARCINOMA

Various histological patterns may be seen in invasive adenocarcinoma of the cervix (see Table 11.1). These patterns are not mutually exclusive, and some tumours may have diverse histological appearances in different parts of the cervix.

Endocervical cell type

This is the most common type of cervical tumour, accounting for up to 90% in some series. The glands are of variable sizes and shapes, showing budding and branching. The epithelium generally resembles normal endocervical epithelium (Fig. 11.11).

Adenoma malignum

The terms 'adenoma malignum' and 'minimal deviation adenocarcinoma' have been used to describe a carcinoma in which the architectural pattern is particularly well differentiated. Moreover, there is virtually no atypia of the epithelial cells, which show normal polarity and very little mitotic activity (Fig. 11.12). Histological features do not reflect the biological behaviour of these tumours, and prognosis is poor.

Mucinous and papillary tumours

These tumours have the appearances that their names imply. The mucinous tumour is composed of cells of enteric type, with abundant mucin-rich cytoplasm and basal nuclei. The papillary pattern is rarely seen as a pure variant, and is usually associated with other patterns; it is composed of complex papillary fronds, supported by fibrovascular cores.

Clear cell carcinoma

This carcinoma is morphologically the same as the more common clear cell tumours of the ovary and endometrium, and has been extensively studied because of its development in the daughters of women who were given diethylstilboestrol in pregnancy. It comprises a variety of different patterns: solid, clear cell, tubulocystic and papillary areas, and 'hobnail' epithelium (Figs 11.13 and 11.14). Only about 2% of cervical carcinomas belong to this category.

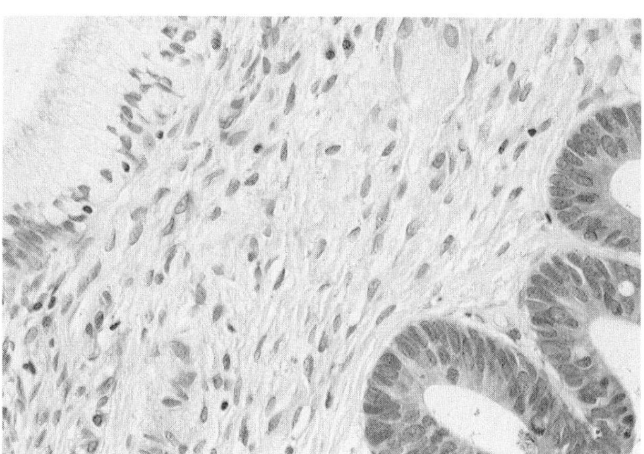

Fig. 11.10 *c-myc* oncogene amplification. Normal columnar epithelium (above left), and high-grade CGIN (below right). Immunoperoxidase staining; reaction product is brown.

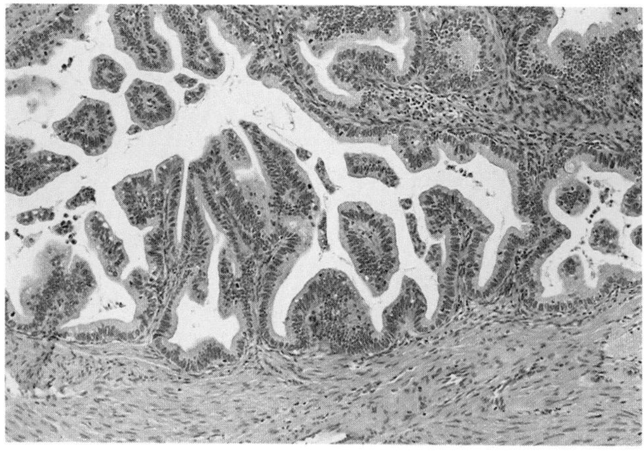

Fig. 11.11 Invasive adenocarcinoma of the cervix: cervical cell type.

Endometrioid carcinoma

This has the same appearances as the common type of endometrial carcinoma. Diagnosis can only be made if the endometrium itself is normal, and is best made on a complete hysterectomy specimen. Also, the distinction is possible only on a fairly well-differentiated tumour.

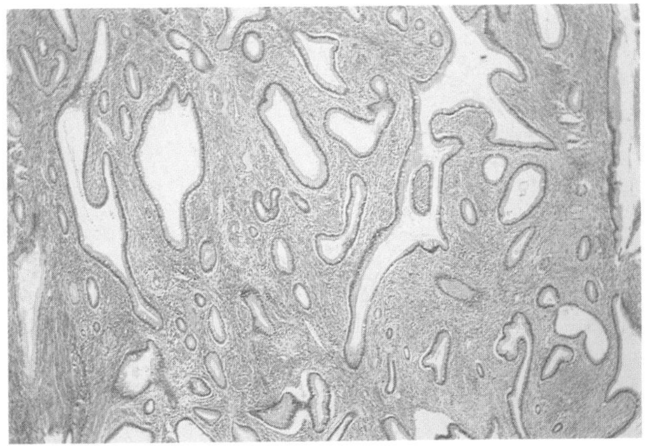

Fig. 11.12 Invasive adenocarcinoma of cervix: minimal deviation type. There is some irregularity of the glandular architecture of the tumour which is deeply invasive. However, the epithelium is indistinguishable from normal epithelium.

CYTOLOGY OF GLANDULAR LESIONS OF THE CERVIX

The cytological assessment of glandular lesions is hampered by a lack of knowledge regarding the significance and natural history of intraepithelial abnormalities, and uncertainty over the earliest stages of invasive disease (see above). The absence of precise histological guidelines in some of these areas also adds to the difficulty of a cytological interpretation.

Adenocarcinoma of the cervix

This is not often recognized by cytologists. The recognition of individual cell changes is difficult. An experienced cytologist will be able to recognize them when the features are pronounced and noticeably at variance with the normal. Furthermore, if changes occur only in the crypts deep to the surface epithelium, the abnormal cells are unlikely to appear in a cervical smear in significant numbers, if at all. When the surface epithelium is involved, the possibility of obtaining the abnormal glandular cells is, of course, improved.

CYTOLOGICAL FEATURES

The cytological features of adenocarcinoma are nuclear pleomorphism, often with hyperchromasia, irregular chromatin distribution, and occasionally prominent nucleoli (Figs 11.15 and 11.16). Sometimes the nuclei may appear very uniform in size and

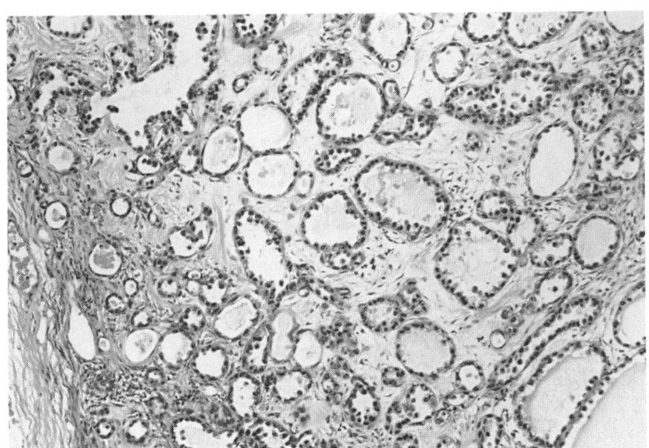

Fig. 11.13 Invasive adenocarcinoma of the cervix: clear cell type. A tubulocystic area is seen, in which 'hobnail' cells are prominent.

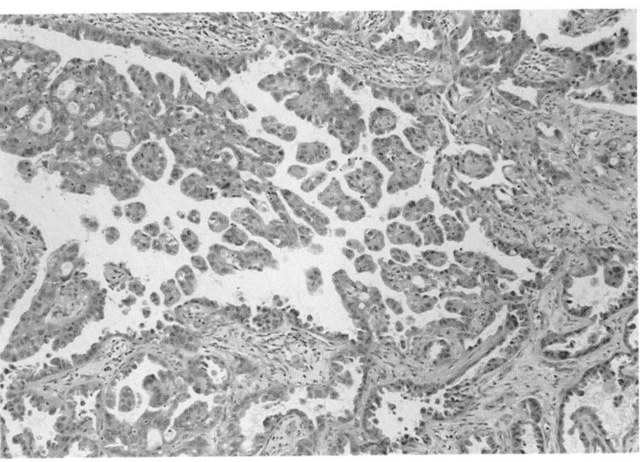

Fig. 11.14 Invasive adenocarcinoma of the cervix: clear cell type. A papillary area is seen.

shape, but one single nucleus may be several times the size of the others (Fig. 11.17).

In a minority of cases, the cells appear as discrete, tightly packed groups with small, densely stained nuclei (Fig. 11.18). The malignant glandular cells most frequently appear in sheets and small groups, sometimes in very large numbers (Fig. 11.19). Occasionally, only discrete single cells or small clusters are seen, known as the 'rosette' formation. Pseudostratification of cells within a group is a common appearance.

The cytoplasm is usually poorly defined, finely vacuolated and granular, and cell borders are indistinct (Fig. 11.20). The cells may have an appreciable amount of cytoplasm or virtually none. Not infrequently, endocervical cells showing the whole spectrum of changes can be observed in a single smear: from cells of normal appearance, through those showing nuclear changes not sufficiently marked to suggest malignancy, to cells showing unequivocal malignant features.

Since a histological distinction between CGIN and invasive adenocarcinoma is made on the architectural features alone, cytologically it is virtually impossible to differentiate between the two. Some authors claim that certain cytological features, namely palisade-like presentation and isolated, often naked, nuclei, showing enlargement without hyperchromasia, can be used to distinguish reliably between *in situ* and invasive adenocarcinoma. However, a diagnosis from

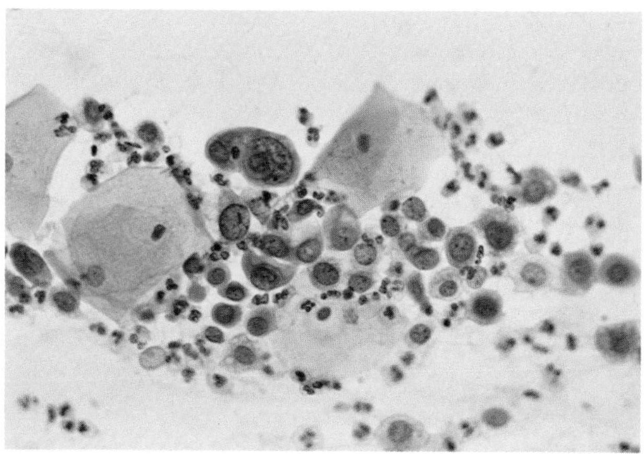

Fig. 11.15 Adenocarcinoma. Cells are showing marked pleomorphism, with obvious nuclear hyperchromasia. The cytoplasm is indistinct and stains blue.

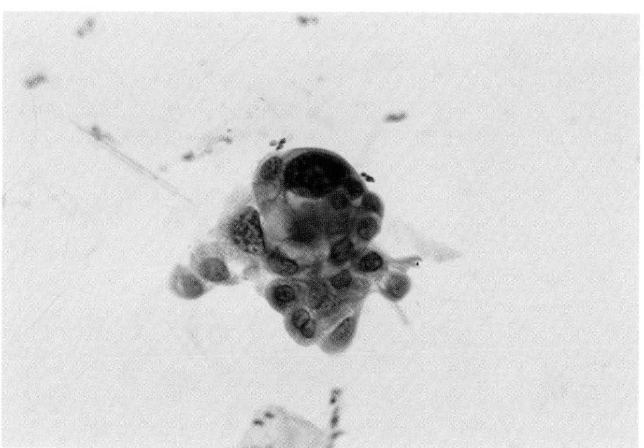

Fig. 11.16 Adenocarcinoma. A small cluster of cells is seen, with obvious pleomorphism and occasional prominent nucleoli. One or two cells retain a distinct columnar shape.

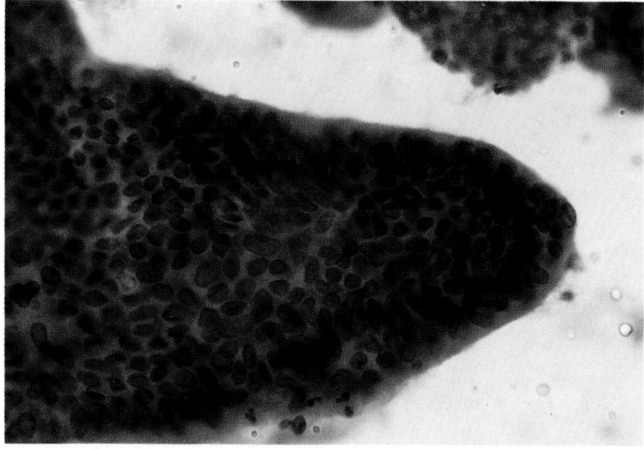

Fig. 11.17 Adenocarcinoma. A tightly packed sheet of cells, with nuclei of much the same shape and intensity of staining, but one or two nuclei in the centre show marked enlargement. The chromatin pattern is grossly abnormal.

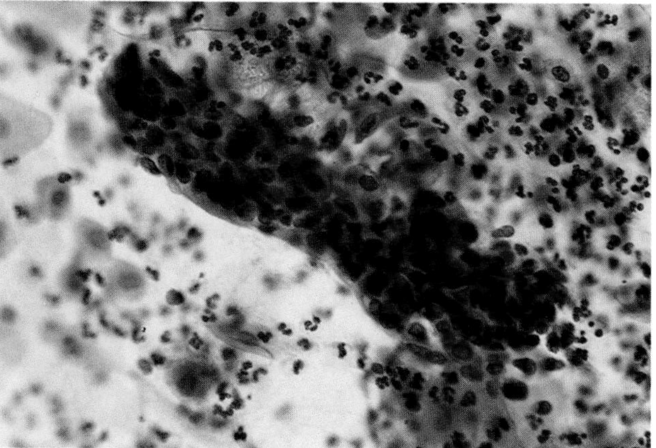

Fig. 11.18 Adenocarcinoma. In this example, a few well-defined groups of malignant cells are seen. Nuclei are small and darkly stained, without obvious pleomorphism, but with pseudostratification.

the appearances in a cervical smear should initially be regarded as suggesting an invasive lesion, and an appropriate diagnostic procedure, usually a cone biopsy, should be undertaken. On rare occasions, the cytological features may be sufficiently obvious to suggest that the malignant cells arise from a mucinous, papillary or endometrioid subtype. However, it is generally not possible to make such distinctions, except perhaps in the case of the clear cell variant which can be recognized cytologically and thus differentiated. This is characterized by a clear zone in the cytoplasm surrounding the nucleus (Fig. 11.21), and by the nucleus containing a prominent nucleolus (Fig. 11.22).

Lesser degrees of glandular abnormality

It is very difficult to recognize cytologically the lesser degree of glandular abnormality, i.e. low-grade CGIN. This needs to be distinguished from high-grade CGIN, as well as from variants of the normal state. The cytological features of this group are generally the same as those described above for adenocarcinoma, but changes are much less marked.

With cytology, it is often possible to recognize and differentiate the minor degrees of glandular atypia; for instance, those associated with intrauterine contraceptive devices (Fig. 11.23) or inflammation

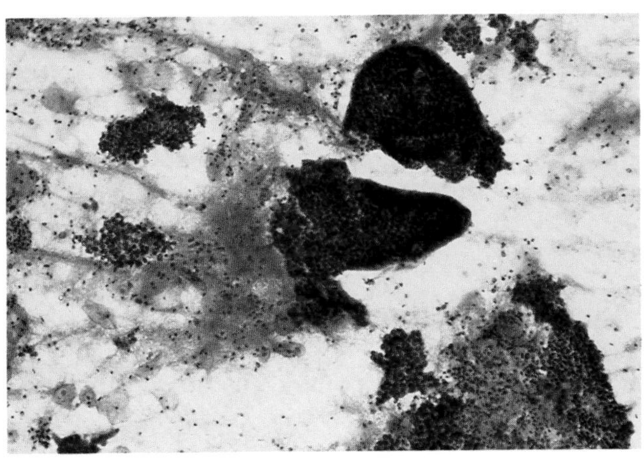

Fig. 11.19 Adenocarcinoma. In this example, large, dense papillary fragments of malignant and benign glandular cells are seen.

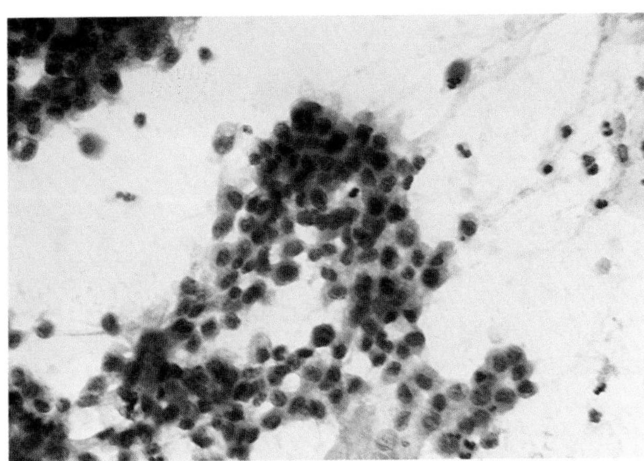

Fig. 11.20 Adenocarcinoma. Small cells with nuclear hyperchromasia and irregular chromatin distribution. The cytoplasm is poorly defined and granular, with indistinct cell borders.

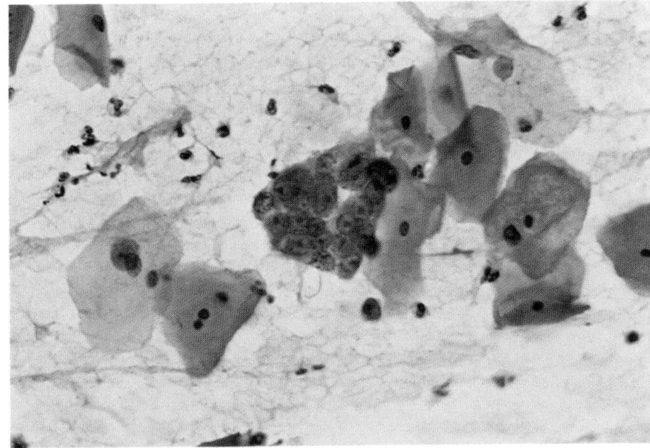

Fig. 11.21 Adenocarcinoma. In the clear cell variant, the cells characteristically appear in small clusters with prominent nucleoli.

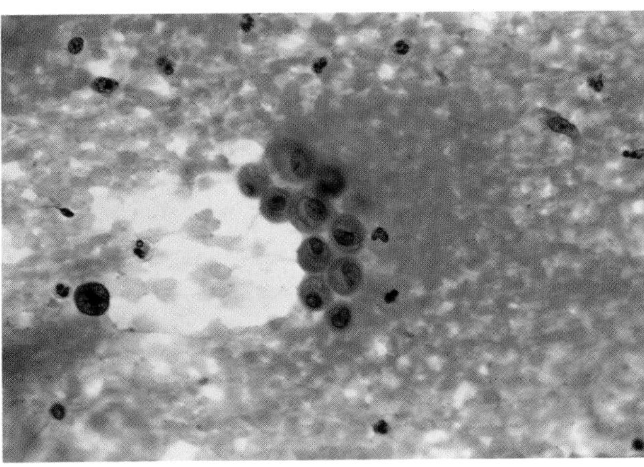

Fig. 11.22 Adenocarcinoma. The clear perinuclear zone, characteristic of clear cell carcinoma, is well shown in this small cluster of cells.

(Fig. 11.24), where the cytoplasm may show eosinophilia and the nuclei are enlarged with some anisonucleosis but minimal chromatin disturbance. Apart from these cases, the role of cytology has yet to be ascertained, as it is in this area that least is known of the significance of abnormalities. A careful study of these minor lesions is needed to establish criteria that can be applied with sufficient confidence in determining management.

The cytology of glandular abnormalities of the cervix remains a poorly defined but challenging area. However, it must be appreciated that, at present, cervical cytology cannot be regarded as a screening method for these changes, although it is fortunate when glandular lesions are detected in the course of screening for squamous abnormalities.

Table 11.4 Differential cytological features of cervical adenocarcinoma and CIN 3

Cervical adenocarcinoma	Cervical intraepithelial neoplasia
1 Indistinct cytoplasm	1 Well-defined cytoplasm
2 Pale-stained nuclei	2 Hyperchromatic nuclei
3 Subtle nuclear changes	3 Gross nuclear changes
4 Small clusters or large sheets	4 Strings of cells

Cytological differential diagnosis

The cytological distinction between severely dyskaryotic squamous cells and cells arising from an adenocarcinoma can be difficult (Fig. 11.25), and on occasions impossible. The main differences are listed in Table 11.4.

Endometrial adenocarcinoma can also be confused with endocervical adenocarcinoma. However, a distinction is often possible as the cells from an endometrial adenocarcinoma tend to be smaller and more densely stained, with a more coarsely clumped chromatin and less cytoplasm than is seen in an endocervical adenocarcinoma (Fig. 11.26). Reference to the patient's age and clinical data may also prove helpful (Table 11.5).

Histologically, microglandular hyperplasia is a recognized entity, but the distinguishing cytological features remain elusive (see Chapter 18).

DIFFERENTIAL DIAGNOSIS OF GLANDULAR LESIONS

A number of glandular 'deviations' may be found in the cervix, and these are shown in Table 11.6. It is

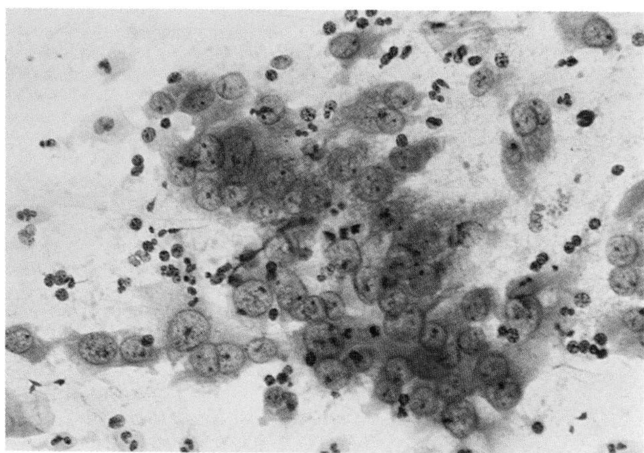

Fig. 11.23 Atypical glandular cells associated with intrauterine contraceptive device. This is nuclear enlargement, with prominent nucleoli and variation in nuclear size. However, the chromatin is regular in distribution and finely granular.

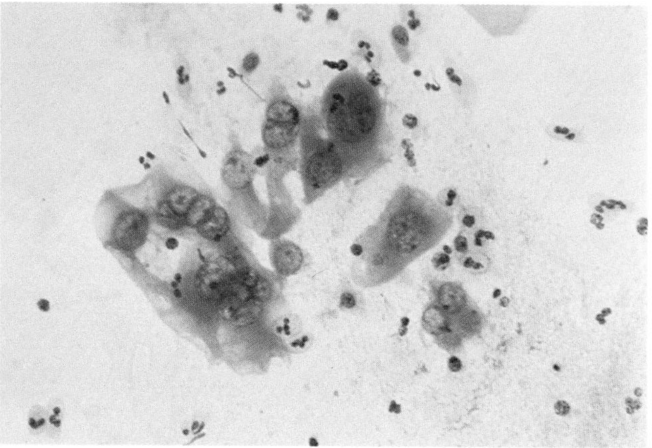

Fig. 11.24 Atypical glandular cells. These are showing binucleation and nuclear enlargement, with prominent nucleoli. There is some eosinophilia and thickening of the cytoplasm, probably reflecting inflammatory changes of little significance.

important that histopathologists, cytologists and colposcopists are aware of these patterns and do not mistake them for malignant change, either intra-epithelial or invasive.

Müllerian 'metaplasias'

The epithelium of the female genital tract, which lines the fallopian tubes, endometrium, endocervix and ectocervix, is derived embryologically from the müllerian (paramesonephric) duct.

Although the typical epithelium of each site is characteristic of that site, apparently inappropriate müllerian epithelium may be found in any position within the tract. Thus, although cervical epithelium is predominantly composed of tall, columnar, mucin-secreting cells with basal nuclei (typical endocervical epithelium), occasional glands, or groups of glands, lined by epithelium of the ciliated (tubal) or endometrial type may be found.

Similarly, ciliated cells may be seen within the fallopian tubes. These variants of müllerian epithelium should not be considered abnormal, or even strictly metaplastic, as they represent only a slightly inappropriate müllerian differentiation.

Examples of ciliated and endometrial epithelium in the endocervix are shown in Figs 11.27–11.30. Both epithelial types run a risk of being misinterpreted as CGIN because of the different arrangement of nuclei within the cells and the overall darker appearance of

Table 11.5 Distinguishing cytological features between endometrial adenocarcinoma and cervical adenocarcinoma

Endometrial	Endocervical
1 Small clusters	1 Large clusters of sheets
2 Little cytoplasm	2 Larger cells
3 Darkly stained, coarse chromatin	3 Less coarsely clumped chromatin
4 Occasional cytoplasmic vacuoles	4 Rarely vacuolated cytoplasm
5 Blood and debris cytoplasm	5 Occasional giant nuclei

Table 11.6 Cervical glandular 'deviations'

Müllerian metaplasias
- Ciliated cell (tubal)
- Endometrial

Inflammatory changes
Tunnel clusters
Microglandular endocervical hyperplasia
Arias-Stella change
Mesonephric remnants

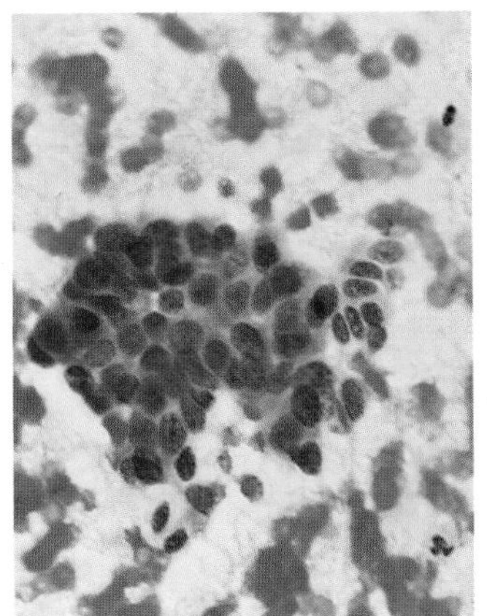
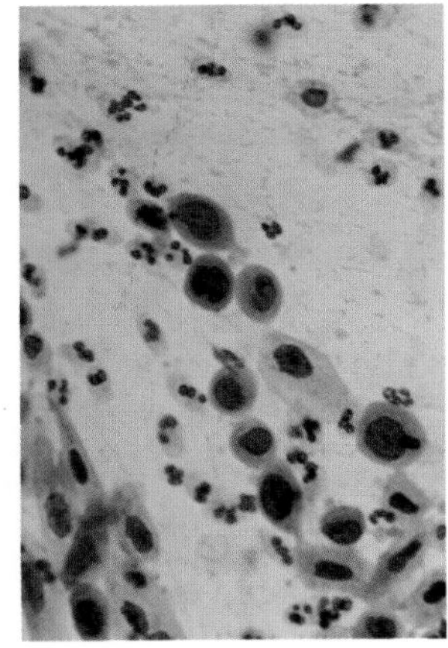

Fig. 11.25 Adenocarcinoma and CIN 3. This illustrates the important differences in shape, size and staining quality between squamous (right) and cervical glandular (left) cells. See also Table 11.4.

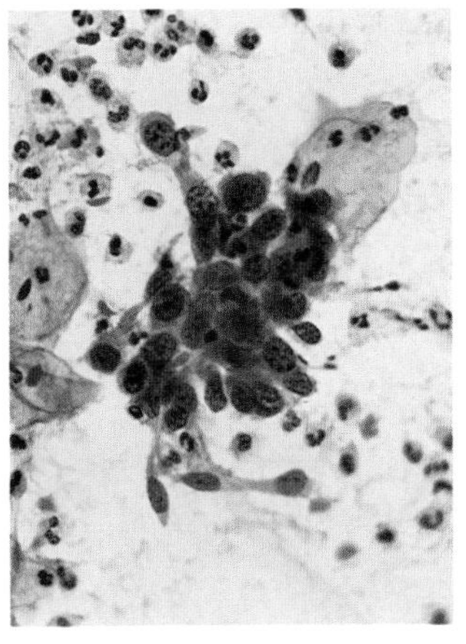
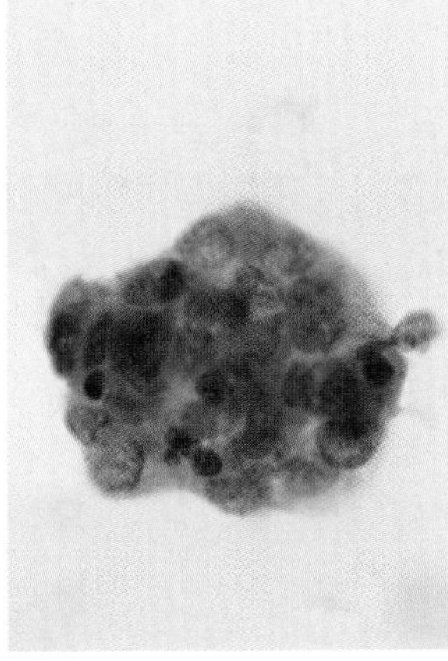

Fig. 11.26 Cervical and endometrial adenocarcinomas. The cell group on the left demonstrates the small, tightly clustered and densely stained endometrial cells associated with endometrial adenocarcinoma. This is in contrast to the larger, less closely associated but obviously glandular-shaped cells of endocervical adenocarcinoma (right).

the epithelium compared with the normal, mucin-secreting endocervical epithelium.

Mitotic activity is not seen in the ciliated epithelium, but it may be found in the endometrial type.

Inflammatory changes

In the presence of severe inflammation in the cervix, the glandular epithelium may show some nuclear changes; in particular, slight nuclear enlargement and pleomorphism (Figs 11.31 and 11.32). These changes may pose serious problems in the distinction from genuine atypia. The changes are usually mild, with no reduction of cytoplasm or mitotic activity.

Tunnel clusters

This histological pattern is common (Figs 11.33 and 11.34). The apparent proliferation of glandular elements, combined with dilatation, gives an appearance that may be confused with hyperplasia or even neoplasia. However, the condition is most probably the result of blockage of the outlet of crypts, and is of no significance; the crypts are generally lined by flattened, inactive epithelium.

Microglandular endocervical hyperplasia

This is a common proliferative state of endocervical epithelium usually associated with pregnancy or

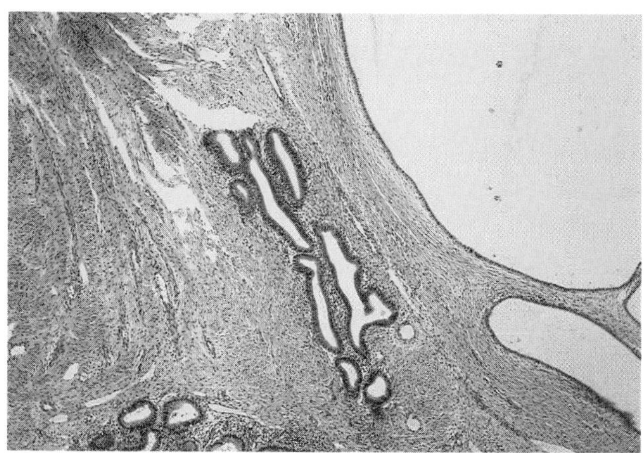

Fig. 11.27 Ciliated cell metaplasia. This usually affects a small group of glands, which appear dark.

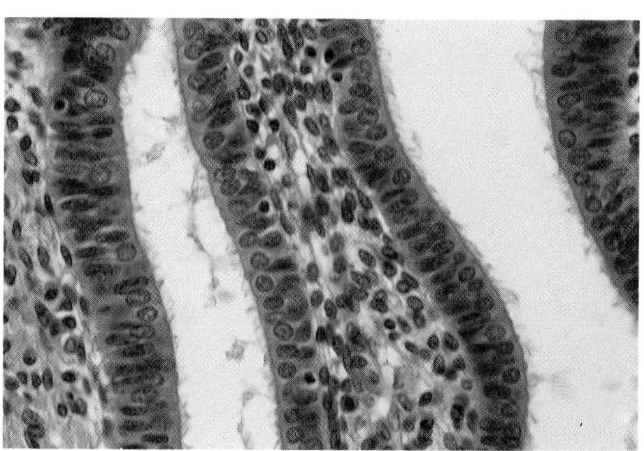

Fig. 11.28 Ciliated cell metaplasia. The benign nature of ciliated cells is apparent at high magnification. The rather haphazard policy of the nuclei may initially cause confusion with CGIN.

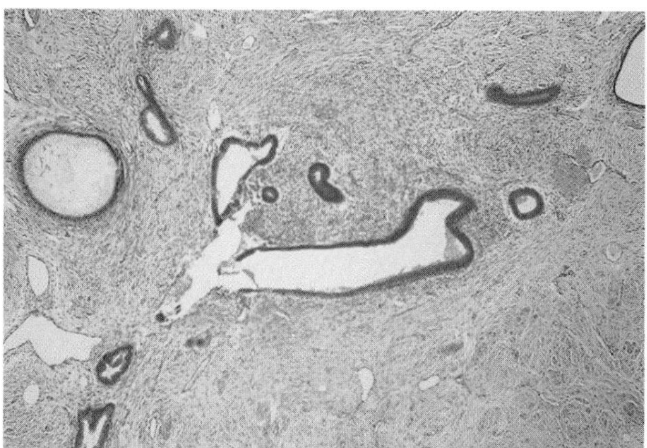

Fig. 11.29 Endometrial 'metaplasia'.

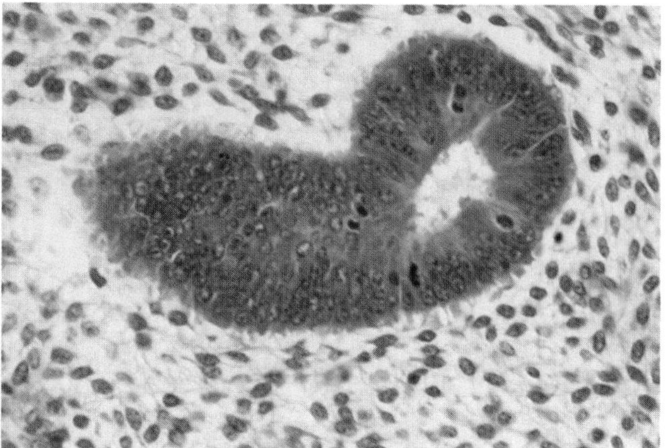

Fig. 11.30 Endometrial 'metaplasia'. The presence of mitotic figures and haphazard polarity of the cells sometimes makes difficult the distinction from CGIN.

progestogen administration. It will be described in detail in Chapter 18.

Arias-Stella change

This is another pregnancy-related phenomenon, and will be described in Chapter 19.

Mesonephric remnants

The remnants of the vestigial mesonephric (wolffian) duct enter the lateral part of the cervix approximately at the level of the internal cervical os. They pass through the cervical mesenchyme and into the vaginal wall, continuing as Gartner's ducts. These may be identified deep within the fibromuscular tissue of the cervix as rather nondescript collections of tubules lined by 'bland' cuboidal cells (Figs 11.35 and 11.36).

On occasion, these mesonephric remnants may become particularly prominent and hyperplastic (Fig. 11.37). It is important that they are recognized as such and not mistaken for malignancy. It is thought that only very rarely do genuine mesonephric carcinomas arise from these structures in the cervix.

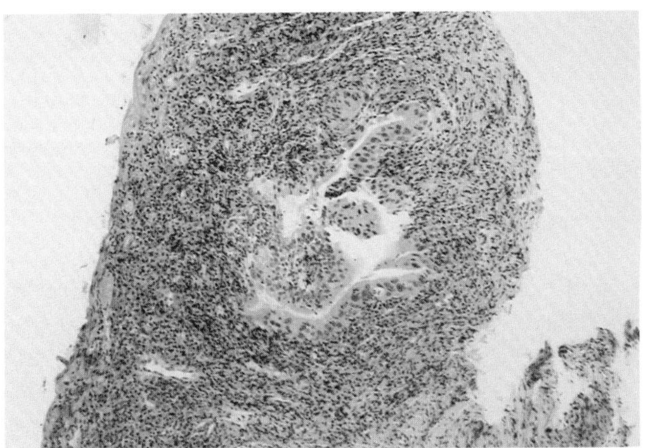

Fig. 11.31 Inflammatory change. An irregular gland is surrounded by stroma which is densely infiltrated by polymorphs and plasma cells.

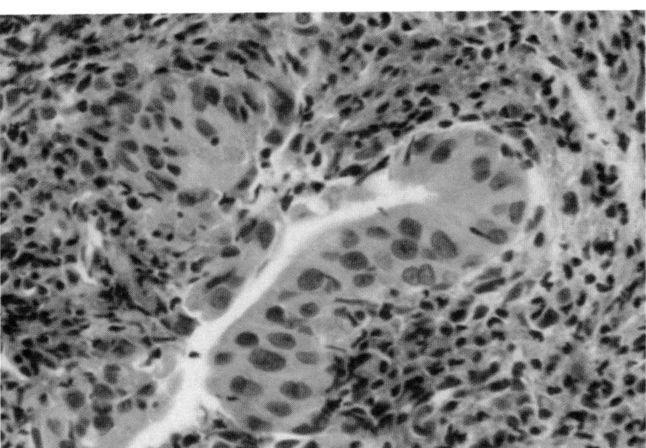

Fig. 11.32 Inflammatory change. The nuclei are enlarged but lack detail. Abundant eosinophilic cytoplasm is present. Mitotic figures are not seen.

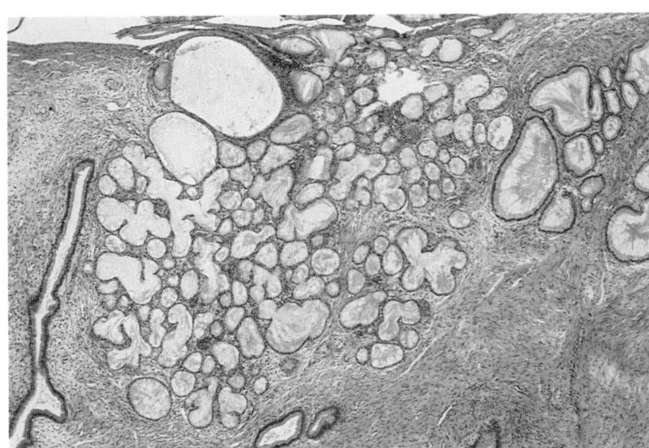

Fig. 11.33 Tunnel clusters. Multiple reduplication of dilated glands is the hallmark of this condition.

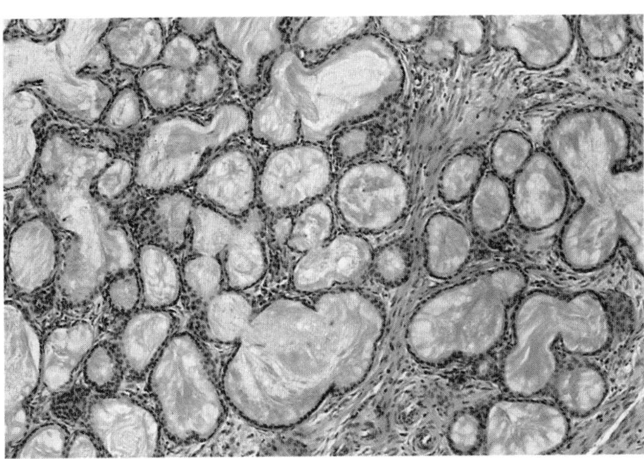

Fig. 11.34 Tunnel clusters. The glands are lined by flattened, inactive epithelium, and contain mucin.

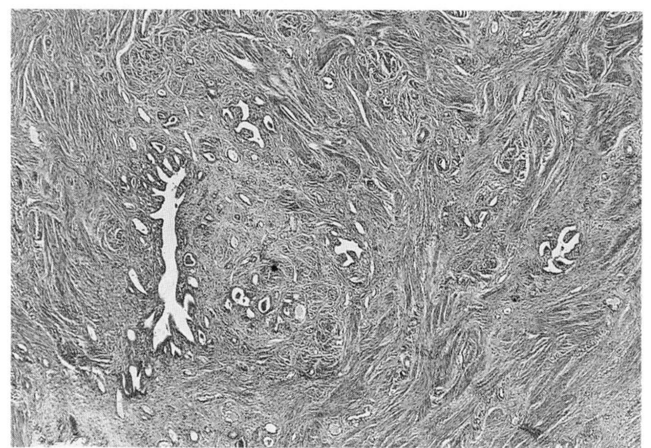

Fig. 11.35 Mesonephric remnants. At low magnification, these are seen as scattered collections of rounded and slightly irregular tubules. Often, as in this example, the main duct is seen as a larger, slit-like space.

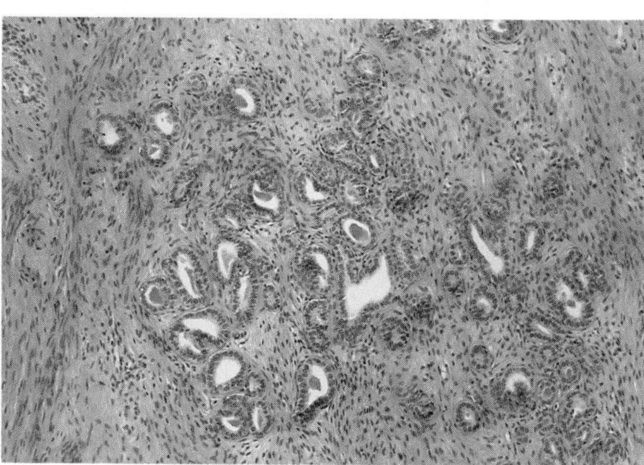

Fig. 11.36 Mesonephric remnants. The round or oval spaces are lined by benign, cuboidal epithelium.

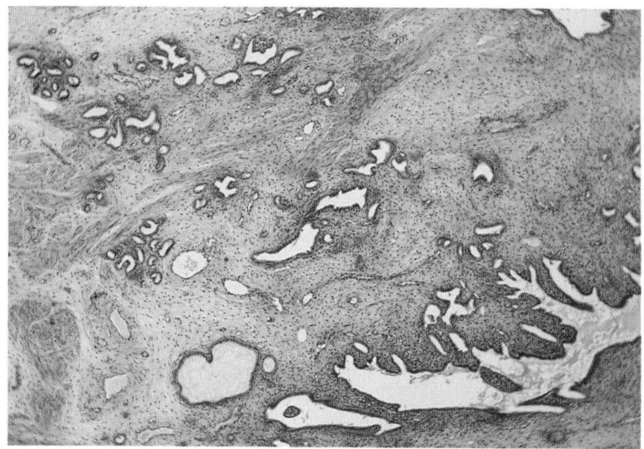

Fig. 11.37 Hyperplasia of mesonephric remnants. Occasionally, these remnants occupy a large area within the cervical fibromuscular stroma.

COLPOSCOPIC ASSESSMENT

Cervical glandular intraepithelial neoplasia

This lesion received increasing attention during the 1980s. Cervical glandular intraepithelial neoplasia has no typical colposcopic appearance. However, some colposcopists have noted that the tips of columnar epithelial villi can appear acetowhite, which may be the first sign, but this is not a constant feature. It has also been observed that CGIN may have a flat and densely acetowhite surface that is remarkably fragile and strips as soon as it is touched during the examination.

Adenocarcinoma

As with invasive squamous carcinoma, this lesion is characterized by atypical vessels, irregularity of the surface, and areas suggestive of ulceration. However, the colposcopist will sometimes also find areas with enlarged columnar villi adherent to each other, giving an appearance somewhat similar to that seen in a papillomavirus-induced exophytic papilloma. A number of such areas on the cervix will give it a 'cauliflower' appearance, and the papillae or villi will be very marked (Figs 11.38–11.40).

Adenosquamous carcinoma

A combined adenosquamous lesion is currently being diagnosed more frequently than it has been in the past, primarily because of pathologists' awareness that squamous invasive carcinoma often has an adenocarcinoma component that can be recognized with the use of appropriate stains. The combined lesion has no characteristic colposcopic appearances.

MANAGEMENT OF GLANDULAR INTRAEPITHELIAL NEOPLASIA

This topic is addressed in Chapter 13.

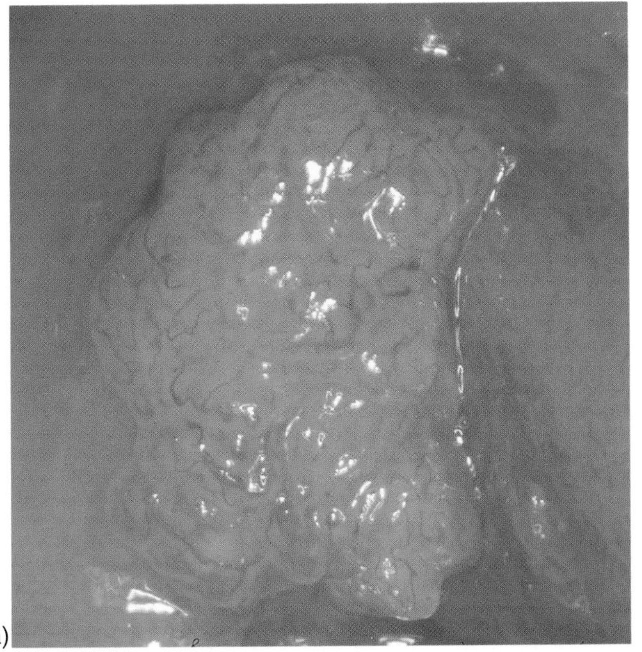

(a)

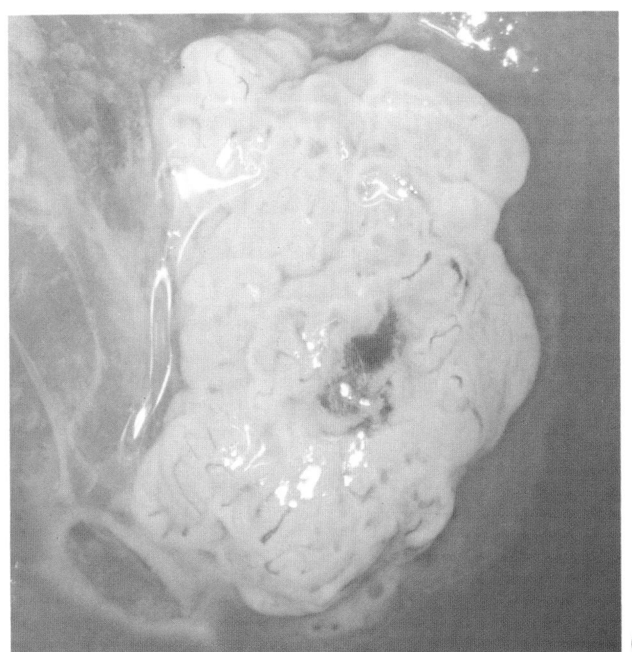

(b)

Fig. 11.38 Adenocarcinoma before (a) and after (b) application of acetic acid. The lesion is relatively small. It is markedly raised and shows atypical vessels. Such a lesion demands a cone biopsy, or at the very least, an excisional biopsy. Squamous carcinoma may exhibit the same features.

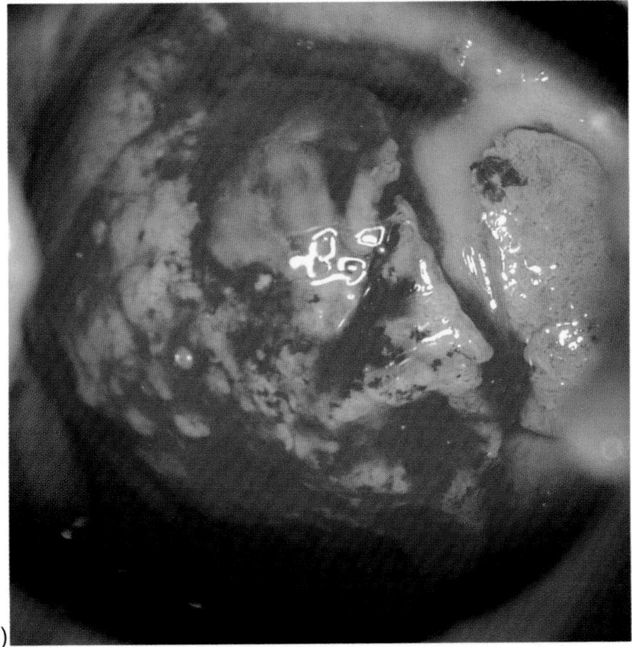

(a)

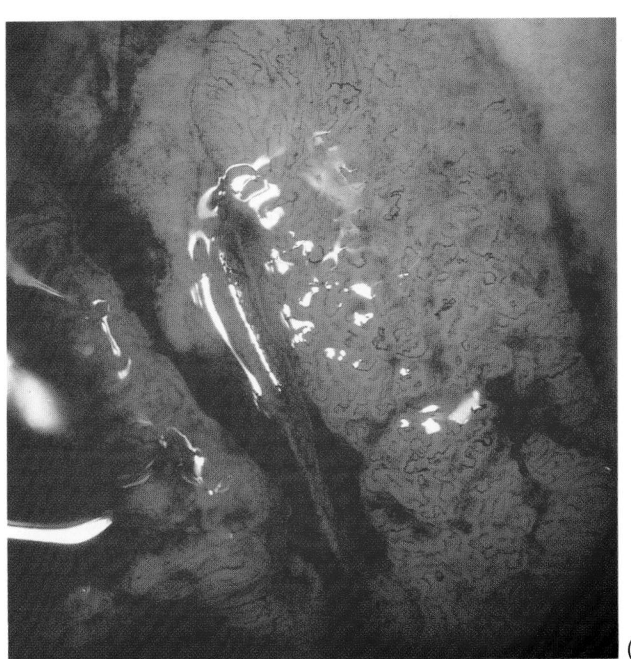

(b)

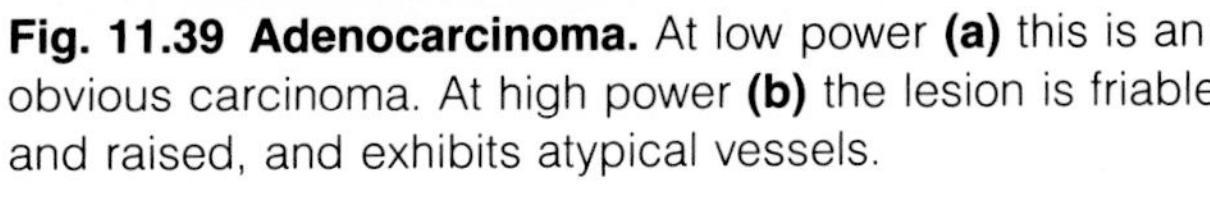

Fig. 11.39 Adenocarcinoma. At low power **(a)** this is an obvious carcinoma. At high power **(b)** the lesion is friable and raised, and exhibits atypical vessels.

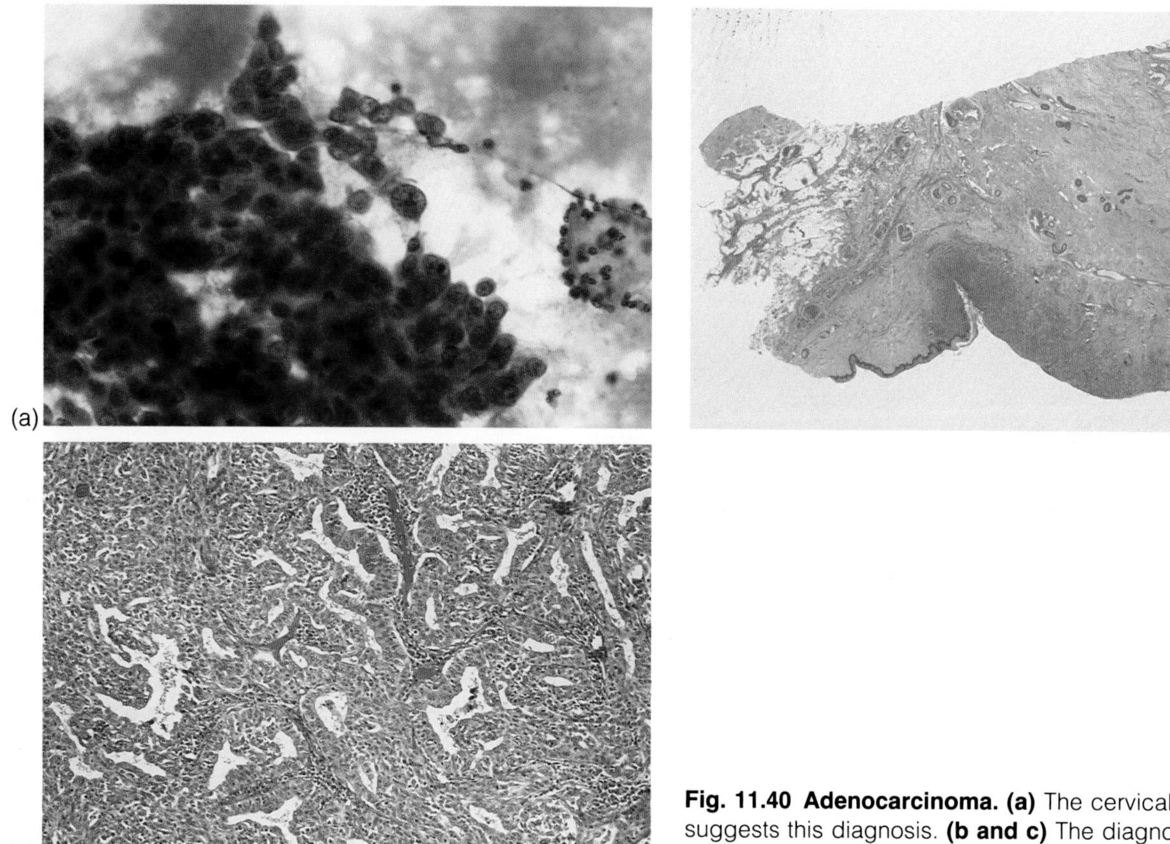

Fig. 11.40 Adenocarcinoma. (a) The cervical cytology suggests this diagnosis. **(b and c)** The diagnosis was confirmed on biopsy.

12. *Inflammatory and infective conditions of the cervix*

CYTOLOGICAL INTRODUCTION

The problems surrounding 'inflammation', perhaps more than any other area of cytology, have given rise to considerable controversy and discussion over recent years. Inflammatory changes in themselves are of little significance. In strictly pathological terms, cells affected by inflammation show cloudy swelling or necrosis as a result of cell damage. These cellular appearances may be accompanied by increased numbers of polymorphonuclear leucocytes or lymphocytes and macrophages, depending on the duration of the condition, and are the same whatever the cause of the inflammatory response.

Table 12.1 Causes of inflammatory and degenerative changes of the cervix

Bacteria
Viruses
Trauma
Surgery
Chemical agents
Radiotherapy
Vitamin deficiency (e.g. folate depletion)

Acute inflammation

In smears taken from an acutely inflamed cervix, an inflammatory exudate is seen with debris and sometimes bacteria, together with numerous polymorphonuclear leucocytes. It is important to exclude physiological causes for the increased polymorphonuclear leucocytes; the pre- and postmenstrual phase, cervical ectropion, pregnancy and the oral contraceptive pill will normally produce an increase in the number of polymorphonuclear leucocytes.

Epithelial cells in inflammation may show enlargement and appear 'bloated' due to cloudy swelling (Fig. 12.1) and necrosis, which appears as pyknosis and karyorrhexis (Fig. 12.2).

Often, the staining reaction will be altered and the smear will show excessive eosinophilia. In smears from premenopausal women there may be increased parabasal cells as a result of sloughing of superficial layers. In postmenopausal women there may also be an increase in intermediate and superficial squamous cells, possibly associated with the increased vascularity.

Nuclear enlargement of the endocervical glandular cells may be seen, with prominent multiple chromocentres and occasionally nucleoli, multinucleation and mitotic figures. The distinction between inflammatory changes and glandular intraepithelial neoplasia is difficult (see Chapter 11 for a more detailed discussion).

Chronic inflammation

Chronic cervicitis is associated with healing and repair; regenerative changes in cells are discussed in Chapter 14. Cytologically, the pattern is mixed, showing the same degenerative changes seen in acute inflammation together with the features of regenera-

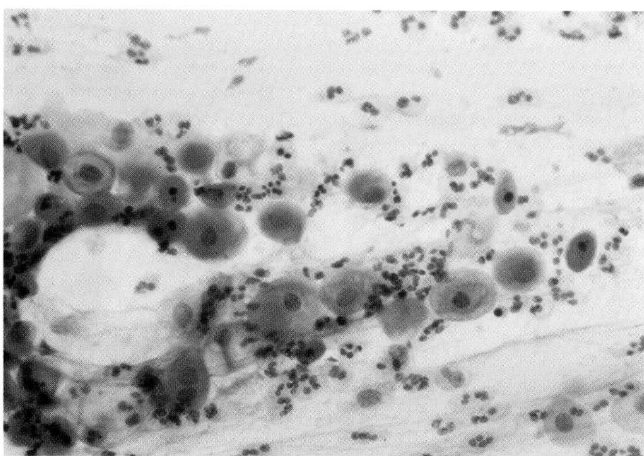

Fig. 12.1 Acute inflammation. Cells are showing cloudy swelling associated with early inflammatory response. The cells appear bloated with eosinophilia.

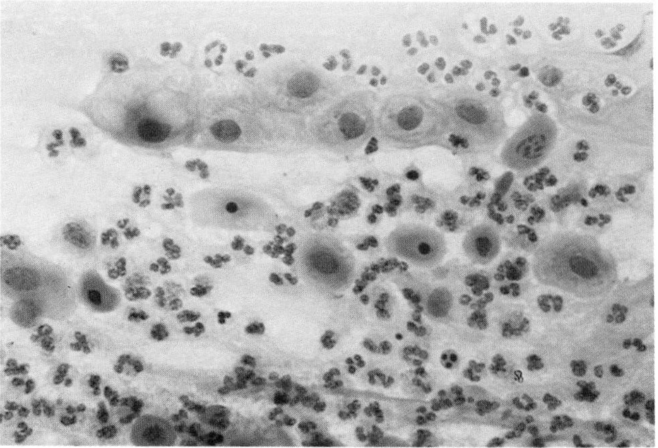

Fig. 12.2 Acute inflammation. Some cells are showing cloudy swelling as in Fig. 12.1. This is pyknosis and karyorrhexis, with cytoplasmic eosinophilia. Polymorphonuclear leucocytes are also present.

tion (Fig. 12.3). Increased numbers of lymphocytes may be seen with polymorphonuclear leucocytes, but the plasma cells that are usually so prominent in the stroma of histological sections are rarely identified in cervical smears. In the cervix, the inflammatory response is most commonly associated with bacterial infections (often a result of the toxins produced, rather than the organisms themselves), or viral infections. However, other situations may give rise to degenerative and inflammatory changes in the cells, and it is important for cytologists to be aware of them (Table 12.1).

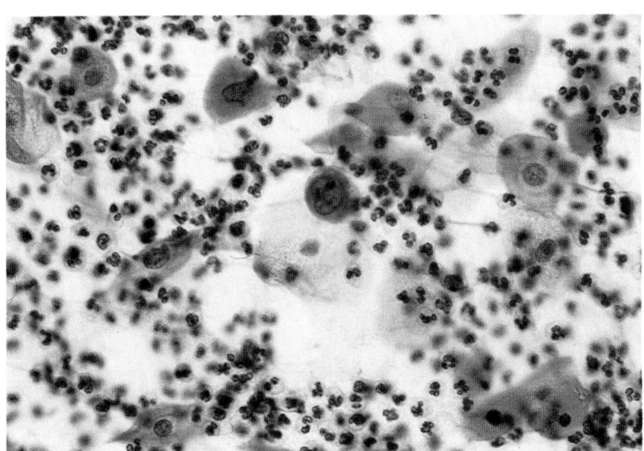

Fig. 12.3 Chronic inflammation. Numerous polymorphonuclear leucocytes are seen, with lymphocytes and degenerative inflammatory changes as in Figs 12.1 and 12.2. The cells in the centre are showing regenerative changes, with enlarged, hyperchromatic nuclei.

HUMAN PAPILLOMAVIRUS

Introduction

Since the mid-1970s, human papillomavirus infection has been proposed as an aetiological agent in cervical neoplasia. This aspect has been fully discussed in Chapter 3, and therefore only the morphological effects of infection with human papillomavirus will be considered here.

The human papillomavirus produces two types of lesion on the cervix: the condyloma acuminatum, and a flat lesion which has been described as a 'flat wart', non-condylomatous cervical papillomavirus infection, or subclinical papillomavirus infection. Colposcopically, the latter is obvious only after application of aqueous acetic acid.

Cytological features

Koilocytic change, a term first used by Koss and Durfee in 1956, is the feature that has been linked most frequently with subclinical papillomavirus infection.

The cytological features associated with human papillomavirus infection are shown in Table 12.2. The koilocyte is generally accepted as being pathognomonic of this infection, but DNA hybridization studies have shown that koilocytes are only identified in 50–70% of these infections.

The koilocyte has an enlarged nucleus which shows an irregular distribution of nuclear chromatin, surrounded by a large, irregularly shaped halo. The margin of the halo shows cytoplasmic condensation

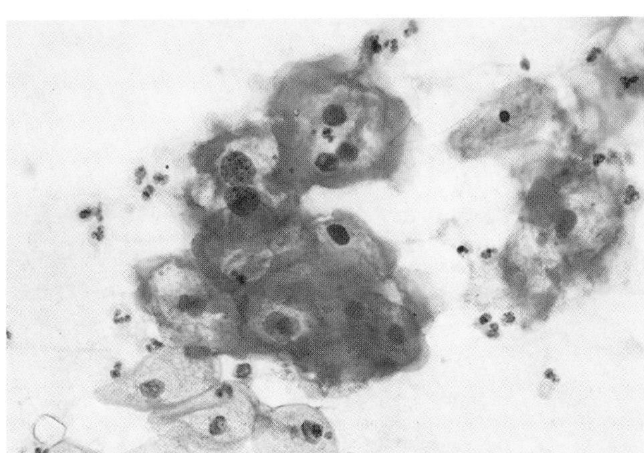

Fig. 12.4 Human papillomavirus infection. A group of koilocytes are showing enlarged nuclei, with minimal chromatin disturbance and prominent perinuclear halos of irregular shapes.

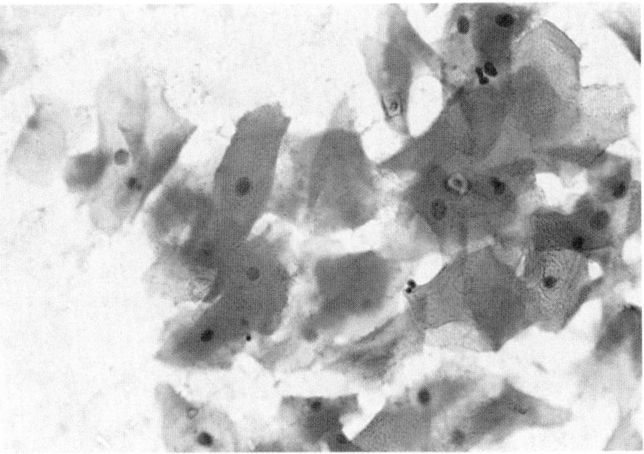

Fig. 12.5 Human papillomavirus infection. Keratinized and anucleate keratinized squamous cells.

and appears more darkly stained, with a well-defined edge (Fig. 12.4).

Keratinized cells, both nucleate and anucleate (Fig. 12.5), are most commonly seen in sheets or plaques with poorly defined cell borders (Fig. 12.6). Although closely associated with human papillomavirus infection, these cells may also be seen in any specific and non-specific inflammatory response.

Multinucleation, most usually binucleation, is frequently seen (Fig. 12.7). Dyskeratosis or individual cell keratinization is another feature (Fig. 12.8); the cells are discrete and often small, with highly keratinized cytoplasm and small, dense nuclei, sometimes showing pyknosis and karyorrhexis.

Overall, the smear may be poorly stained with a 'washed out' appearance (Fig. 12.9), possibly due to acantholysis, and extensive degenerative inflammatory changes. The degree of nuclear aberration may be difficult to assess and differentiate from that of dyskaryotic change. In this instance, the smear should be classified as showing borderline nuclear change. Even so, the interpretation of nuclear changes can give rise to difficulties of over- and underdiagnosis, and the recommended policy of referral for colposcopy after two smears showing borderline change should be adhered to. With careful evaluation and application of criteria, an accurate assessment can be made in most instances; therefore, a distinction between changes associated with human papillomavirus infection and those of cervical intra-

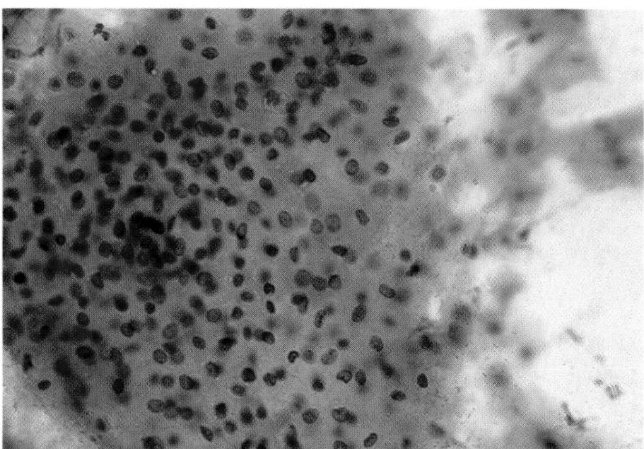

Fig. 12.6 Human papillomavirus infection. Keratinized squamous cells, showing minimal nuclear changes and poorly defined cell borders.

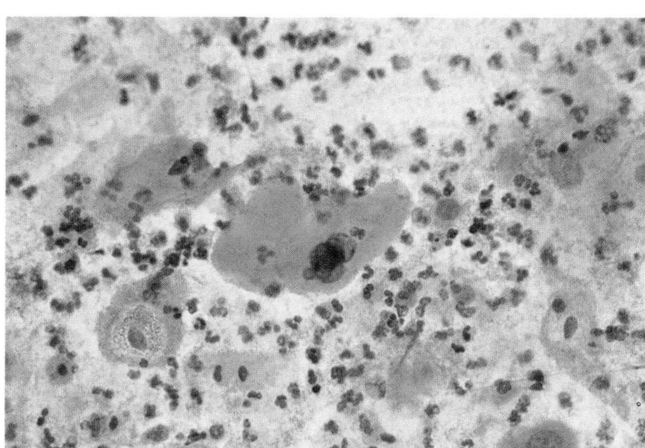

Fig. 12.7 Human papillomavirus infection. A single multinucleated squamous cell is seen, of the type frequently associated with this infection. Note that the nuclei may touch or overlap but without moulding one another, as opposed to herpes simplex virus.

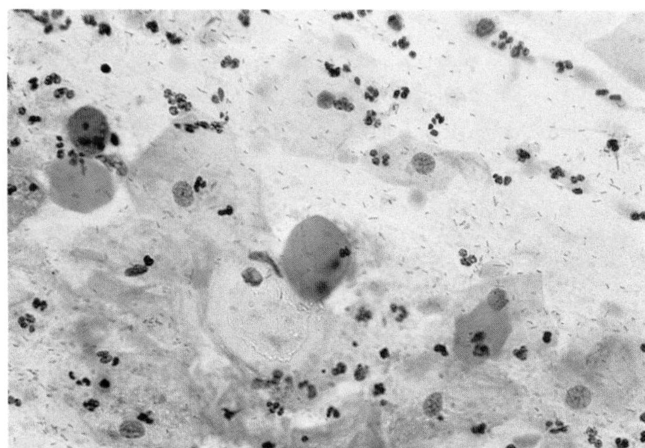

Fig. 12.8 Human papillomavirus infection. Discrete, highly keratinized or dyskeratotic cells, with pyknotic and karyorrhexic nuclei.

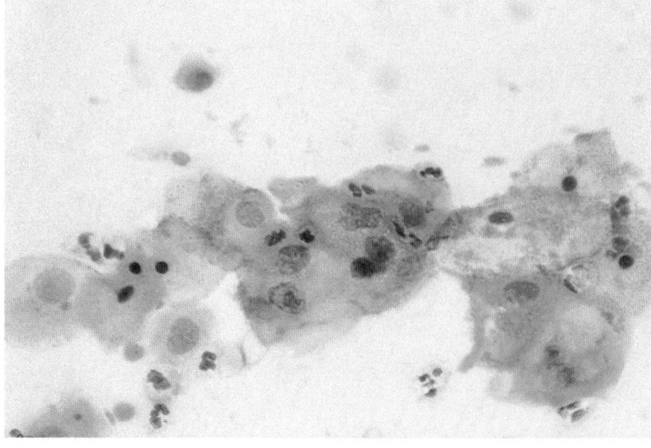

Fig. 12.9 Koilocytes and multinucleated cells, showing an overall 'washed out' appearance.

epithelial neoplasia is possible. It is important to grade a smear in terms of the degree of dyskaryotic change present, and to recommend management accordingly.

Condyloma acuminatum

HISTOLOGY

In the past, condylomata acuminata of the cervix were considered rare. However, in recent years, and particularly with the increasing use of colposcopy, these lesions have been frequently seen but are still not regarded as common.

Characteristically, condylomata are multiple, and examination will reveal further, perhaps very small, lesions on the cervix, vagina or vulva. Histological examination shows papillomatosis, acanthosis, parakeratosis and hyperkeratosis (Fig. 12.10). At a higher magnification (Fig. 12.11), koilocytic change is a usual feature, as is individual cell keratinization (dyskeratosis) and multinucleation. Often there is a chronic inflammatory infiltrate in the underlying cervical stroma.

Condylomata are frequently associated with cervical intraepithelial neoplasia, and therefore histological examination should include an assessment of atypia in the lesion itself, as well as in the surrounding epithelium; it is not uncommon for a condyloma to contain cells with sufficient atypia to warrant a diagnosis of CIN 2.

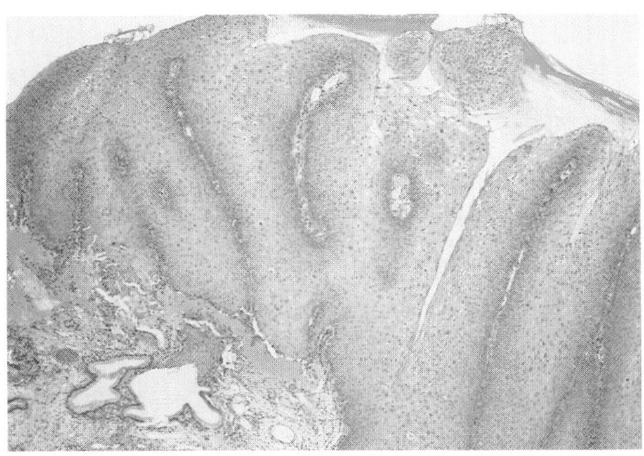

Fig. 12.10 Cervical condyloma acuminatum, affecting the transformation zone. The striking acanthosis and papillomatosis are apparent. Each frond bears a central capillary.

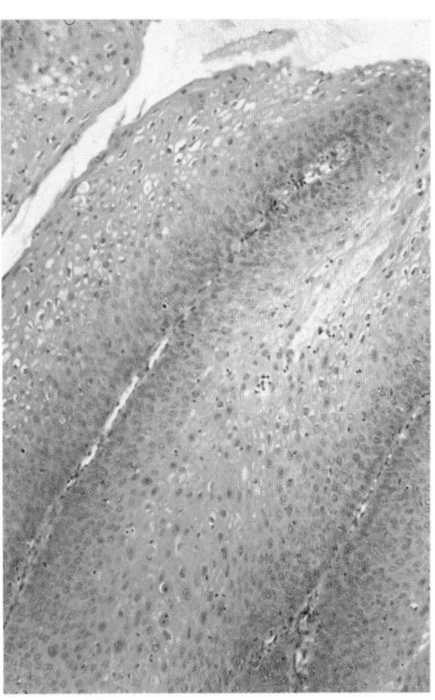

Fig. 12.11 Cervical condyloma acuminatum. Koilocytic change is present in groups of superficial cells; the basal cells in this example show no atypia.

(a) 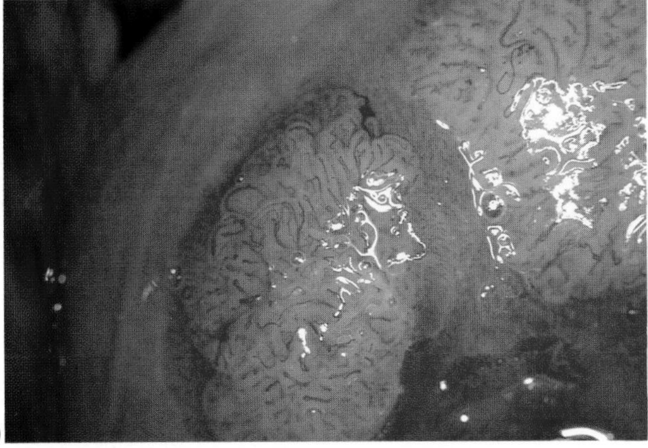

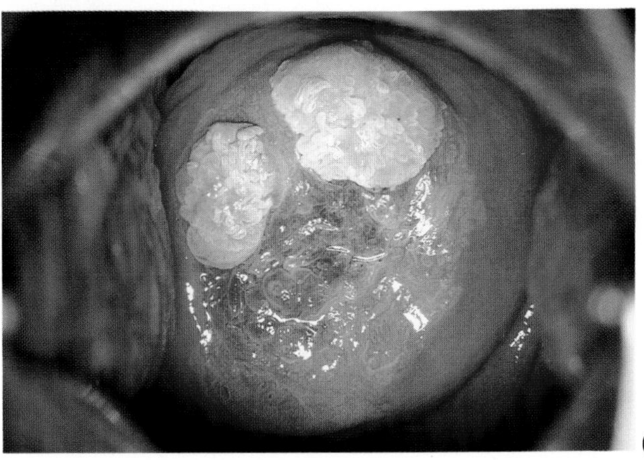 (b)

Fig. 12.12 Cervical condylomata acuminata. (a) Before application of acetic acid. Finger-like projections with a central capillary are seen. **(b)** After application of acetic acid. Pronounced acetowhite change is seen.

COLPOSCOPY

Condylomata are exophytic and, depending on their size, they may be obvious to the naked eye. They usually present as soft, pink or white vascular tumours with multiple, fine, finger-like projections on the surface (Fig. 12.12).

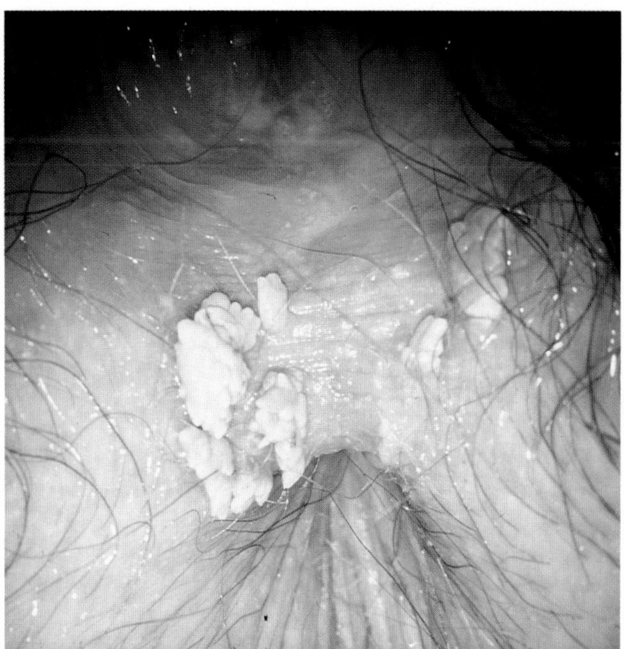

Fig. 12.13 Perianal condylomata acuminata.

Genital human papillomavirus should be viewed as a field change, involving a large area of similarly derived squamous epithelium. As well as the entire length of the female lower genital tract, the epithelium most at risk extends posteriorly to include the perianal, anal and rectal regions (Fig 12.13).

Presentation is not uncommonly multicentric, involving any combination or even all of these sites which must be examined to prevent reinfection from undiagnosed lesions. The vulva is most commonly involved (Fig. 12.14(a)), and exophytic cervical condyloma acuminatum will be seen in 5–10% of such cases (Fig. 12.14(b)). Moreover, women with vulval warts are at increased risk of associated cervical intraepithelial neoplasia: colposcopic differentiation of the effects of human papillomavirus and those of cervical intraepithelial neoplasia at all sites may be difficult (see below). Cervical cytology and colposcopy are, therefore, mandatory in the management of women with warts in the lower genital tract, or indeed in the perianal/rectal region. Because of the sexually transmissible nature of this infection, cytology and colposcopy should, if possible, also be offered to the female partners of men with penile warts.

Under the colposcope, cervical condylomata have a typical appearance, with a vascular papilliferous or frond-like surface, each element of which contains a central capillary (Fig. 12.15). After application of acetic acid, there is blanching of the surface and usually definitive acetowhite change, which may

(a)

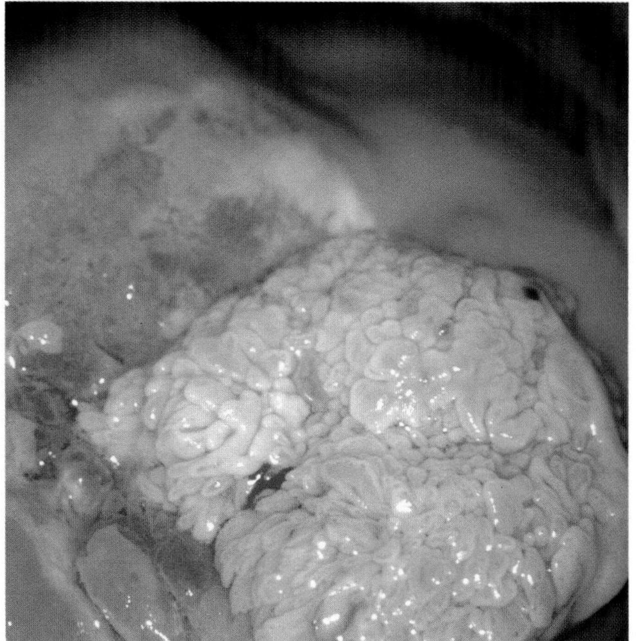

(b)

Fig. 12.14 (a) Vulval warts. (b) Extended colposcopy, showing a large cervical wart and subclinical papillomavirus infection after application of acetic acid.

persist for some time (see Fig. 12.12). The lesion may be single or multiple, and may be located within or outside the transformation zone (Fig. 12.16).

Occasionally, the surface of the condyloma may have a whorled, heaped-up appearance resembling the cerebral cortex, known as *encephaloid* (Fig. 12.17), or the surface of the lesion may be overtly hyperkeratotic (Fig. 12.18). It should be stressed that a histological diagnosis should be obtained in every case. Sometimes, these lesions may be mimicked by a carcinoma (Fig. 12.19) or, rarely, by a verrucous carcinoma (Fig. 12.20).

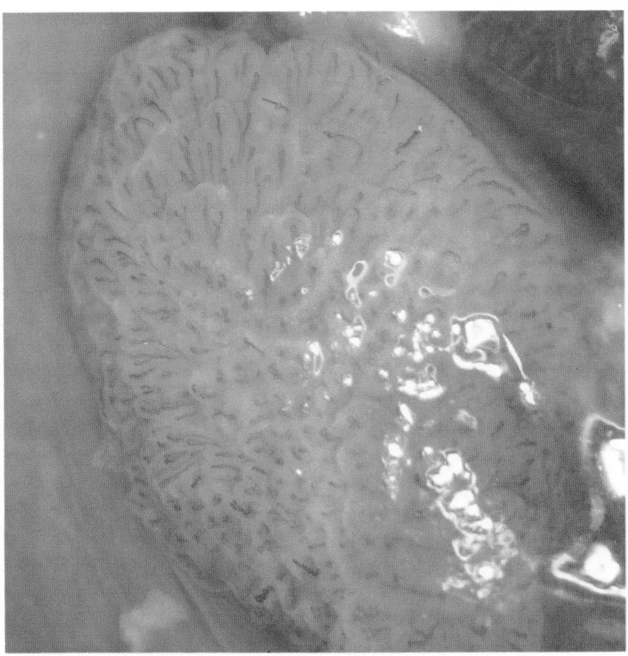

Fig. 12.15 Cervical condyloma. Before application of acetic acid: finger-like projections with central capillary loop are seen.

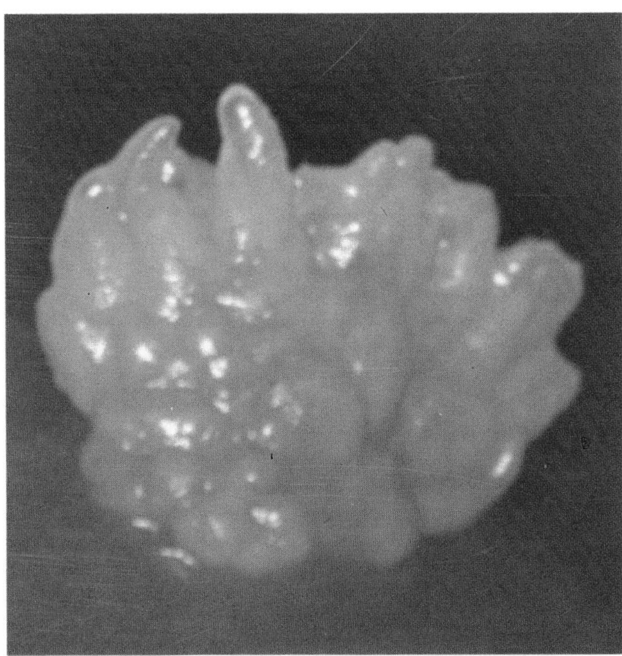

Fig. 12.16 Small, solitary cervical condyloma.

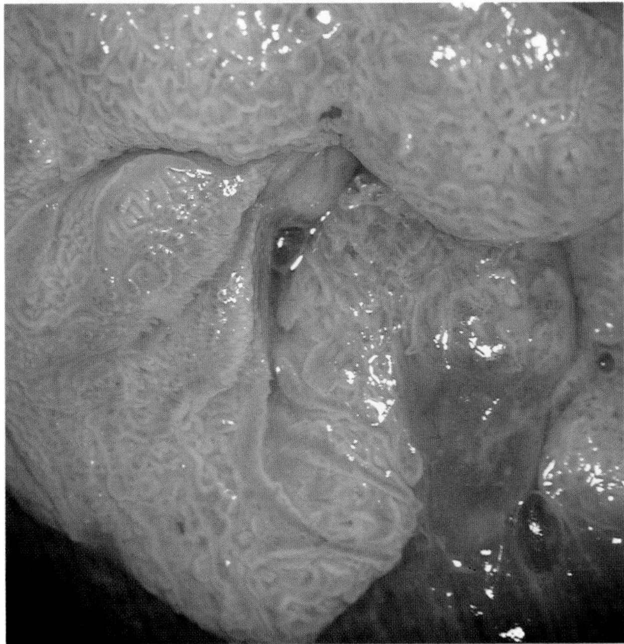

Fig. 12.17 Brain-like texture of a cervical condyloma, of the 'encephaloid' type.

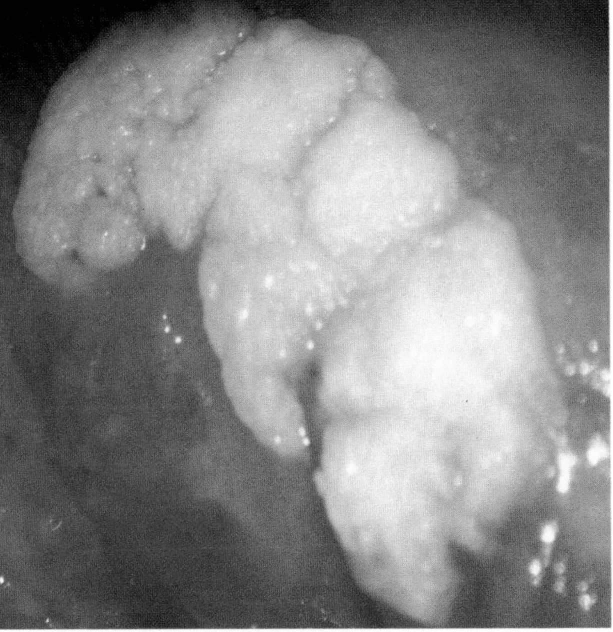

Fig. 12.18 Cervical condyloma, with a dense hyperkeratotic surface. No application of acetic acid.

Subclinical papillomavirus infection

HISTOLOGY

Subclinical papillomavirus infection presents as flat lesions which cannot usually be detected at naked-eye examination. The histological features are listed in Table 12.2, and are illustrated in Figs 12.21–12.23.

The koilocyte is a cell which has a prominent space around the nucleus, with extensive margination of the cytoplasm, giving a sharp edge to the halo. The nuclei of these cells are irregular and hyperchromatic, and those near the surface show wrinkling of the nuclear membrane. The nuclei are usually larger than those of the adjacent, non-ballooned cells (see Fig. 12.22).

It is important that koilocytic change is not confused with the 'basket weave' pattern of the normal, mature squamous epithelium. The two other main histological features of subclinical papillomavirus infection are individual cell keratinization (dyskeratosis) and multinucleation (usually binucleation; see Fig. 12.23).

Other features which have been described are parakeratosis, frequent mitotic figures, acanthosis, prominent rete pegs and blood vessels surrounded by a little stroma reaching up to the surface.

The histological features of subclinical papillomavirus infection and cervical intraepithelial neoplasia may be combined in two ways (Figs 12.24–12.26): first, both conditions may occur separately in adjacent areas of the epithelium, a

Table 12.2 Histological and cytological features of human papillomavirus infection

Koilocytic change
Multinucleation (usually binucleation)
Dyskeratosis (individual cell keratinization)
Parakeratosis
Acanthosis
Papillomatosis
Appearances possibly due to acantholysis
Keratinized squamous cells
Anucleate keratinized squamous cells

(a)
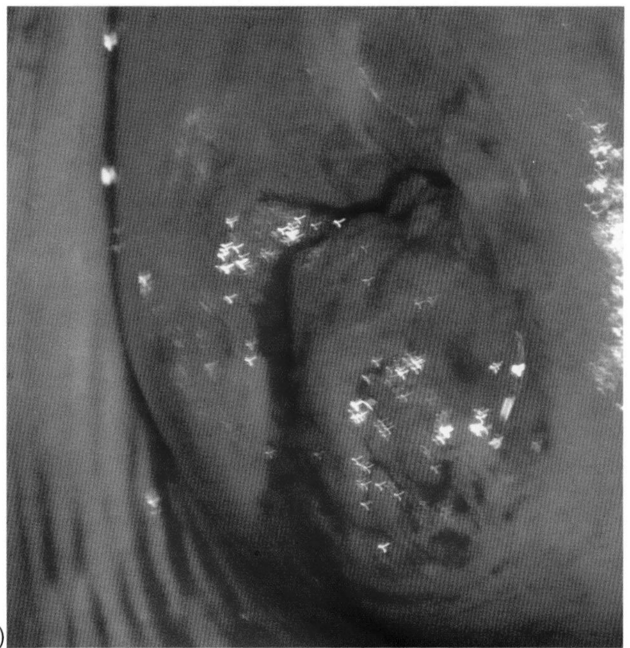

(b)
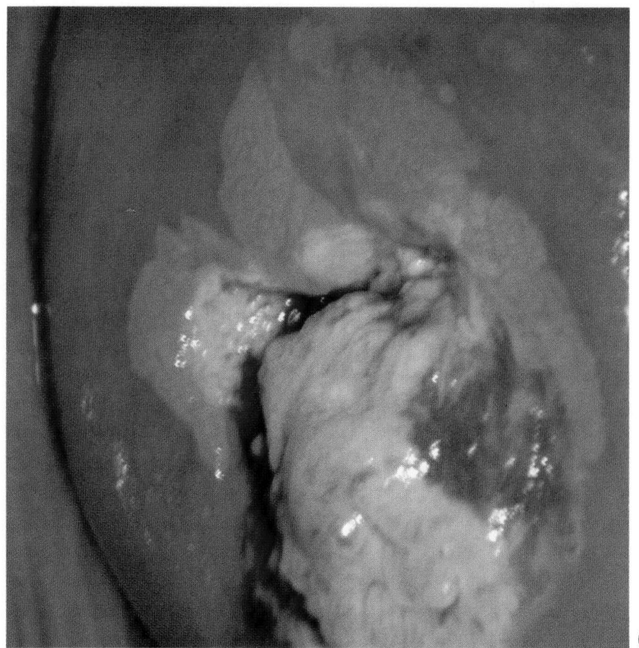

Fig. 12.19 Raised lesion on the posterior lip of the cervix; cervical carcinoma. (a) Before application of acetic acid. (b) After application of acetic acid. The typical features of invasion are seen, with a halo of cervical intraepithelial neoplasia and microinvasive disease anteriorly.

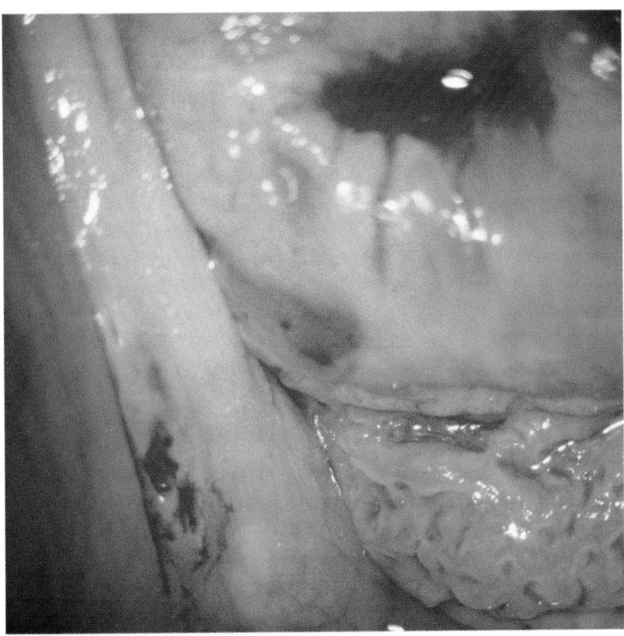

Fig. 12.20 Rare verrucous carcinoma in the posterior fornix. This patient had been treated for CIN 3. The lesion could be easily confused with an encephaloid condyloma.

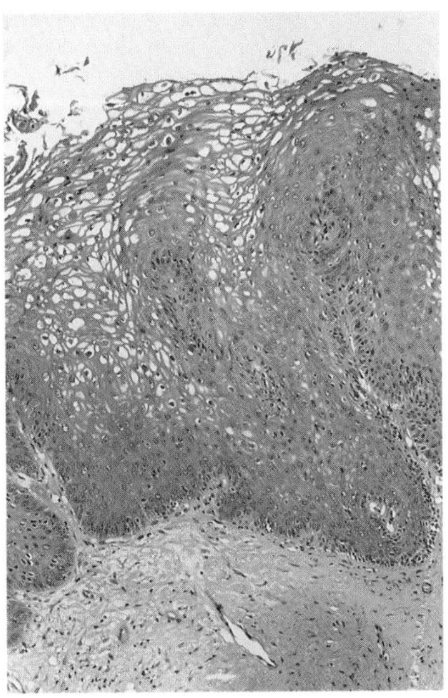

Fig. 12.21 Subclinical papillomavirus infection. Although not a clinical condyloma, this example shows acanthosis with some papillomatosis. Even at this low magnification, koilocytic change is obvious.

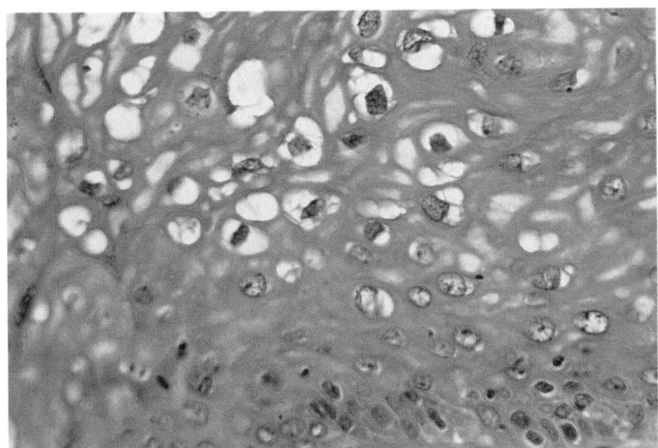

Fig. 12.22 Koilocytic change. A group of cells contain irregular, hyperchromatic, slightly enlarged nuclei which are surrounded by a clear halo.

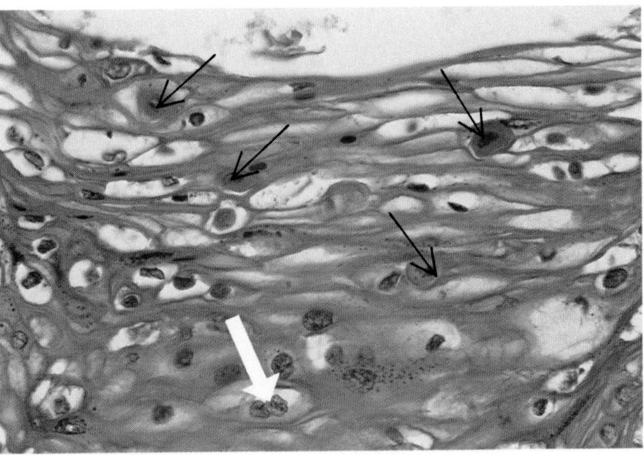

Fig. 12.23 Individual cell keratinization and multinucleation. In addition to koilocytic change, four cells are showing individual cell keratinization (solid arrows), and a further cell is binucleate (open arrow).

pattern frequently seen colposcopically (see Fig. 12.24). Secondly, an epithelium may show the features of both subclinical papillomavirus infection and cervical intraepithelial neoplasia in the same area. Therefore, koilocytic change, multinucleation and individual cell keratinization may occur in conjunction with the changes of cervical intraepithelial neoplasia (see Figs 12.25 and 12.26).

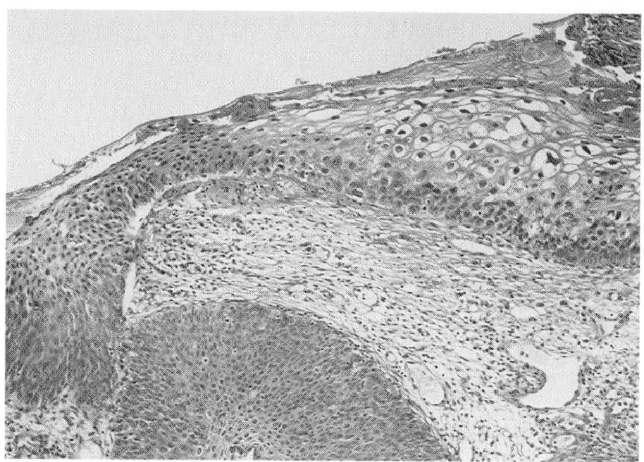

Fig. 12.24 Coexistent subclinical papillomavirus infection and cervical intraepithelial neoplasia. Subclinical papillomavirus infection is affecting the surface epithelium on the right, and cervical intraepithelial neoplasia is affecting both the surface epithelium on the left and part of the gland crypt on the lower part of the field.

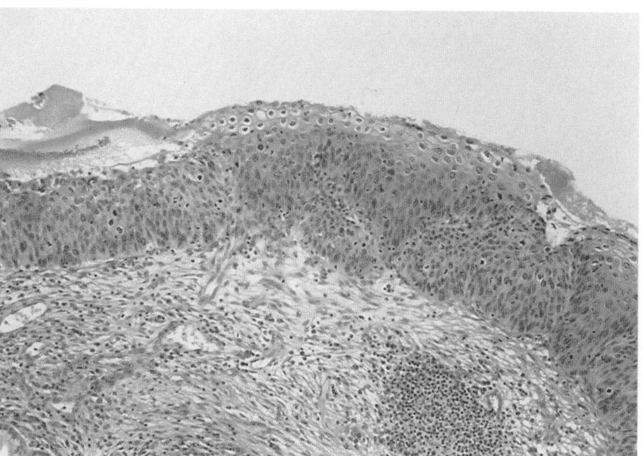

Fig. 12.25 Combined cervical intraepithelial neoplasia and subclinical papillomavirus infection. The epithelium is showing all the features of cervical intraepithelial neoplasia, together with koilocytic change of the superficial cells.

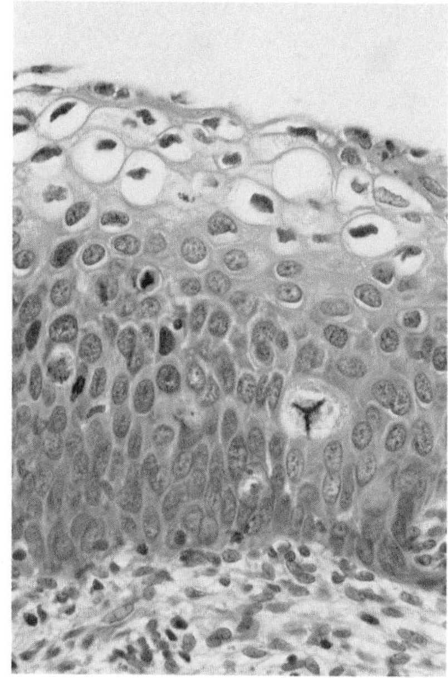

Fig. 12.26 Combined cervical intraepithelial neoplasia and subclinical papillomavirus infection. Superficial cells are showing prominent koilocytic change, but in the lower two-thirds of the epithelium the features of CIN 3 are apparent. Note the tripolar mitotic figure.

COLPOSCOPY

Colposcopically, subclinical papillomavirus lesions are best assessed after application of acetic acid (Fig. 12.27). The changes seen are: a shiny, snow-white lesion (Fig. 12.28); an irregular outline with jagged, angular or feathered margins (Fig. 12.29); and the presence of satellite lesions extending beyond the transformation zone (see Fig. 12.29).

Apart from acetowhite changes, subclinical papillomavirus infection is also assessed on the basis of the vascular pattern of the lesion, and response to Lugol's iodine applied in the Schiller's test. Strong or partial uptake (Fig. 12.30) of the dye by the affected epithelium denotes glycogenation, which may be present in subclinical papillomavirus infection, compared with the negative staining response usually shown by significant degrees of cervical intraepithelial neoplasia.

Capillary patterns may be pronounced and could be confused with, or be difficult to differentiate from, the mosaic and punctation patterns characteristic of cervical intraepithelial neoplasia. Reid has described the vascular pattern of subclinical papillomavirus infection as consisting of uniform, fine vessels, loosely and randomly arranged, often as a horizontal mesh reminiscent of bizarre spider's webs. Non-dilated capillary loops may also run vertically towards the epithelial surface, with a uniform calibre throughout their course (Fig. 12.31).

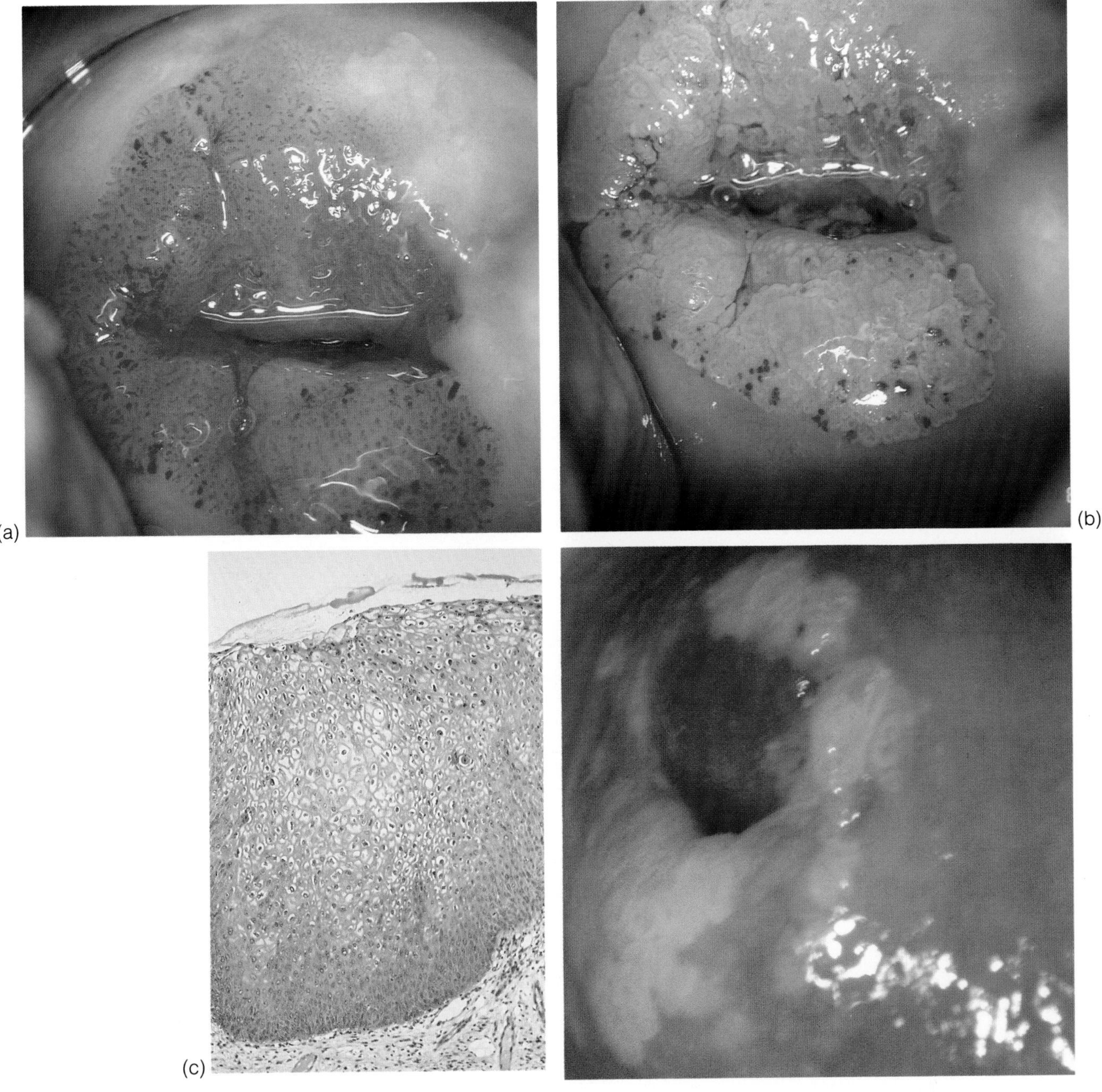

Fig. 12.27 Subclinical papillomavirus infection. (a) Before application of acetic acid. **(b)** After application of acetic acid; the lesion is now obvious, with acetowhite change. **(c)** A biopsy confirms the diagnosis.

Fig. 12.28 Subclinical papillomavirus infection. A shiny, snow-white lesion is apparent.

It is relatively difficult to distinguish between subclinical papillomavirus infection and cervical intraepithelial neoplasia. Several groups of workers have attempted to produce scoring methods for establishing a differential diagnosis, with varying degrees of success. In routine practice, a final diagnosis will depend on histological assessment of the biopsy material, and the biopsy report will usually be the final arbiter. This is particularly true where a combination of both conditions is observed. In these circumstances, diagnosis will depend on the histology of biopsies from each area (see Fig. 12.31). Nevertheless, some degree of colposcopic assessment is required if punch biopsy is to be directed to the area of significant disease.

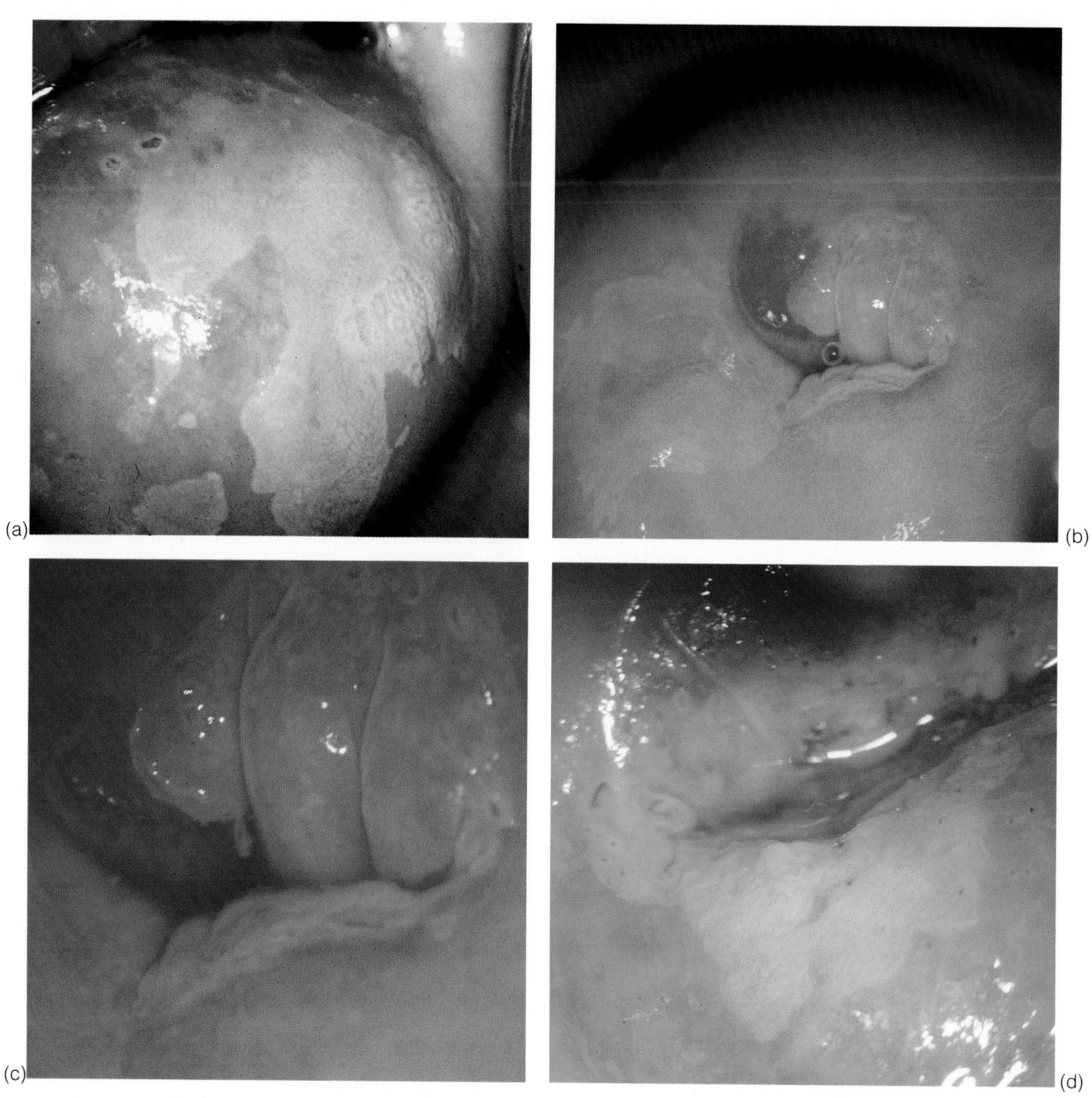

Fig. 12.29 Subclinical papillomavirus infection. (a) Multifocal acetowhite lesions, irregular outline with angular shapes and satellite lesions beyond the transformation zone. Note the encephaloid surface. Courtesy of Professor A Singer. **(b)** Low-power view of minor acetowhite HPV lesion, and **(c)** higher-power view of same. **(d)** Acetowhite change within the transformation zone. Viral features only on biopsy.

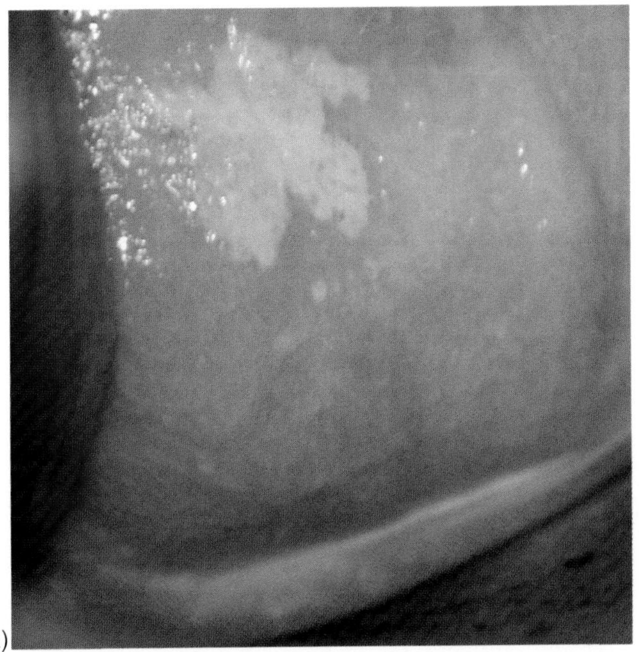

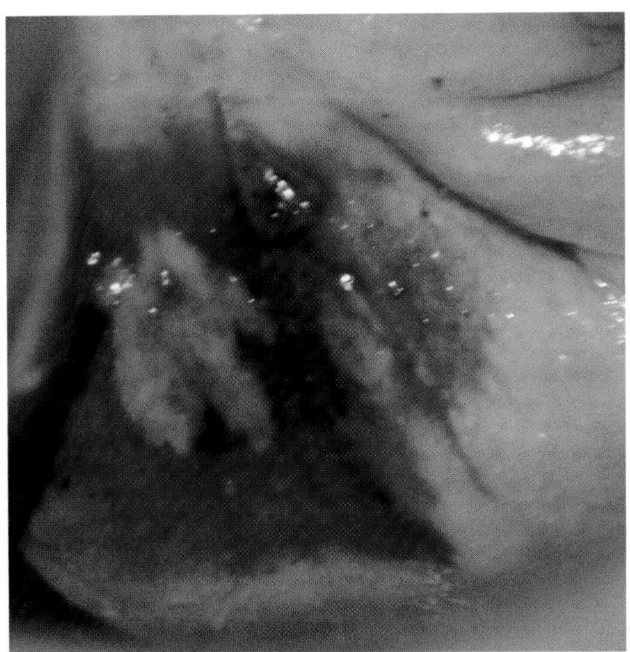

(a) (b)

Fig. 12.30 Cervical subclinical papillomavirus infection, extending beyond the transformation zone. (a) After application of acetic acid. **(b)** After application of Lugol's iodine, with partial uptake of dye by the lesion.

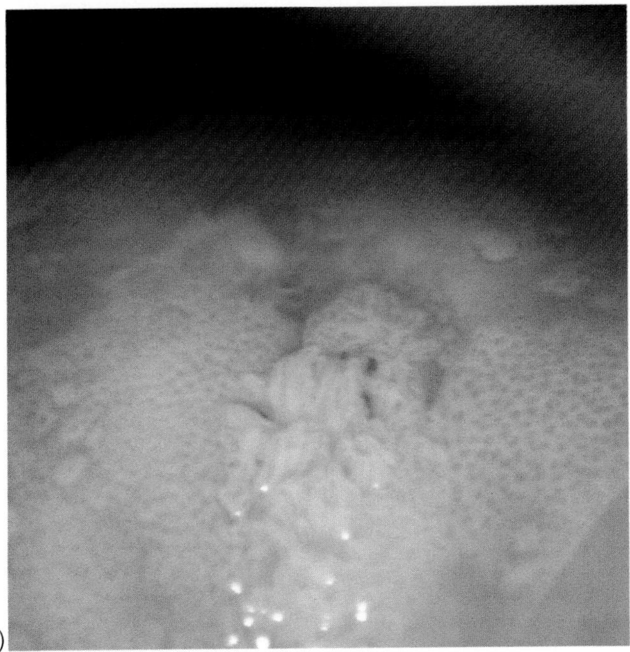

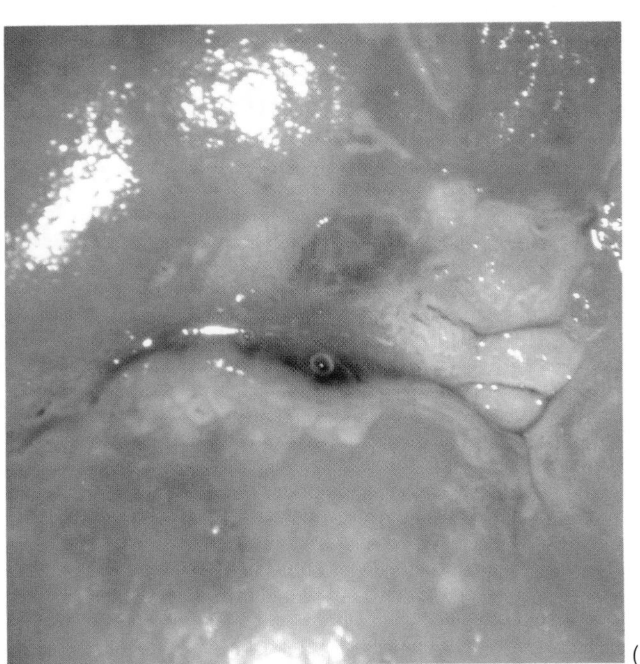

(a) (b)

Fig. 12.31 (a) Mixed condylomatous and subclinical papillomavirus infection lesions with cervical intraepithelial neoplasia on the cervix. The variety of vessel patterns for each lesion are clearly seen. Only multiple biopsies unravel the problem. **(b)** Mixed CIN/HPV lesion. Multifocal acetowhite lesions. Canal involved. Note satellite lesions.

MANAGEMENT OF HUMAN PAPILLOMAVIRUS INFECTION

Should an attempt be made to treat all patients with human papillomavirus infection? Some authorities argue that all such cases should be treated because of the potentially carcinogenic effect of the virus, but this raises the question of how treatment should be carried out. Exophytic warts can be recognized and dealt with fairly simply. However, recent evidence shows that up to 80% of all women have HPV-16 DNA in cervical, vaginal and vulval epithelium. Therefore, how can HPV-16 DNA be eliminated from the entire lower genital tract, including the vulva?

Exophytic warts can be treated quite simply with podophyllin, trichloroacetic acid, diathermy, cryocautery or laser. More recently, the use of local or systemic injection of interferon has been reported. Exophytic warts on the vulva will be distressing to the patient, but when planning management the clinician should be aware that up to 10% of such lesions disappear within 12 months without treatment.

Also, the colposcopist should remember that such warts may be associated with premalignant disease and should look specifically for any evidence of concurrent premalignancy: if present, it should be treated on its merits.

Cervical and vaginal warts are usually relatively easy to treat, as indeed are vulval warts when present in small numbers. However, it is difficult to eradicate very extensive exophytic warts that involve not only the vulva, but frequently the perineum and perianal areas. The colposcopist should look for evidence of intraepithelial neoplasia in these lesions, taking multiple biopsies before treatment is instituted. Laser vaporization (and, in the future, possibly interferon) would seem to be the treatment of choice. Frequently, further areas of exophytic warts will develop, but usually these are well localized and can be treated fairly simply.

If extensive warts are associated with intraepithelial neoplasia, local treatment will often be ineffective and excision should be considered. Because of the large areas involved, especially if the perianal area is affected, the optimal treatment may be local excision of all affected tissue, immediately followed by skin grafting. Where the perianal area is involved, a preoperative colostomy may be necessary; this can be closed a few weeks postoperatively.

Since patients with subclinical papillomavirus lesions will have HPV-16 DNA affecting the rest of the lower genital tract, it is debatable whether any form of treatment is likely to eradicate the disease. However, if subclinical papillomavirus is associated with intraepithelial neoplasia, a different approach will have to be considered. According to some authorities, CIN 1 is no more than a change induced by human papillomavirus, and indeed some workers have shown that up to 50% of lesions that feature human papillomavirus and CIN 1 will disappear spontaneously within 12 months. However, because other lesions progress, some authorities would advocate that all cases should be treated.

If, indeed, all of these lesions are treated, some women will undoubtedly receive unnecessary treatment. Therefore, if the colposcopist is certain that neither cytology, colposcopy nor histology raises the suspicion of invasive disease, consideration should be given to allowing the patient to proceed without treatment, provided that follow-up can be assured. If follow-up is doubtful, then a strong case can be made for treating at that particular time. However, human papillomavirus in association with CIN 3 should always be treated. As a general rule, if the colposcopist decides to treat human papillomavirus seen in association with cervical intraepithelial neoplasia, treatment should be exactly the same as for that degree of intraepithelial neoplasia.

Since changes in the cervix are occasionally associated with changes in the vagina and vulva, a full inspection of the lower genital tract should always take place. Subclinical papillomavirus infection of the vulva may present as 'burning vulva' syndrome. Colposcopic examination will show diagnostic microscopic changes, but before embarking on any form of treatment other causes of vulval burning and discomfort should be excluded. If treatment is thought necessary, superficial laser vulvectomy may be performed, but long-term results of this procedure are proving disappointing.

HERPES SIMPLEX VIRUS

Histology

The histological appearances of a cervix infected with herpes simplex virus type 2 depend upon the stage of the disease. Biopsies are very rarely taken at an early stage of the disease, and therefore examples of the early stages are rarely available for study. Changes start in the parabasal cells of the squamous epithelium, with nuclear enlargement and development of multinucleate cells. The characteristic nuclear moulding without overlapping is a feature more easily appreciated in cytological preparations. Intranuclear inclusions are uncommon.

Vesicle formation and ulceration follow within approximately 36 hours. At this time, multinucleate giant cells may be identified at the edges of vesicles and in their bases, with a polymorphonuclear leucocyte infiltration and, often, basal cell hyperplasia of the adjacent epithelium. Once ulceration has occurred and secondary infection has supervened, changes are those of a non-specific, acute necrotizing cervicitis (Fig. 12.32). A very dense stromal infiltrate of acute and chronic inflammatory cells extends into the granulation tissue at the base of the ulcer.

Cytology

The cytological features of herpes simplex virus infection are easily recognized. The cells are characteristically large, with multiple nuclei which mould one another and show emargination of chromatin and empty nuclei (Fig. 12.33). Occasionally, large intranuclear inclusions may be seen (Fig. 12.34), and this is believed to represent an early stage of infection.

If infection presents as a necrotizing cervicitis, the

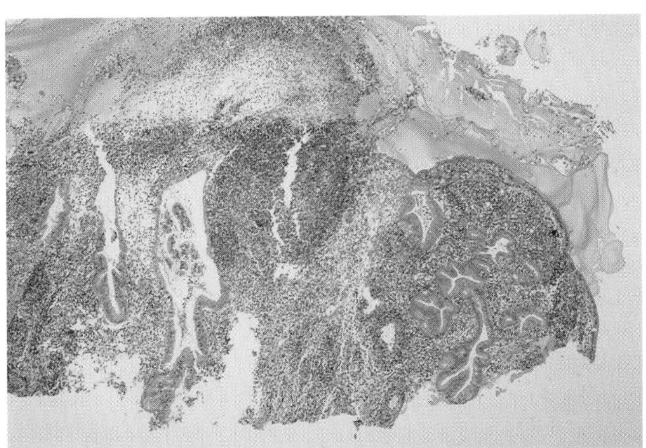

Fig. 12.32 A cervical biopsy, showing acute necrotizing cervicitis in a woman with herpetic cervicitis. This is the same patient as shown in Fig. 12.38. Much of the surface epithelium is lost, apart from the right side of the biopsy. The stroma is densely infiltrated by acute inflammatory cells, with crumbling. An inflammatory exudate is present on the surface.

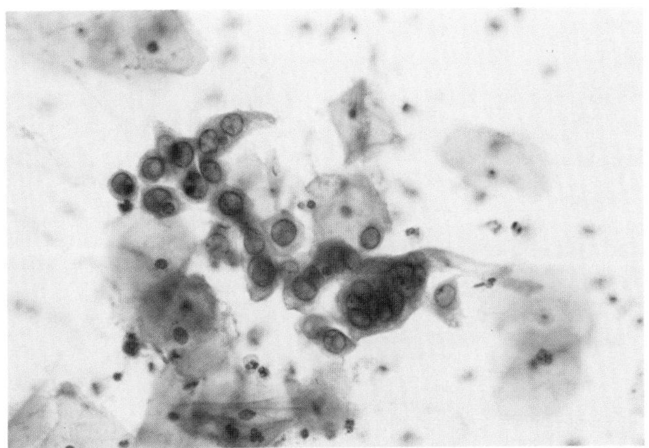

Fig. 12.33 Herpes simplex virus infection. A large, multinucleated cell, showing moulding of nuclei with emargination of chromatin.

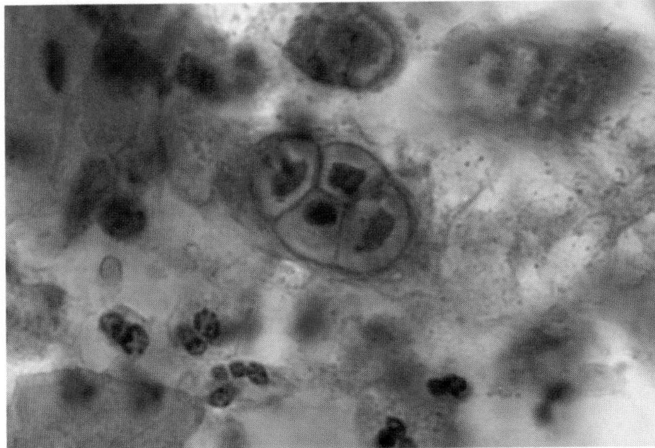

Fig. 12.34 Herpes simplex virus infection. Multinucleated cells, showing moulding of nuclei and large central inclusions.

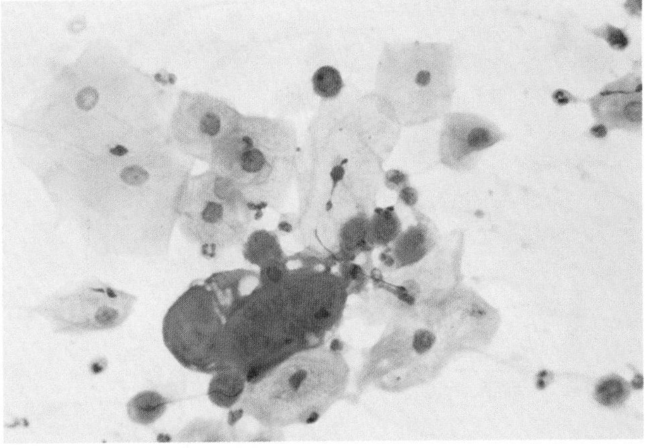

Fig. 12.35 Herpes simplex virus infection. These cells are showing multinucleation, but the nuclear features are poorly defined as a result of necrosis.

cells appear degenerate and necrotic, with only the ghosts of nuclei being barely visible (Fig. 12.35). With experience, the cytologist can recognize the characteristic nuclear features in mononuclear and binuclear cells (Fig. 12.36), and it is unlikely that cellular changes would be misinterpreted.

The inexperienced or unwary cytologist may confuse the appearances in the necrotic stage with invasive squamous cell carcinoma (also an area of clinical difficulty), or cervical intraepithelial neoplasia.

Colposcopy

Normally, the colposcopist will see herpetic changes only if the patient has vulval herpes and presents with vulval pain. Occasionally, the cervix will also be infected and should be examined, unless vulval pain is so severe that examination is impossible. If herpes is confined to the cervix, the patient will usually present with profuse vaginal discharge of sudden onset. Epithelial changes begin in the form of one or more vesicles which are of short duration and usually not visible. This stage is followed by ulceration within 24–36 hours (Fig. 12.37).

Sometimes the damage is so extensive that the areas of ulceration coalesce, and the cervix becomes the seat of one large ulcer with some of the appearances of invasive carcinoma (Figs 12.38 and 12.39).

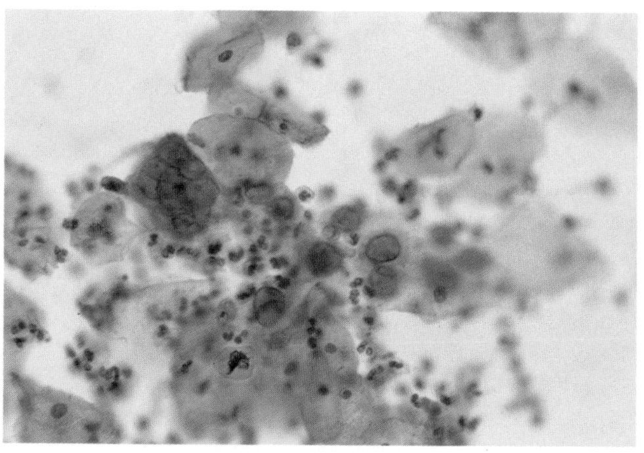

Fig. 12.36 Herpes simplex virus infection. Several cells with single nuclei, showing emargination of chromatin and empty nuclei. These changes are identical to those seen in the nuclei of the characteristic, large, multinucleated cell on the left.

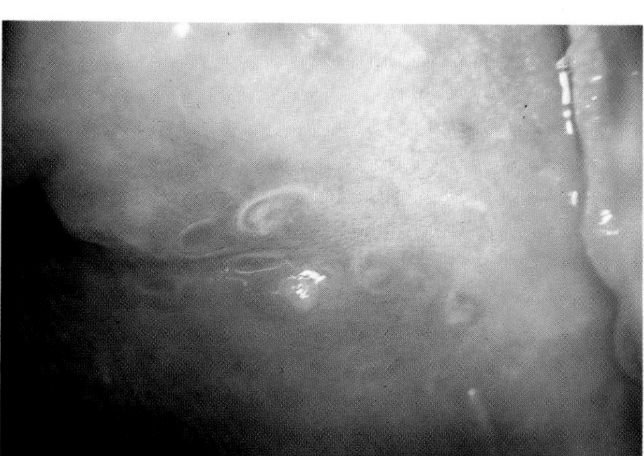

Fig. 12.37 Areas of early herpetic vesicles.

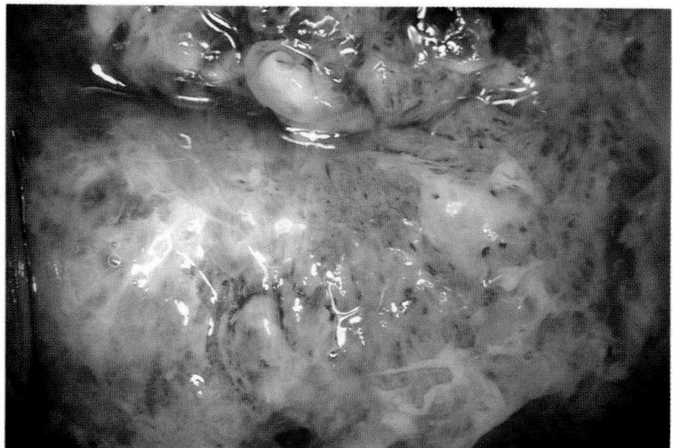

Fig. 12.38 Gross herpetic ulceration and acute inflammatory changes.

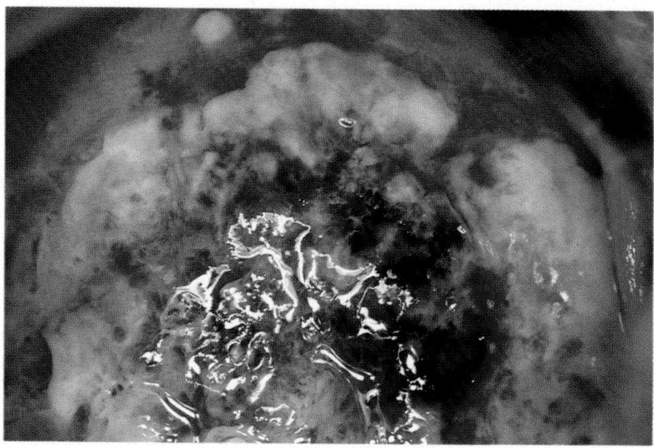

Fig. 12.39 Gross herpetic ulceration and acute inflammatory changes.

TRICHOMONIASIS

Cytology

This common protozoan infestation may be easily identified in cervical smears. The trichomonad appears as a small, blue-grey, poorly defined body with an elongated nucleus (Fig. 12.40); this must be identified in order to differentiate the protozoan from cell debris or mucus. The presence of the protozoan does not always give rise to active infection; some women are carriers, but on occasion the infection may be accompanied by a severe inflammatory reaction, with extensive cell necrosis. Trichomonas can rarely be associated with *Leptothrix vaginalis*, a filamentous organism which seems to be non-pathogenic (Fig. 12.41).

Colposcopy

The cervix appears red, due to hyperaemia occurring as a reaction to the trichomonas infection. Close examination shows that the cervix is covered by a

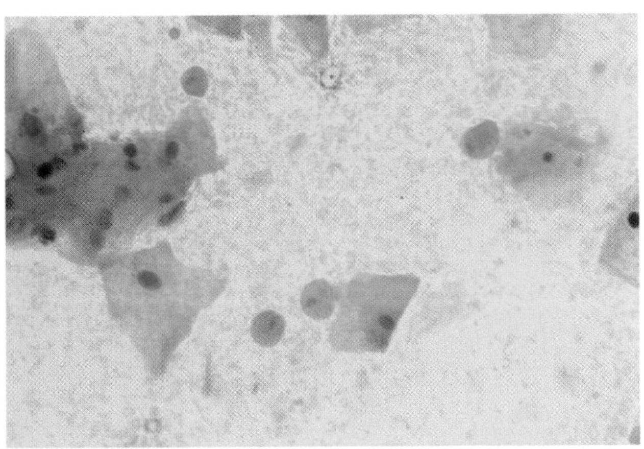

Fig. 12.40 Specific infection. *Trichomonas vaginalis* is recognized by the elongated or slit nucleus in the pale blue, indistinct bodies

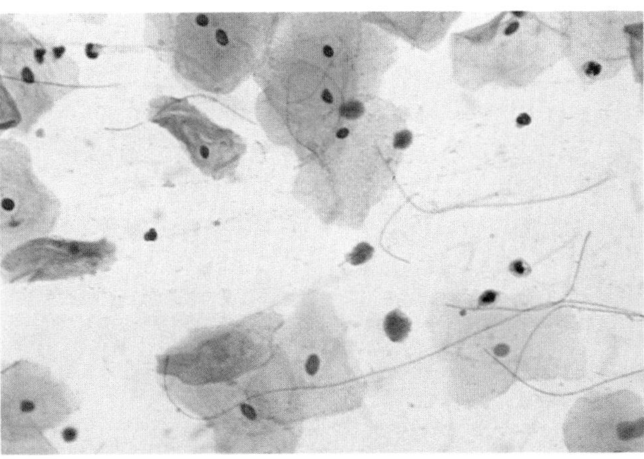

Fig. 12.41 Specific infection. *Trichomonas vaginalis* is sometimes associated with the filamentous organism *Leptothrix*, seen here as hair-like strands.

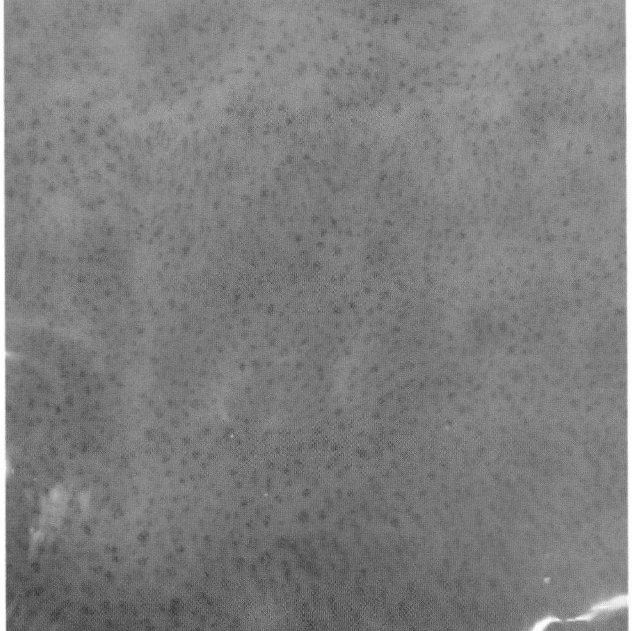

Fig. 12.42 Small red spots due to *Trichomonas* infection.

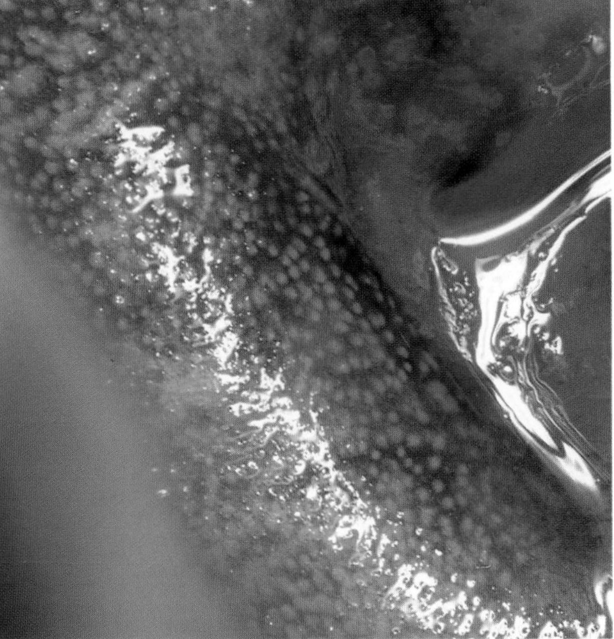

Fig. 12.43 *Trichomonas* changes following application of Lugol's iodine.

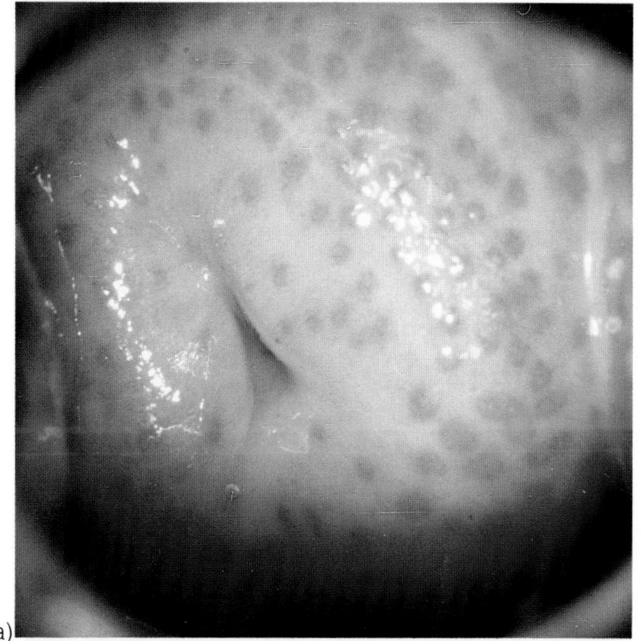
(a)

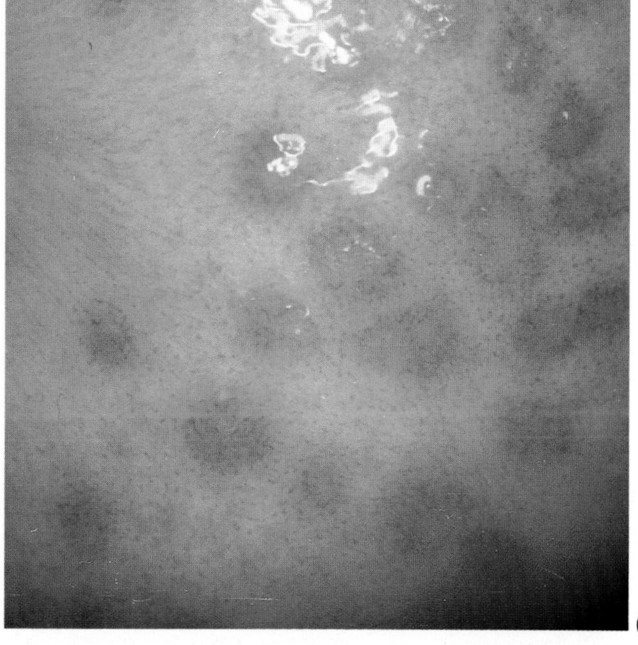
(b)

(c)

Fig. 12.44 'Strawberry' patches due to *Trichomonas* infection (a) Low power. **(b)** High power. **(c)** Following application of Lugol's iodine.

multitude of tiny red dots, each of which is the tip of a dilated subepithelial capillary reaching almost to the surface (Fig. 12.42).

When this is compounded by the fact that some of the superficial squamous cells desquamate, relatively few cells remain between the tip of the capillary and surface; these cells are poorly glycogenated, and as a result application of Lugol's iodine shows a multitude of tiny non-staining areas (Fig. 12.43).

Occasionally, the cervix has a typical 'strawberry' appearance: large collections of capillaries are grouped together, to form a red spot which is visible to the naked eye (Fig. 12.44(a,b)). Subsequent application of Schiller's iodine will reveal that the epithelium covering each red spot is non-glycogenated, and consequently the cervix has a speckled appearance due to the non-staining areas (Fig. 12.44(c)).

Candida albicans

The spores and hyphae of *Candida albicans* are easily identified, usually staining pink, although their colour can vary from almost colourless to pale blue or orange (Fig. 12.45).

Candidiasis may be frequently present without an associated inflammatory response, but in some instances degenerative cellular changes (see page 137) may be seen despite the lack of response.

Actinomyces israeli

Actinomyces is an anaerobic bacterium, most commonly seen as small aggregates (Fig. 12.46) in the cervical smears of women using intrauterine contraceptive devices, although occasionally large and multiple aggregates are present. Other bacteria and increased polymorphonuclear leucocytes are frequently seen in association with the *Actinomyces* organisms.

BACTERIAL INFECTIONS

Cervical smears often contain large numbers of bacteria which can be differentiated from the commensal *Lactobacillus*. If such bacteria are apparent in large numbers, both in the background of a smear and clustering on the surface of epithelial cells (Fig. 12.47), there is a very high probability that they represent a pathogenic infection. The presence of increased numbers of polymorphonuclear leucocytes (Fig. 12.48), histiocytes, occasionally lymphocytes and rarely plasma cells, increases this probability. The distinction between lactobacilli (Döderlein) and treatable bacterial infections is essential in terms of management (Fig. 12.49; see Chapter 5).

Although cytology cannot differentiate between the various bacterial infections, it is useful to alert the clinician to the presence of excessive numbers of bacteria which may render the smear unsatisfactory or give rise to problems of interpretation (Fig. 12.50). Microbiological screening, followed by appropriate treatment, may be advisable before another smear is taken.

Bacterial infections most commonly associated with cervicitis are *Chlamydia trachomatis*, bacterial vaginosis and *Neisseria gonorrhoeae*.

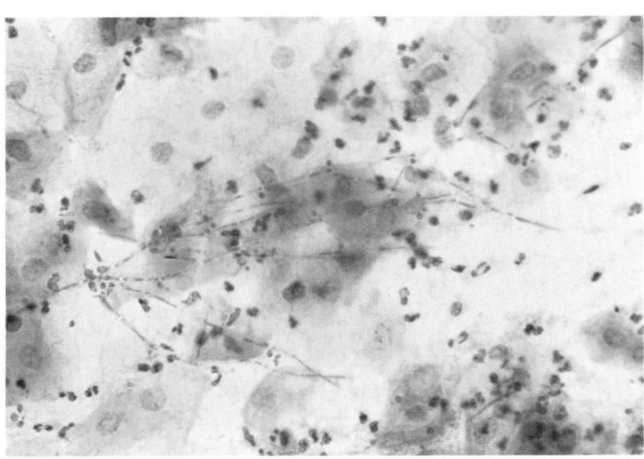

Fig. 12.45 Specific infection. The pink-staining, spore-bearing hyphae of *Candida albicans* can be seen overlying the central group of squamous cells.

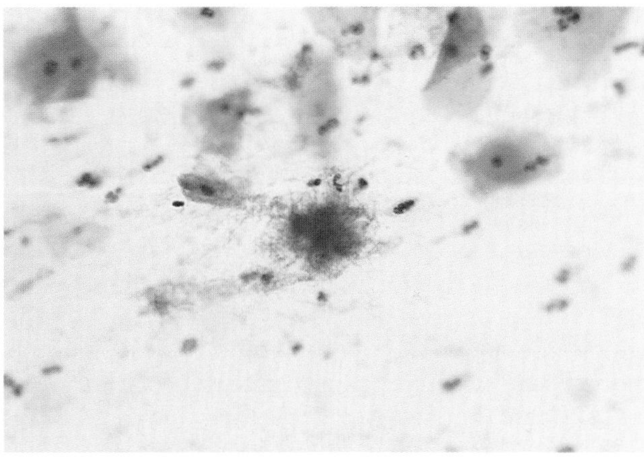

Fig. 12.46 Specific infection. A small bacterial aggregate is shown, with a dense central area. The club-like filamentous projections, characteristic of *Actinomyces israeli*, can be clearly seen.

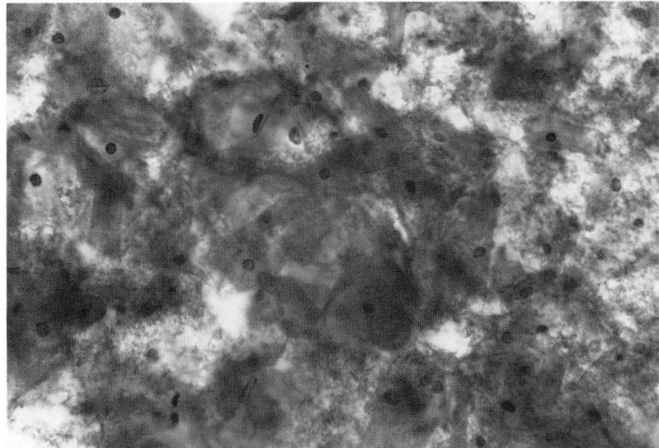

Fig. 12.47 Bacterial infection. Large numbers of bacteria can be seen in the background and overlying the surface of squamous cells, partially obscuring the cellular detail.

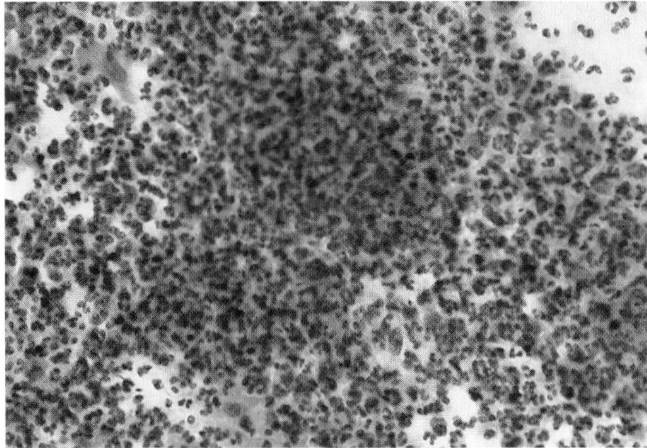

Fig. 12.48 Bacterial infection. In this case, epithelial cells are completely obscured by polymorphonuclear leucocytes and lymphocytes with bacteria in the background.

Follicular cervicitis

Follicular cervicitis may be associated with chlamydial infection; in cervical smears, large numbers of lymphocytes are characteristically seen (Fig. 12.51), often in wide streaks.

Once the pattern has been diagnosed, it is unlikely to cause diagnostic problems in the future. However, the differential diagnosis between follicular cervicitis and cervical intraepithelial neoplasia may be difficult for the inexperienced cytologist. The possibility of a lymphoma or endometrial adenocarcinoma should also be considered in the diagnosis.

BORDERLINE CHANGES

The 'inflammatory' smear

The term 'inflammatory smear' is, regrettably, widely used in cytological reports. However, this term probably makes sense only to the cytologist responsible for such a report, as it is open to individual interpretation by the recipient clinician.

Cytologists need to give a great deal of thought to the identification of inflammatory responses in cervical smears, in relation to both cellular changes and background appearances, as well as to the way in which the patterns are combined. These features require careful analysis in an attempt to clarify and discriminate between unimportant and significant elements. While some studies have suggested that women with 'inflammatory smear' reports harbour a high incidence of cytologically unrecognized cervical intraepithelial neoplasia, or even invasive disease, other studies have shown that up to 70% do not have significant cervical disease and therefore do not require colposcopy.

A conservative approach, identifying a treatable infection and repeating cytology after treatment, is probably all that is required in the majority of women in this category. Referral for colposcopy should be reserved for the minority who have recalcitrant infection or show persistent nuclear changes after a second or third smear.

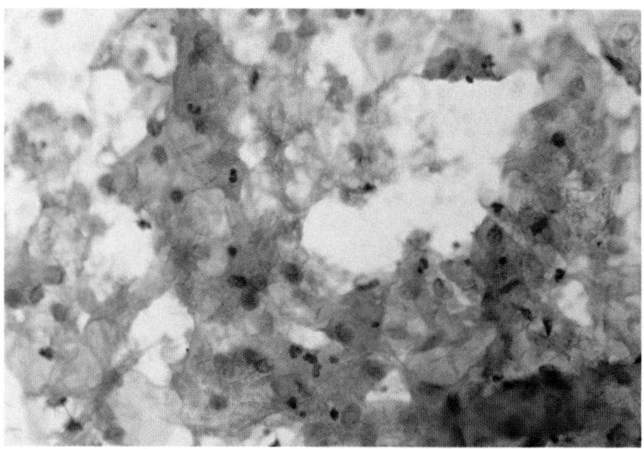

Fig. 12.49 Bacterial infection. At first glance, this pattern appears similar to that seen in Fig. 12.47, but closer inspection shows that these bacteria are the rod-like Doederlein bacilli which are non-pathogenic.

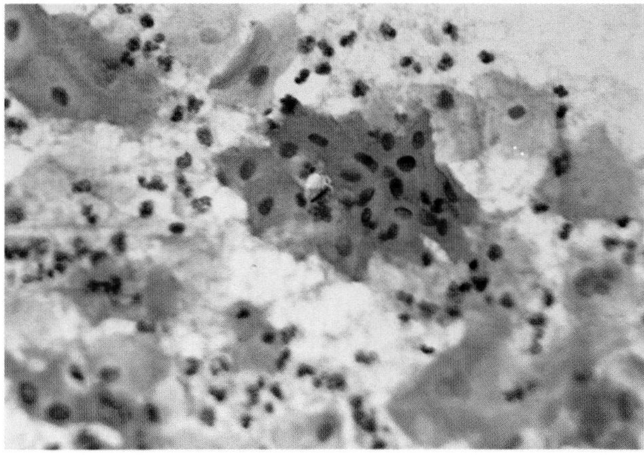

Fig. 12.50 Degenerative inflammatory change. The squamous cells show nuclear enlargement with minimal chromatin change. These probably represent degenerative inflammatory change associated with bacterial infection or human papillomavirus infection. However, mild dyskaryosis cannot be confidently excluded.

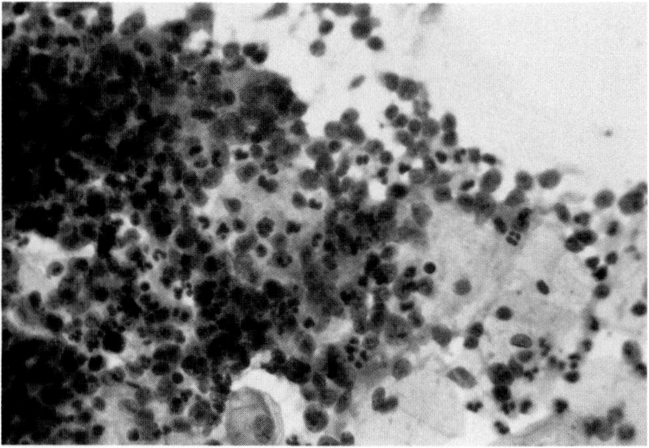

Fig. 12.51 Follicular cervicitis. Numerous lymphocytes, often in large sheets or streaks, are seen when a lymphocytic follicle is scraped with the spatula during sampling.

Nuclear changes bordering on mild dyskaryosis

The introduction of this category was an attempt by the British Society for Clinical Cytology to assist in clarifying this area of uncertainty, both in terms of actual cell appearance and, more importantly, in linking the language and terminology used by cytologists (including the term 'inflammatory' smear) to a management policy. In this way, it was hoped that the small minority of women with cervical intraepithelial neoplasia or early invasive disease, whose smears fall into this category, would be followed up with cytology and referred after a short period for subsequent colposcopic management.

To some extent this has succeeded in abolishing many meaningless terms, but the arguments presented for 'inflammatory smears' still apply no clear cytological criteria, and therefore a great deal of subjectivity remains. Furthermore, there is a temptation, especially for the inexperienced cytologist lacking in confidence, to use this category as a convenient 'dumping ground' without addressing the basic issues. The biological potential of 'borderline' lesions at the bottom end of the scale of abnormality (which is the context in which this phrase is used here and is the generally accepted interpretation) is not known. With regard to their management, the consensus of opinion in the UK at present is to wait and see, rather than refer immediately for colposcopy. Since this may not resolve the situation and indeed may be detrimental to the well-being of the woman concerned, referral is reserved for cases of persistent abnormality following a repeat smear at six months.

Organized, long-term, case-controlled studies are being set up to evaluate the significance of these lesions in terms of progression rates and optimal treatment regimens. In the meantime, strenuous attempts should be made by cytologists to agree on reproducible criteria, so that reliable management decisions can be taken. Adherence to the recommendations of the British Society for Clinical Cytology for colposcopic referral of patients should minimize the risk of not treating the proportion of women with significant disease (see Chapter 5). Cytologists have a responsibility to address the issue of 'inflammatory' and borderline smears, and should appreciate the importance of evaluating smears as being genuinely unsatisfactory for a reliable assessment. Equally, care must be exercised in identifying features of specific infections which indicate the appropriate treatment, and in critically evaluating cellular changes which do represent dyskaryosis or malignancy. A better understanding of the cause and effect of an inflammatory response in a cervical smear, together with a growing awareness of diagnostic pitfalls, should help to improve both cytological and clinical expertise in this area.

The whole area of borderline nuclear changes has been addressed by a joint working party with members drawn from the British Society for Clinical Cytology and the Royal College of Pathologists; helpful guidelines for the recognition and management of these changes have been published

UNUSUAL INFECTIVE LESIONS OF THE LOWER GENITAL TRACT

Introduction

Particularly in developing countries, there are a number of unusual conditions of the cervix, vagina and vulva which may be encountered. These are important as disease entities in their own right. For the colposcopist practising in such countries, familiarity with the following conditions is important as from time to time **these lesions may mimic invasive cancer**, even to the naked eye or examining finger. The essential role of diagnostic biopsy, and microbiological investigation where appropriate, cannot be stressed too much. No patient should be treated on only a clinical suspicion of lower genital tract cancer. Confirmatory biopsy should be obligatory.

Conditions to be considered in the differential diagnosis of cervical cancer in developing (and developed!) countries include chancroid, tuberculosis, lymphogranuloma venereum, amoebiasis, schistosomiasis (bilharzia), and syphilitic ulcers. A full account of these diseases is beyond the scope of this book, and reference will be limited largely to those areas of pertinence to colposcopy.

Pitfalls for the cytologist

This account is adapted from Bloch, Dehaeck and Soeters (1995), with permission (see Bibliography).

ATYPICAL REPAIR

Sheets of cells with prominent nucleoli are frequently seen in association with inflammatory conditions of the cervix. At times these changes may be difficult to differentiate from dyskaryosis when in addition there is significant nuclear atypia (see Chapter 14; Figs. 14.5 and 14.6).

TUBERCULOSIS

Tuberculosis may affect the female genital tract and because of the associated necrosis of tissue with chronic inflammation, may mimic carcinoma cytologically as well as clinically. Identification of epithelioid cell granulomas is necessary for diagnosis, and these are not seen on cytology. Smears from women with cervical tuberculosis may sometimes contain multinucleate giant cells, rarely identifiable as Langhan's type (Fig. 12.52), but these are not pathognomonic and can be found in a number of other conditions.

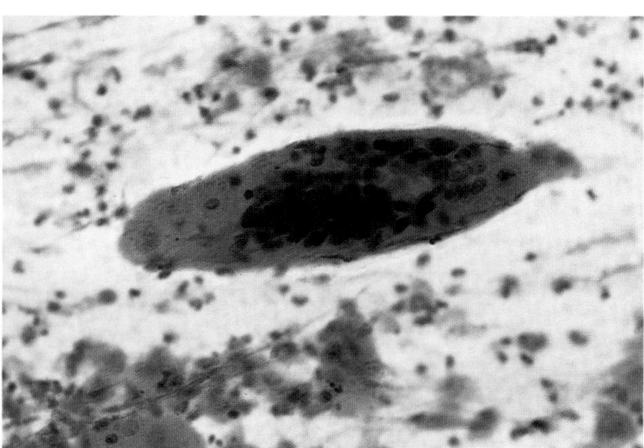

Fig. 12.52 Tuberculosis of the cervix. A smear from a woman with cervical tuberculosis, showing a multinucleated giant cell. There is the hint of a peripheral arrangement of the nuclei, suggesting that this may be a Langhan's-type giant cell (see Fig. 12.54).

AMOEBIASIS

Similar features to the above may be noted in cervical amoebiasis. Classical amoebae within the necrotic tissue may be difficult to identify

SCHISTOSOMIASIS

Extensive fibrosis and chronic inflammatory changes are associated with this condition. Again the condition may mimic carcinoma cytologically as well as clinically. The ova occasionally may be found on cervical smears (Fig. 12.53).

Genital tuberculosis

AETIOLOGY

Despite early recognition and effective treatment, tuberculosis of the female genital tract is common in those communities where pulmonary or other forms of extragenital tuberculosis are prevalent. Genital tuberculosis is nearly always secondary to a focus elsewhere in the body, but the spread takes place at a very early stage of the disease, usually in adolescence or early maturity. By the time the genital lesion

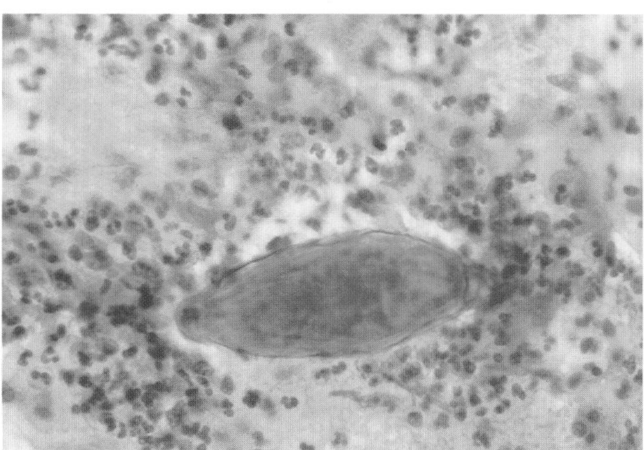

Fig. 12.53 Cervical schistosomiasis. An ovum of *Schistosoma haematobium* is seen in a characteristic background of red blood cells and polymorphonuclear leucocytes.

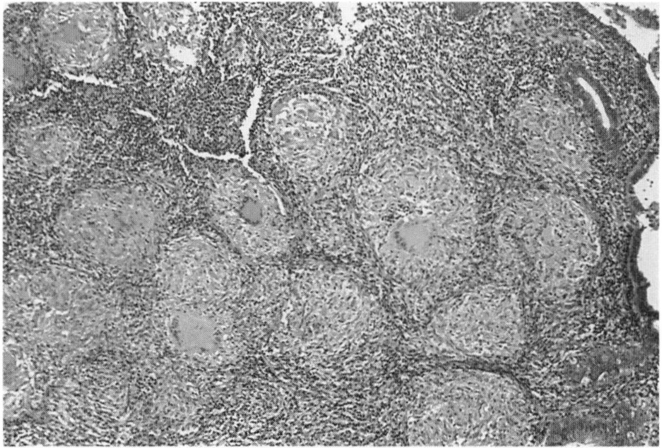

Fig. 12.54 Endometrial tuberculosis. Numerous well-formed epithelioid cell granulomas are seen against a chronic inflammatory background. Langhan's-type giant cells have multiple nuclei arranged in the form of a horseshoe around the periphery of the cell and are present in the centres of several granulomas.

is found, which can be at any age, the primary lesion is often healed and inconspicuous. Nevertheless, many affected women give a past history of an extragenital infection, and a further number can recall, if questioned closely, contact with the disease in childhood or adolescence.

The tubercle bacilli may reach the genital tract from the primary focus by one of the following mechanisms. Spread by the bloodstream accounts for at least 90% of cases, the primary focus being most often situated in the lungs, lymph nodes, urinary tract, bones and joints. In descending spread the infection reaches the pelvic organs by direct or lymphatic spread from infected adjacent organs such as the peritoneum, bowel and mesenteric nodes. Ascending spread is a theoretical possibility in which a few cases of tuberculosis of the vulva and vagina, and of primary tuberculosis of the cervix, may be explained by children sitting unclothed where an infected person has spat or coughed, or by a woman having coitus with a male suffering from urogenital tuberculosis.

PATHOLOGY AND BACTERIOLOGY

When the pelvic disease is secondary to tuberculous peritonitis, or when the primary focus is in the lymph nodes or bowel, the bovine bacillus (*Mycobacterium tuberculosis bovis*) is likely to be involved. In all other cases it is generally the human bacillus (*M. tuberculosis*) which is the causative agent. So, in those countries where cattle or their milk are relatively free from the tubercle bacillus, the human bacillus is found in 95% of cases of genital tract infection.

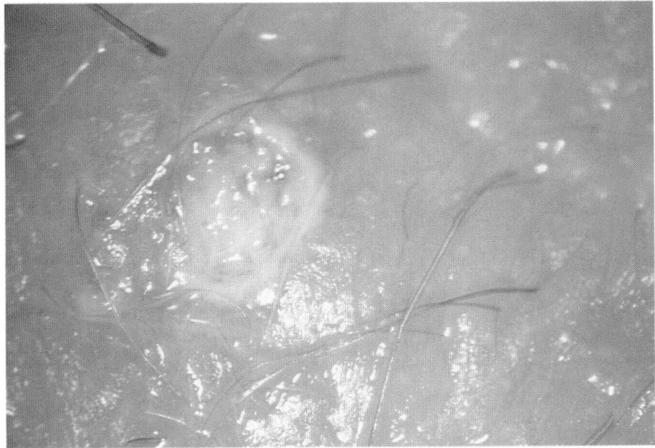

Fig. 12.55 Tuberculosis of the vulva. Note small shallow ulcer with early undermining of the lower edge.

Any part of the genital tract can be affected but the common sites are the fallopian tubes and the endometrium (Fig. 12.54). The tubes are involved in at least 90% of cases and the organism probably arrives there by bloodstream spread. Spread to the endometrium may then occur. The finding of endometrial tuberculosis almost always means that the tubes are infected, but tuberculous salpingitis can exist without associated endometritis.

Genital infection can be an acute and fulminating disease but is mostly indolent. There are several cases reported in which the disease appeared to commence, or to become violently active, immediately after pregnancy. In such circumstances fatal miliary spread is not uncommon.

Vulva and vagina

These sites may concern the colposcopist. Tuberculosis of the vulva and vagina usually takes the form of shallow, superficial, indolent ulcers with undermined edges (Fig. 12.55). The ulceration tends to spread slowly, healing in some areas with the formation of scar tissue. A vulval hypertrophic lesion is less common and mostly represents inflammatory induration and oedema resulting from fibrosis and lymphatic obstruction. Vulval lesions are usually painful and tender. Vaginal ulcers, unless sited at the introitus, are painless. Both often cause a bloodstained purulent discharge.

Cervix

Clinically recognizable tuberculosis of the cervix can be ulcerative but more often appears as a bright red papillary erosion which bleeds easily (Fig. 12.56). It can be confused with carcinoma (Fig 12.57). As a histological finding, cervical tuberculosis is not uncommon in cases of endometrial tuberculosis. Overt tuberculosis of the cervix is painless but also causes a bloodstained, purulent discharge and also postcoital bleeding.

Diagnosis

So far as the colposcopist is concerned, if tuberculosis is suspected, the lesion is accessible (as in cervix, vagina and vulva), and the diagnosis is made by examining biopsy material both bacteriologically and histologically. The finding of epithelioid cell granulomas with Langhan's-type giant cells (Fig. 12. 57) is highly suggestive but is not conclusive evidence unless tubercle bacilli can also be demonstrated in Ziehl–Neelsen-stained preparations (Fig 12.58) or there is a positive culture.

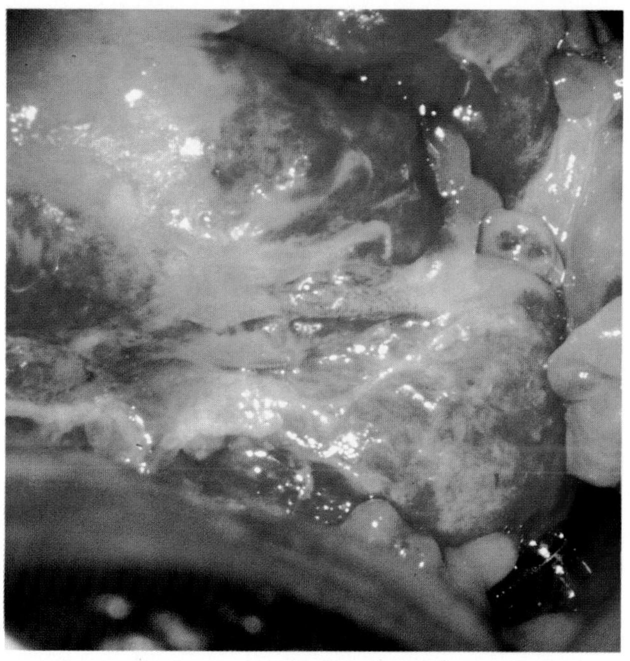
(a)

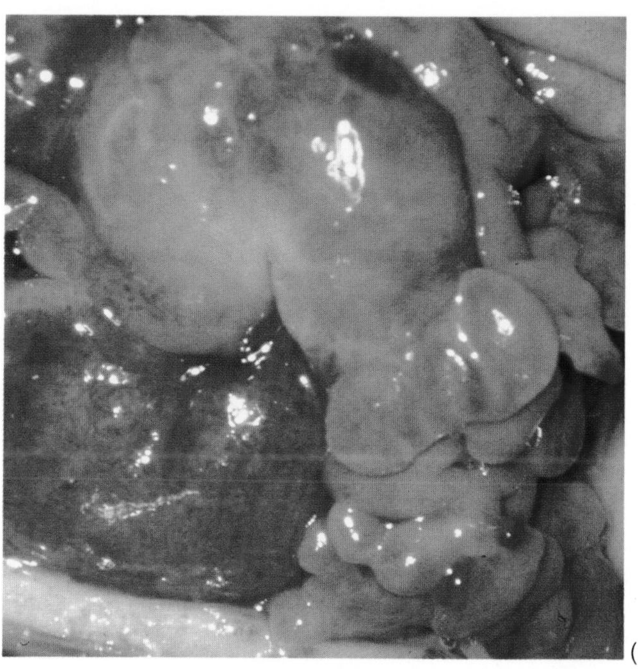
(b)

Fig. 12.56 Tuberculous cervicitis in pregnancy. (a) Low-power view showing eroded area with contact bleeding. Histology showed tuberculous cervicitis with atypical reserve cell hyperplasia. **(b)** Higher-power view. Courtesy of Professor Ernst Sonnendecker.

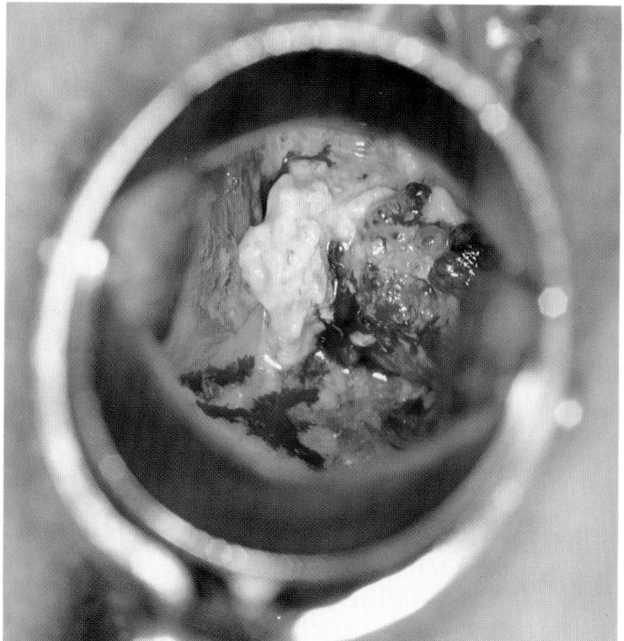

Fig. 12.57 Cervical tuberculosis. This lesion could readily be mistaken for invasive carcinoma. Courtesy of Professor Ernst Sonnendecker.

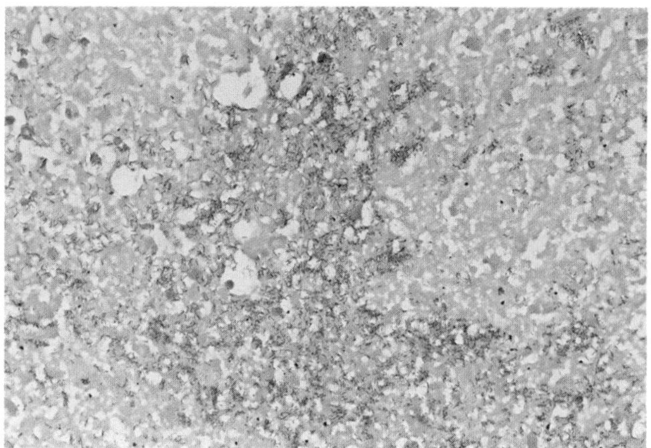

Fig. 12.58 Positive Ziehl–Neelsen stain in pulmonary tuberculosis. A very large number of acid-fast bacilli are present and stain deep red. Only occasionally are isolated organisms found in genital tuberculosis; more often the Z–N stain is negative and the diagnosis depends on a positive culture.

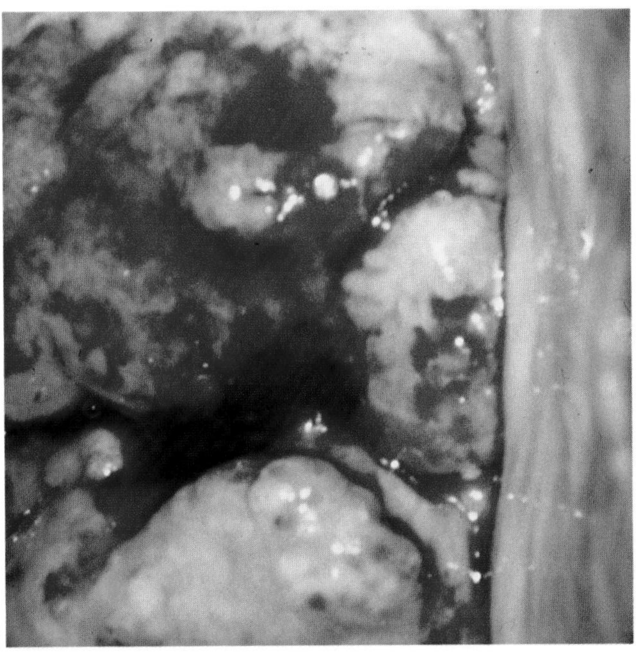

(a)

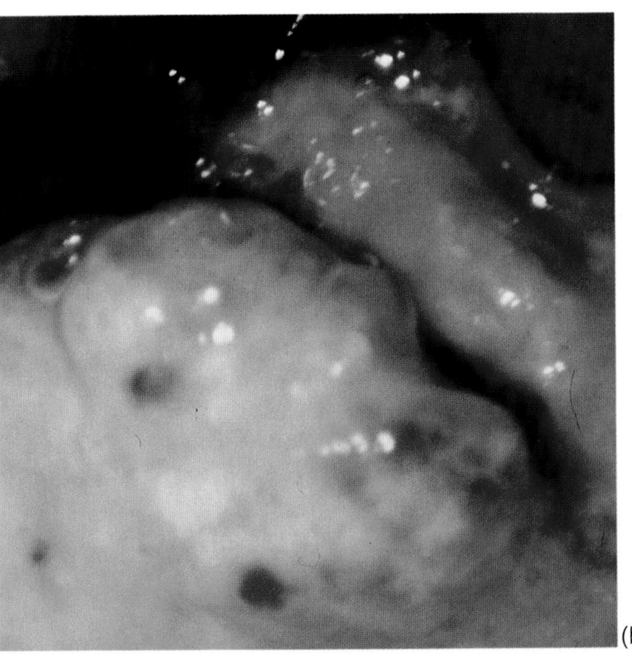

(b)

Fig. 12.59 Schistosomiasis of the cervix. (a) Exfoliative haemorrhagic appearance of the cervix. **(b)** Higher power-view of posterior lip showing craggy surface simulating invasive cancer. Courtesy of Professor Ernst Sonnendecker.

Schistosomiasis (bilharzia)

Genital schistosomiasis is seen in all tropical and subtropical countries, including Egypt, other countries in Africa, India, Malaysia, Indo-China, and Central and Southern America, where the causal worm and its immediate host, a water snail, are prevalent. The worm, *Schistosoma haematobium*, having entered the skin from infested water, spreads by the bloodstream to invade the tissues, where it deposits ova which cause local inflammatory reactions. Adult *S. haematobium* worms live in the genitourinary veins. The lesions are predominantly in hollow viscera, especially the bladder and rectum, but any part of the genital tract from the vulva to the ovaries can be involved. The most common genital site is the cervix (Fig 12.59). Vulval lesions are mostly seen in children. The infestation is chronic and can persist for a lifetime, the carrier continually excreting ova to contaminate the environment.

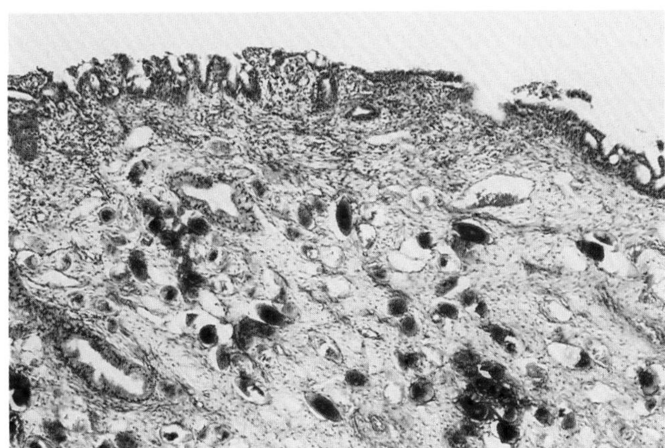

Fig. 12.60 Schistosomiasis of the cervix. Numerous ova are present in the endocervix. In this example, there is little accompanying inflammation. Courtesy of Professor Andrew Tiltman.

The inflammatory reaction may be a severe one with each ovum being surrounded by a giant cell, epithelial cells, lymphocytes and eosinophils (Fig. 12.60). In some respects the microscopic appearances can resemble those of tuberculosis.

Bladder and bowel symptoms predominate and the discomforts referred to the reproductive organs vary with the site infected. Schistosomiasis of the vagina and cervix can cause discharge, bleeding and dyspareunia; it also favours sterility in that antibodies to the disease are spermatotoxic.

To the naked eye the disease appears in the form of nodules, plaques, ulcers or papillomas with surrounding induration. On the cervix the disease can

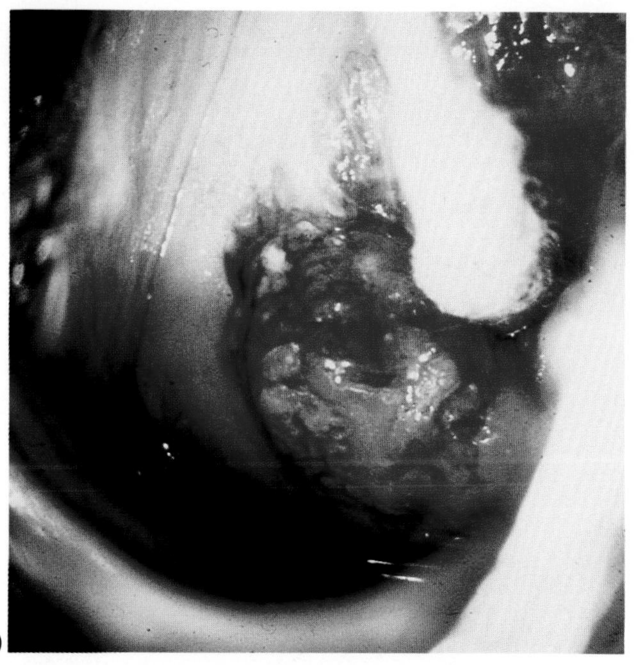

(a)

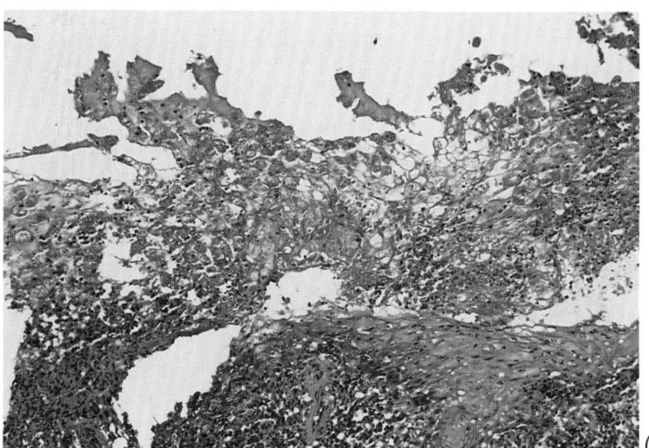

(b)

Fig. 12.61 Amoebiasis of the cervix. (a) Amoeboma of the posterior lip of the cervix. The lesion mimics cancer. **(b)** Histology. There is non-specific severe inflammation with partial dissolution of the surface epithelium. The trophozoites of *Entamoeba hystolytica* may sometimes be identified using a periodic acid–Schiff stain. Courtesy of Professor Andrew Tiltman.

simulate cancer, as it may any site. It is suggested that schistosomiasis may occasionally contribute to oncogenesis.

The prognosis is good for treatment in the early stage but poor in the late stages of the disease.

Amoebiasis

Amoebiasis of the genital tract occurs at any age and wherever intestinal infection is common. It is prevalent among the less-privileged communities living in warm climates. The parasite, *Entamoeba histolytica,* spreads from the lower bowel when standards of hygiene are poor. It causes ulcerative lesions in the vagina, cervix (Fig. 12.61) and endometrium and these can be mistaken for cancer on naked-eye examination.

Apart from any bowel symptoms the patient complains of a bloodstained purulent vaginal discharge. The diagnosis is made by the microscopic demonstration of the parasites in stools, vaginal discharge and tissue sections; the finding of the organism incidentally during cervical cytology is also described. A negative gel diffusion precipitation test, or amoebic latex agglutination test, carried out on serum, excludes active disease but a positive finding may only mean a previous infection.

13. *Management of premalignant and early malignant disease of the cervix*

INTRODUCTION

The treatment of squamous cervical intraepithelial neoplasia, microinvasive carcinoma and glandular intraepithelial neoplasia (cervical glandular atypia and adenocarcinoma *in situ*) should be tailored to meet the needs of individual patients and particular lesions. The place of cone biopsy, hysterectomy and the more recent conservative methods of local destruction in the current management of these lesions will be outlined. Newer approaches to improving the cone biopsy technique and efficiency, and reducing morbidity, will also be considered.

Glandular lesions will be considered separately, as they constitute a peculiar problem in that their natural history is less well understood, and occasionally they may involve the whole length of the endocervical canal.

KNIFE CONE BIOPSY

No woman with abnormal cervical cytology should be treated without prior colposcopic assessment. This applies to the primary surgical methods of management of cervical intraepithelial neoplasia, whether the choice of treatment is excision or ablation. It is logical to assume that the efficacy of a chosen method of treatment will be maximized when the topography of the individual lesion is known.

The terms 'cone biopsy' and 'conization' (see Chapter 9) are often used synonymously for a variety of surgical procedures, ranging from standardized biopsies with specially designed instruments, to large shaped cone/amputations of the cervix. Although originally cone biopsies were aimed at women with suspected early cancer, many of the early cones were used to treat benign cervical conditions. In 1938, Martzloff used cervical biopsy to detect the presence of premalignancy, which he described as 'carcinomatoid'.

Cone biopsy in the management of cervical intraepithelial neoplasia should always aim to achieve a combined diagnostic and therapeutic effect. Optimally, the tissue removed by the cone should include not only the abnormal epithelium, but also the whole transformation zone, including its caudal and cranial limits; that is, the original and new squamocolumnar junctions. Only in this way can a cone biopsy be deemed diagnostic and in turn therapeutic.

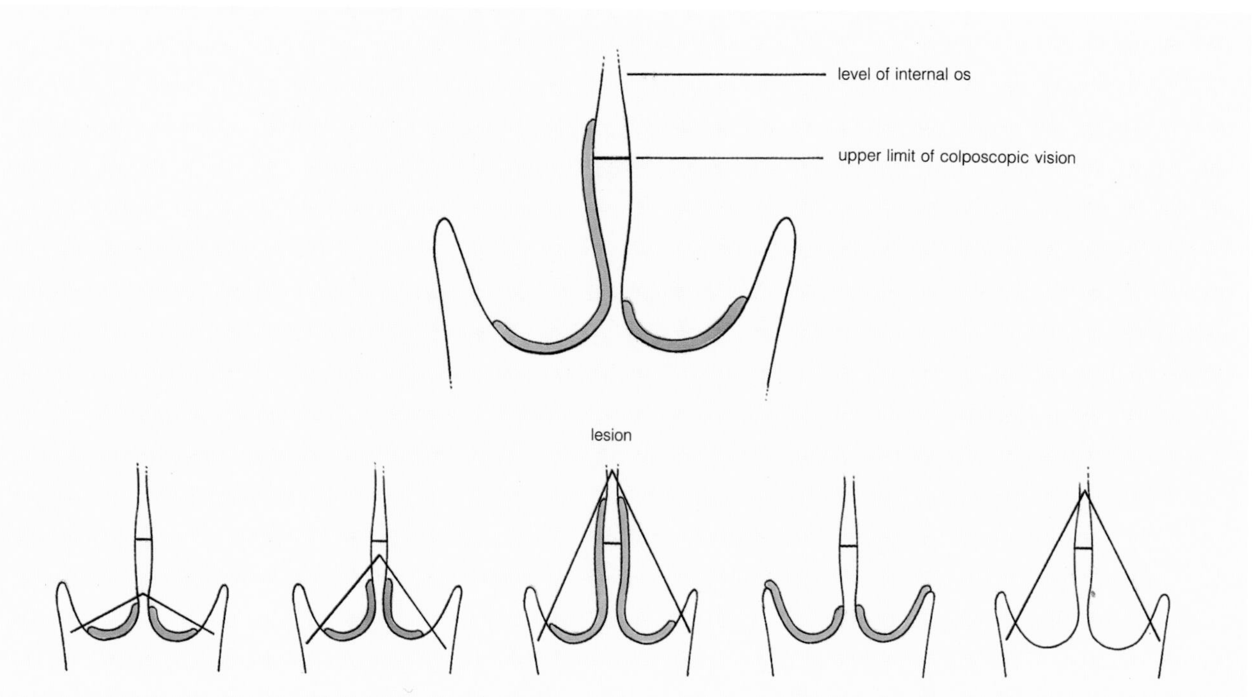

Fig. 13.1 Diagrammatic representation of classification of lesion topography after colposcopy. Lesion represented by bold line.

Indications for cone biopsy after colposcopy

In a majority of cases, colposcopic assessment in the presence of abnormal squamous cytology will allow accurate definition of the topography of the underlying lesion. Colposcopic findings will fall into one of the following categories (Fig. 13.1):

(a) The entire lesion and transformation zone will be visible with or without the aid of an endocervical speculum.
(b) The lesion will be located within the transformation zone, but its endocervical limit will extend into the cervical canal, within or without colposcopic vision.
(c) Either (a) or (b), together with vaginal extension of the lesion.
(d) There is no lesion detectable to account for the abnormal cytology.

The examination may have revealed colposcopic appearances not only consistent with cervical intraepithelial neoplasia, but also raising a suspicion of breach of the basement membrane due to microinvasive or frankly invasive carcinoma. Moreover, in a minority of cases the primary cervical lesion may be part of multifocal intraepithelial neoplastic change involving the vagina, vulva or perianal region.

In all categories, a histological diagnosis is essential before treatment or as part of it if an excisional biopsy is involved. Where an expert colposcopy service is available, lesions in category (a) are suited to target or punch biopsy, followed by local destruction (see below). Lesions in category (b) carry a risk of hidden invasive disease in the non-visible portion lying within the endocervical canal.

The main indications for diagnostic cone biopsy after colposcopic assessment are as follows:

1. The lesion and/or transformation zone extends into the cervical canal, outside the range of colposcopic appraisal.
2. There is repeated abnormal cytology, suggestive of neoplasia in the absence of colposcopic abnormality.
3. Cytology suggests a graver lesion than that seen at colposcopy.
4. Any suggestion of invasive disease from cytology, colposcopy or directed biopsy.
5. There are atypical glandular cells in the index cytology, indicating the possibility of glandular intraepithelial neoplasia or adenocarcinoma.
6. Abnormal histology of endocervical curettings.

Where the entire transformation zone and the abnormality itself are visible, a small, colposcopically tailored cone biopsy may be preferred to a locally destructive technique, as it carries the advantage of rendering all abnormal tissue available for histological study. In such cases, excision may be performed with the cold knife, carbon dioxide laser or large diathermy loop (LLETZ: large loop excision of the transformation zone; page 167).

Technique of knife cone biopsy

The optimal cone biopsy should remove the entire transformation zone. In all cases, colposcopy should allow accurate placing of the ectocervical circumferential incision, encompassing the lesion and all squamous epithelium containing evidence of underlying glandular activity, namely surface gland openings or Nabothian follicles. In most cases, the line of the old squamocolumnar junction may correspond to the outer edge of an acetowhite lesion. Sometimes, Schiller's test is used to define this ectocervical limit of an intraepithelial neoplastic lesion. However, it should be borne in mind that this test is associated with false positive and false negative correlations, as for example in cases of severe inflammation or oestrogen deficiency.

The major problem in cone biopsy is when the

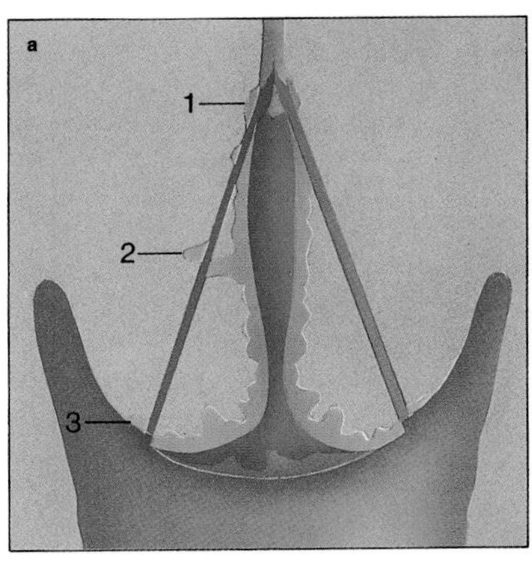

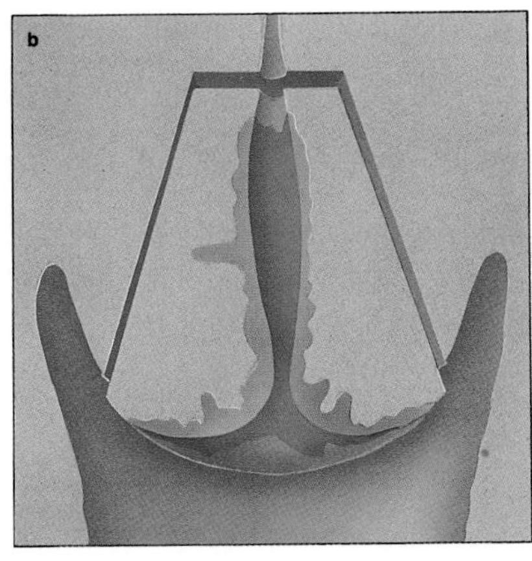

Fig. 13.2 (a) Possible sites for incomplete excision of cervical intraepithelial neoplasia. 1. Cone apex; 2. Glands in the stroma near the apex; 3. Ectocervical limit. **(b)** A truncated cone or cylinder should reduce problems at 2.

upper limit of the transformation zone or lesion is outside colposcopic vision, even with the aid of an endocervical speculum. In these circumstances, the actual length of the cervical canal requiring removal can only be a matter of conjecture.

Furthermore, cervical intraepithelial neoplasia may involve gland crypts to a depth of 4 mm on average below the surface of any aspect of the epithelium of the transformation zone. Therefore, if the apex of the cone is fashioned too narrowly, gland crypts affected by cervical intraepithelial neoplasia may be transected, leaving residual disease in the stroma of the cone bed. In theory, this may be avoided by removal of a cylindrical block of tissue or a truncated cone (Fig. 13.2).

OPERATIVE TECHNIQUE

This is an in-patient procedure, requiring general anaesthesia. There is little to be gained by prolonged postoperative hospitalization, and most patients are able to leave hospital soon after surgery. A number of surgical variations have been described; the following is a common approach.

Preliminary ligation of the cervical branches of the uterine arteries is achieved by placing lateral sutures deep on each side in the substance of the cervix. Anterior and posterior sutures may also be used. The ectocervical circumferential incision is then made with a Beaver blade, ensuring several millimetres of clearance of the outer limit of the transformation zone.

Handling the surface epithelium must be avoided. Focal bleeding points are individually ligated, or diathermy is applied. No attempt is made to cover the cone bed by any form of suturing of the cut edges, thus minimizing the risk of burying residual abnormal epithelium where removal of the primary lesion is subsequently seen to be incomplete. Apart from the removal of the whole length of the cervical canal at biopsy, any decision regarding optimal cone length to ensure complete removal of the transformation zone on its endocervical aspect, where the new squamocolumnar junction lies out of sight in the canal, can only be arbitrary. This is unless more recent approaches to visualization are employed (see below).

If adequate haemostasis has not been achieved, it is best to avoid suturing. The cone bed may be packed with a 5 cm-wide ribbon gauze, the tip of which has been soaked in proflavine in glycerine, or alternatively in Monsel's solution (see page 66). In a series of cone biopsies performed at the Northern General Hospital, Sheffield, Monsel's solution was the sole method of haemostasis, with no increase in haemorrhagic complications. The pack is removed on the following day, and the patient is discharged.

When the biopsy is completely removed without traumatizing the epithelium, a marker suture may be placed in the stroma at the '12 o'clock' position (Fig. 13.3) to allow orientation, and the biopsy is placed in fixative in a container prelabelled with the patient's name (see Chapter 9).

IMPROVING TECHNIQUE AND EFFICACY, REDUCING MORBIDITY: NEW APPROACHES

In some cases where cervical intraepithelial neoplasia extends into the endocervical canal, beyond the limits of colposcopic vision even with the aid of an endocervical speculum, cone biopsy that removes the entire length of the canal may be required. However, as cervical intraepithelial neoplasia often does not extend far into the canal, this approach may be excessively radical, especially for patients in the reproductive age group.

Moreover, large cone biopsies are associated with increased short- and long-term complications. Appropriate, individually tailored cone biopsies could be performed in these patients, where it is possible to assess the extent of involvement of the canal by cervical intraepithelial neoplasia. This would increase the efficacy of the operation, and reduce morbidity.

MICROCOLPOHYSTEROSCOPIC ASSESSMENT OF THE CANAL

The Hamou microcolpohysteroscope (Storz, supplied by Rimmer Bros, London, UK) has been used to determine the extent of involvement of the endocervical canal in patients undergoing cone biopsy (Figs 13.4 and 13.5). With this technique, the epithelium

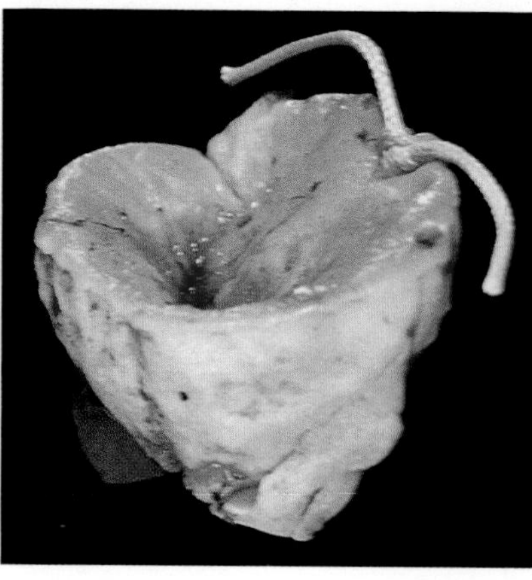

Fig. 13.3 Cone biopsy specimen with orientating marker stitch at '12 o'clock'.

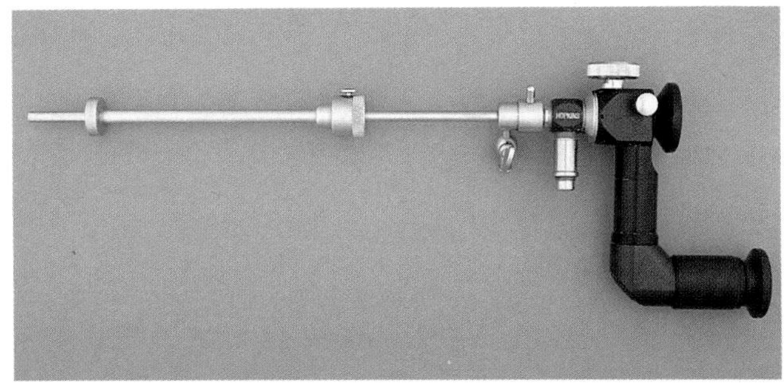

Fig. 13.4 Hamou microcolpohysteroscope, with additional metal sleeve to aid measurement of the distance to the squamocolumnar junction (see also Fig. 13.5). Reproduced by kind permission of the *British Journal of Obstetrics and Gynaecology*.

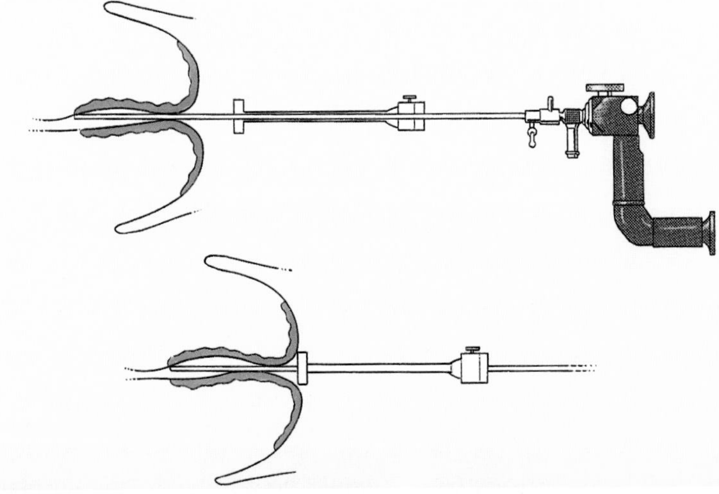

Fig. 13.5 Microcolpohysteroscopic measurement of the distance to the squamocolumnar junction. The junction is identified within the endocervical canal, and the metal sleeve is then pushed gently along the hysteroscope until the plastic washer is just resting on the cervix. Reproduced by kind permission of the *British Journal of Obstetrics and Gynaecology*.

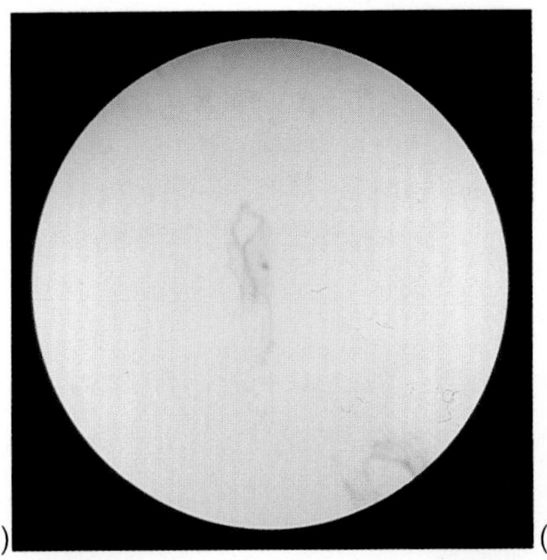

(a)

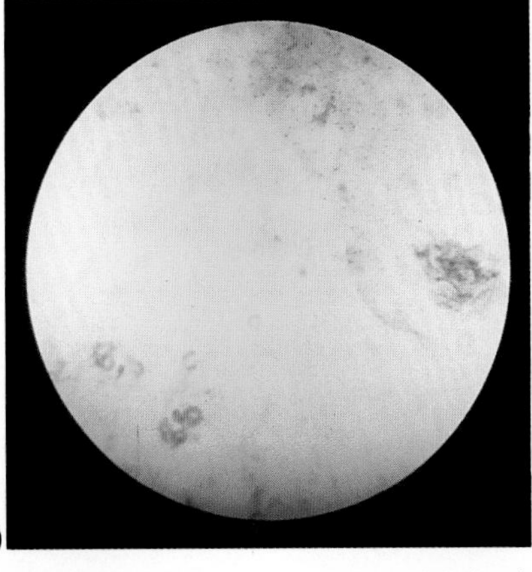

(b)

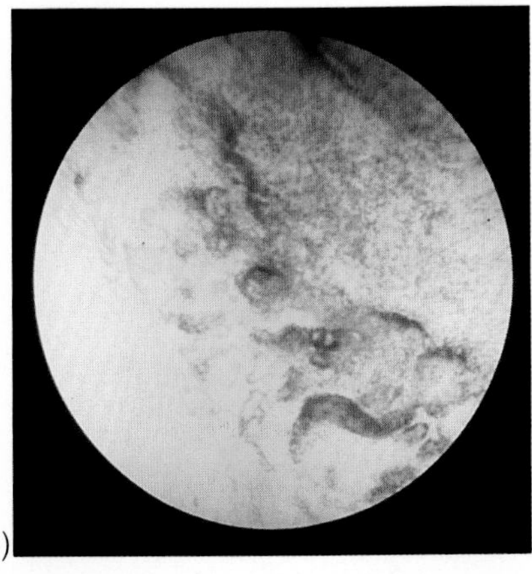

(c)

Fig. 13.6 Microcolpohysteroscopic in contact mode. (a) Looped capillaries in a single villus; note the absence of blue-stained squamous epithelium. **(b)** Normal squamous epithelium, top right; group of looped capillaries (indicating villi), bottom left; clear squamocolumnar junction visible. **(c)** Dyskaryotic squamous epithelium on the right; villi immediately to the left, indicating true squamocolumnar junction. Reproduced by kind permission of *Colposcopy and Gynecologic Laser Surgery*.

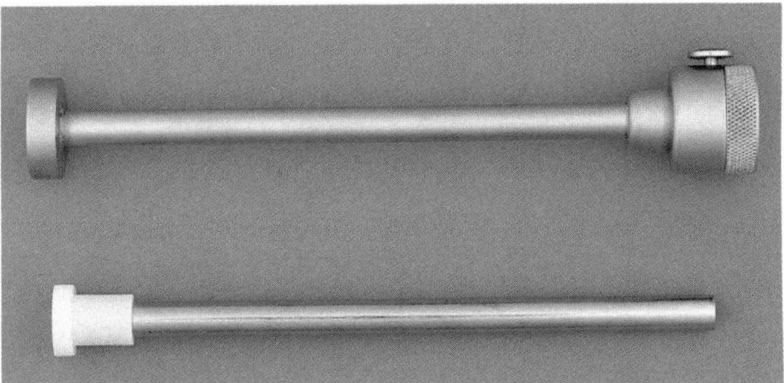

Fig. 13.7 Metal sleeves for use in microcolpohysteroscopic measurements: prototype (below) and commercially available type (Scaife endocervicometer) (above).

is first stained with Waterman's blue ink which, *in vivo*, is taken up only by squamous cells. The blue-stained epithelium is then visualized with the microcolpohysteroscope in the contact mode, with a 60-fold magnification and a resolution of 2 μm (Fig. 13.6).

When the highest point of the squamocolumnar junction within the canal is identified, its distance from the anatomical external os can be measured with the aid of a special sleeve with an expanded distal end (Fig. 13.7). Good correlation has been obtained between these measurements and subsequent histological assessment of the excised cone specimen. A considerable reduction in incomplete excision of neoplastic lesions is achieved, especially at the apex of the cone, when this method is employed to determine the appropriate cone length required in a given case.

LASER EXCISIONAL CONE BIOPSY

Knife excisional cone biopsy carries inherent morbidity, such as haemorrhage (primary and secondary) and cervical stenosis. One approach to minimizing these complications is to use the carbon dioxide laser, usually mounted on a colposcope, and with the micromanipulator as the cutting modality (Fig. 13.8(a)). Lateral cervical sutures may or may not be used to assist haemostasis.

Smaller excisional cones may be performed in this way on an out-patient basis, where a local anaesthetic is infiltrated under the cervical epithelium outside the lateral boundaries of the lesion (Fig. 13.8(b)). As a substitute for laser vaporization cone (see below), the excisional approach carries the advantage of preserving tissue for histopathological appraisal (Fig. 13.8(c)), which would be a safeguard against inadvertent vaporization of an unsuspected microinvasive lesion. In skilled hands, thermal artefact in the margins of the laser-excised cone specimen does not interfere with histopathological interpretation.

Haemorrhage, infection and cervical stenosis are not reported as a problem, and the reformed squamocolumnar junction is visible at colposcopic follow-up in a high percentage of cases; this is a clear advantage if residual disease is to be detected. In addition, laser excision cone may be combined with more superficial vaporization of the extension of the main central lesion beyond the acquired transformation zone, even so far as the vaginal fornices. Usually, such an extensive procedure would require general anaesthesia, and it would be difficult to contemplate this with the cold knife. The Nd:YAG laser, transmitted through a fine fibreoptic cable attached distally to an artificial sapphire tip which is contrived like a scalpel, has also been used as the cutting modality for excisional cones. This wavelength of laser light has a useful coagulative effect, and

(a)

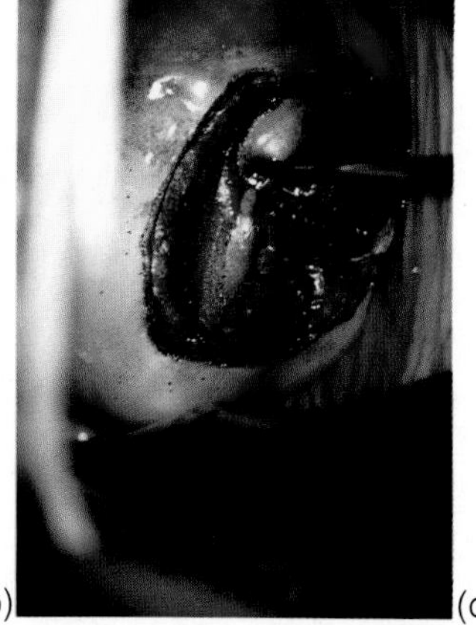
(b)

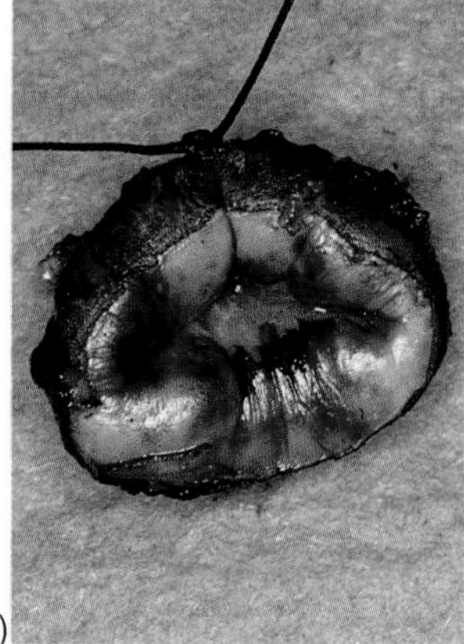
(c)

Fig. 13.8 (a) Carbon dioxide laser and colposcope combination. (b) Carbon dioxide excisional cone in progress. This shows the manipulating hook on the cervix which is stained with Waterman's blue for preoperative microcolpohysteroscopy. **(c)** Excised cone specimen showing minimal thermal trauma and marker stitch in place.

theoretically it should be associated with less intraoperative bleeding. However, the equipment is vastly expensive, safety aspects of its operation require meticulous care, and the method seems unlikely to find a place in routine conization except in the hands of a few enthusiasts.

LARGE LOOP EXCISION OF THE TRANSFORMATION ZONE

Excision of abnormal cervical epithelium by diathermy loop is based on an idea of Cartier who used a small diathermy loop to remove small pieces of cervical tissue for biopsy. The technique described by Prendiville, Cullimore and Norman (1989) involved a much larger loop which removed relatively large areas of cervical epithelium. The advantages of this procedure are outlined below:

1. Usually the procedure can be carried out on an out-patient basis, using local anaesthesia and a vasoconstrictor.
2. Bleeding is minimal.
3. Healing is rapid, with minimal fibrosis or stenosis.
4. The whole specimen can be sent for histological assessment, to discover any unsuspected invasive disease. This is an advantage, compared with the destructive methods which rely on a colposcopically directed biopsy or biopsies excluding areas of invasion before the destruction is carried out. However, while this is rarely a problem for the experienced colposcopist, for the less experienced the loop provides a very valuable safeguard against missing unsuspected invasion.
5. The histological specimen is processed in exactly the same way as a cone biopsy. Damage by the diathermy loop to the cut surface of the specimen is minimal and does not pose a problem to the pathologist.
6. The cost of the apparatus is relatively low; many operating theatres already possess diathermy equipment that would be suitable for this type of procedure (Fig. 13.9), and therefore the only expenditure would be that of the diathermy loops (Fig. 13.10).
7. The procedure can, if necessary, be carried out at the time of the first visit to a colposcopy clinic, thereby minimizing the number of visits the patient has to make and the hospital has to provide.

The technique of diathermy loop excision is very simple and can be summarized as follows (Figs 13.11 and 13.12): the cervix is visualized using a standard laser-adapted speculum, allowing smoke evacuation. The colposcopist delineates the area of abnormality to be removed. The local anaesthetic, combined with a vasoconstrictor, is injected at four points ('2, 5, 8 and 11 o'clock'). It usually takes about three minutes for the effects to take place; a useful endpoint is when the puncture marks caused by the needle stop bleeding. A loop is selected according to the size of the area to be excised. The loop is pushed into the normal tissue immediately lateral to the abnormality, at approximately '9 o'clock', and advanced to a depth of about 7–10 mm. The loop is then removed transversely from left to right, and exited on the other side of the cervix at a point lateral to the area to be excised. The base of the resulting crater is then coagulated by ball diathermy.

The wound is left open and the patient advised to

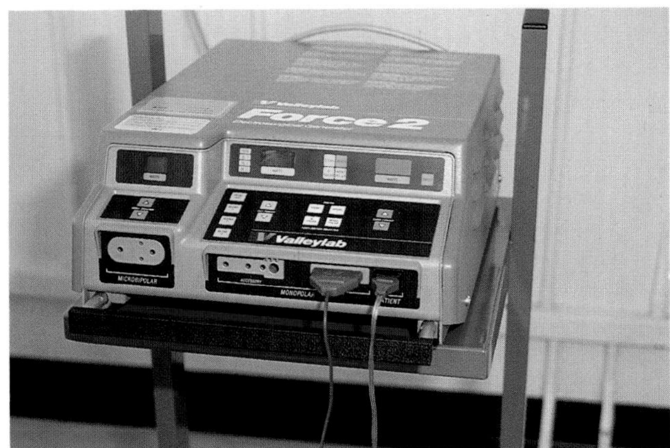

Fig. 13.9 Diathermy/coagulator console, suitable for diathermy loop excision.

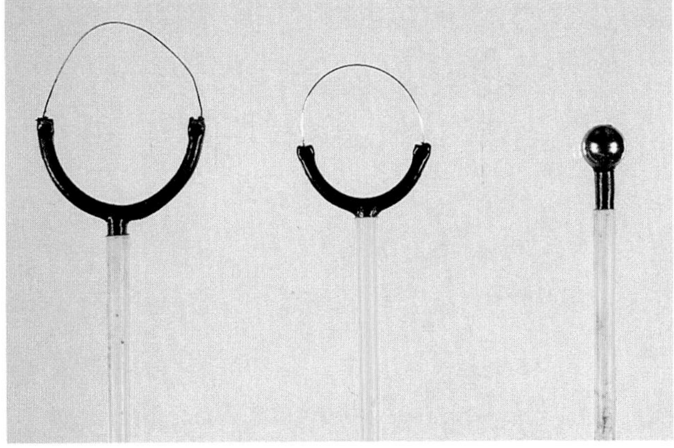

Fig. 13.10 Two sizes of diathermy loop for excision of the transformation zone, and a coagulation ball. Courtesy of Valleylab UK.

avoid intercourse or the use of tampons and douches for three weeks. It is rarely necessary to use a pack or haemostatic agent.

Excision of a transformation zone too large to be accommodated by a single sweep of the largest available loop can be achieved with several systematic sweeps.

Hysterectomy and treatment of cervical intraepithelial neoplasia

Currently, routine hysterectomy in the primary management of cervical intraepithelial neoplasia is rarely practised. Indications for the procedure are mainly relative: coexisting benign gynaecological problems, such as dysfunctional uterine bleeding, fibroids, uterovaginal prolapse, or patient request for sterilization. Histological confirmation of neoplasia by punch or cone biopsy should be obtained before hysterectomy.

In selected cases, hysterectomy may be decided upon where the resection margins of a cone biopsy specimen show significant abnormality. Follow-up cytology may indicate residual disease. However, even in such circumstances residual disease could be successfully treated with further cone biopsy or local destruction.

The lesion may extend on to the vaginal wall. Although a combined surgical and destructive technique may be used, hysterectomy may be the appropriate therapy in many cases. Colposcopy is essential to define the limits of the lesion and to establish the size of the vaginal cuff to be removed.

HYSTERECTOMY IN THE PRESENCE OF CERVICAL INTRAEPITHELIAL NEOPLASIA

Invasive carcinoma should first be excluded by colposcopically directed biopsy. The colposcopy allows clear characterization of the atypical transforma-

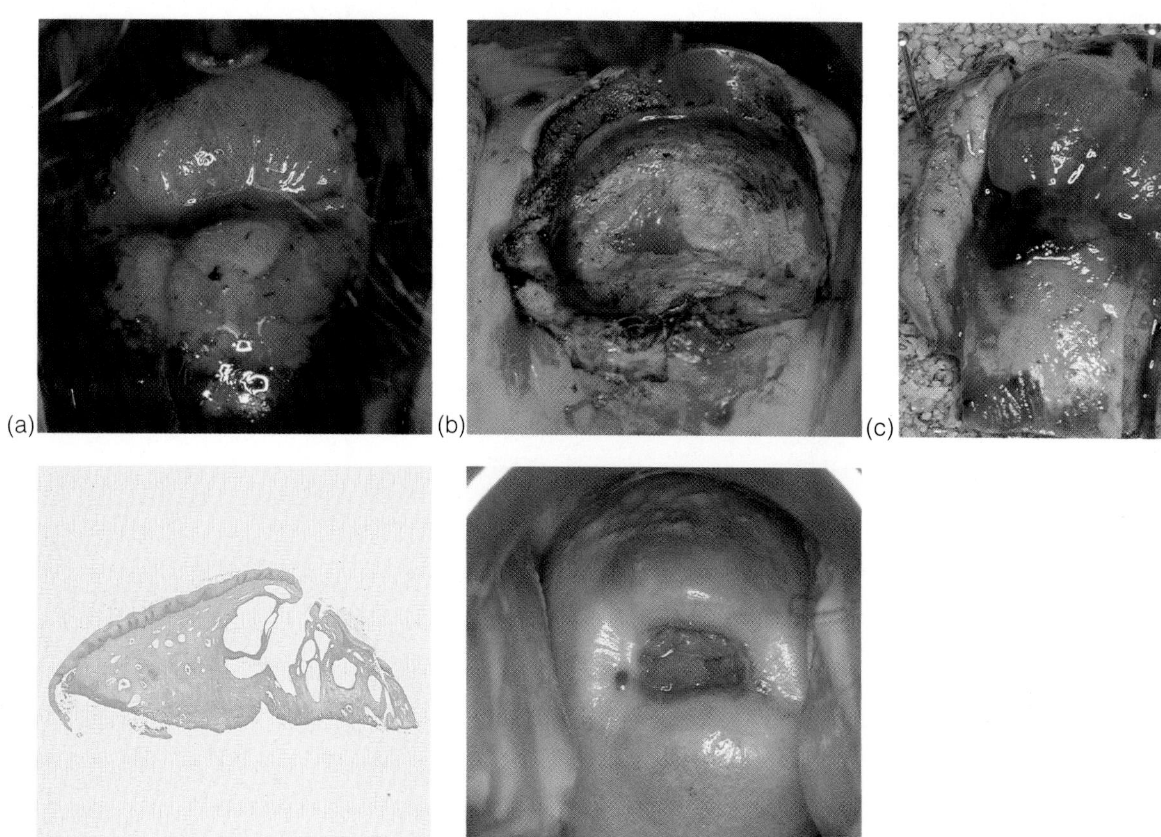

Fig. 13.11 Large loop excision of the transformation zone (LLETZ). (a) Cervix before LLETZ, with abnormal transformation zone highlighted with Lugol's iodine. **(b)** Completed LLETZ; large and deep cylindrical defect after four sweeps of the loop. **(c)** Loop biopsies reorientated and pinned to cork support. **(d)** Histopathological preparation of loop-excised tissue, showing good clearance of glands to 1 cm depth. **(e)** Same cervix four months after treatment. Well-healed cervix, with easily visible new squamocolumnar junction.

tion zone, which may extend on to the vaginal vault. This has been reported in 5–10% of cases. Preoperative histological assessment of such vaginal changes should be obtained by biopsy. Although the epithelium may show acetowhite change or exhibit non-staining in Schiller's test, it is frequently histologically benign.

If the cone biopsy precedes the hysterectomy, it may be best to defer the operation for about six weeks because of reported increased morbidity if the ab-

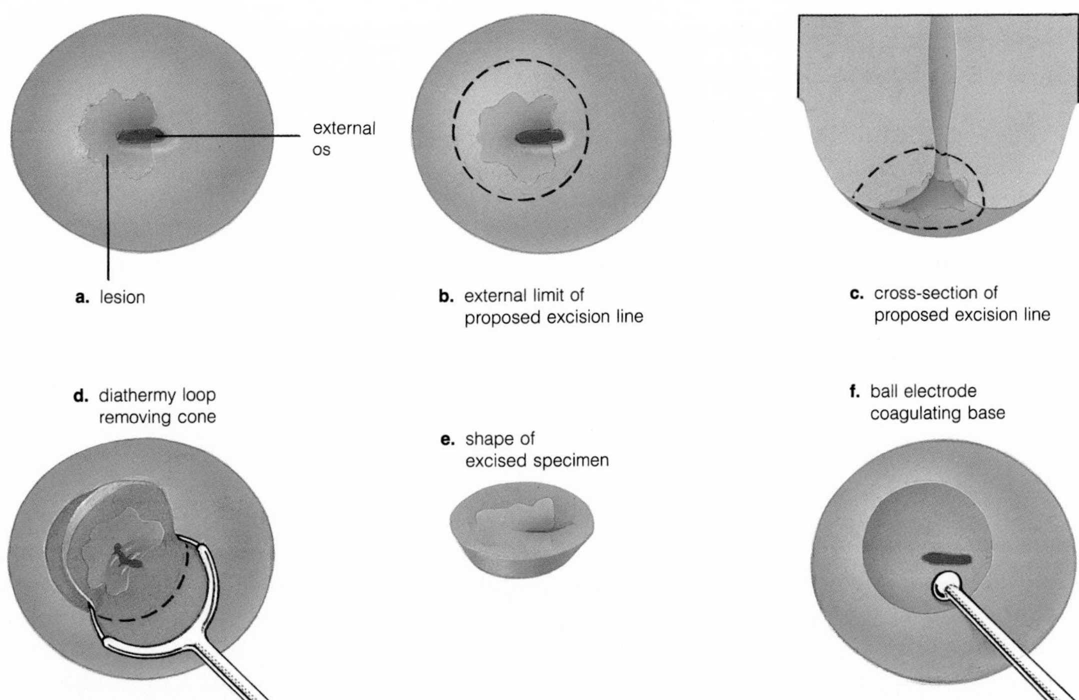

Fig. 13.12 Diagrammatic representation of LLETZ. (a) Lesion in red. **(b)** External limit of proposed excision. **(c)** Depth and contour of tissue to be excised. **(d)** Excision in progress. **(e)** Excised specimen. **(f)** Ball electrode coagulating base.

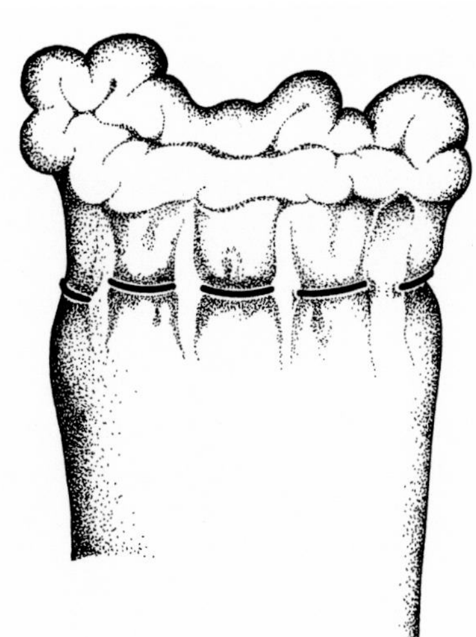

Fig. 13.13 Commonly used closure of the vaginal vault at hysterectomy using the mattress technique. There is a danger of burying sheets of cords of intraepithelial cells.

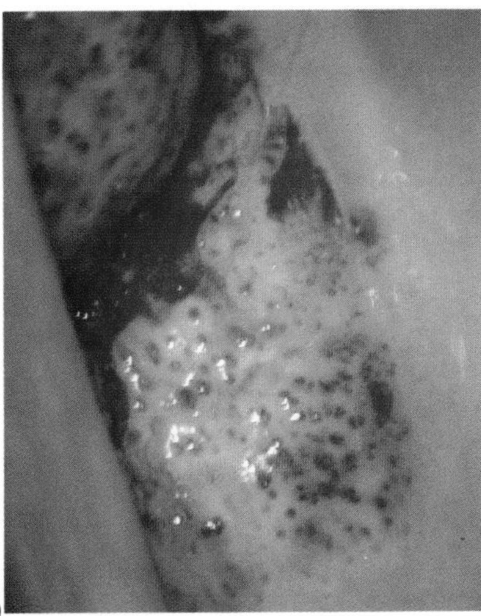
(a)

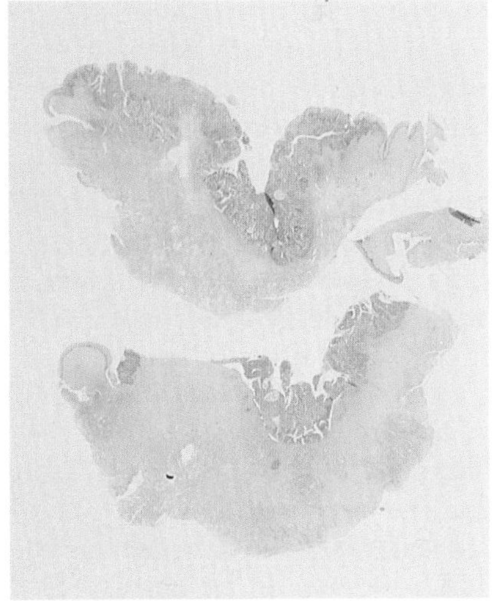
(b)

Fig. 13.14 (a) Acetowhite change with punctation around and in the old suture dimple at the reconstructed vaginal angle following hysterectomy. **(b)** Photomicrograph of excised dimples in (a), showing residual vaginal intraepithelial neoplasia extending to 7 mm below the surface.

dominal route is followed. If the vaginal route is chosen, the post-cone interval does not appear to matter. The route is a matter of personal choice or individual patient circumstances. In the majority of cases, simple hysterectomy is sufficient therapy, with or without removal of a cuff of vagina tailored to the individual lesion.

Several authors have emphasized the importance of the technique of closure of the vaginal vault. Mattress suturing of the vaginal edges (Fig. 13.13) and angles may result in any residual atypical epithelium being buried in the suture line, with colposcopic and cytological appraisal at follow-up rendered difficult or impossible (Fig. 13.14). While it is obviously important to ensure haemostasis, it is essential that the epithelium at the vault and angles after healing remain available for inspection. Invasive cancer has been reported to develop in these circumstances, where buried residual disease after hysterectomy remained.

Table 13.1 Selection criteria for local destruction

Assessment by skilled colposcopist
The whole transformation zone should be visible
Histopathology of punch biopsy from the most severe area of change should be available
No suspicion of invasive disease from cytology, colposcopy or histopathology
No suspicion of atypical glandular cells in the smear (i.e. suspected glandular intraepithelial neoplasia or carcinoma)

METHODS OF LOCAL DESTRUCTION

The introduction of diagnostic colposcopy allows the topography of a lesion to be defined (see Fig. 13.1) and, where appropriate, the epithelium bearing the most severe change to be biopsied and the lesion to be histologically characterized. The technique has also contributed to improved cure rates of treatment by the traditional surgical approach of cone biopsy and hysterectomy. In addition, it has allowed the introduction of more conservative methods of treatment of cervical intraepithelial neoplasia, which are especially relevant in the younger women who constitute a significant proportion of presenting patients. Furthermore, these newer techniques offer the advantage of being predominantly out-patient procedures, and may be carried out under local anaesthesia.

By definition, cervical intraepithelial neoplasia is a local disease. It does not involve the underlying stroma or the lymphatics. The concept of applying a local biophysical method to destroy the epithelium is attractive, provided that the three-dimensional nature of these intraepithelial lesions is borne in mind (i.e. the degree of potential gland involvement by the process), as well as the fact that the entire transformation zone should be destroyed, as all its squamous epithelial cells may have been at risk of exposure to the carcinogenic process. In effect, these biophysical methods must seek to produce the equivalent of a small, colposcopically directed excisional cone.

Selection of patients

Over the years, strict selection criteria have evolved and should be observed (Table 13.1). It is safer to manage patients or lesions not conforming to this checklist by excisional cone biopsy (see above). It should be noted that almost four in five women over the age of 45 years will have a transformation zone out of sight inside the canal, and therefore are likely to require excisional cone.

Methods of local destruction

Methods of local destruction presently available for the treatment of cervical squamous premalignancy are radical diathermy (the longest-established method), cryotherapy, laser vaporization cone, and cold coagulation. As already mentioned, all of these methods seek to achieve the same effect, and it is imperative that the rigorous selection criteria are applied in each case. Two other methods of treatment (see above), although not locally destructive as such, are also finding favour: (i) the laser excisional cone, and (ii) the large loop diathermy excision of the transformation zone. Both yield bulk tissue for histological examination, which is a clear advantage, especially in the exclusion of unsuspected microinvasive disease. Both methods may be used as out-patient alternatives to local destruction of the transformation zone in selected cases.

RADICAL ELECTROCOAGULATION DIATHERMY

Historically, this is the oldest of the local destructive techniques, developed by the Melbourne group under Chanen and Rome (1983). Its main drawback is that its radicality demands general anaesthesia or regional block, usually on an in-patient or day-case basis, although recently Chanen (1989) has reported a successful feasibility study of the method carried out under local anaesthesia.

After induction of anaesthesia, the patient is examined in the lithotomy position and the colposcopy repeated to confirm the original findings. Chanen recommends dilatation and curettage at this stage. Dilatation should help to counteract any tendency to post-treatment stenosis. The cervix is painted with Lugol's iodine (Fig. 13.15(a)). The needle electrode is then used to outline the transformation zone, with a series of insertions 2–3 mm beyond the iodine non-staining area. The entire transformation zone is then 'pepper-potted' with similar needle insertions at approximately 2 mm intervals (Fig. 13.15(b)). The needle is inserted to a depth of some 7–8 mm on each occasion, ensuring adequate destruction in depth to clear gland involvement.

On completion, the ball electrode is applied systematically to the entire surface of the circumscribed area (Fig. 13.15(c)). As considerable local heat is generated in the process, it is advisable to stop the procedure once or twice and douche the vagina and cervix with ice-cold saline.

It should be stressed that this radical destruction cannot be substituted by superficial diathermy or electrocautery, which will not guarantee a sufficiently deep destruction.

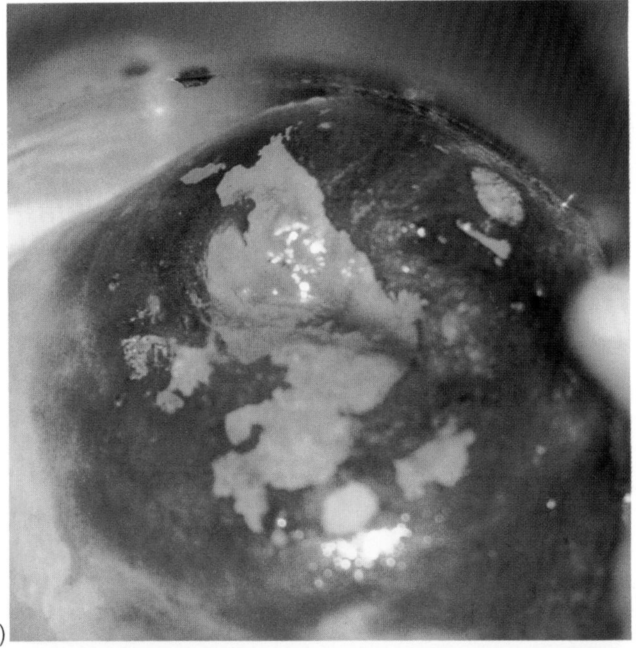
(a)

Fig. 13.15 Radical electrocoagulation diathermy. (a) Multifocal lesion highlighted with Lugol's iodine. **(b)** Transformation zone after multiple applications of needle electrode to 8 mm. **(c)** Procedure completed (after application of ball electrode).

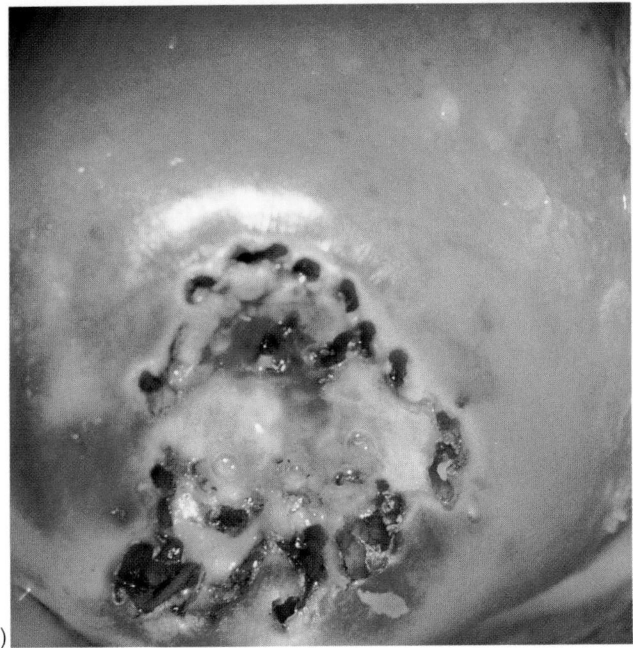
(b)

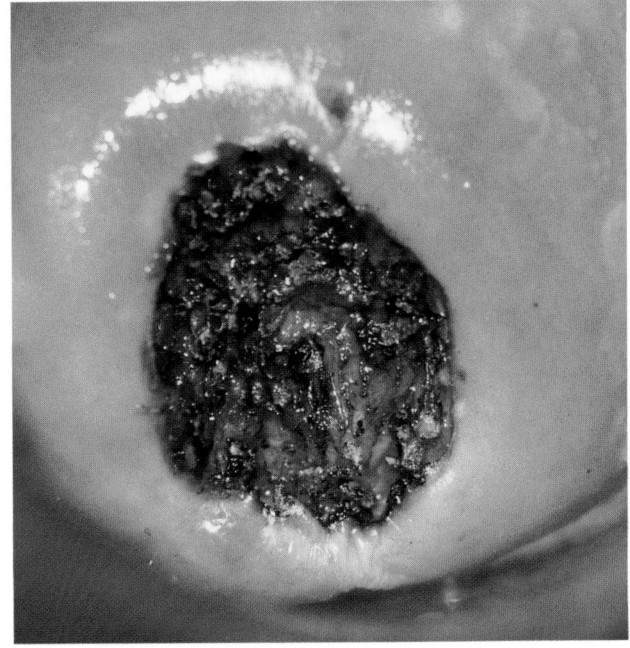
(c)

CRYOTHERAPY

Cryotherapy has also been used as a local destructive treatment for approximately two decades. The procedure is carried out on an out-patient basis, usually requiring no anaesthesia. The cervix is exposed, the earlier findings confirmed and the selected shape of cryoprobe applied and then freeze-generated (Fig. 13.16(a)), until the resultant iceball extends 4–5 mm beyond the periphery of the probe (Fig. 13.16(b)). Usually, a three-minute freeze followed by a five-minute thaw and a further three-minute freeze is recommended.

Reported cure rates with this method have been inferior to those of radical diathermy. In particular, the technique seems unsuitable for larger lesions (occupying half or more of the cervix) and high-grade lesions (CIN 3). Another less significant drawback is the complaint of a watery discharge which may persist for several weeks after treatment.

CARBON DIOXIDE LASER VAPORIZATION CONE

Carbon dioxide laser light is especially well suited to local destruction of cervical intraepithelial neoplasia. With a wavelength of 10.6 μm, it is predominantly absorbed by tissue water, either intra- or extracellular, with little reflection or transmission through the tissue as forward scatter. By the use of appropriate power density at a focal point equivalent to that of the colposcope used to direct the beam, vaporization of tissue is achieved with a coagulative effect. An articulated arm brings the energy from the laser console to a precision micromanipulator which is attached to the front of the colposcope, and the carbon dioxide beam (invisible to the naked eye) is directed over the epithelial surface to be vaporized, with the aid of a visible red helium neon aiming beam.

The treatment is well tolerated, with a local anaesthetic injected subepithelially beyond the boundary of the lesion, and is performed under direct colposcopic control. Carbon dioxide laser vaporization offers the maximum degree of precision in tissue destruction, as the diameter of the beam is around 1.5–2 mm.

A cylinder of tissue is vaporized to the desired depth, which is usually 8–10 mm (Fig. 13.17). On completion, the depth of the crater can be measured with precision, which is not possible with any of the other methods of local destruction and is a clear advantage. Another positive feature of this technique is the ability to continue the vaporization process more superficially, to include any extension of the lesion on to the vaginal fornices. Healing is swift, with some epithelial covering present after three weeks. There is little or no necrotic debris, and therefore post-treatment discharge is minimal.

(a)
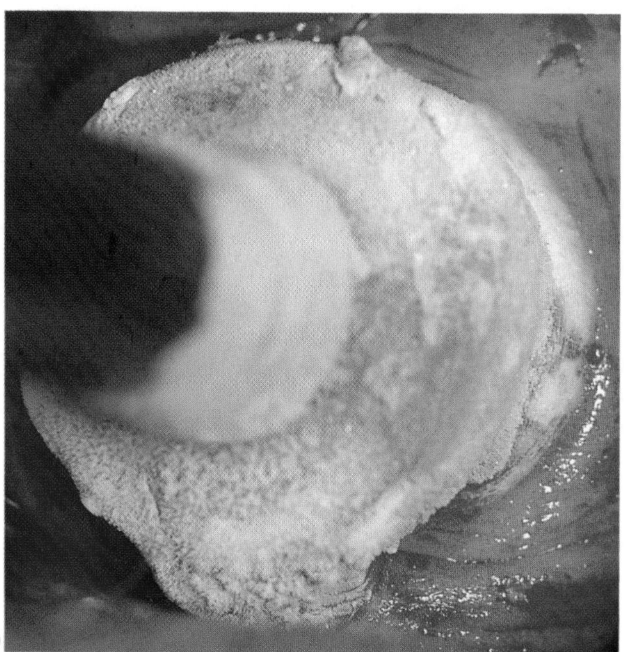

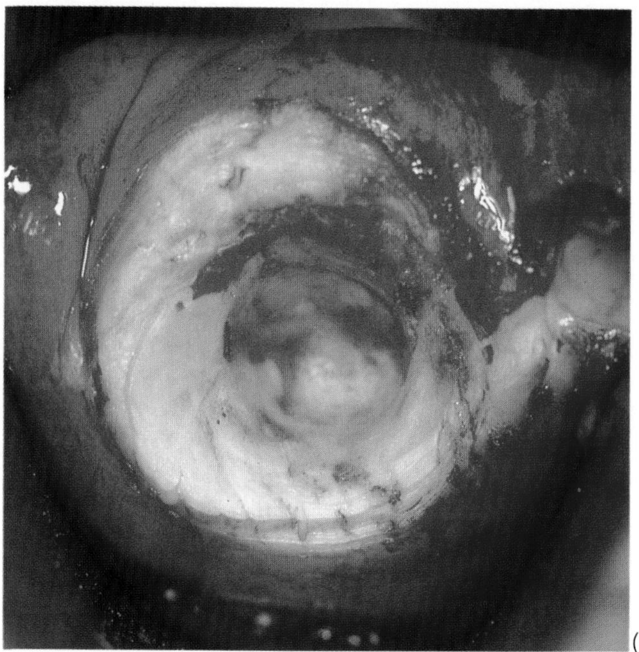
(b)

Fig. 13.16 Cryosurgical destruction of the transformation zone. (a) Probe applied and cryofreeze in progress. **(b)** Iceball effect following removal of probe upon completion.

COLD COAGULATION

The original cold coagulation apparatus was designed and used by Semm to treat benign lesions. The name 'cold coagulator' (Fig. 13.18(a)) is a misnomer, as the Teflon-coated thermosounds are heated to a temperature of 100°C. Various sizes and shapes of sound or probe are available to suit the macroanatomy of individual cervices and topography of lesions (Fig. 13.18(b)).

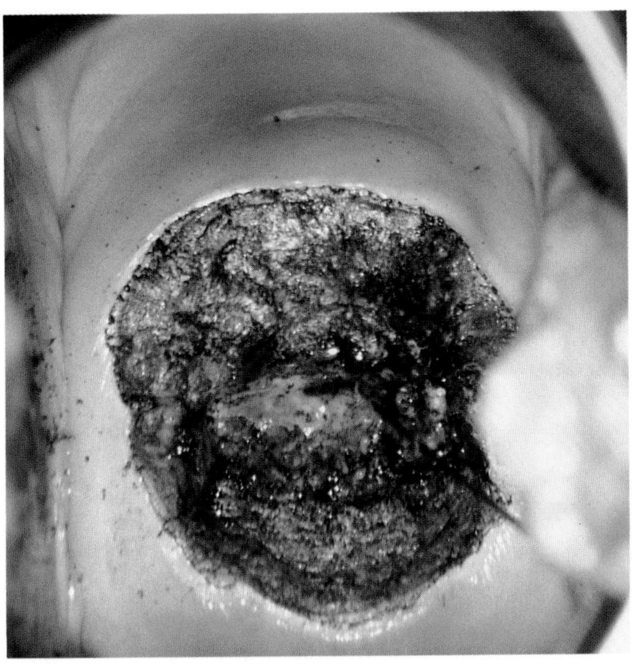

Fig. 13.17 Cylindrical defect on cervix upon completion of carbon dioxide laser vaporization cone for cervical intraepithelial neoplasia.

The procedure is performed on an out-patient basis, is well tolerated and usually requires no local anaesthesia, although some pelvic cramp-like discomfort may be experienced. The aim is to destroy the entire transformation zone (Fig. 13.19(a)), using overlapping areas of coagulation if required, and including the lower endocervix. The average treatment time is 100 seconds, with each application of the probe lasting 20 seconds. When the probe is removed, a blistered appearance is noted and the superficial overlying epithelium is usually detached (Fig. 13.19(b)). As a result, it is virtually impossible to quantify the true depth of destruction achieved (Fig. 13.19(c)), which is a serious disadvantage of the method. In addition, there is postoperative discharge from the slough that is created by this process.

Results of local destruction

The success of locally destructive methods in 'curing' cervical intraepithelial neoplasia, based on relatively short-term evidence of lack of residual or recurrent intraepithelial disease, seems to be very similar for the different techniques; it is in excess of 90%, and over 95% in some series. This compares favourably with the results of cold knife excisional biopsy and even simple hysterectomy. However, it would be a mistake to compare data from such dissimilar methods. Women subjected to treatment with local destruction represent a very carefully selected group. Most series report long-term results of the traditional surgical excisional methods dating from the days when all women and all cervical lesions were similarly treated. Moreover, a 'cure' is considered real when there is long-term evidence that

(a)

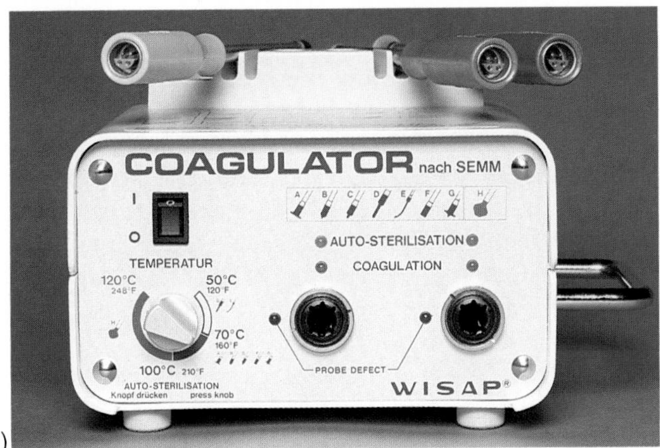

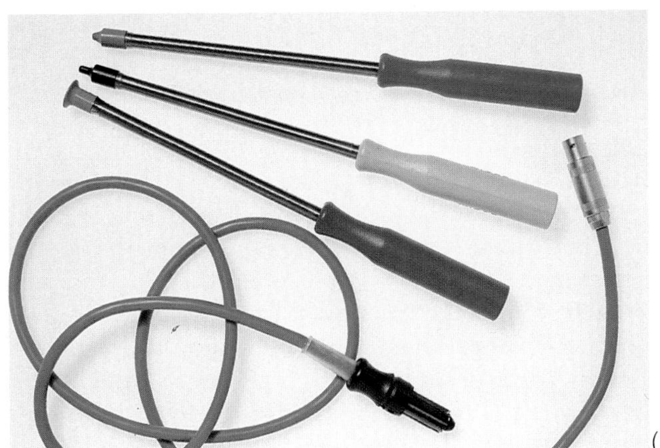

(b)

Fig. 13.18 (a) Semm cold coagulator. (b) Various shapes of Teflon-coated thermosounds for use with Semm cold coagulator.

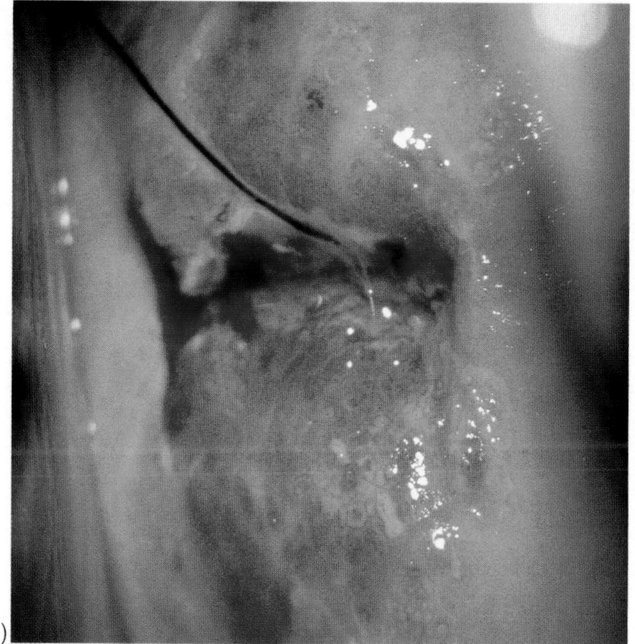

(a)

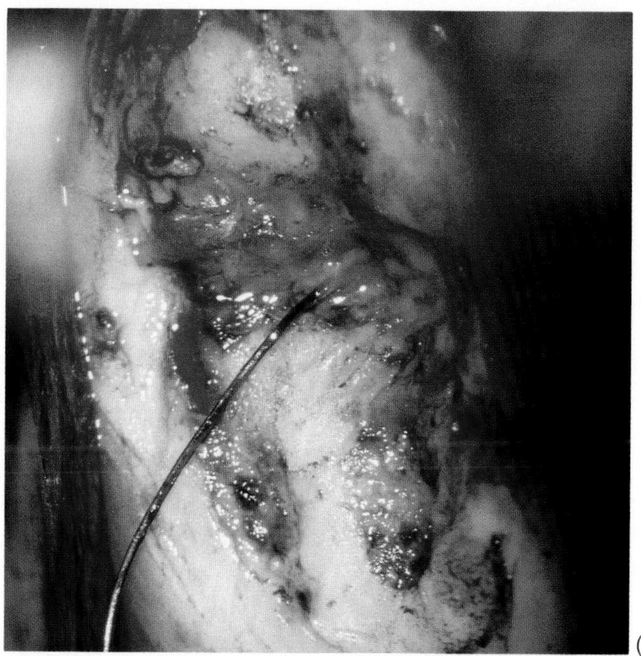

(b)

Fig. 13.19 Local destruction of cervical intraepithelial neoplasia using Semm cold coagulator. (a) Pre-treatment transformation zone; note the intrauterine contraceptive device *in situ*. **(b)** Coagulated transformation zone upon completion of treatment; note that the area is denuded of epithelium which has blistered off. **(c)** Same cervix after healing. Courtesy of Dr I D Duncan.

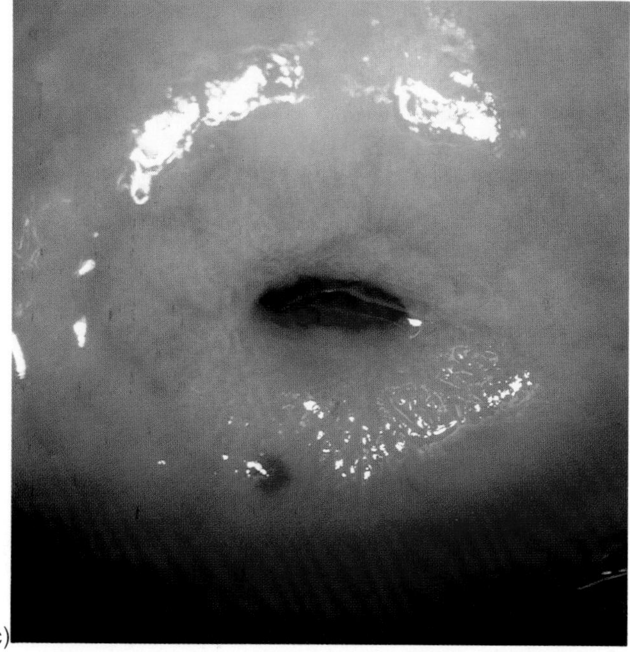

(c)

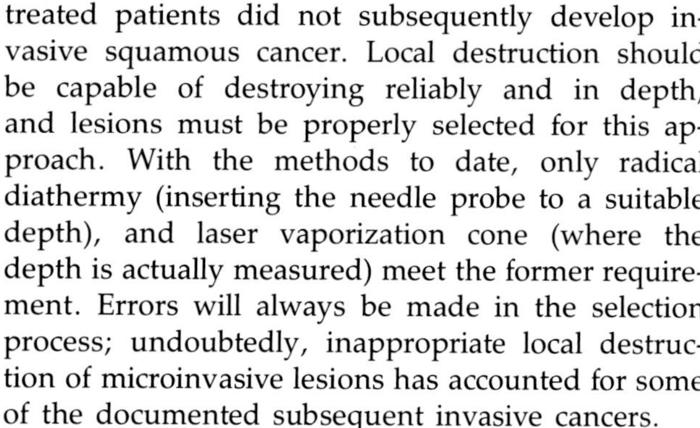

treated patients did not subsequently develop invasive squamous cancer. Local destruction should be capable of destroying reliably and in depth, and lesions must be properly selected for this approach. With the methods to date, only radical diathermy (inserting the needle probe to a suitable depth), and laser vaporization cone (where the depth is actually measured) meet the former requirement. Errors will always be made in the selection process; undoubtedly, inappropriate local destruction of microinvasive lesions has accounted for some of the documented subsequent invasive cancers.

Reports are beginning to appear of invasive cancer following all local destructive methods. Fortunately, at present, the incidence seems no greater than for cone biopsy or even hysterectomy. Nevertheless, these cases underline the need for continuing vigilance, adherence to strict selection criteria and proper evaluation of new methods before they can be widely applied on a routine basis.

Where local destructive methods fail, as evidenced by cytological, colposcopic or histological suspicion of residual disease, there is a current view that the next step should be excision rather than further destruction. This trend is based on accumulating experience of repeat treatments and subsequent development of invasion.

In spite of these difficulties, it seems clear from studies to date that, with locally destructive methods, it is possible to retain the cervix and its function in a woman of reproductive age, without reducing the efficacy of treatment for cervical intraepithelial neoplasia.

EXCISION OR DESTRUCTION?

Excision of CIN using hysterectomy and then cone biopsy formed the basis of treatment for a good number of years. The place for these procedures at the present time has been elaborated earlier. The newer treatment techniques have brought considerable advantage to the patient, being by and large out-patient procedures performed under local anaesthesia, and with reduced complications. They achieve their effect by either **destruction** or **excision** of the atypical transformation zone, along with any associated underlying gland involvement by CIN, much in the manner of knife cone biopsy, in carefully selected circumstances, particularly when destruction is chosen (Table 13.1).

The major criticism of local destructive techniques, however, is that full histopathological appraisal of the lesion is not possible, especially the exclusion of any previously unsuspected early invasive process. Some maintain that cytology, colposcopy and colposcopically directed biopsy cannot with certainty always exclude invasion, and advocate the use of an excisional method where treatment is planned. There is some evidence that colposcopic awareness of the presence of microinvasion is dependent upon the depth of invasion, the figure of 1 mm being critical, as up to this depth the lesion is more likely to go undetected. Whether this is of any importance in the long-term objective of preventing frankly invasive disease, were the atypical transformation zone to be destroyed, would be virtually impossible to study in a proper scientific, prospective randomized controlled trial.

Any method of treatment of CIN carries a small risk of the subsequent development of frankly invasive cancer, whether the method is destructive or excisional. The destructive methods described above have been in use for some considerable time, and cancers developing after such treatment have been described. At the present time this event does not appear to occur any more frequently than after knife cone biopsy. Cancer after LLETZ for CIN has also been described, although the technique has been in use for a relatively short time, and it is not yet possible to assess what the final incidence of cancer after such treatment will be. Regardless, the debate as to whether any excisional method, such as LLETZ or laser excisional cone, is preferable to destruction continues. While these two excisional methods are readily performed as an out-patient procedure, it is not surprising that they are being performed with increasing frequency.

Cervical squamous intraepithelial neoplasia is known sometimes to be associated with coexisting cervical intraglandular neoplasia. If the latter is suspected also from the index cytology report, then an adequate knife cone biopsy is indicated. If the glandular element of the disease is unsuspected, then use of an excisional method as opposed to a locally destructive one might be advantageous, by yielding a specimen for full histopathological appraisal.

MANAGEMENT OF MICROINVASIVE SQUAMOUS DISEASE

The difficulties over the histopathological aspects of stage Ia or microinvasive carcinoma of the cervix have already been discussed in Chapter 10. Microinvasive carcinomas are paradoxical in that they have all the hallmarks of invasive disease with breach of the basement membrane, and yet they are rarely associated with metastases.

In selecting women for less radical treatment, Coppleson holds that it is possible to recognize the odd case where spread may already have occurred by an integration of colposcopic observations into the pretreatment protocol. Before conservative treatment is employed, the following criteria should be met:

1. The lesion should not be colposcopically overt.
2. The colposcopic survey should be adequate.
3. The lesion should not present with atypical vessels, large tumour area or deep histological penetration and vascular space involvement.
4. Frank, crumbling tumour of the cervical canal should be excluded by endocervical curettage.

Conservative, simple hysterectomy, belonging to the less radical procedures, can be recommended in most cases. The ovaries need not be removed in the interests of curing the cancer. There is no strong case in favour of vaginal over abdominal approaches, although some gynaecologists may prefer the latter as it gives the opportunity of detecting any enlarged draining lymph nodes, although this is unlikely. There is no indication for extending the operation to remove a cuff of vagina, except in the unusual case where extension of the cervical lesion on to the vaginal fornix has occurred, and this should have been recognized at the preoperative colposcopic assessment. In such a case, particular care must be taken over the histopathological measurements, as the large surface area may exclude the lesion from the category of microinvasion.

While the above approach has been shown to be satisfactory, it would be of great disadvantage to the younger woman who still plans to start or increase her family. There is mounting evidence that, in these circumstances, a large cone biopsy, at least 2 cm long, may be safely considered as adequate therapy.

Alternatively, amputation of the cervix has been suggested, but this has no advantage over conization, provided that the latter has achieved eradication of disease, i.e. the cone margins have been shown to be free of disease, both intraepithelial and invasive. In this group of women, the use of preconization microcolpohysteroscopic evaluation of the degree of canal involvement, with tailoring of the length of the cone to suit particular requirements, would be an advantage (see above).

MANAGEMENT OF CERVICAL GLANDULAR INTRAEPITHELIAL NEOPLASIA

The management of cervical gladular intraepithelial neoplasia (CGIN), presents as difficult a challenge to

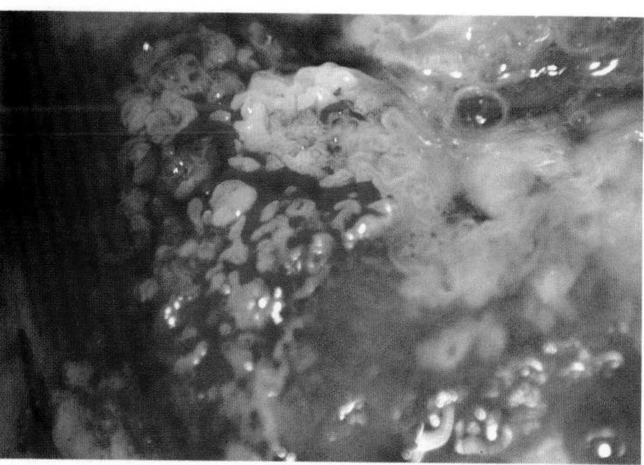

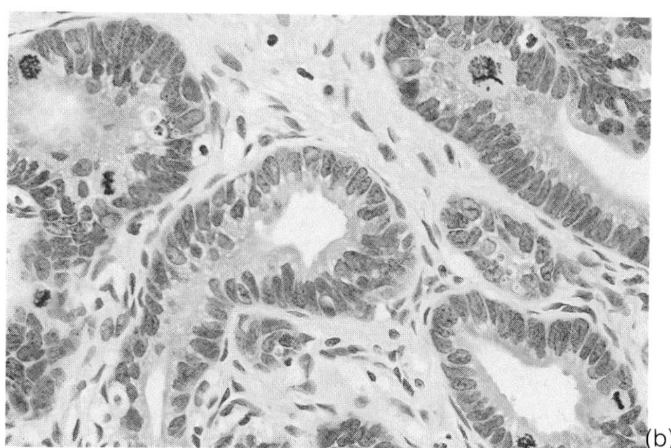

Fig. 13.20 (a) Colposcopic findings in a case of squamous dyskaryosis in a smear. Note acetowhite change in the transformation zone (right), along with large hypertrophic villi with some showing acetowhite change and contact bleeding (left). **(b)** Histopathology of the same cervix showing high-grade cervical glandular intraepithelial neoplasia. Mitotic figures are numerous and one is of abnormal configuration.

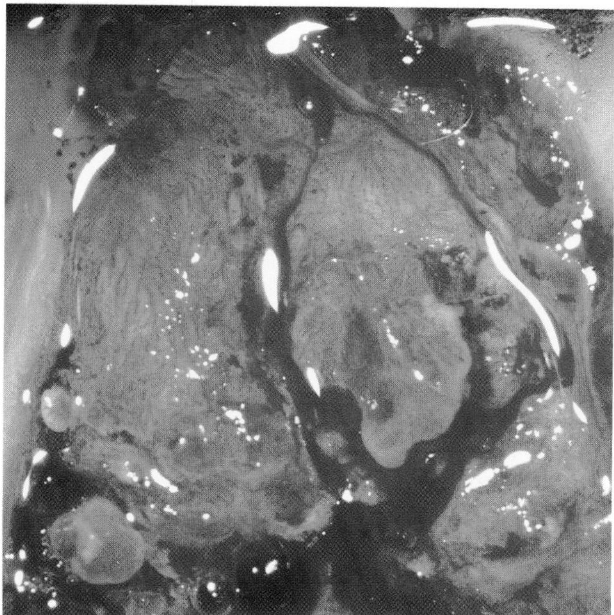

Fig. 13.21 Colposcopy reveals large, hypertrophic, partly fused villi in the external os, with contact bleeding. Histopathology showed adenocarcinoma *in situ* with early invasion.

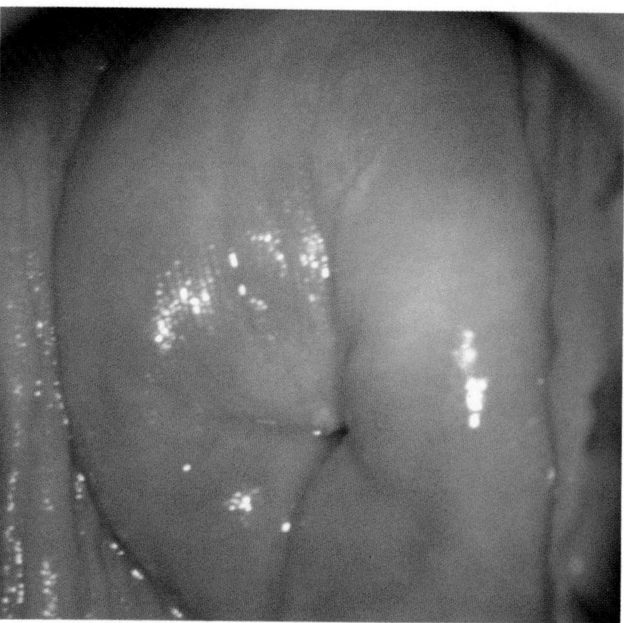

Fig. 13.22 Marked stenosis of the external os following cone biopsy. This renders endocervical cytology sampling difficult.

the clinician as does their detection and histological definition to the cytologist and pathologist. Undoubtedly, many cases of CGIN are detected incidentally in cone biopsy specimens performed for suspected squamous neoplasia (Fig. 13.20). In addition, cytologists seem to have an increased awareness of exfoliated atypical glandular cells in screening smears.

Management

These premalignant lesions will be located in the field of cervical columnar epithelium. This includes columnar epithelium lying in the depths of crypts, or beneath squamous metaplastic epithelium in the glands of the transformation zone, and from the squamocolumnar junction to the upper limit of the endocervical canal at the internal os.

The abnormal epithelium may lie substantially beneath the surface. Thus, it is impossible to scrutinize colposcopically the entire target epithelium; indeed, any visible columnar epithelium is likely to represent a very small fraction of the whole. Furthermore, even on rare occasions where a glandular colposcopic abnormality is identified (Fig. 13.21), it is not possible to confirm whether the whole problem is a single focus, as a multifocal disposition is also described.

It is clear that the only way of fully investigating the target epithelium is to have the entire length of the endocervical canal along with the transformation zone available for histological examination. This would involve a large cone biopsy removing the entire length of the canal, or alternatively a hysterectomy specimen, neither of which may always be appropriate. Therefore, the questions are raised as to whether a smaller cone biopsy which identifies a source lesion (or lesions) and whose excision margins are free of disease may be considered adequate treatment; or whether hysterectomy with excision of the whole cervical canal should be an obligatory next step.

The management dilemma hinges on our incomplete knowledge of the natural history of CGIN; the inappropriateness of total extirpation of the uterus for younger women who undoubtedly are now presenting with the problem; and our uncertainty over the adequacy of cytology to identify ongoing exfoliation of abnormal glandular cells, especially if there are potential sampling difficulties (i.e. due to stenosis following an antecedent cone).

In the latter circumstances it would seem prudent to use one of the newer sampling devices, such as the Cytobrush or the Aylesbury spatula (see page 54), for optimal collection of large numbers of columnar cells from the cervical canal, provided that this is readily accessible (see page 182).

Sometimes it may not be unreasonable to follow a conservative approach of observation without treatment, for example in the elderly or medically unfit patient. Also, where some additional gynaecological problem of a benign nature accompanies the CGIN (such as fibroids, dysfunctional uterine bleeding or a request for sterilization), it may be wiser to proceed to hysterectomy, following the index cone biopsy that defined the premalignant nature of the disease and excluded invasion.

The same may apply to the older woman who has completed her family, although even in these circumstances removal of the uterus may be excessive. It is in relation to the younger woman that the real management dilemma arises. Here, the information from clinical studies is not available to allow clear recommendations. At present, the following seems a reasonable approach.

Regardless of age, in the presence of atypical glandular cells in the smear, a diagnostic cone biopsy is indicated following colposcopy which, although unlikely to be helpful with the glandular lesion, may help to exclude any coincident cervical intraepithelial neoplasia. In the younger woman with a vested interest in future child bearing, this may be limited to removing 2 cm of the canal. It is unlikely that middle trimester abortion or preterm delivery in subsequent pregnancy is associated with this procedure. If the margins of the excision are free of the CGIN, then no immediate further treatment is recommended, provided that follow-up smears remain free of atypical glandular cells.

Where cone margins are involved, and the disease is apparently multifocal, hysterectomy would be indicated in the older woman, and seriously considered in the younger, although repeat cone biopsy may be a reasonable first option.

The mainstay of follow-up is cytology, frequently in the first two years (four-monthly) and annually thereafter. After cone biopsy, both ectocervical and endocervical specimens are advisable (Fig. 13.22). Even after hysterectomy, vault smears at the same intervals are suggested. If atypical glandular cells reappear (see Fig. 11.24), further biopsy is indicated in the form of a repeat cone, hysterectomy, or full-thickness biopsy from the vault if the uterus has already been removed.

Clarification of these difficult management issues will only come from appropriate clinical studies. These must be based on multicentre protocols so that sufficient numbers of cases are available for proper analysis. Finally, detection of a *de novo* primary lesion and of persistent or recurrent disease would be improved if a suitable cytological marker for the atypical glandular cell could be found in these selected cases.

14. *Follow-up after treatment of cervical disease*

REGENERATING/HEALING EPITHELIUM

Histological features

Re-epithelialization may take place in a variety of ways following treatment of cervical intraepithelial neoplasia, in spite of whether ablation or excision was the mode employed. Ideally, the treated surface will be covered by mature squamous epithelium within three weeks. Initially, this epithelium is of an important type, and consists of cells migrating from both edges of the treated area as well as from residual gland crypts (Fig. 14.1).

In an acid environment, differentiation and maturation into squamous epithelium will be encouraged. Quite often the maturation process of this new squamous epithelium will be impaired, and thus 'healing' epithelium, morphologically similar to immature squamous epithelium, will cover a small or large part of the treated area (Figs 14.2 and 14.3).

Consequently, the histopathologist is likely to encounter exactly the same difficulties in arriving at a differential diagnosis between healing epithelium and residual cervical intraepithelial neoplasia (see page 34), as in distinguishing between mature metaplastic squamous epithelium and cervical intra-

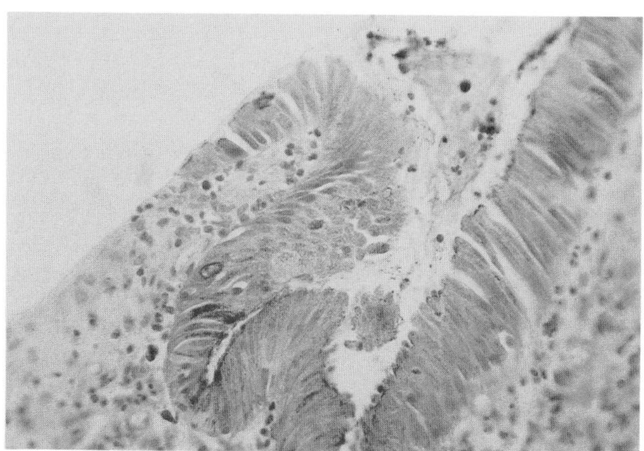

Fig. 14.1 Cervix healing after laser vaporization cone. Regeneration of squamous epithelium by metaplasia from columnar epithelium in gland crypts in the cone bed.

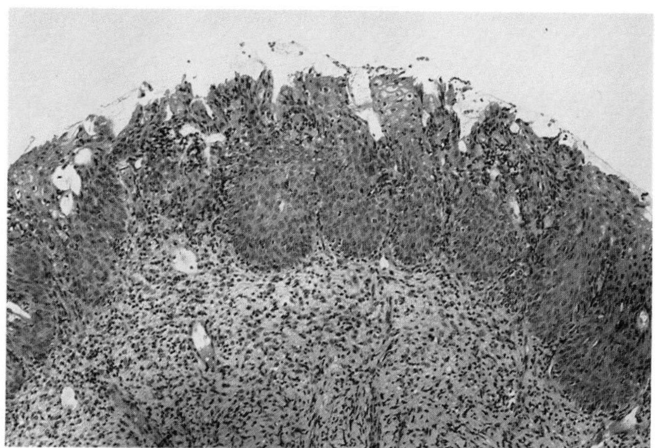

Fig. 14.2 Healing epithelium following laser vaporization. The epithelium shows virtually no maturation; the appearances are very similar to those of immature squamous metaplasia.

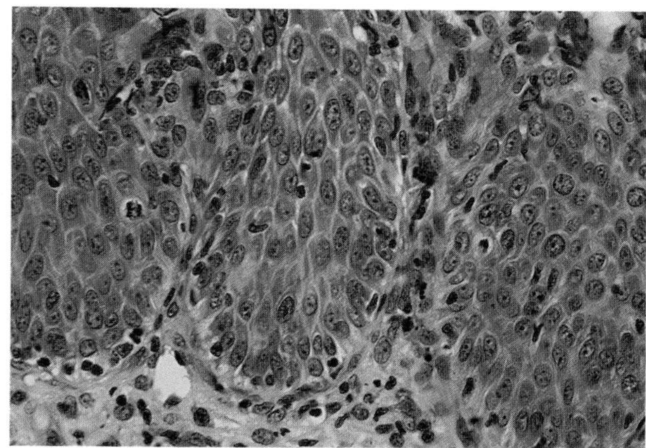

Fig. 14.3 Healing epithelium following laser vaporization. The nuclei are enlarged and show prominent nucleoli. They are uniform in shape, size and staining. Mitotic figures are infrequent and normal in configuration.

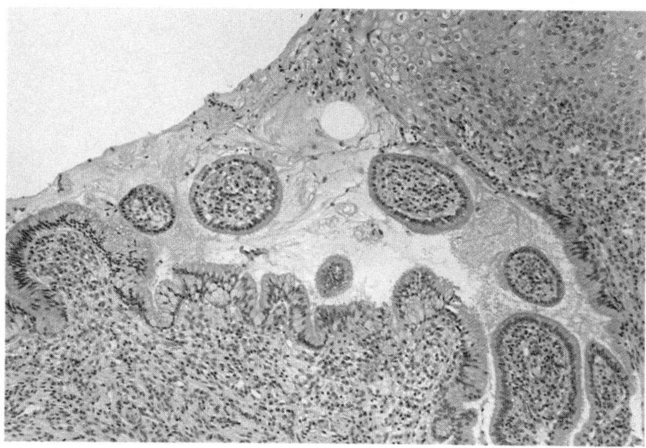

Fig. 14.4 Columnar epithelium growing far out on the ectocervix, following laser vaporization of a large area.

epithelial neoplasia. This difficulty is compounded by the colposcopic impression that this epithelium, which is frequently acetowhite, represents residual disease (see below).

In circumstances that encourage an alkaline environment, the epithelium will frequently heal with islands of granulation on the surface. This is more likely to occur if very large areas are treated, where islands of villous, columnar, endocervical-type epithelium may be found on the ectocervix, or in the vaginal fornices, amounting almost to an iatrogenic vaginal adenosis. Biopsy of these areas will show inflamed but otherwise normal 'endocervical' tissue (Fig. 14.4).

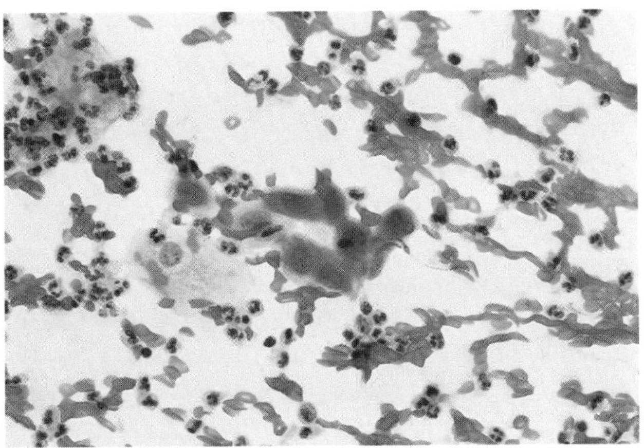

Fig. 14.5 Regeneration and healing. The cells in the centre are showing enlarged nuclei with some hyperchromasia but an even chromatin pattern and granular, pink-staining cytoplasm, similar to the appearances seen in squamous metaplasia.

Cytological features

On most occasions, the cellular changes associated with regeneration and healing are easily recognized since the features are similar to those of immature squamous metaplasia, and in most instances it may be difficult to make a cytological distinction (Fig. 14.5).

Healing following ablation of cervical intraepithelial neoplasia, particularly if laser vaporization has been used, can be rapid. The cytologist is faced with difficulties in making a differential diagnosis between healing or regenerating epithelium and residual intraepithelial neoplasia (Fig. 14.6), as are the histopathologist and colposcopist. The difficulties are compounded where the regenerative process is part of a chronic inflammatory response. This is probably one of the most significant areas where serious errors can be made in cytology, by failing to make the correct differential diagnosis between regenerative change and severe dyskaryosis or even invasive carcinoma (Fig. 14.7).

The cells may show nuclear enlargement with hyperchromasia and a prominent chromatin pattern. There is a homogeneous appearance to the cytoplasm, which appears blue or green in immature cells and pink in the more mature forms.

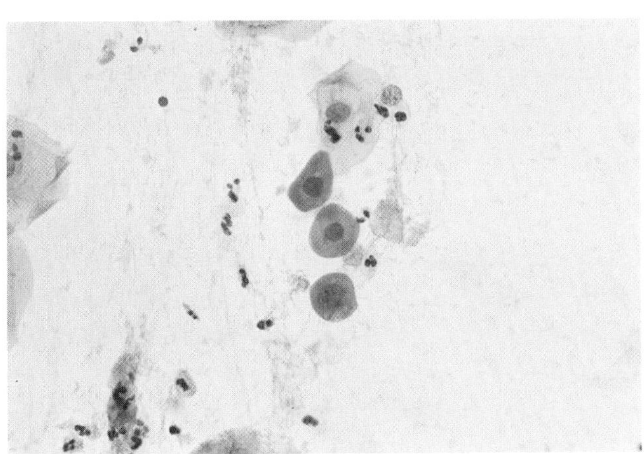

Fig. 14.6 Regeneration and healing. In this example, the nuclei are showing a marked hyperchromasia with coarse chromatin and dense blue–green cytoplasm. The distinction from dyskaryosis can be difficult.

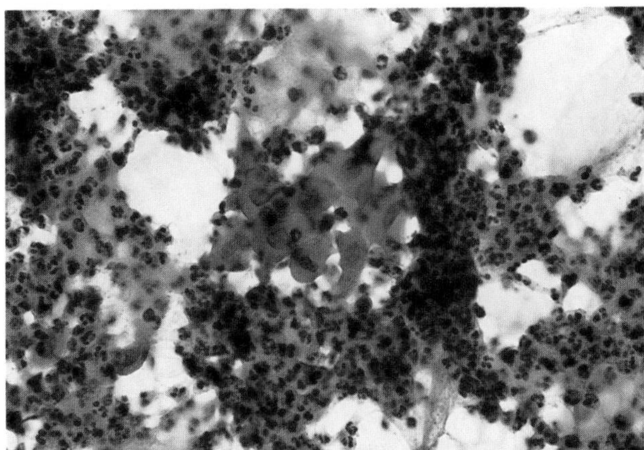

Fig. 14.7 Regeneration and healing. The cells in the centre show a pale-stained but irregular chromatin pattern. There is evidence of a chronic inflammatory response.

HEALING COMPLICATIONS

Stenosis

Cervical stenosis is reported after knife cone biopsy in about 1–4% of cases (Fig. 14.8). This is a much underrated complication, which may present as menstrual dysfunction or dysmenorrhoea. In severe cases, where occlusion of the canal is total (Fig. 14.9), amenorrhoea will result. This may be more common in women over 35 years of age as a result of the greater endocervical involvement by cervical intraepithelial neoplasia in this group, necessitating a larger cone biopsy to effect cure. Apart from the symptoms of stenosis, there is a further problem in following up the treated intraepithelial neoplasia: poor cell sampling may be obtained by the cytology spatula, and it may not even be possible to pass a fine endocervical brush if the os is too tight. The implications of not detecting residual disease are obvious, and if the os is completely sealed the patient may be at considerable potential risk in this respect. In women of child-bearing age, severe grades of stenosis may cause dystocia in subsequent pregnancy and labour. In older women, or where child bearing is complete, resorting to hysterectomy may be necessary in order to deal with the problem.

The traditional approach to the treatment of cervical stenosis involves vigorous dilatation of the cervix under general anaesthesia. However, this is often ineffective as stenosis tends to recur with time. More recently, the procedure of carbon dioxide laser endocervicectomy has been described, where the stenotic segment of the lower canal, often limited to only a few millimetres, is excised using the precision afforded by this modality. The results of this procedure seem fairly successful, as restenosis has been less frequently observed.

Stenosis has also been reported after local destruction for cervical intraepithelial neoplasia. It is recognized after cryotherapy and electrocoagulation diathermy (less than 1% of cases in Chanen's series), but is seen less after laser vaporization and excisional cones.

Data for cold coagulation do not suggest an excess of the complication, and information regarding stenosis after large loop excision of the transformation zone is not yet available. The problem in these circumstances may be managed in the same way as was described for following cone biopsy.

Squamocolumnar junction

Following treatment of cervical intraepithelial neoplasia by local destruction or excision, the squamocolumnar junction may (Fig. 14.11) or may not (Fig. 14.10) be visible and available for

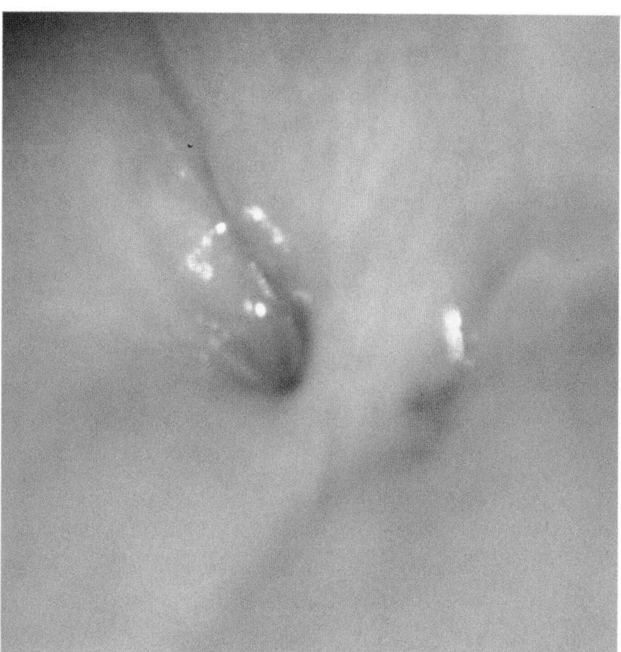

Fig. 14.8 Cervical stenosis after knife cone biopsy. The new squamocolumnar junction lies out of sight beyond the tiny os.

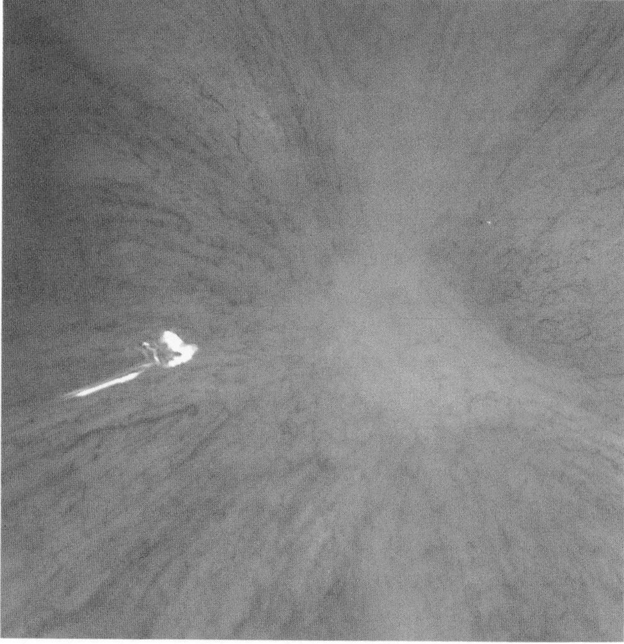

Fig. 14.9 Total stenosis of new external os after treatment.

Where significant disease is suspected from cytology, with no colposcopically overt lesion identified, then an excisional cone would be prudent. Occasionally, in the face of subsequent disease after a primary cone in the postmenopausal woman, further conization may be deemed technically impossible as the cervical remnant may be too small. In these circumstances, although harbouring the risk that unsuspected invasive disease may be encountered, hysterectomy may be the only feasible recourse.

Where subsequent disease arises after local destruction of cervical intraepithelial neoplasia, another attempt with this method may be permissible if the lesion is visible and confirmed on biopsy, and invasion has been excluded. In all cases considered for repeat local destruction, the lesion should be subjected to the same selection criteria used at the initial choice of the method.

Another problem is the continued exfoliation of dyskaryotic cells seen in vaginal vault smears, where hysterectomy had been the treatment of choice for cervical intraepithelial neoplasia: one of the main difficulties is to exclude buried vaginal intraepithelial neoplasia or invasive disease within the vault scar tissue. This question is addressed in Chapter 15.

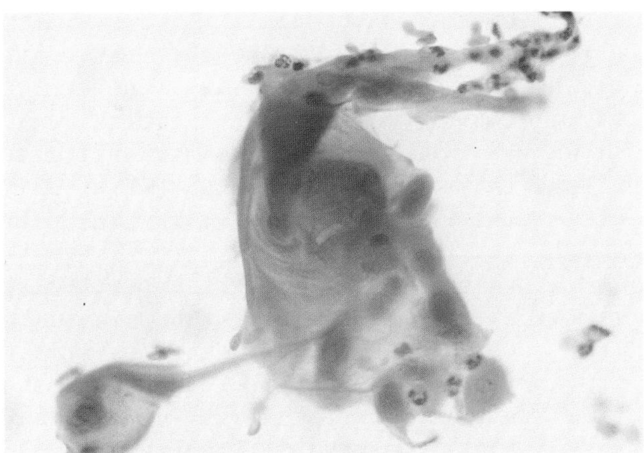

Fig. 14.20 Radiation changes. The cells are showing gross enlargement and variation in shape. The large cells appear bloated, and although the nuclei are enlarged the chromatin has a bland appearance. The cytoplasm is showing vacuolization characteristic of radiation change.

POST-RADIATION CHANGES

Cytology

Treatment by radiotherapy is not appropriate for the majority of conditions dealt with in this book. However, occasionally smears will be taken from women who have had radiotherapy in the recent past, and it is relevant to mention at this point the cellular changes that may be seen.

Changes associated with radiation, which can be seen in non-neoplastic squamous epithelial cells, include multinucleation and bizarre forms with gross cellular enlargement. Frequently, the nuclei are pale-stained and have a characteristic wrinkled appearance (Fig. 14.20). It is important that the cytologist is alerted to the fact that radiation treatment had been employed, as these features can be confused with dyskaryosis or malignancy.

Colposcopy

Following radiotherapy, the epithelium becomes relatively thin and atrophic, so that the subepithelial

Fig. 14.21 Radiation changes. Note the prominent but regularly branching vessels.

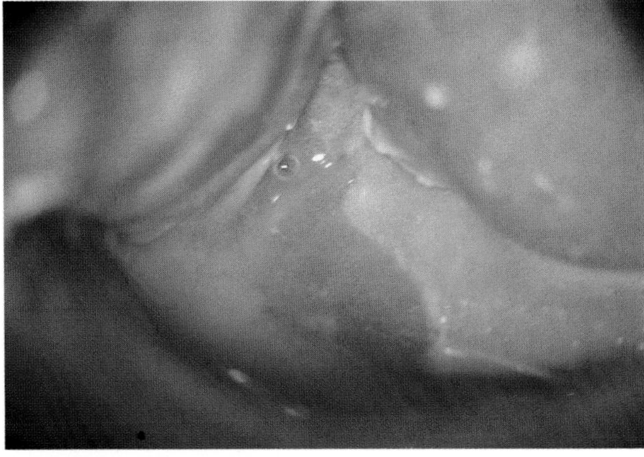

Fig. 14.22 Post-radiation. Avascular necrosis is seen at the vaginal vault.

vessels may become clearly visible. The smaller vessels occasionally disappear, leaving only the larger vessels. The latter may be irregular and tortuous, and are sometimes dilated such that the inexperienced colposcopist may mistake them for vessels suggestive of invasive disease (Fig. 14.21). This misinterpretation is even more likely if the cytologist has already reported the presence of abnormal cells. Occasionally there may even be an avascular necrosis (Fig. 14.22).

TIMING OF VISITS

It is traditional for patients to be seen for a postoperative review approximately six weeks following gynaecological surgery, but after treatment for cervical intraepithelial neoplasia this can be counterproductive. If the patient is examined within a few weeks of treatment, regenerating cervical epithelium may have cytological and colposcopic features suggestive of persistent disease, whereas over a further few weeks these changes will disappear leaving a perfectly normal, mature squamous epithelium.

Another consideration is that visits to the clinic that are more frequent than necessary may cause concern and inconvenience to the patient, also generating extra work for the hospital and clinic staff. Many centres have shown that for the average patient there is nothing to be gained by following up too soon or too frequently. However, if the first visit is delayed for a very long time, the colposcopist may miss persistent disease that requires further treatment. In the case of cervical intraepithelial neoplasia there is usually no major problem, but if the persistent disease is unsuspected invasive carcinoma or adenocarcinoma *in situ*, a delay could prove serious.

A number of centres arrange the first follow-up visit at four to six months, or approximately one year after surgery, followed by annual smears. The subsequent frequency at which the patient is seen depends on local circumstances and will vary between one- and three-year intervals. Ideally, at the time of follow-up visits particular care must be taken to obtain cytology samples from the endocervical canal as well as from the ectocervix, especially if the pathologist has reported a suspicion of incomplete excision of the lesion.

Place of colposcopy

Combined colposcopic and cytological follow-up will allow the colposcopist to detect persistent or recurrent disease with great accuracy. It has been estimated that a single cervical smear will prove to be a false negative in approximately 10–20% of cases, and the same applies to colposcopy. However, with the two techniques combined, the false negative rate drops to 2–3%. Although it would seem ideal to combine cytology with colposcopy at each follow-up visit, the sheer weight of numbers of patients attending most colposcopy clinics makes this an unattainable goal, and a compromise may have to be reached.

In the case of cervical intraepithelial neoplasia, a combined cytological and colposcopic assessment at four months (and afterwards perhaps once a year) can be followed by cytology alone, with the proviso that if an abnormal smear is obtained at any time in the future, colposcopic examination should be instigated. This follow-up regimen also presupposes that the colposcopist can visualize the cervix adequately and, if necessary, take an endocervical sample.

If the original lesion is thought to have been incompletely excised, or where features of early stromal invasion or microinvasion are detected, a combined cytological and colposcopic assessment should be considered for the first five years.

15. *Vaginal intraepithelial neoplasia*

HISTOLOGY

Vaginal intraepithelial neoplasia (VAIN) is far less common than its cervical counterpart. It is most frequently seen in association with cervical intraepithelial neoplasia, sometimes as an extension of it. More usually, it is seen in the vaginal vault following hysterectomy for treatment of cervical intraepithelial neoplasia, where the line of excision has not been sufficiently wide to remove an unsuspected vaginal extension of it.

Less frequently, vaginal intraepithelial neoplasia may be found in the vagina at a site distant from the cervix; the cervix itself may be entirely normal.

The histological features (Figs 15.1–15.3) are very similar to those of cervical intraepithelial neoplasia. All possible variants are seen in the vagina, such

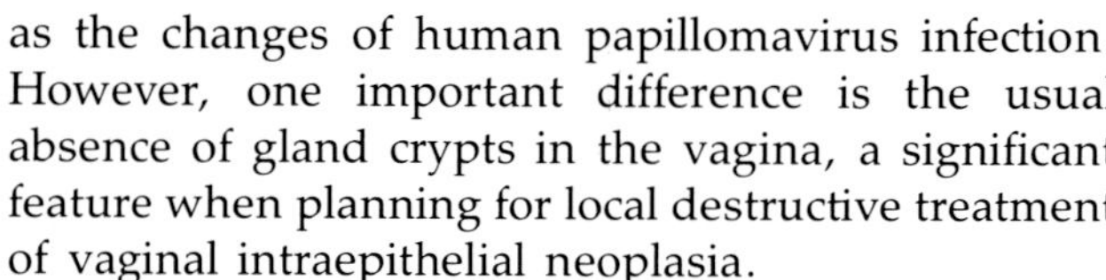

as the changes of human papillomavirus infection. However, one important difference is the usual absence of gland crypts in the vagina, a significant feature when planning for local destructive treatment of vaginal intraepithelial neoplasia.

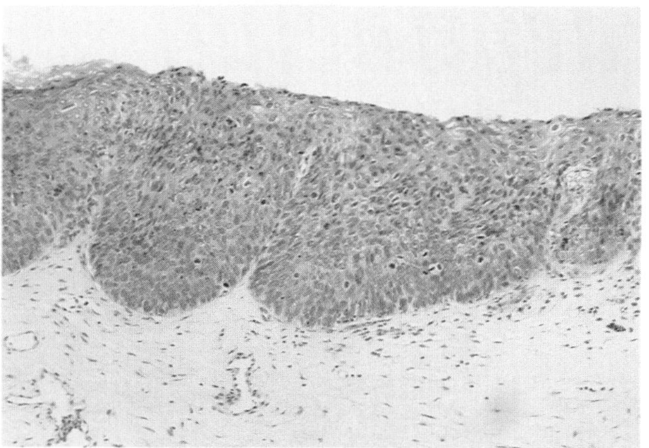

Fig. 15.1 VAIN 3. The appearances are identical to those of CIN 3, with loss of differentiation and nuclear abnormalities.

CYTOLOGY

The cytological features are similar to those of cervical intraepithelial neoplasia. The changes associated with human papillomavirus may also be seen, either alone or in combination with vaginal intraepithelial neoplasia (Figs 15.4–15.7).

COLPOSCOPY

When assessing a patient with a cervical intraepithelial lesion, the colposcopist must always consider whether the lesion extends beyond the cervix into the vagina. Vaginal extension of cervical intraepithelial neoplasia will occur in approximately 1.5% of cases, and should be taken into consideration when planning treatment. Once vaginal extension is recognized, treatment will be straightforward. However, the presence of vaginal intraepithelial neoplasia following hysterectomy is a much more difficult clinical problem.

The colposcopic features of vaginal and cervical intraepithelial neoplasia are identical, and their interpretation usually presents little difficulty (Figs 15.8 and 15.9). In order to minimize the possibility of overlooking vaginal intraepithelial neoplasia, the inexperienced colposcopist is advised to use Lugol's

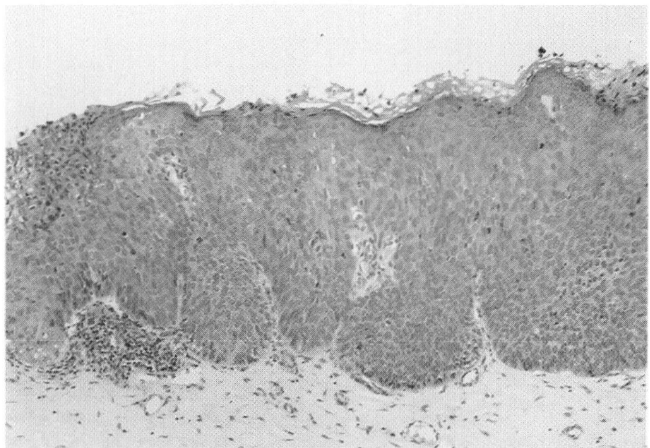

Fig. 15.2 VAIN 3. This example is showing irregular, bulky downgrowths and a little keratinization.

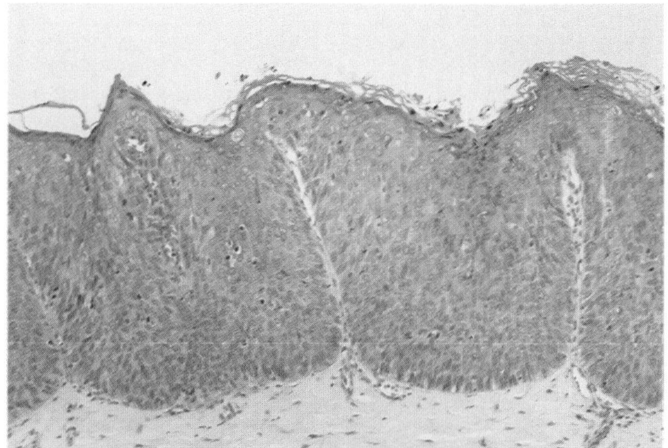

Fig. 15.3 VAIN 3. Slight papillomatosis and hyperkeratosis are seen.

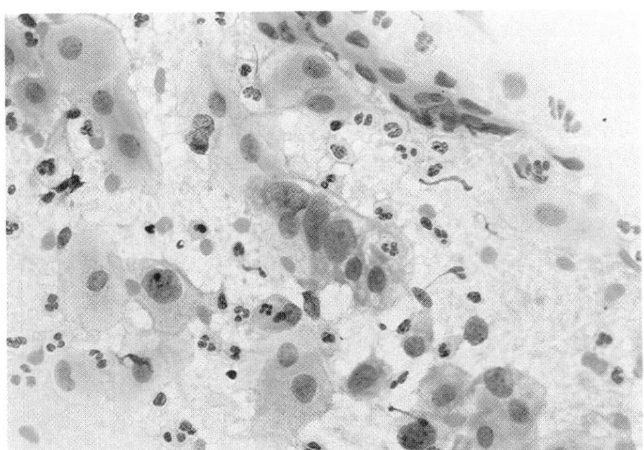

Fig. 15.4 Vaginal intraepithelial neoplasia. Cells are showing mild, moderate and severe dyskaryosis. The nuclei are showing all the features of dyskaryotic change, except marked hyperchromasia.

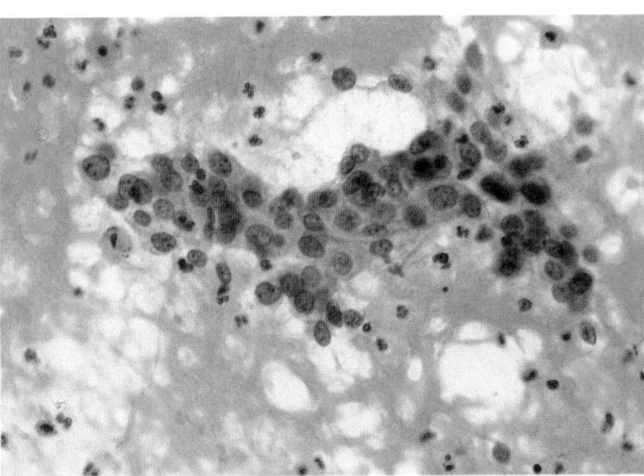

Fig. 15.5 Vaginal intraepithelial neoplasia. This is a sheet of severely dyskaryotic cells, showing anisonucleosis and hyperchromasia. Numerous red cells are present.

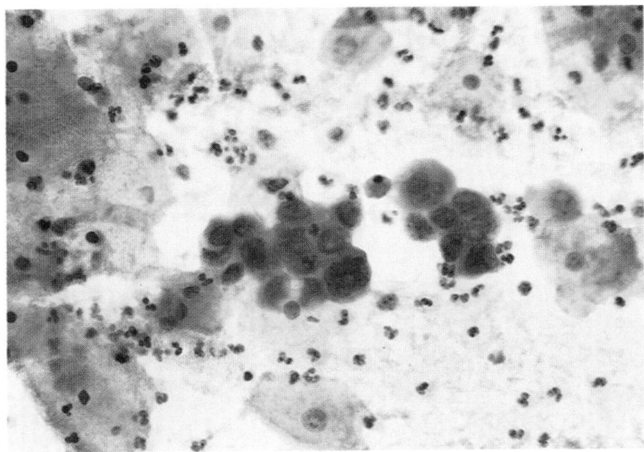

Fig. 15.6 Vaginal intraepithelial neoplasia. A number of severely dyskaryotic nuclei are present, showing hyperchromasia, pleomorphism and irregularly clumped chromatin.

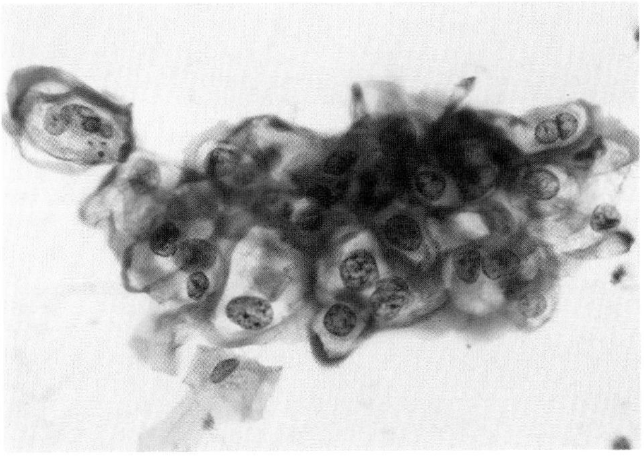

Fig. 15.7 Vaginal intraepithelial neoplasia. A well-defined group of squamous cells is showing prominent koilocytic change with binucleation, features associated with human papillomavirus infection.

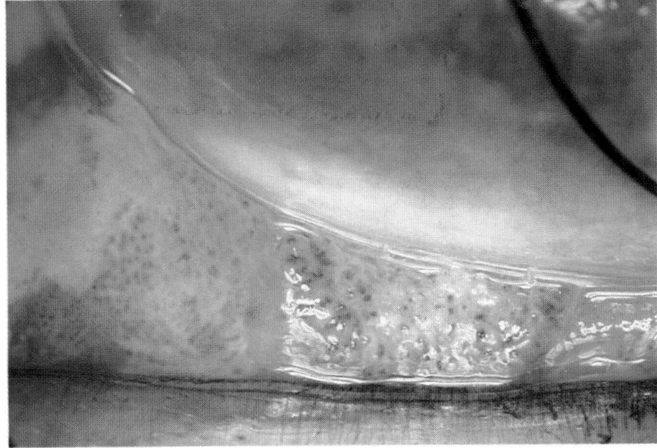

Fig. 15.8 A coarse punctation pattern, extending from the cervix on to the posterior vaginal wall.

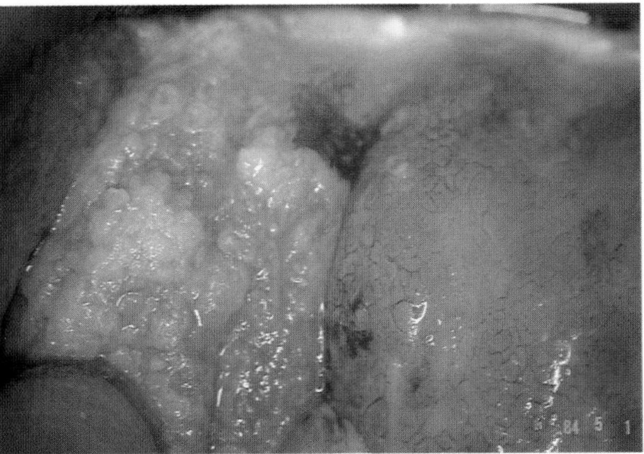

Fig. 15.9 Cervix exhibiting a mosaic pattern. The lesion is extending on to the right lateral vaginal wall, showing leucoplakia and gland openings. Biopsy revealed vaginal intraepithelial neoplasia.

iodine at the completion of every colposcopic assessment (Fig. 15.10).

It should also be borne in mind that the presence of vaginal intraepithelial neoplasia may be falsely suspected in a congenital transformation zone which frequently involves the vagina and has the colposcopic appearances of cervical intraepithelial neoplasia. Moreover, vaginal adenosis, whether or not associated with diethylstilboestrol *in utero*, undergoes physiological metaplasia which can be confused with vaginal intraepithelial neoplasia (see Fig. 20.7, page 242).

For these reasons, it is important to establish a histological diagnosis before attempting to

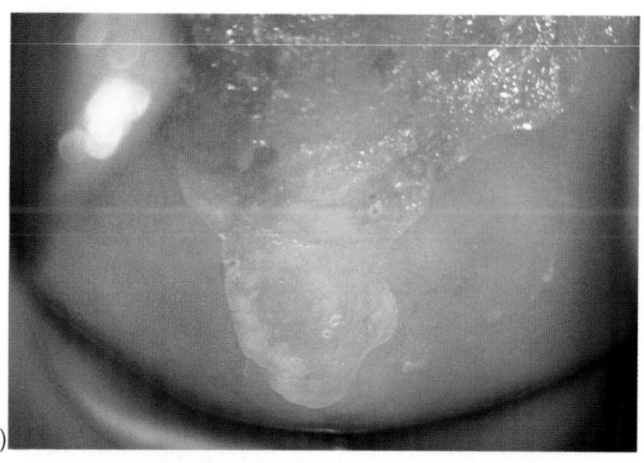
(a)

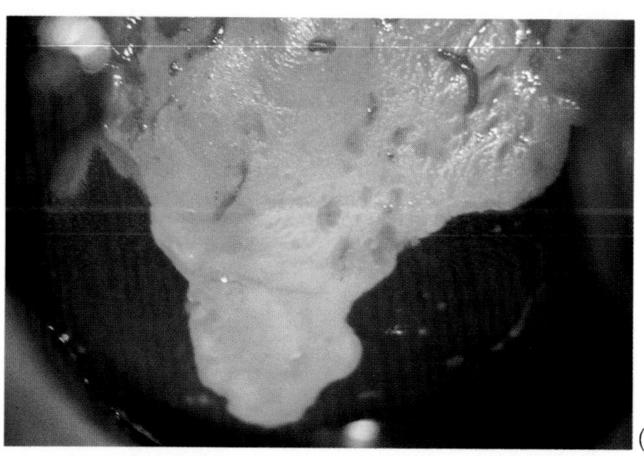
(b)

Fig. 15.10 Vaginal intraepithelial neoplasia in the posterior vaginal fornix. This is in continuity with cervical intraepithelial neoplasia. **(a)** After application of acetic acid, mild acetowhite demarcated lesion is seen, with waxy leucoplakia. **(b)** Following Schiller's test.

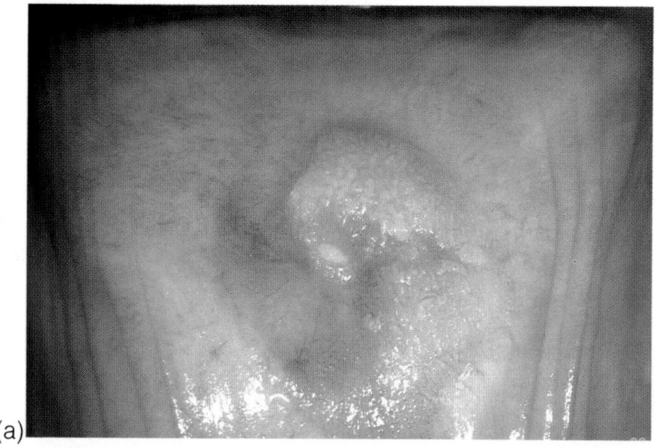
(a)

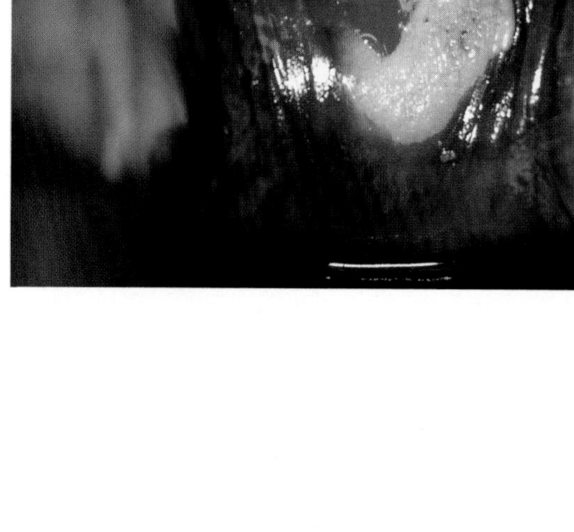
(b)

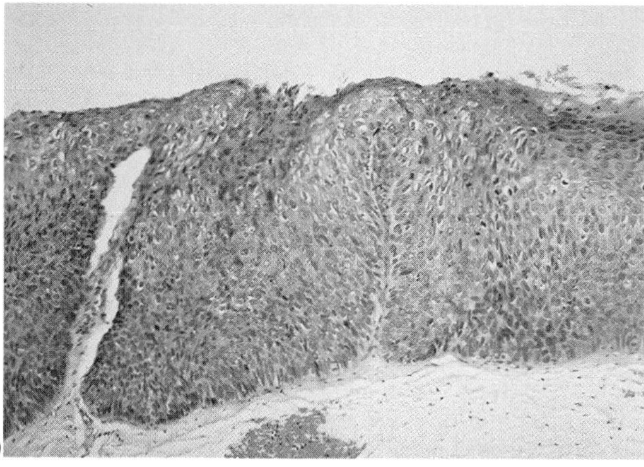
(c)

Fig. 15.11 Residual vaginal intraepithelial neoplasia in the midpoint of the vaginal vault, after hysterectomy. (a) Following application of acetic acid. **(b)** Following application of Lugol's iodine, showing the biopsy site. **(c)** Biopsy showing VAIN 3.

remove what appears to be vaginal intraepithelial neoplasia.

Vaginal intraepithelial neoplasia following hysterectomy is usually suspected because of abnormal cytology, but when present it is usually easy to identify (Fig. 15.11). Care should be taken to inspect the vaginal angles, where a 'pocket' will often be found; this pocket may be exposed using skin hooks or an endocervical speculum (Fig. 15.12).

Acetowhite epithelium, suggestive of vaginal intraepithelial neoplasia following hysterectomy, may sometimes be due to human papillomavirus infection (Fig. 15.13); it is therefore important that an adequate histological diagnosis is made before treatment is planned.

Figure 15.14 shows an unusual example of VAIN 3 developing following amputation of the cervix as treatment for CIN 3. The site was repaired using Sturmdorf sutures. In the postmenopausal patient interpretation may be more difficult, and a six- to eight-week course of oral or intravaginal oestrogen could prove helpful.

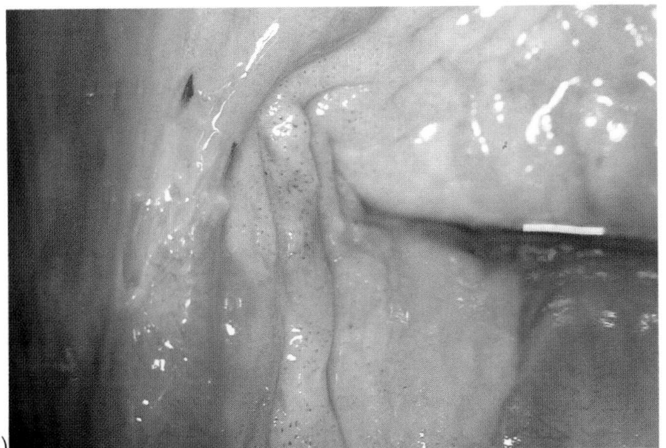
(a)

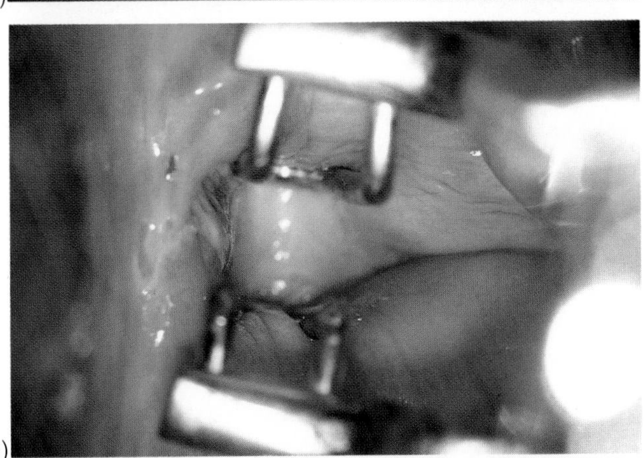
(b)

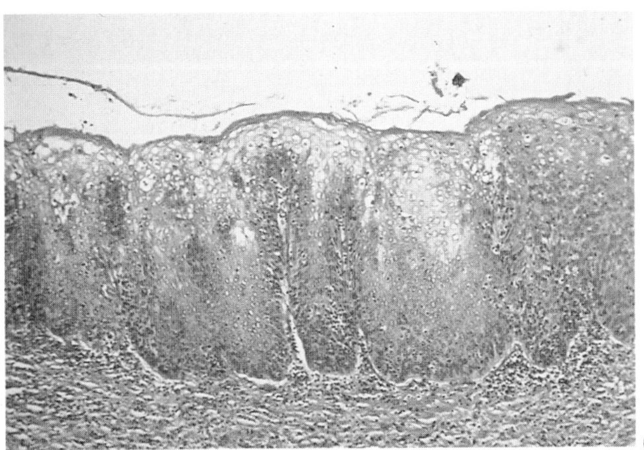
(c)

Fig. 15.12 Residual vaginal intraepithelial neoplasia at the right vaginal angle, after hysterectomy. (a) Acetowhite epithelium disappearing into the 'pocket' at right-angle. **(b)** Vaginal angle pocket, opened with an endocervical speculum. **(c)** Biopsy from the lesion, confirming the presence of vagina intraepithelial neoplasia with human papillomavirus change.

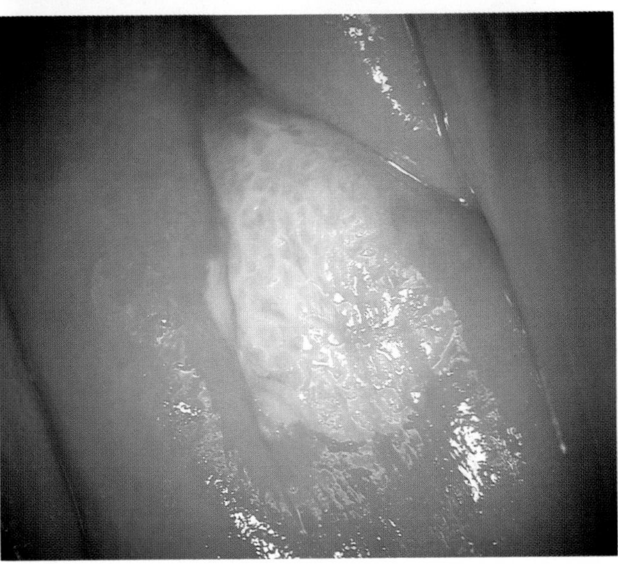

Fig. 15.13 Acetowhite epithelium suggestive of vaginal intraepithelial neoplasia following hysterectomy. This may often be due to human papillomavirus infection.

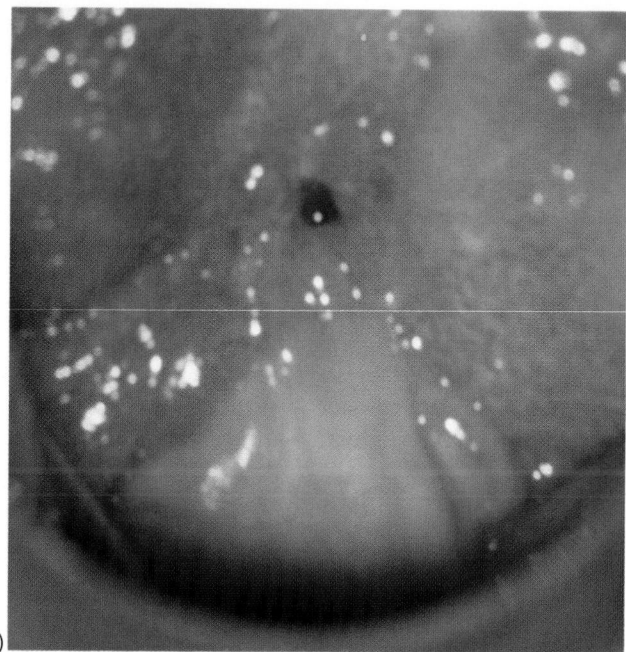

(a)

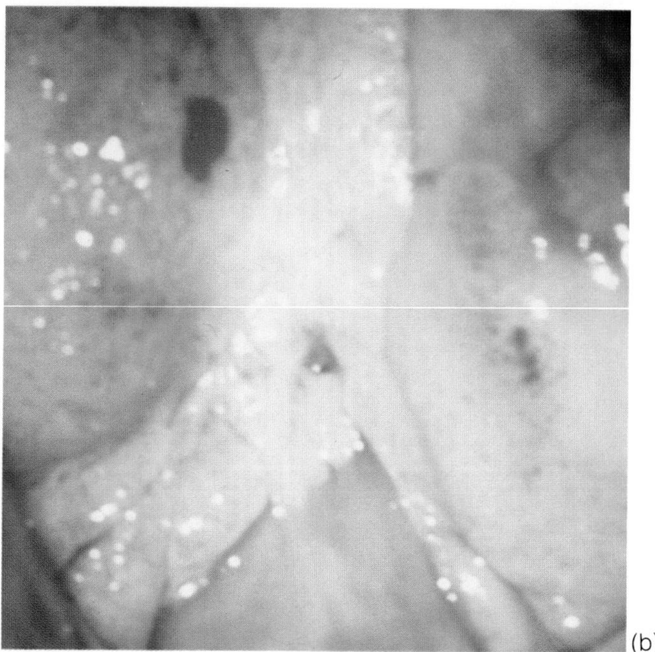

(b)

Fig. 15.14 An unusual case of VAIN 3. Previous amputation of cervix for CIN 3, repaired using Sturmdorf stitch. Recurrent intraepithelial neoplasia in the vaginal epithelium covering the cervical stump. **(a)** Slightly raised, reddened epithelium with punctation before applying acetic acid. **(b)** Marked acetowhite change in the same area.

MANAGEMENT

With uterus present

There are several treatment options to be followed, but each must be based on colposcopic assessment. These options involve methods of local destruction and surgical excision. When planning treatment by a destructive method, i.e. cryocautery, electrodiathermy or carbon dioxide laser, the gynaecologist should be aware of the proximity of the bladder, rectum and urethra in the operation field. In the postmenopausal patient the epithelium will usually be atrophic, and therefore it is advisable to prescribe a six-week course of oestrogen before proceeding with local destructive methods.

Laser vaporization is probably the best mode of treatment. The operator must follow the same rules that apply in the local destruction of cervical intraepithelial neoplasia. It should also be remembered that vaginal epithelium has no crypts or clefts, and destruction to a depth of 2–3 mm will be perfectly adequate. Any associated cervical lesion can be treated on its own merits, by local destruction or excision.

In the case of associated menorrhagia, fibroid uterus or uterine prolapse, hysterectomy may be indicated, with removal of the appropriate cuff of vagina as determined by the colposcopic assessment of the lesion. Alternatively, it is possible to destroy the vaginal lesion first, and provided that at follow-up the gynaecologist is satisfied that the vaginal lesion has been adequately dealt with, a simple hysterectomy may be performed.

Following hysterectomy

When planning treatment for vaginal intraepithelial neoplasia at the reconstructed vaginal vault following hysterectomy, the colposcopist should remember that the detected lesion is not a simple superficial lesion, as it is impossible to determine the amount of vaginal tissue remaining above the vault suture line (see Fig. 13.13, page 169). Failure to recognize this fact will often lead to inadequate treatment. When the carbon dioxide laser was first introduced into gynaecology, it was thought that laser vaporization was the perfect way to treat these lesions. However, long-term follow-up showed that the failure rate was relatively high, and some patients subsequently presented with invasive carcinoma.

The reasons for this failure are quite obvious: the operator does not know how deep the laser destruction should be, being aware of the presence of other structures above, in front of and behind the vaginal vault. Furthermore, vaporization must be preceded by an adequate biopsy, to exclude unsuspected invasive disease.

Alternatively, the colposcopically localized lesion may be surgically excised: small lesions can be adequately removed by local excision biopsy, lesions involving most of the vaginal vault by partial vaginectomy, and those involving most or all of the vagina by total vaginectomy (with or without reconstruction of an artificial vagina). However, the problem of not knowing how much vaginal tissue lies above the vaginal vault, especially in the lateral vaginal angles, remains; any attempt to remove tissue deeply in this region carries the risk of damage to the bladder or ureters. Therefore, the abdominal approach may be considered more appropriate.

Because of these difficulties, treatment by radiotherapy has been advocated, offering excellent results. Before radiotherapy, the patient should have a colposcopically directed biopsy performed under general anaesthesia, aiming to exclude unsuspected invasive carcinoma. This is followed by insertion of one or two cylinders, each containing 15–20 mg of radium. The duration of insertion is between 72 and

(a)

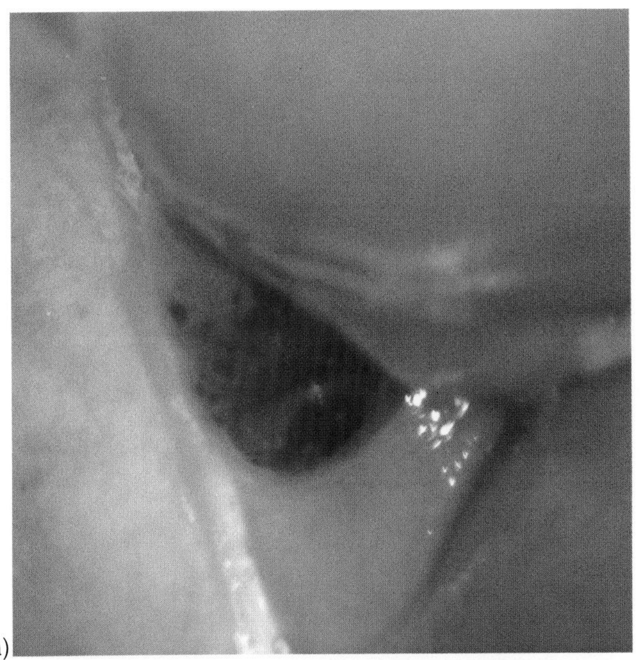

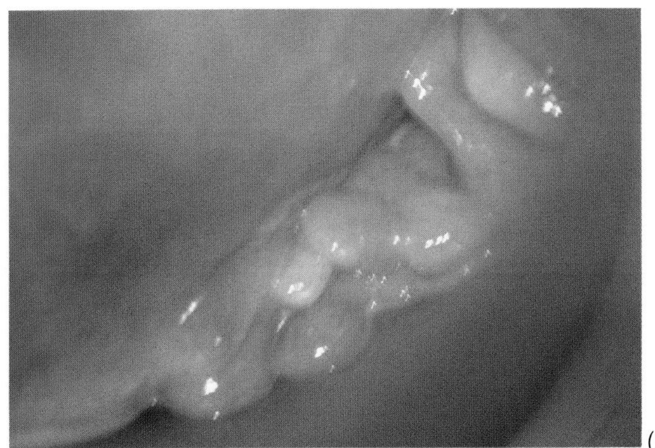

(b)

Fig. 15.15 Endometriosis in vaginal fornices. (a) Endometrioma; cervix above. **(b)** Endometriotic scarring in the left posterolateral fornix; cervix above and to the left.

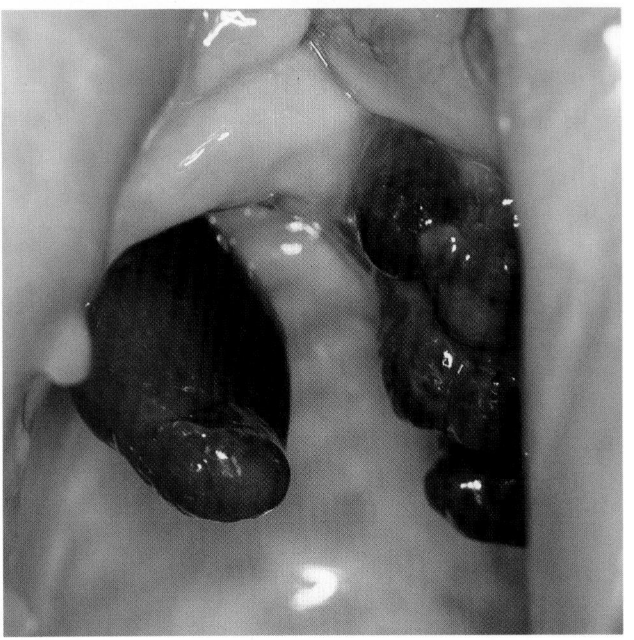

Fig. 15.16 Recurrent malignant melanoma of the lower third of the vagina. Colposcopy has little to offer in this instance.

100 hours, depending on the amount of radium used and the patient's tolerance to the procedure. The patient is discharged on the same day of treatment and instructed to start using a vaginal dilator daily, resuming normal sexual activity after four weeks. With this method, vaginal stenosis and dyspareunia are not usually a problem. In the premenopausal patient, ovarian function may cease, which is a clear disadvantage; in this case, oestrogen replacement therapy should be prescribed.

Intravaginal 5-fluorouracil cream has also been used in the treatment of supravaginal lesions. It is not well tolerated, and there have been mixed reports as to its efficacy in destroying these lesions.

MISCELLANEOUS VAGINAL LESIONS

Other than vaginal intraepithelial neoplasia, the most common vaginal lesions likely to be encountered are those induced by the human papillomavirus, discussed in Chapters 12 and 16.

A less common condition, occasionally seen at colposcopy, is endometriosis affecting the vaginal fornices (Fig. 15.15). Pigmented lesions of the vaginal epithelium are very uncommon, for instance clinically overt, pedunculated lesions of recurrent malignant melanoma, arising from the lower third of the vagina (Fig. 15.16). Colposcopy has little to add to their assessment.

16. *Vulval disease and vulval intraepithelial neoplasia*

CLASSIFICATION OF VULVAL DISEASE

The epithelial abnormalities of the vulva fall into three categories: the non-neoplastic epithelial disorders (previously known as dystrophies), papillomavirus infection and intraepithelial neoplasia (Table 16.1). In addition, because the vulva is an area of skin, general dermatological conditions, including psoriasis, eczema, pemphigus, lichen simplex and lichen planus, must be borne in mind. However, a detailed account of these is beyond the scope of this book.

Non-neoplastic epithelial disorders

This is a group of skin conditions of unknown aetiology, and many terms have been used to describe them in the past. The current classification is shown in Table 16.2. Terms such as kraurosis vulvae, leucoplakia, leucoplakic vulvitis, atrophic leucoplakia, neurodermatitis, hyperplastic vulvitis and, most recently, dystrophy have been removed from the terminology of vulval disease; the term 'hyperplastic dystrophy' has been replaced by squamous hyperplasia.

Although the non-neoplastic epithelial disorders are presented in this classification as apparently distinct entities, it is probable that they are best thought of as a spectrum of disease, with the most hyperplastic forms at one end of the spectrum, and lichen sclerosus at the other.

Table 16.1 Relationship between VIN, NNED and HPV

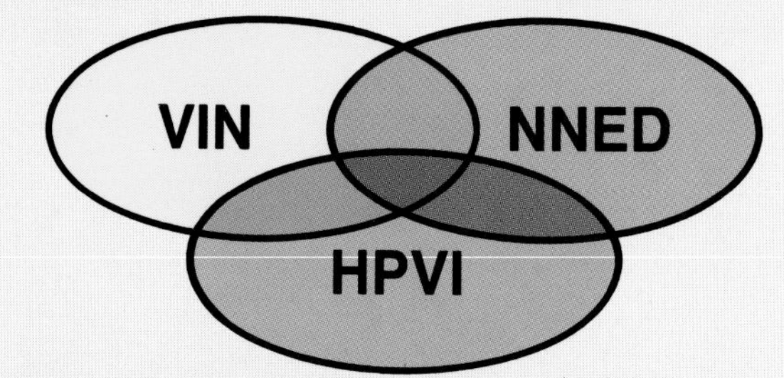

VIN Vulva intraepithelial neoplasia
NNED Non-neoplastic epithelial disorders
HPVI Human papillomavirus infection

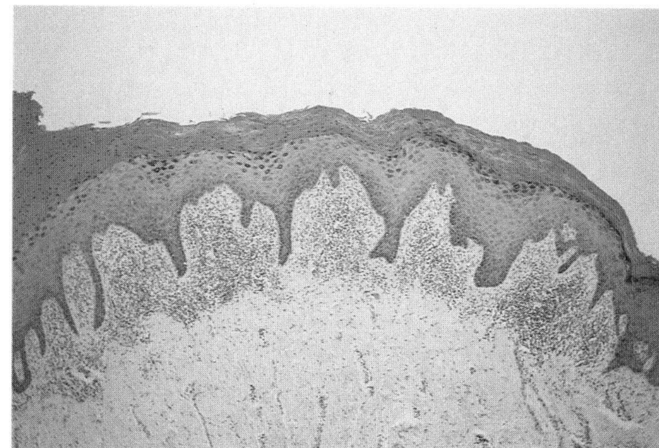

Fig. 16.1 Squamous hyperplasia of the vulva. The thickening of the epidermis, with irregular prolongation of rete ridges, is apparent. The band-like, chronic inflammatory infiltrate hugging the lower surface of the epidermis is well shown.

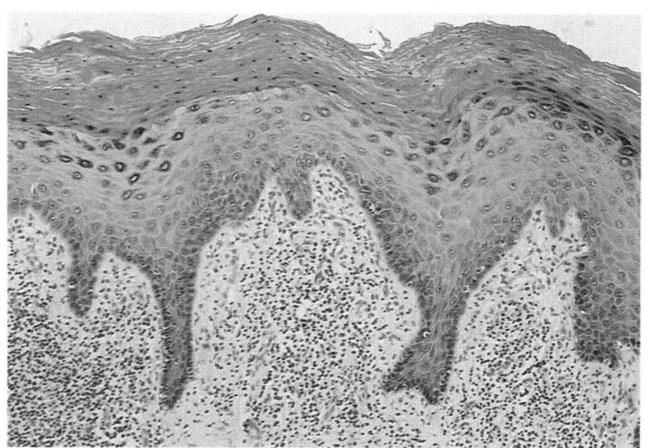

Fig. 16.2 Squamous hyperplasia of the vulva. Parakeratosis and a striking granular layer are seen.

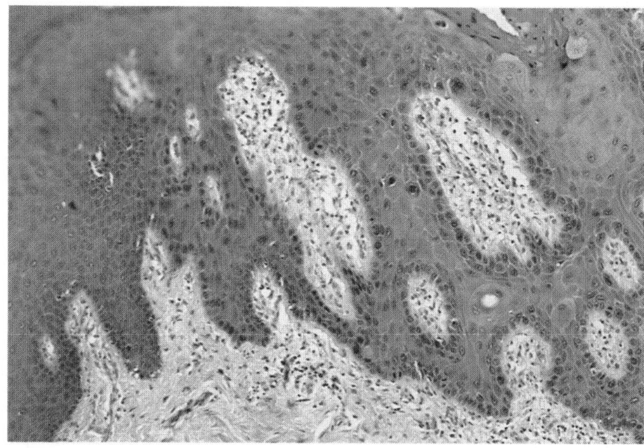

Fig. 16.3 Squamous hyperplasia of the vulva. An area showing slight atypia of the basal cells, with increased mitotic activity and some nuclear enlargement and hyperchromasia.

Table 16.2 Non-neoplastic epithelial disorders of skin and mucosa of the vulva

1 Lichen sclerosus
(lichen sclerosus et atrophicus)

2 Squamous cell hyperplasia
(formerly hyperplastic dystrophy)

3 Other dermatoses

SQUAMOUS CELL HYPERPLASIA

This term characterizes the chronic vulval dermatosis which clinically has formerly been known as 'leucoplakia'. It is most commonly seen in postmenopausal women. The disease usually presents as vulval itching. The clinical appearances are of raised, white plaques on the vulva, which may involve both the labia majora and labia minora. Cracks and fissures appear, and from time to time red areas are seen.

The histological features are epithelial thickening with acanthosis, hyperkeratosis, parakeratosis and irregular prolongation of the rete ridges (Figs 16.1 and 16.2). As leucoplakia is associated with hyperkeratosis, there is usually a prominent granular layer. The superficial dermis contains an infiltrate mainly of lymphocytes, but with some plasma cells and macrophages closely underneath the epidermis. When atypia is present, it is seen as enlarged, hyperchromatic nuclei with chromatin clumping, mitotic figures and individual cell keratinization (Fig. 16.3).

LICHEN SCLEROSUS

This is a benign cutaneous disease of unknown aetiology, which is also encountered on the skin of the trunk, neck and extremities. It can affect any age group; the median age is just under 60 years, and approximately 60% of affected women are postmenopausal, although the condition may be seen in childhood.

The histological changes in lichen sclerosus of the vulva are the same as those seen at the extragenital sites. The most prominent feature is a broad zone of hyalinization and oedema in the papillary and reticular dermis (Fig. 16.4). The usual fibrillary pattern of the dermal collagen is lost, and elastic stains show a marked decrease in elastic fibres. Sometimes the oedema beneath the epidermis is so great that vesicles are formed. The epidermis is thinned, with flattening of the rete ridges (Fig. 16.5), and there may be liquefactive degeneration of the basal layer. There is always hyperkeratosis, with the keratin layer often being thicker than the epidermis itself.

MIXED EPITHELIAL DISORDERS

Squamous cell hyperplasia and lichen sclerosus may be mixed in two ways: first, it is not uncommon to encounter a vulval lesion which has adjacent areas of each type of abnormality. Secondly, an area may show some of the features of both forms of epithelial disorder, such that the epidermis is thickened, with

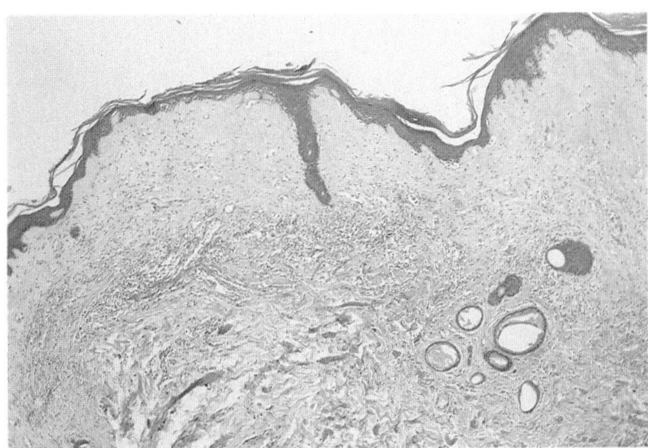

Fig. 16.4 Lichen sclerosus. The epidermis is markedly thinned, with 'flaky' hyperkeratosis. The hallmark of the condition is a clear, hyaline, oedematous band in the superficial dermis, beneath which there is an inflammatory infiltrate (rather sparse in this example).

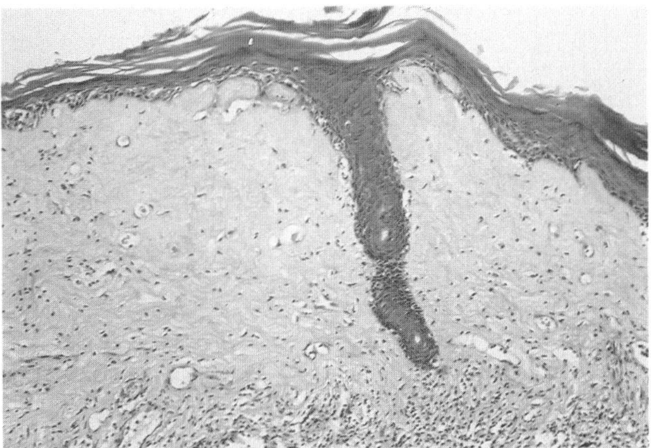

Fig. 16.5 Lichen sclerosus. The epidermis is markedly thinned, and the skin appendage is compressed by the sclerotic superficial dermis.

hyperkeratosis and irregular elongation of the rete ridges, but with the superficial dermis showing the characteristic oedema and hyalinization of lichen sclerosus.

Papillomavirus infection

CONDYLOMA ACUMINATUM

The most striking feature of condyloma acuminatum is papillomatosis; in the absence of this feature, a diagnosis cannot be made. In addition, the lesion will show acanthosis, elongation of rete pegs, koilocytosis and, in some cases, a dermal inflammatory infiltrate (Fig. 16.6). Parakeratosis will very often be seen at the surface of the epithelium, and less frequently hyperkeratosis will be present. Nuclear abnormalities are not apparent; the nuclei are uniform and show no hyperchromasia. Mitotic activity is often increased, but the mitotic figures are not abnormal.

SUBCLINICAL PAPILLOMAVIRUS INFECTION

The exophytic condyloma described above is not the only manifestation of papillomavirus infection of the vulva; 'flat warts' are also encountered. The term 'subclinical papillomavirus infection' is preferred, as it brings the terminology into line with that used for the cervix.

These lesions are not as frequently seen on the vulva as they are on the cervix. It seems that wart infection of the vulva is more usually associated with exophytic warts or intraepithelial neoplasia, whereas in the cervix the infection most commonly results in subclinical papillomavirus infection, or it is associated with intraepithelial neoplasia, with the exophytic condyloma being a relatively less common manifestation.

Vulval subclinical papillomavirus infection has the features of papillomavirus infection (see pages 143, 144), koilocytosis being the most prominent. As in the cervix, this constellation of features may be seen in epithelium that also carries the features of intraepithelial neoplasia (Fig. 16.7).

Vulval intraepithelial neoplasia (VIN)

For many years, the terminology of premalignant conditions of the vulva has been confused by the number and complexity of the terms used. In the past few years, the accepted terminology has been modified to bring the concept of preinvasive malignant disease of the vulva into line with that of the cervix. As a result, a system of nomenclature has evolved that uses the term 'vulval intraepithelial neoplasia' expressed as grades 1, 2 and 3.

Even though this system of terminology is gaining general acceptance, it seems that application of the concept of a continuous spectrum of disease may be rather less appropriate in the vulva than it is in the cervix. The difficulty is compounded by the phenomenon of non-neoplastic epithelial disorders with which vulval intraepithelial neoplasia appears to overlap at the mild end of its spectrum.

Moreover, many more cases of VIN 3 seem to be

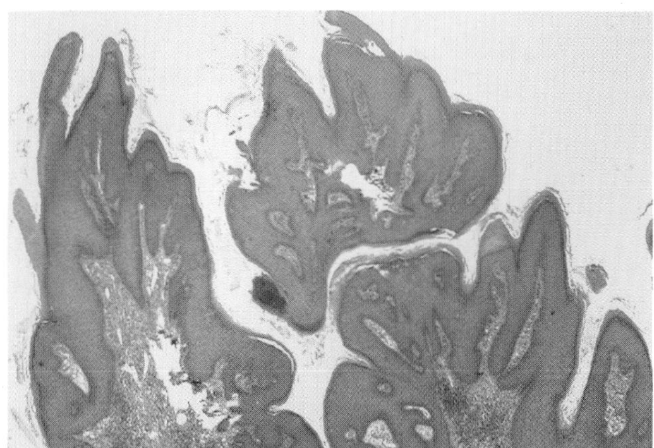

Fig. 16.6 Condyloma acuminatum, showing marked papillomatosis. Keratin is present on the surface, and a patchy, chronic inflammatory infiltrate is seen in the dermal core.

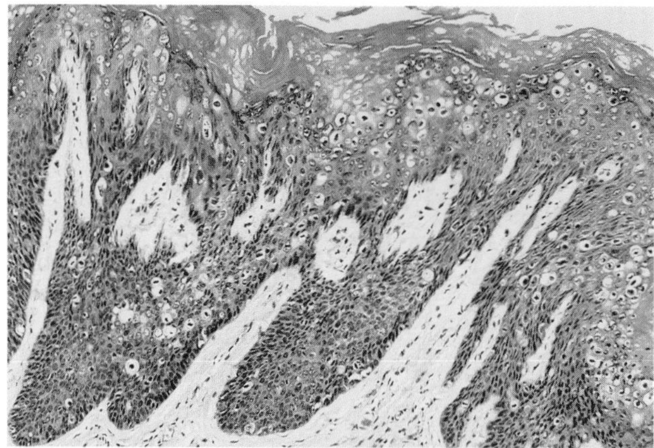

Fig. 16.7 VIN 3 with evidence of papillomavirus infection. The cells in the lower part of the epidermis are showing the features of VIN 3, but nearer the surface koilocytic change and individual cell keratinization are prominent.

diagnosed than the less severe forms, which would not be expected if the disease was a spectrum of change, with the milder forms either progressing towards the more severe forms, or regressing (as is thought to happen in cervical intraepithelial neoplasia). However, this difference may lie in an inability to detect cases of lesser degrees of vulval intraepithelial neoplasia, which are usually asymptomatic.

HISTOLOGY

In general, the diagnosis of vulval intraepithelial neoplasia is histologically very similar to that of cervical intraepithelial neoplasia (Figs 16.7–16.12): it depends upon arrest of differentiation, maturation

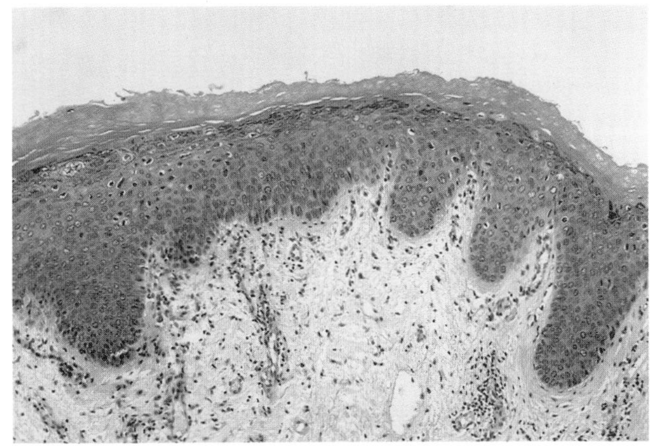

Fig. 16.8 VIN 1. The epidermis is showing slight hyperkeratosis and some arrest of maturation. Nuclear enlargement and mitotic activity are slight. Koilocytic change is present in this example.

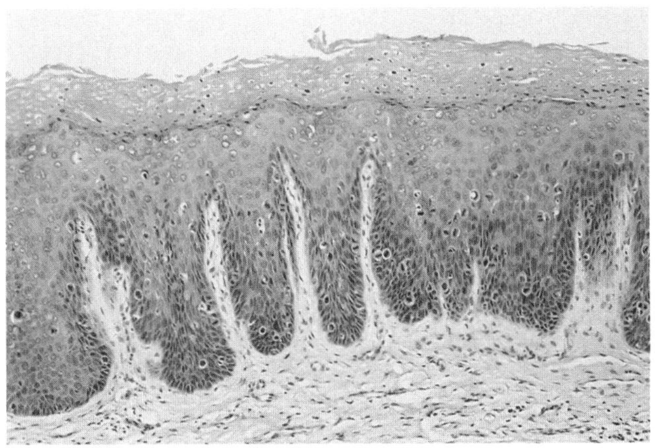

Fig. 16.9 VIN 2. Mitotic activity and nuclear enlargement are in this example confined to the lower third of the epithelium.

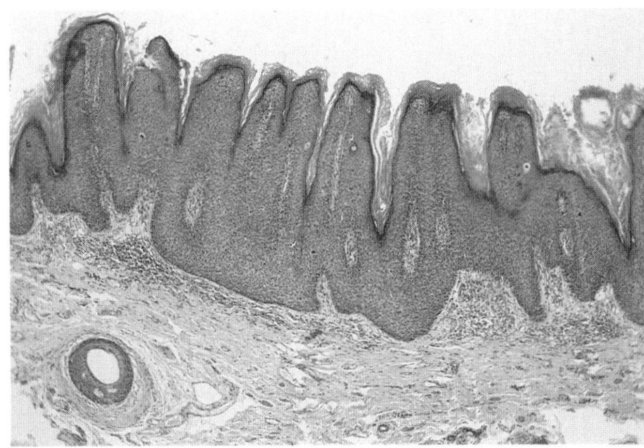

Fig. 16.10 VIN 3. In this example there is considerable thickening of the epithelium, with striking papillomatosis. There is almost total arrest of maturation until the keratinized layer is reached.

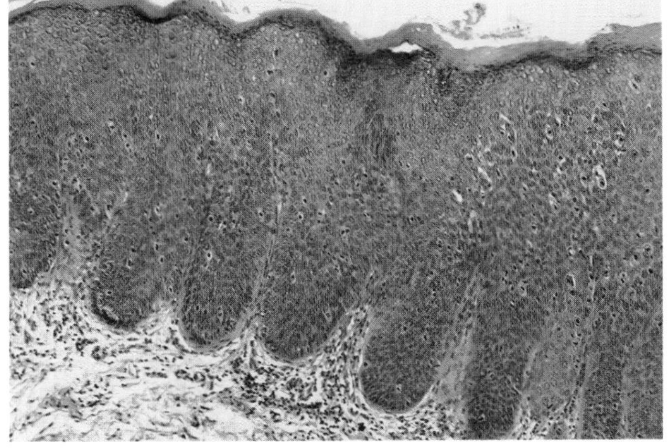

Fig. 16.11 VIN 3. The cells of most of the thickness of the epithelium are showing nuclear enlargement, and mitotic activity is scattered throughout.

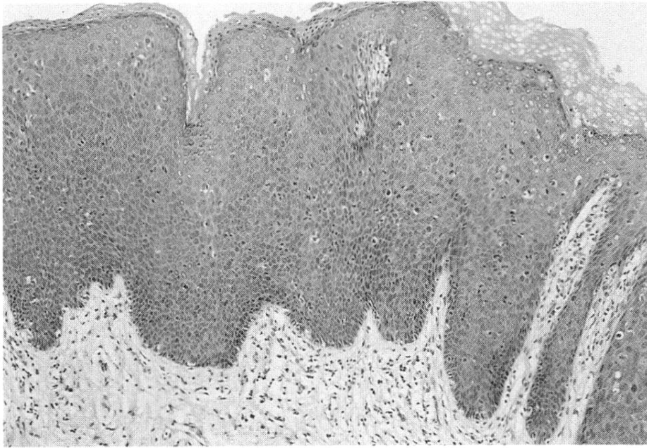

Fig. 16.12 VIN 3. Note the abnormal mitotic figure.

and stratification, nuclear abnormalities and mitotic activity (see Chapter 2).

As the grade of neoplasia advances, the proportion of epithelium showing differentiation decreases, the degree of nuclear pleomorphism increases, and mitotic figures are more numerous and are found at a higher level in the epithelium. Abnormal forms of mitotic figures are more common in the higher grades of disease. There is usually some degree of hyperkeratosis/parakeratosis, although this is not invariable.

The changes of vulval intraepithelial neoplasia may affect not only the surface epithelium; the pilosebaceous units can also be involved (Fig. 16.13). These may be as deep as 10 mm, a feature that must be taken into account when treatment is being planned. Involvement of skin appendages of the labia minora is very uncommon. A case of the duct of a sweat gland being affected by vulval intraepithelial neoplasia is illustrated in Fig. 16.14.

CYTOLOGY

Vulval cytology is limited mainly to those situations where cervical intraepithelial neoplasia is known to be present, or where colposcopic or clinical ex-

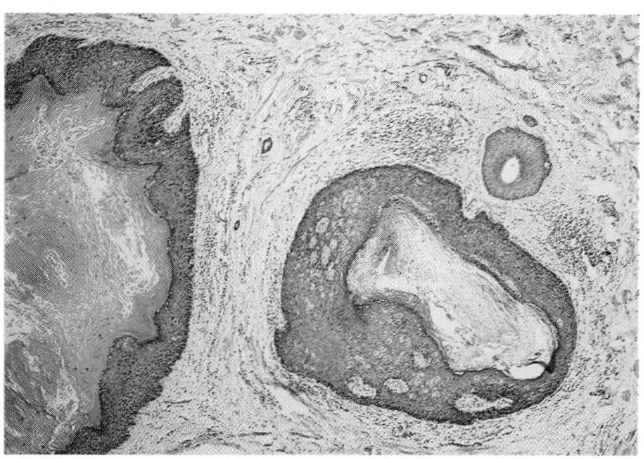

Fig. 16.13 VIN 3 affecting a pilosebaceous unit deep to the surface epithelium of the labium majus. Involvement of the skin appendage on the labium minus is uncommon.

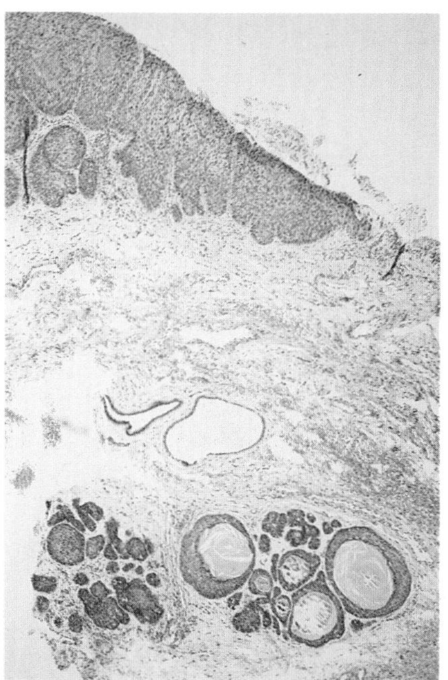

Fig. 16.14 VIN 3 affecting a sweat gland deep to the surface epithelium on the labium minus. Involvement of the skin appendage on the labium minus is uncommon. H&E, x12.8

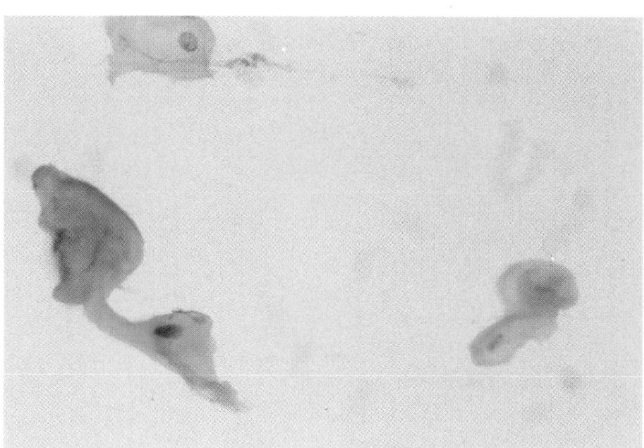

Fig. 16.15 Invasive squamous cell carcinoma of the vulva. Large, bizarre, highly keratinized squamous cells are present, one of which is anucleate.

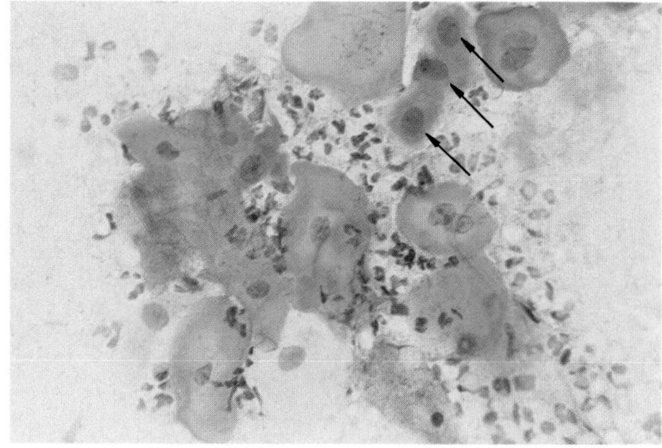

Fig. 16.16 VIN 3. The central groups of cells are showing a keratinized cytoplasm. The nuclei are showing varying degrees of abnormality, amounting to severe dyskaryosis in three cells (arrows). Other cells are binucleate, suggesting the possibility of papillomavirus infection.

amination has identified a vulval lesion. In the majority of cases the smears are scanty and require careful evaluation. The cytological features of vulval dyskaryosis are essentially the same as those described for cervical intraepithelial neoplasia (see Chapter 2).

However, vulval smears will contain predominantly keratinized squamous cells; indeed, sometimes it is the number and configuration of these highly keratinizing and bizarre shaped, anucleate cells which will lead to the diagnosis (Fig. 16.15).

The nuclei of dyskaryotic and malignant cells may not appear hyperchromatic; on the contrary, they are frequently pale-stained, and very few cells may be present (Fig. 16.16). The large, pale-staining cells with clear cytoplasm associated with Paget's disease may occasionally be identified.

Occasionally, vulval smears from benign conditions are seen, and these are mainly composed of superficial squamous cells with some anucleate cells of normal shape and size. The features associated with human papillomavirus infection, already described, can sometimes be identified on vulval smears. In most cases, there are no reliable cytological criteria that can be applied to distinguish between VIN 3 and invasive squamous cell carcinoma. Vulval candidiasis may be identified by the presence of spores and hyphae in smears.

COLPOSCOPY OF THE VULVA

Conditions other than vulval intraepithelial neoplasia and human papillomavirus-related disease should not be overlooked when a woman with vulval symptoms or a definite vulval lesion is referred for colposcopy. Where appropriate, the help of a colleague specializing in dermatology or genitourinary medicine should be sought (Figs 16.17 and 16.18).

Indeed, consideration should be given to setting up a specialist combined clinic for vulval disease, staffed by a colposcopist/gynaecologist, a dermatologist and even a histopathologist, all with a special interest, if the referral rate of vulval conditions to the colposcopy clinic is sufficiently large to justify it.

Colposcopy has not been found to be particularly useful in the examination of vulval lesions, compared with lesions of the vagina and cervix. For cervicovaginal lesions, topography can be defined and some approximation of the degree of severity made, and the same approach may be employed to identify lesions on the vulva. This may be easier in the vestibule and on the medial aspects of the labia minora, where the epithelium is relatively thin (Fig. 16.19) or less keratinized.

However, keratinization interferes to a greater or lesser degree with the filter effect upon which grading colposcopic images on the cervix or vagina

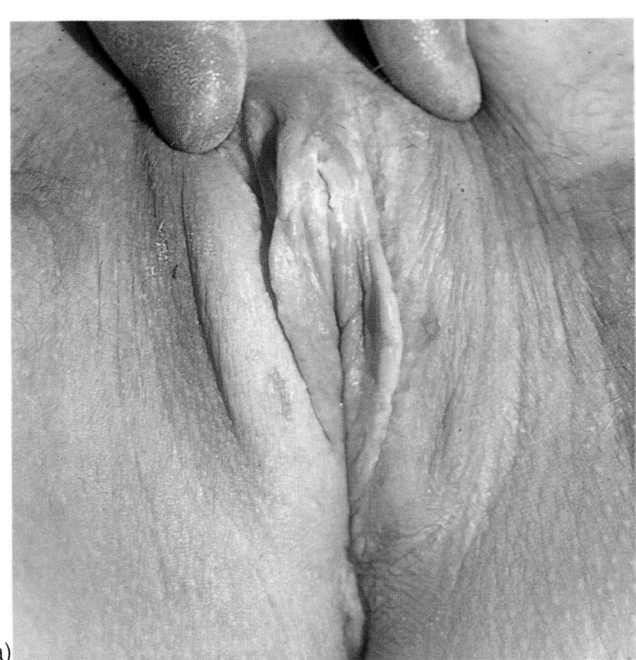

(a)

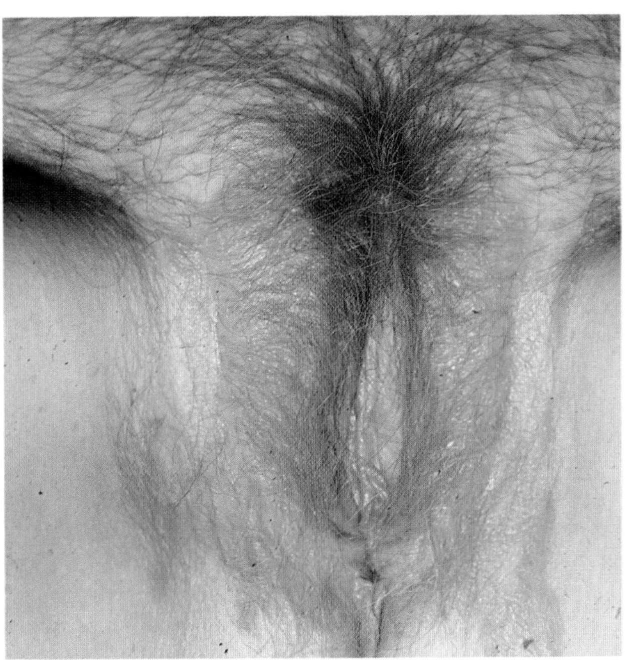

(b)

Fig. 16.17 Two common vulval conditions: (a) lichen sclerosus et atrophicus; **(b)** psoriasis. In these cases colposcopy has little or no place, and a dermatologist's opinion is essential.

depends. Keratin is opaque, making evaluation of thickness of the affected epithelium difficult. Also, the vascular aberrations of punctation and mosaic are less commonly seen on the vulva, and if present they tend to be observed in lesions occupying the vestibule.

Elsewhere, the vascular patterns may underlie but be obscured by keratinization. Ultimately, the colposcopist has to rely upon vulval biopsy to establish the true nature and severity of the lesion. Where vulval disease is multifocal, the colposcope may be invaluable in identifying the individual components, both for biopsy and treatment purposes.

Techniques of vulval colposcopy

The patient is examined in the lithotomy position. First, the vulva is inspected with the naked eye. Vulval intraepithelial neoplasia may appear as patches of white change, red or pigmented areas, or there may be an isolated or associated warty appearance. Using low-power magnification (six-fold), the vulva is again scrutinized. Some of the obscuring effect of keratinization may be alleviated by thinly smearing a water-soluble lubricant over areas of interest to assist visualization of abnormal vessels. This is equivalent to the saline method for visualization of the cervix and vagina.

The junction between the glycogen-bearing vaginal epithelium and keratin-producing vulval epithelium is considered at high risk for intraepithelial neoplasia, and demands special attention. However, all areas of vulval epithelium should be systematically examined: the vestibule; urethral meatus; both aspects of the labia minora; the clitoris, prepuce and glans; the interlabial sulcus; the hair-bearing areas and perineal skin; concluding with the perianal skin and its mucocutaneous junction.

If a lubricant has been used, it should be removed with a dry gauze swab before using acetic acid on the vulva. This is best done by applying gauze swabs soaked in the 3–5% acetic acid, arranged so as to be in contact with the affected skin and left in place for approximately three minutes. After removing the swabs, a systematic scrutiny through the colposcope

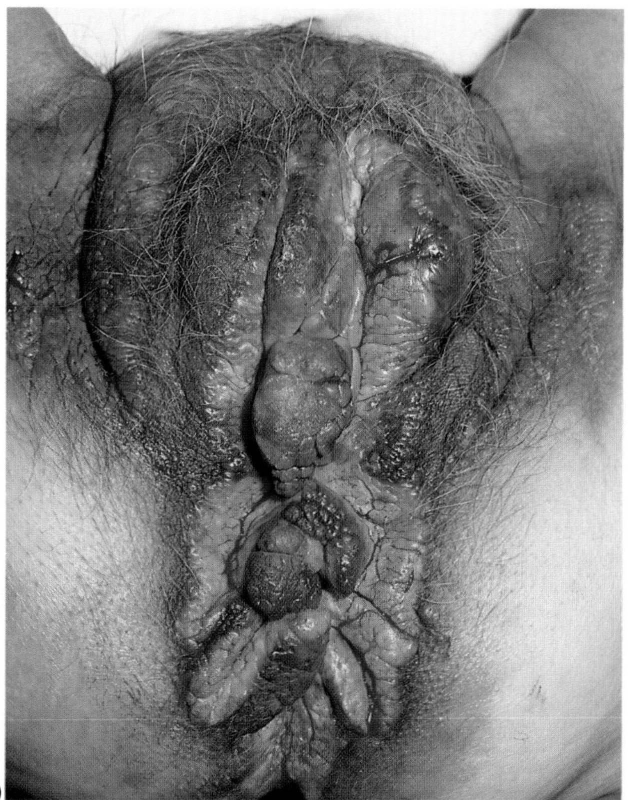

(a)

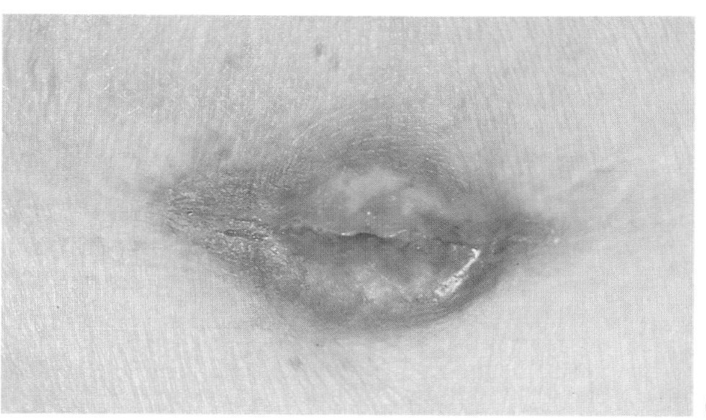

(b)

Fig. 16.18 A rare dermatological condition of the vulva, which could be confused with cancer. Pemphigus vegetans of **(a)** the vulva and **(b)** umbilicus, showing similar change. In this case, colposcopy was of no diagnostic help.

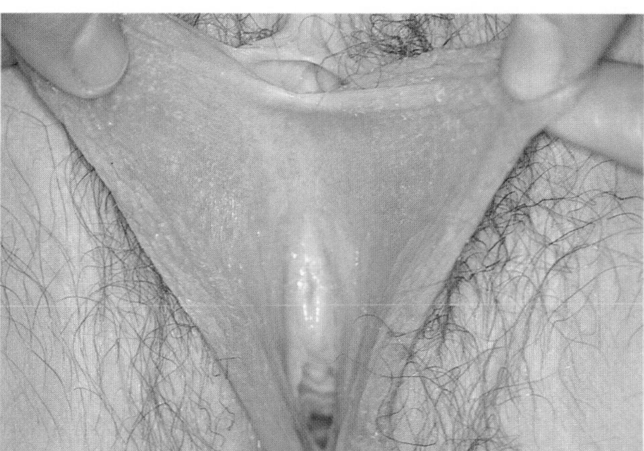

Fig. 16.19 Vulva showing thin epithelial covering, with minimal keratinization over the vestibule and medial aspects of labia minora.

is repeated, using higher magnifications where appropriate. Areas of acetowhite change are noted.

Staining the epithelium with toluidine blue is thought to help in the identification of certain lesions, especially if these are red in appearance due to lack of keratin. Excess blue dye is washed away by further application of acetic acid before an interpretation is made. Unfortunately, the dye is also taken up by fissures and excoriated skin. Not all colposcopists feel they can rely on this test, and some do not employ it at all. It may also be wise to carry out a colposcopic examination of the anal canal, if the patient is tolerant of such examination. This can be performed with the aid of a proctoscope, and a device with a side-viewing slot is particularly useful. Direct visualization through the colposcope before and after application of acetic acid will be required.

If vulval intraepithelial neoplasia or human papillomavirus lesions are suspected, it is obligatory to proceed to a colposcopic examination of the cervix and vagina, if this has not already been done, including collection of a cervical smear for cytology.

Techniques of vulval biopsy

Histopathological confirmation of the nature and severity of lesions should be obtained from appropriate biopsy material. This may be by excision biopsy with a scalpel; by target biopsy (single or multiple), using the Keye's punch; or by wider excision of larger tracts of vulval skin. If required, closure with one or more sutures may be necessary, and depending on the circumstances the procedure is carried out under local or general anaesthesia, on an out-patient, day case or in-patient basis.

EXCISION BIOPSY

This type of biopsy is suitable where the lesion is small. A local anaesthetic block is injected subcutaneously, and the lesion is removed as an ellipse of full thickness skin, with several millimetres of clearance around the lesion (Fig. 16.20). A skin hook is preferable for handling the specimen in order to minimize crush artefact; this is introduced subcutaneously. Suturing with fine plain catgut is employed, as necessary.

DIRECTED BIOPSY WITH KEYE'S PUNCH

This standard dermatological biopsy instrument (Fig. 16.21) has a circular cutting edge, and a 3–5 mm diameter, and it may also be obtained as a disposable for single use. It allows targeting of the biopsy from the centre of a lesion, and is also valuable where multiple biopsies are to be taken in multifocal disease (Fig. 16.22).

LARGE KNIFE BIOPSIES

In some cases, especially where the lesion is widespread, multifocal and confluent, a larger biopsy may be required and obtained under general anaesthesia. This procedure is designed to be excisional and curative.

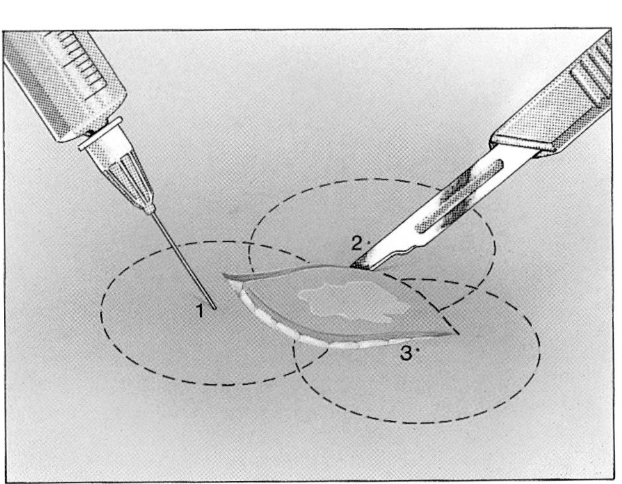

Fig. 16.20 Diagrammatic representation of full-thickness excision biopsy of vulval lesion. This would be carried out under local anaesthesia.

(a)
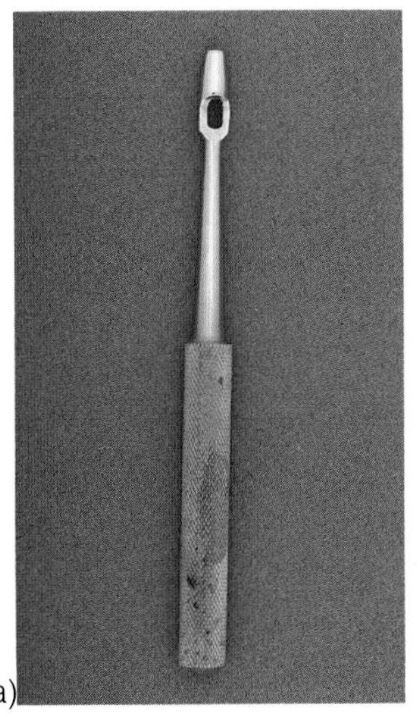

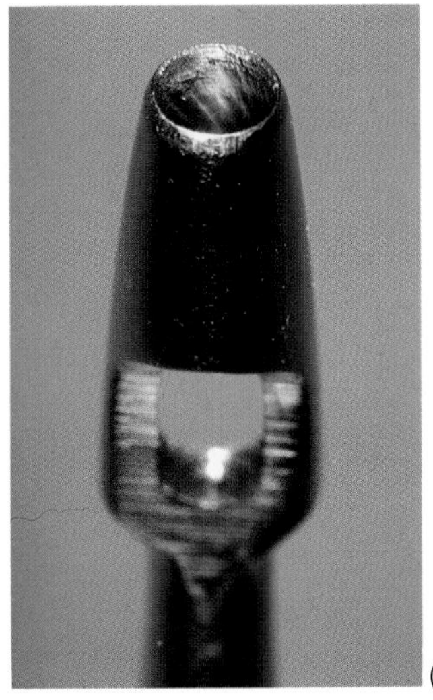
(b)

Fig. 16.21 (a) Keye's punch for vulval biopsy. (b) Magnified view of circular cutting edge (3–5 mm in diameter).

The biopsy will be full thickness, ensuring that any skin appendage involvement by the intraepithelial neoplastic process is cleared (see above). Sometimes with extensive disease it is not possible to be certain that invasion is not present without resorting to removal of a large tract of vulval skin. Closure with sutures will be necessary. This type of biopsy results in a variant of partial or total 'skinning' vulvectomy. In some cases, split skin grafting may also be required (see below).

VULVAL INTRAEPITHELIAL NEOPLASIA

As indicated above, intraepithelial neoplastic lesions of the vulva may be unifocal or multifocal. To the naked eye and through the colposcope they may appear white (leucoplakia; Fig. 16.23), red (Fig. 16.24), or pigmented (Figs 16.25 to 16.27), and after a prolonged soak in acetic acid they may present by acetowhite change (Fig. 16.28).

Dense, keratinized areas may be a feature (Fig.

(a)

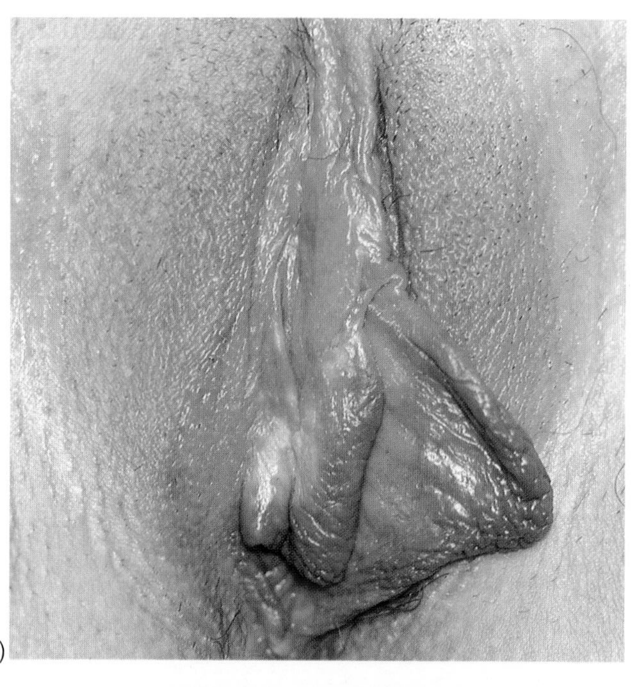

(b)

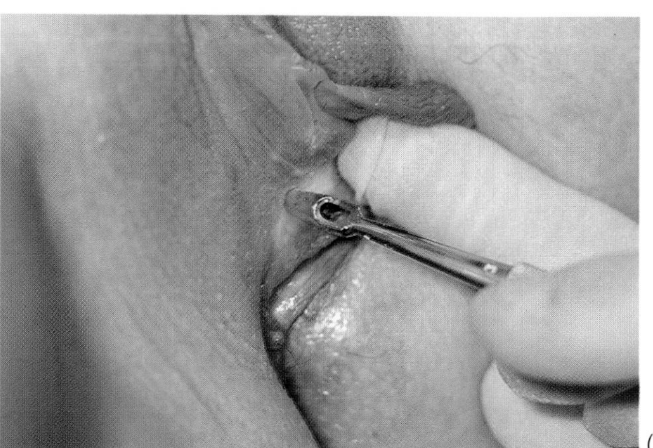

(c)

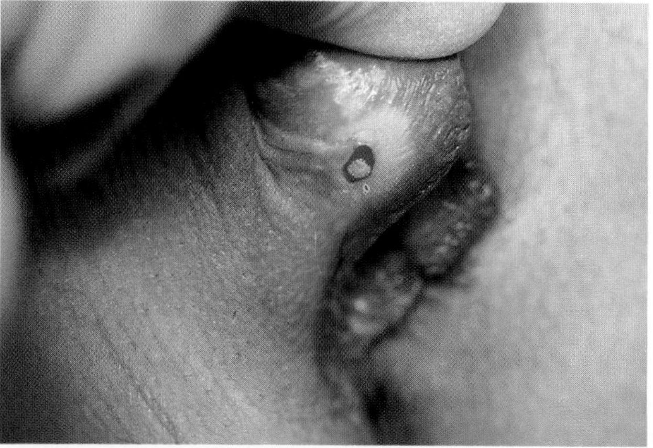

(d)

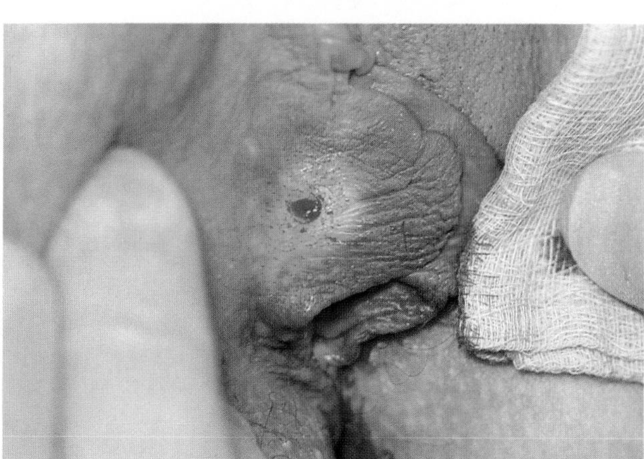

(e)

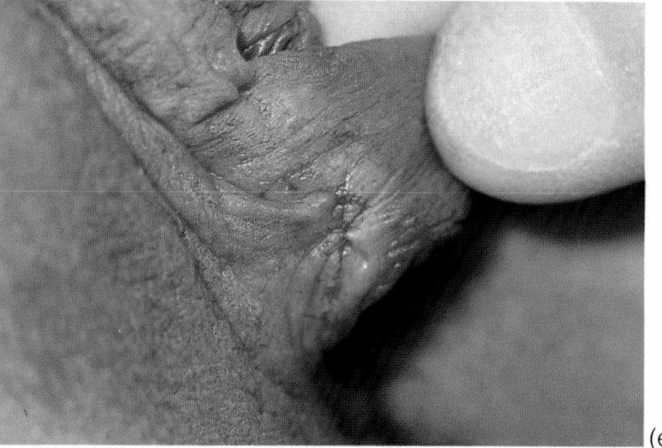

Fig. 16.22 Technique of vulval biopsy using Keye's punch. (a) A solitary white lesion on the outer aspect of the (R) labium minus. **(b)** Punch applied with a circular motion. **(c)** Circular incision on removal of punch. **(d)** Biopsy bed after removal of specimen by undercutting with scalpel. **(e)** Haemostasis achieved with a single plain catgut suture.

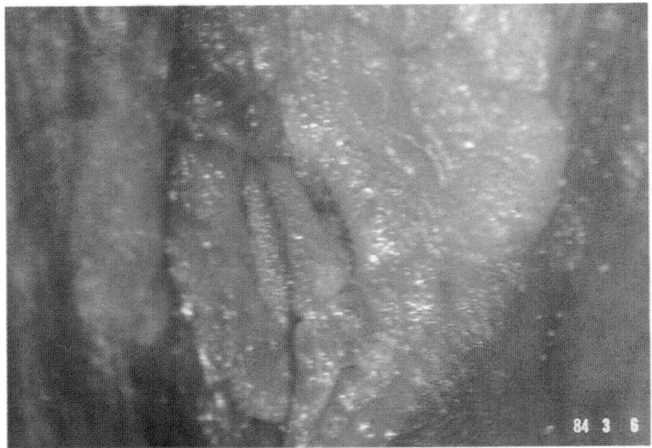

Fig. 16.23 **Vulva intraepithelial neoplasia.** A white lesion before application of acetic acid. A thick superficial keratin layer is seen.

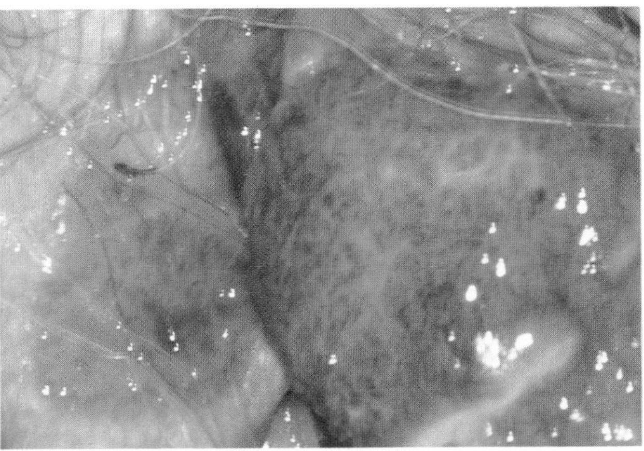

Fig. 16.24 Vulva, before application of acetic acid, showing flat red lesions (VIN 3) on the left. On the right there is an adjacent, raised, irregular vascular lesion, with a linear area of thick white keratin (invasive squamous carcinoma).

(a)

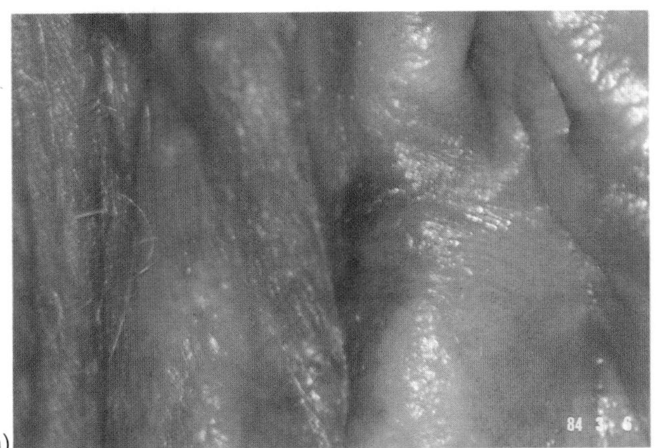

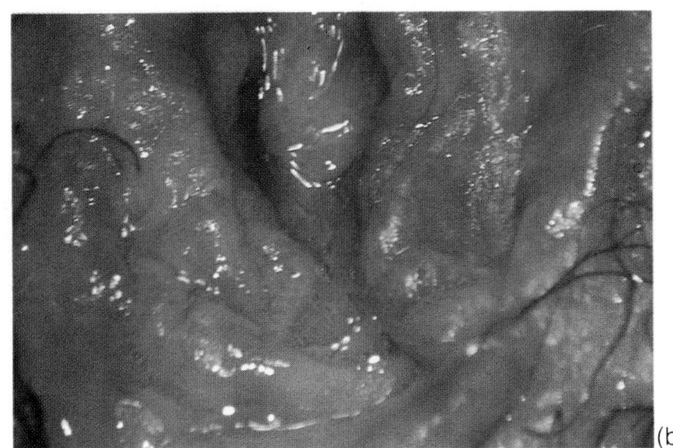

(b)

Fig. 16.25 Vulva intraepithelial neoplasia. Pigmented lesions on the anterior vulva **(a)** and posterior vulva at fourchette **(b)**.

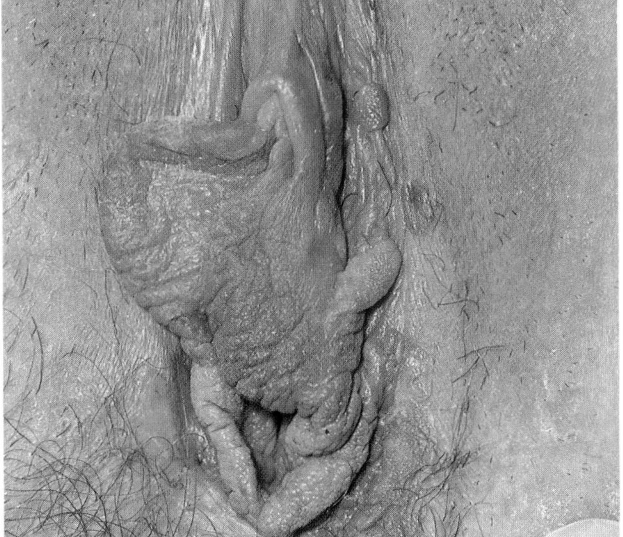

Fig. 16.26 Pigmented multifocal/multicentric intraepithelial neoplasia. Both vulva and perianal skin bear lesions overt to the naked eye.

16.29), and a thin smear of lubricant may assist in visualizing an underlying abnormal vascular pattern, although this may not always be successful. Approximately 15% of intraepithelial neoplastic lesions are associated with previous or concurrent human papillomavirus infection, and an overlay of colposcopic features of the latter may be present as overt condylomatous change or subclinical papillomavirus infection. This may be easily confused with the raised, irregular surface of invasive disease, stressing the need for an appropriate biopsy in all cases.

As already discussed, the abnormal vascular patterns of punctation and mosaic or atypical vessels, so often a readily recognized feature of cervical and vaginal intraepithelial neoplasia or early invasive lesions at these sites, are not commonly seen in vulval lesions; this is partly due to the obscuring effect of keratin or indeed hyperkeratosis.

The naked-eye appearance of the vulva in a case of chronic itching is seen in Fig. 16.29(a). The clitoral area looks thickened, and there is an area of white change. At medium colposcopic magnification (Fig. 16.29(b)), with the aid of a lubricant and before application of acetic acid, the abnormal vascular pattern is obvious, along with dense white patches. These features are even more overt at higher colposcopic magnification (Fig. 16.29(c)). A full-thickness biopsy revealed an extensive VIN 3 with early invasion in several areas, as well as a thick, keratinized surface corresponding to the white patches. In Fig. 16.30, highly atypical vessels are seen at maximum colposcopic magnification, aided by lubrication only, in a case of recurrent invasive carcinoma of the vulva. Vessels are also seen running in 'corkscrew' fashion, parallel to the overlying epithelial surface, along with irregular dilatation

(a) 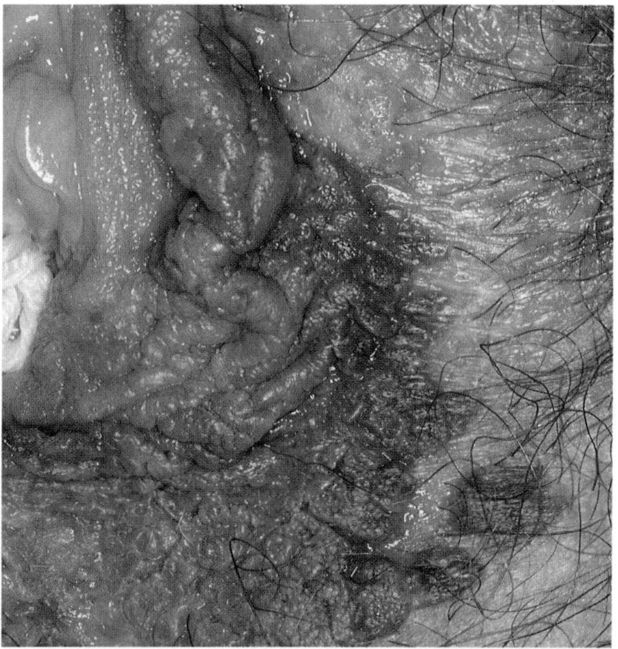

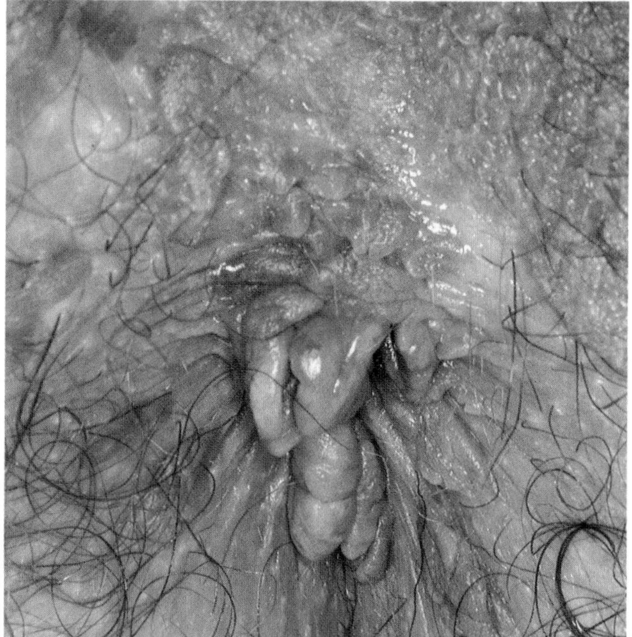 (b)

Fig. 16.27 Pigmented multifocal intraepithelial neoplasia. (a) Raised warty pigmented lesions on the right posterior vulva, and **(b)** similar lesions around anus. High-grade VIN and AIN on mapping biopsies.

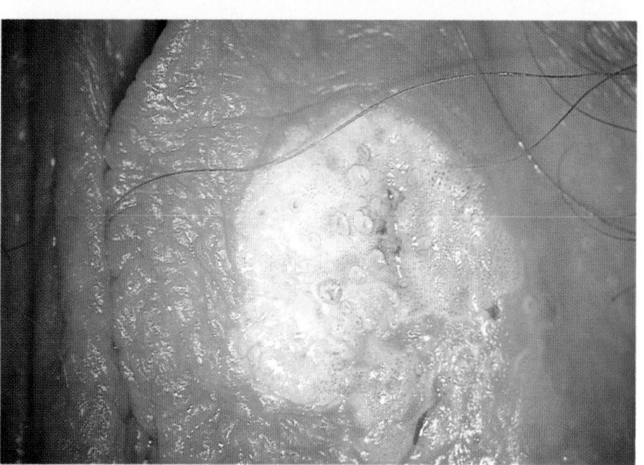

Fig. 16.28 Vulva intraepithelial neoplasia. A raised acetowhite lesion is seen on the outer aspect of labium minus and interlabial sulcus.

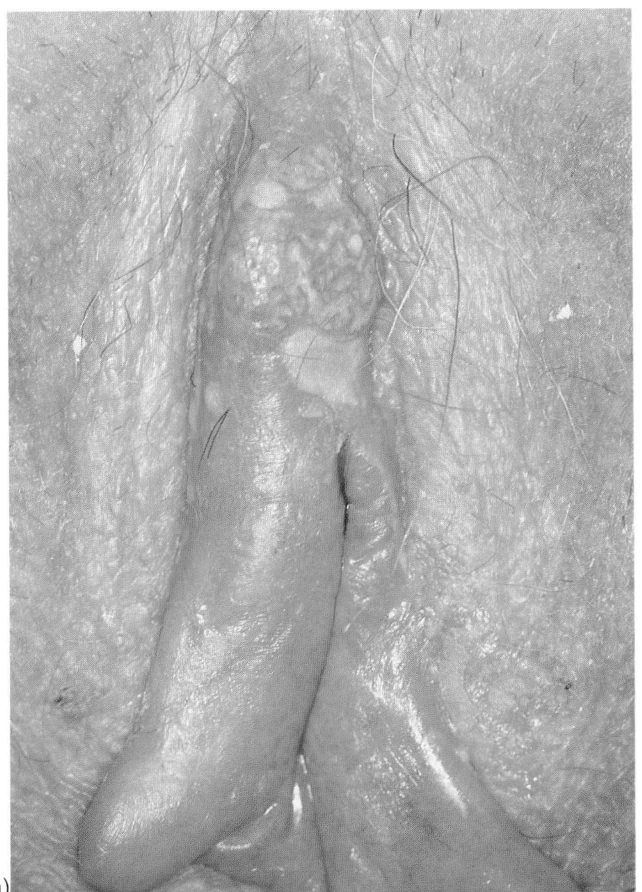

(a)

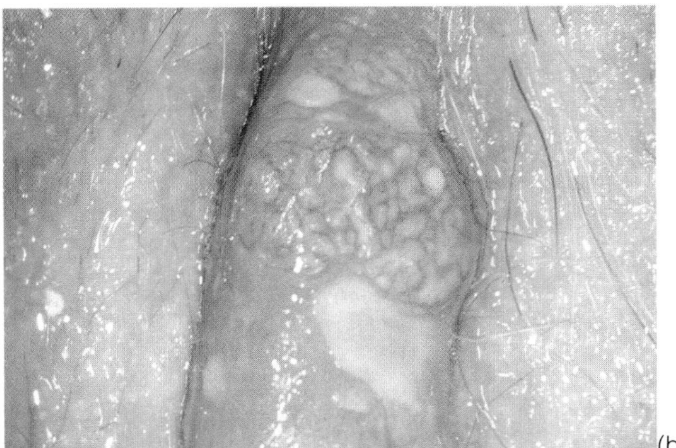

(b)

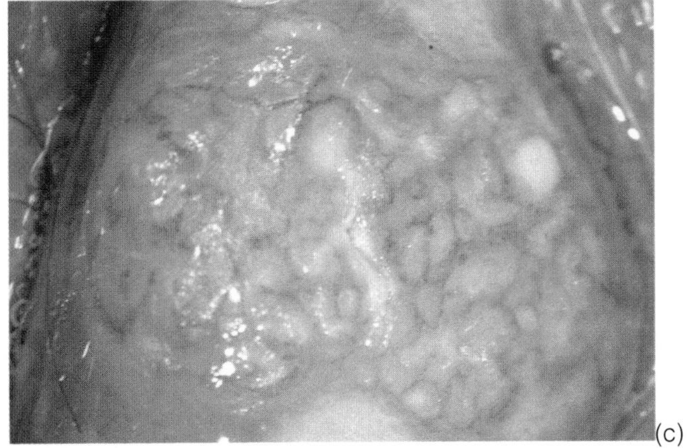

(c)

Fig. 16.29 (a) Naked-eye view of clitoral VIN 3, with areas of microinvasion. (b) Medium colposcopic magnification, showing abnormal vascular pattern and white keratotic patches. Examination was with lubrication only, on application of acetic acid. **(c)** Vascular pattern seen at higher magnification.

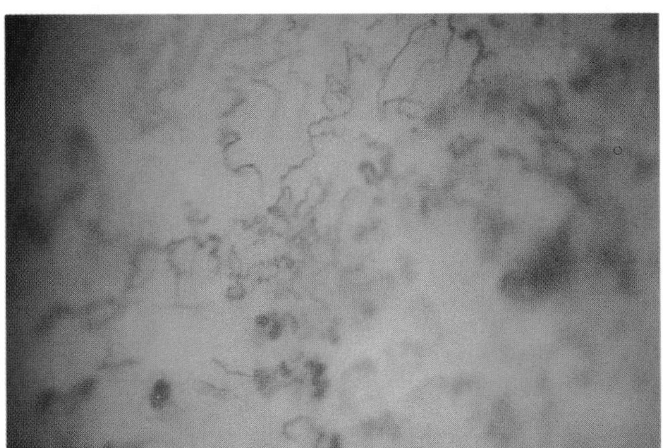

Fig. 16.30 Recurrence of vulval carcinoma. Highly atypical vessels are seen with lubrication only; no application of acetic acid.

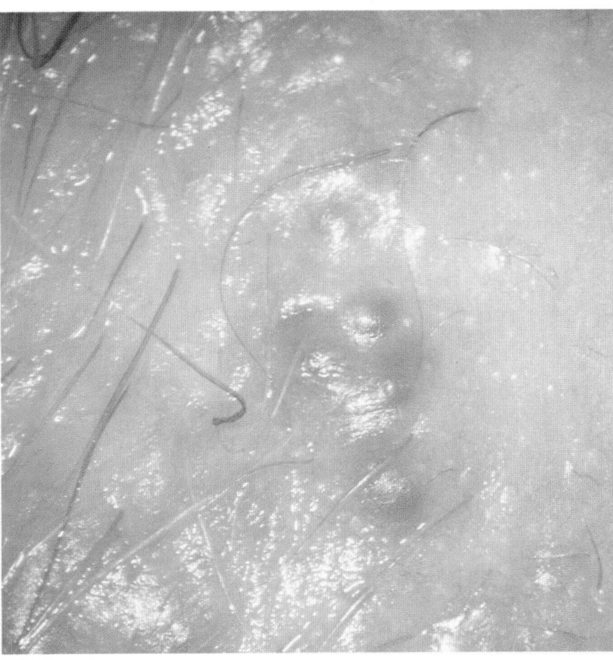

Fig. 16.31 Secondary vulval deposits. Original lesion was primary cervical cancer. Patient presented with recurrent disseminated disease.

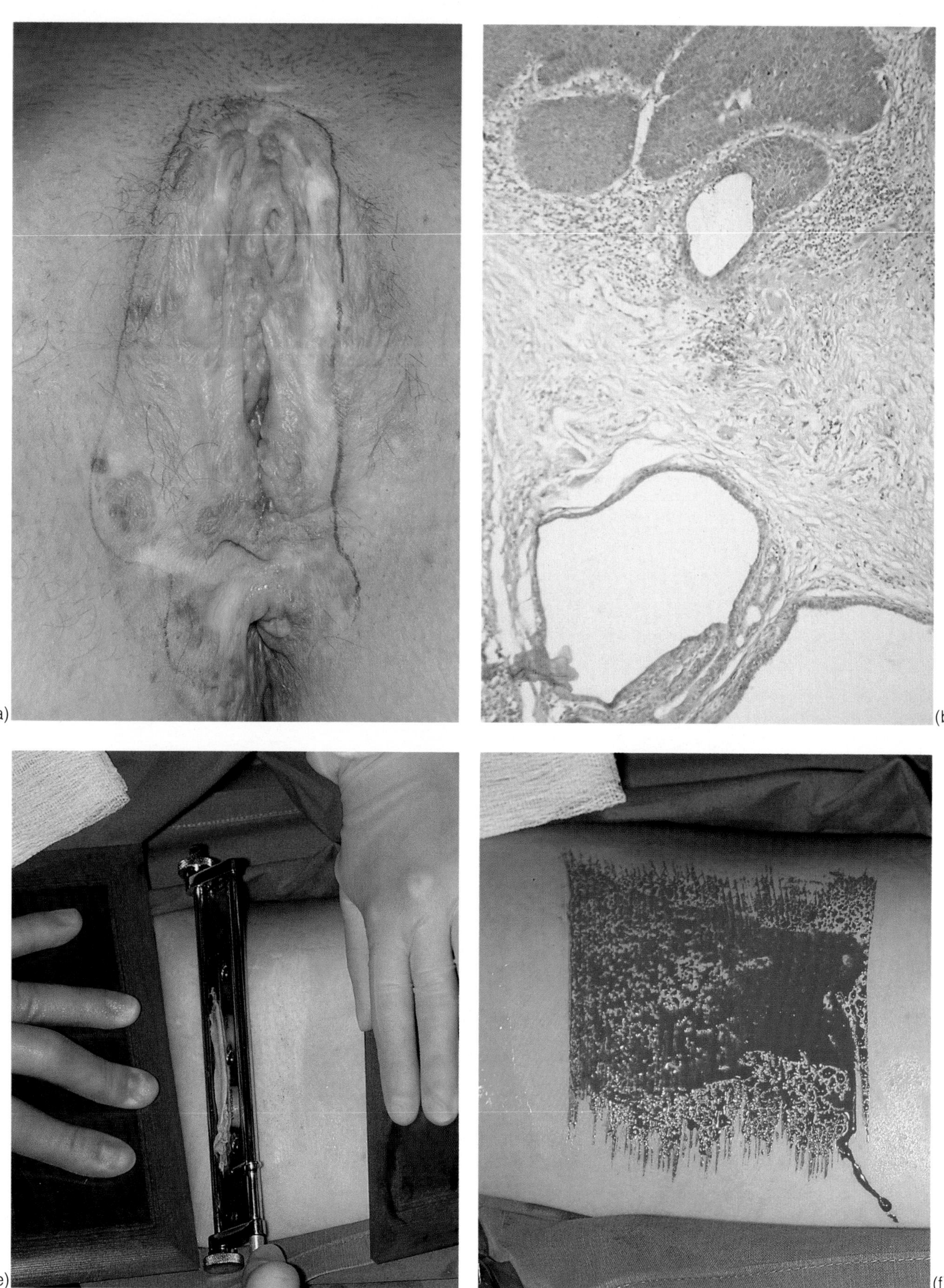
(a)
(b)
(e)
(f)

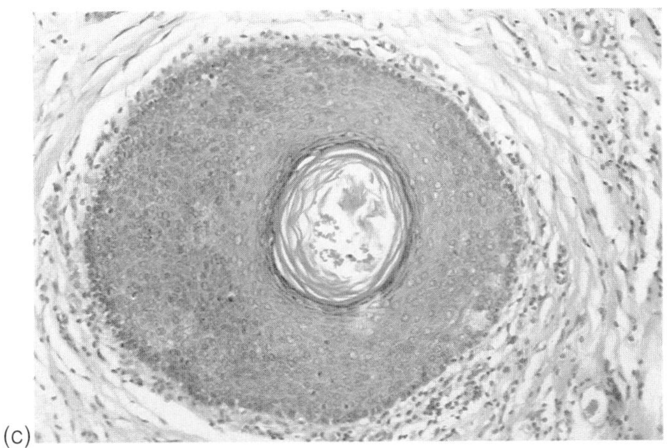

(c)

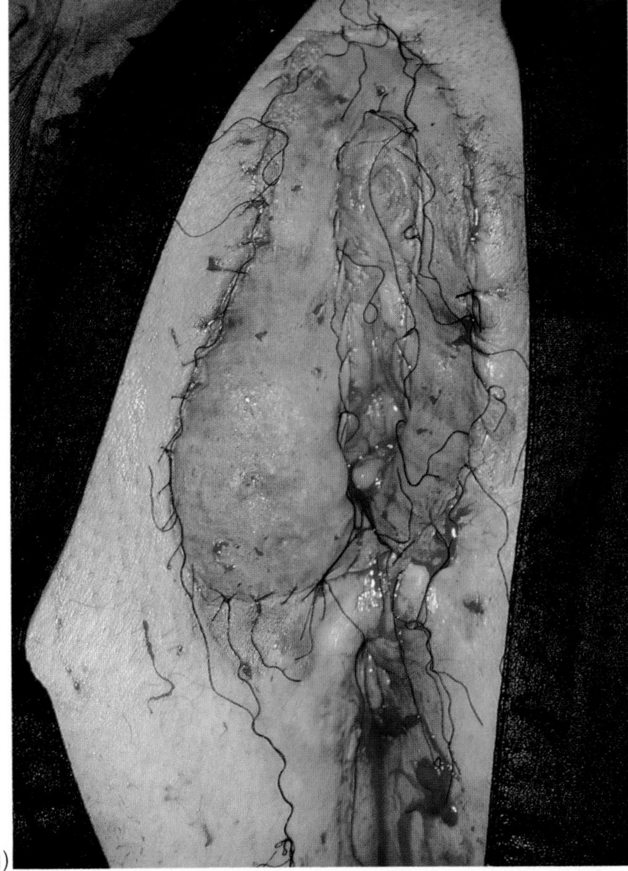

(g)

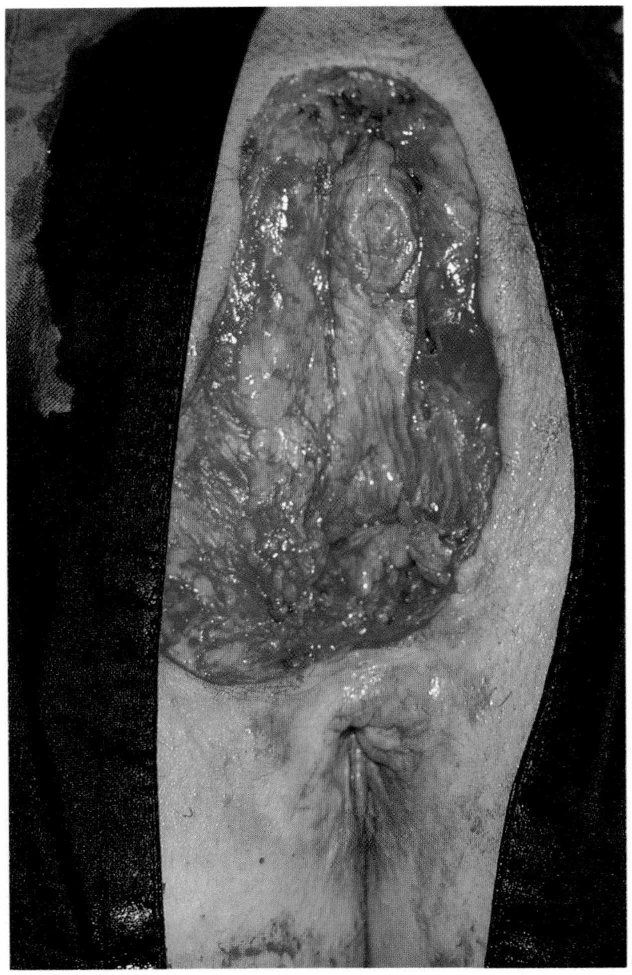

(d)

Fig. 16.32 Extensive recurrent VIN 3. Previous treatment was by local excision, laser vaporization and 5-fluorouracil, but all methods failed. **(a)** Widespread red and pigmented lesions with areas of white change, partly due to scarring. **(b)** Preliminary vulval biopsy shows VIN 3 within the sweat gland ducts (above). **(c)** Preliminary biopsy shows hair shaft involvement by vulval intraepithelial neoplasia (dark-staining haematoxylinophilic crescent on the left of shaft). **(d)** Superficial skinning of vulvectomy completed, conserving the clitoris. **(e)** Fashioning split skin graft from donor site on the thigh. **(f)** Donor site on completion. **(g)** Completion of grafting on the vulvectomy bed.

producing a beading effect. It should be stressed that where an invasive element is suspected, as elsewhere in the lower genital tract, a full-thickness biopsy is mandatory for a proper histopathological evaluation.

Metastatic tumour deposits may very occasionally be seen in the vulva (Fig. 16.31).

Management options

All cases of suspected vulval intraepithelial neoplasia must be diagnosed by biopsy, following the criteria elaborated above. The question of possible skin appendage involvement by the disease process must be taken into account in every case. Hair-bearing vulval skin may be a particular problem in this respect. Adequate biopsy should exclude or define this when present, ruling out microinvasive or frankly invasive disease. The preliminary colposcopy will also have helped in defining the topographical distribution of the lesion(s) on the surface.

Before outlining the available options for treatment, one further consideration must be borne in mind: with cervical intraepithelial neoplasia, some recent long-term observations suggest that as many as one-third of high-grade lesions that continue to exfoliate dyskaryotic cells after the index biopsy may develop into invasive disease in time; however, the same data are not available for vulval intraepithelial neoplasia. In other words, at present our knowledge of the natural history of vulval intraepithelial neoplasia and invasive squamous carcinoma of the vulva is lacking. Nevertheless, it seems likely that we are dealing with similar processes and possibly a similar aetiology.

Observation without treatment

The question may be asked, what happens to high-grade vulval intraepithelial neoplasia if the lesions are simply observed? Some patients have been observed without therapy, and in one report five out of 50 (10%) cases of VIN 3 regressed spontaneously, even in the presence of aneuploidy in the lesion. Progression to invasive disease is also noted, although perhaps with a lesser frequency than might have been expected. However, care must be taken in drawing conclusions from such reports, in view of the relatively short periods of observation. More data are required in these areas, but clearly these will not be forthcoming quickly if long-term studies are required to deal with this problem. In the meantime, there may be occasions where observation without treatment may be justified, for example in the case of elderly and frail patients.

Surgery

The traditional treatment for vulval carcinoma *in situ*, as advocated by Knight, has been wide local excision. Many gynaecologists have preferred to remove the entire vulva on the grounds that the disease was premalignant and often multifocal. This approach reflects the time when diagnostic colposcopy was not widely practised, and is akin to very large cone biopsy without colposcopic control for cervical intraepithelial neoplasia.

In addition, there is greater postoperative morbidity, and loss of the clitoris may render the patient anorgasmic; this may be a particularly important consideration for the younger age groups in whom the disease seems to be more prevalent. Also, total vulvectomy is regarded as disfiguring by a number of treated women, irrespective of age.

These problems have led to the development of a more shallow excisional vulvectomy procedure, with conservation of the clitoris, if possible, and followed by split-thickness skin grafting of the vulva using tissue from the thigh (Fig. 16.32).

Cryotherapy has also been advocated, and it may have a place in very small, isolated lesions without appendage involvement. However, it seems likely that such lesions will be more efficiently removed by excision biopsy in the first instance. Extensive freezing of large areas of vulval skin is likely to be followed by total sloughing, and painful and protracted healing, and is therefore not recommended.

Carbon dioxide laser

Carbon dioxide laser vaporization of the affected or all vulval skin in widespread disease has also been tried, with apparently good results following on from its success in the treatment of cervical and vaginal intraepithelial neoplasia. With this technique, intense, precisely controlled thermal destruction of the epithelium is possible under colposcopic control (Fig. 16.33). Reid (1985) has described four surgical planes of the vulval skin, and claims to be able to destroy the target tissue to the following depths (planes):

1. First plane: surface epithelium.
2. Second plane: dermal papillae.
3. Third plane: pilosebaceous ducts.
4. Fourth plane: depths of pilosebaceous unit.

It is feasible to achieve a depth of laser destruction to the first and fourth planes, as described. However, it is uncertain whether the same is possible for the intervening two planes. Healing of the vulva after superficial laser vulvectomy is protracted but with a satisfactory end result.

Vaporization to the depths of the entire pilosebaceous unit should not be undertaken without split skin grafting.

Chemotherapy

Topical 5-fluorouracil has also been used for vulval intraepithelial neoplasia. Overall response rates, as evidenced from published series, seem to be in the region of less than 50%. Local application is extended over six weeks, producing ulceration and sloughing. Pain may be intense, with significant non-compliance of patients. Remarkably, healing is associated with little scarring.

Treatment using sensitization to 2,4-dinitrochlorobenzene (DNCB) has also been described, producing ulceration followed by healing, as seen with 5-fluorouracil.

Treatment rationalization

Proper colposcopic and histopathological evaluation is a prerequisite for any form of treatment selected, with particular consideration of the need to exclude microinvasive and occult invasive disease and skin appendage involvement.

All destructive methods (cryotherapy, laser vaporization, 5-fluorouracil and DNCB) are limited by the disadvantage of not providing a total tissue specimen for histological appraisal. It is also doubtful and unproven whether 5-fluorouracil or DNCB sensitization can deal adequately with appendage disease. Although uncommon, early invasion may be present in some cases of apparent VIN 3, as is the case with CIN 3. If foci are recognized and adequately removed, prognosis is likely to be excellent.

Likewise, there are at present several studies quantitating the observed depth of appendage involvement by vulval intraepithelial neoplasia. Normal pilosebaceous units may project as deep as 10 mm below the skin surface, although it would seem unusual for the preneoplastic process to reach this depth.

For single or multiple lesions limited to the surface area, a wide local excision biopsy with or without suturing will probably suffice, both as treatment and for histopathological characterization. Lesions in the non-hair-bearing skin of the vestibule and medial aspects of the labia minora, i.e. near the mucocutaneous junction, are suited to superficial carbon dioxide vaporization. The technique is also useful for small and multiple lesions in other parts of the vulva, provided that the histological criteria have been met.

Suspect invasion, biopsy-proven appendage involvement, or very extensive disease are best dealt with by wide excision; in effect, this may represent hemivulvectomy or sometimes superficial excision of the whole vulva. In these circumstances, split skin grafting is indicated. The clitoris should not be removed unless it is clearly involved. Total vulvectomy carrying the dissection to deep planes is rarely indicated; the patient would most likely be elderly.

Irrespective of the treatment method applied, the recurrence rate of vulval intraepithelial neoplasia may be in the region of 15–20%, and close monitoring with colposcopy will be necessary. Any recurrent lesion must be biopsied and further treatment planned along the above lines. Follow-up examination must exclude any *de novo* cervical, vaginal, urethral or anal lesions.

VULVAL PAPILLOMAVIRUS DISEASE

This can be subdivided into clinically overt lesions (condylomata acuminata and pigmented or non-pigmented papules), and subclinical disease, consisting of vestibular papillae, fused papillae and acetowhite epithelium. These will now be discussed with particular reference to colposcopic appearances; perianal and anal disease will also be addressed.

VULVAL CONDYLOMATA ACUMINATA

Condylomata acuminata of the vulva represent one level of a potentially multilevel sexually transmitted disease, with cervix, vagina and anal/perianal sites also likely to be involved.

Genital warts are now one of the most common sexually transmitted diseases, the reported prevalence having increased substantially in Western

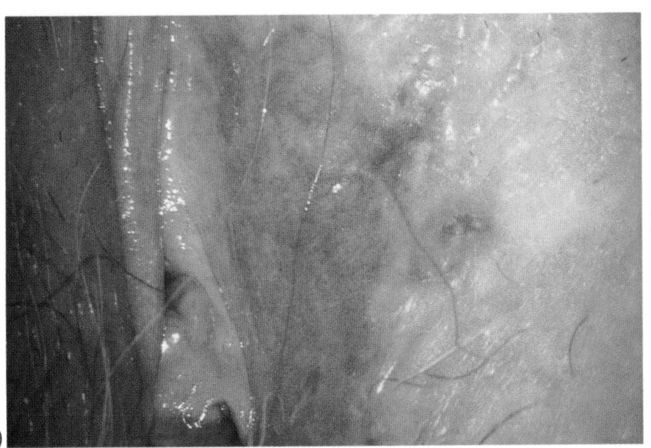

(a)

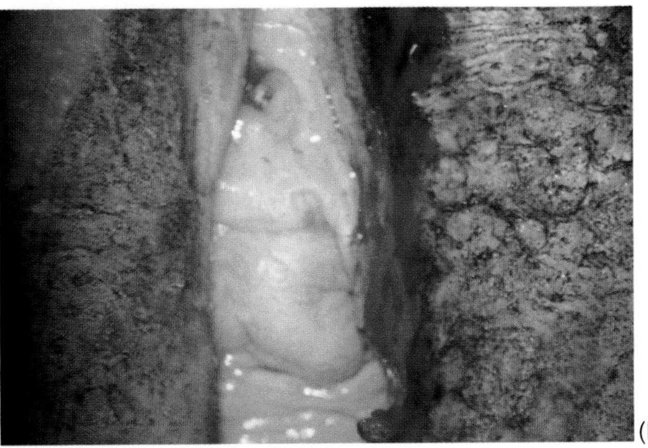

(b)

Fig. 16.33 Vulva intraepithelial neoplasia. Superficial vulvectomy by carbon dioxide laser vaporization. **(a)** Before treatment, a red lesion is seen in the interlabial sulcus. **(b)** Vulva on completion of vaporization (Reid's second surgical plane).

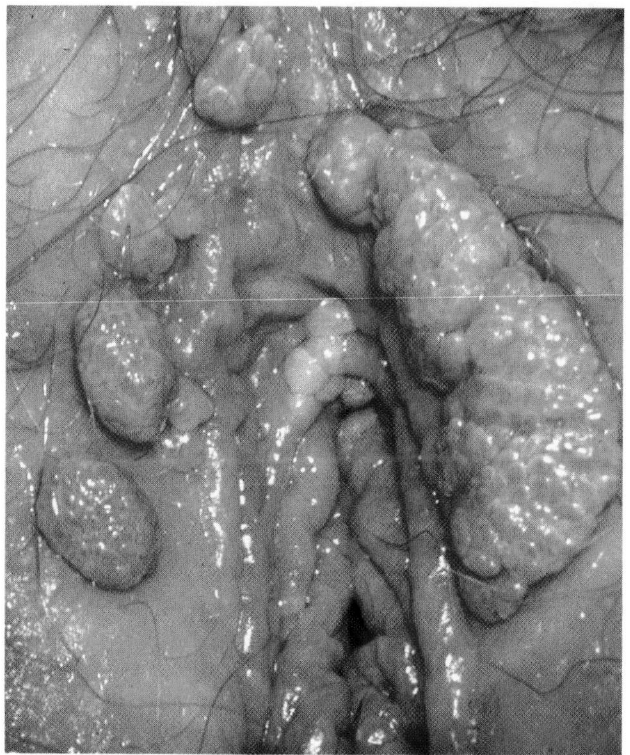

Fig. 16.34 Vulval condylomata acuminata.

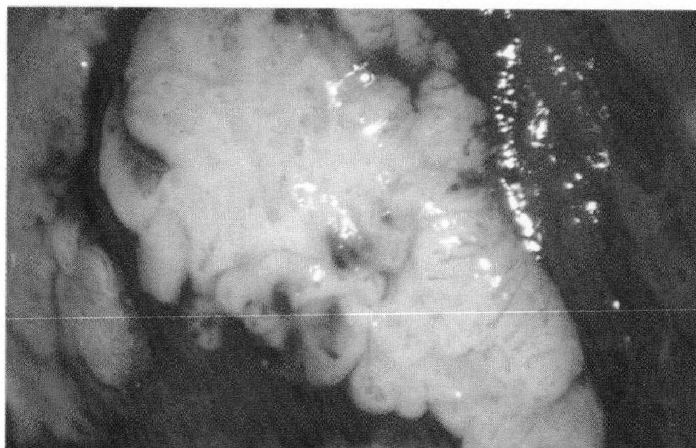

Fig. 16.35 Vulval condyloma after application of acetic acid. Marked acetowhite change and single capillary loop seen in individual fronds.

countries over the past two decades. The majority of exophytic condylomata acuminata are induced by HPV-6 or HPV-11. More than 60% of sexual partners of infected individuals are reported to develop lesions after an incubation period of one to three months. Progression of genital warts to invasive cancer is well documented, although the relative risk is very low.

The naked-eye appearance of condylomata at the vulval site is familiar (Fig. 16.34). Under higher magnification and after application of acetic acid, the agglomerated papilliferous acetowhite nature of the surface is obvious, each element containing an individual capillary loop (Fig. 16.35). Regardless of the apparently obvious naked-eye or colposcopic diagnosis, a biopsy should be taken for confirmation.

HUMAN PAPILLOMAVIRUS-INDUCED VULVAL PAPULES

Clinically overt, pigmented or non-pigmented papules may also be seen in human papillomavirus infection. These are raised, smooth and flat, and about 3–7 mm in diameter. The surface is often slightly glistening. Pigmentation may be present or absent. Less commonly, in negroid women, the papules may be associated with depigmentation. Lesions are frequently multiple and may coalesce. A biopsy would be necessary.

SUBCLINICAL HUMAN PAPILLOMAVIRUS INFECTION

This has been described in association with three types of lesion: vestibular papillae, fused papillae and acetowhite epithelium.

Vestibular papillae are multiple, small, spike-like projections of the vulval epithelium (Fig. 16.36), and as their name implies they are largely confined to the posterior fourchette, introitus and medial aspects of the labia minora. However, the external urethral meatus, the opening of Bartholin's gland ducts, minor vestibular gland ducts and Skene's glands are also reported as common sites.

The individual spike-like projections may occasionally appear to fuse or merge (Fig. 16.37), especially on the medial aspects of the labia minora, hence the name 'fused papillae'. This may result in a granular or velvety appearance, turning white after application of acetic acid. It has been claimed that these papilliferous lesions may be responsible for local pruritus or a burning sensation. For a time, an association between vestibular papillae, discrete or fused, and human papillomavirus was presumed. However, recent studies challenge this, and suggest that these appearances may be a variant of normal.

Finally, and less controversially, areas of vulval epithelium that turn white after application of acetic acid may be noted in otherwise apparently normal, flat vulval skin (Fig. 16.38). These acetowhite changes may affect any area, well keratinized or otherwise, hair-bearing or not. Biopsy will be required to give some indication of whether human papillomavirus or vulval intraepithelial neoplasia are implicated.

PERIANAL AND ANAL LESIONS

Both intraepithelial neoplastic processes and human papillomavirus infection of the vulva may extend and involve the perianal region and anal canal. The appearance of such lesions is similar to those described above under vulval disease. Firm lateral pressure on both buttocks may evert the anal canal to some degree, to reveal abnormality (Fig. 16.39).

However, proper exclusion or confirmation of disease in the anal canal requires the use of a proctoscope combined with a standard colposcopic technique, including application of acetic acid. If this is not tolerated in the out-patient setting, then day-case anaesthesia may be considered. Any lesion identified should be biopsied using a standard colposcopic punch instrument with a small bite.

Treatment of human papillomavirus lesions

Vulval condylomata acuminata vary from small, readily treatable lesions to extensive superficial growths affecting substantial areas of skin, with a tendency to local recurrence that may become an almost intractable process.

Biophysical methods of eradication are usually employed, such as application of surface electrodiathermy, diathermy excision of larger masses, cryotherapy and carbon dioxide laser vaporization or excision (Fig. 16.40). Success in part relates to the fastidiousness with which similar lesions at the other common adjacent sites are

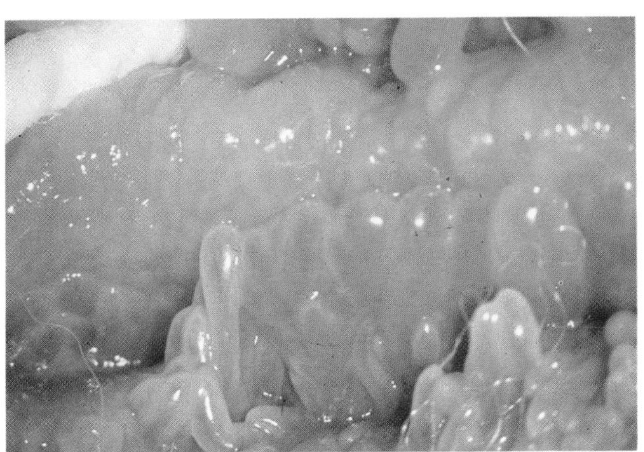

Fig. 16.36 Vestibular papillae. The multiple, small, spike-like projections are clearly seen.

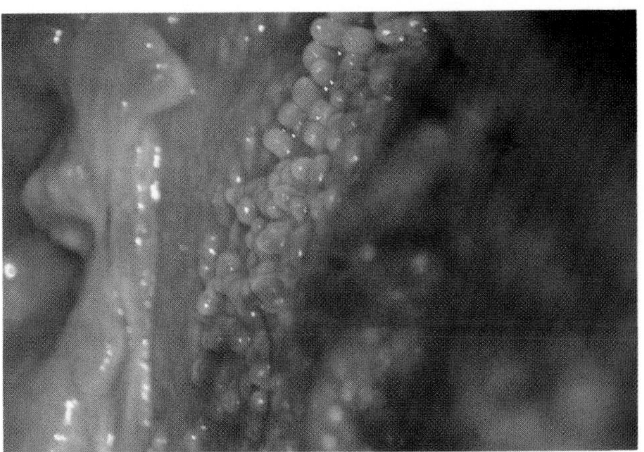

Fig. 16.37 Fused papillae in the posterior lateral vestibule. These give rise to a naked-eye velvety appearance.

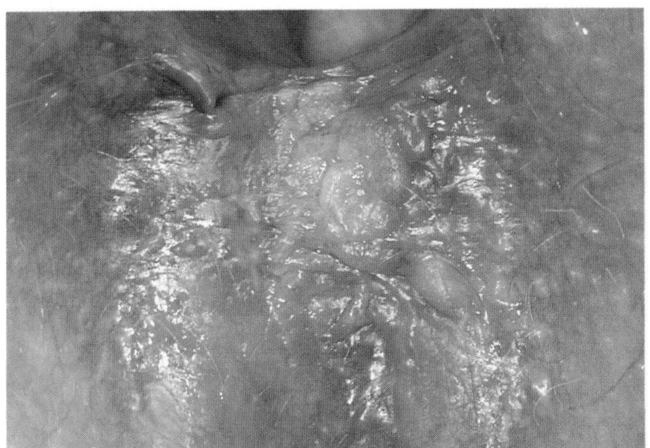

Fig. 16.38 Acetowhite change associated with human papillomavirus infection. Vulva, over the perineal body posterior to fourchette.

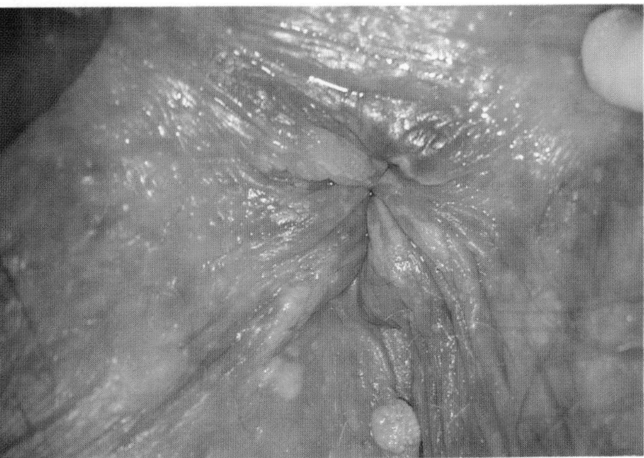

Fig. 16.39 Human papillomavirus-induced anal lesions. Patchy, fairly well-defined acetowhite islands (subclinical papillomavirus infection) are seen, together with a small discrete condyloma.

identified and treated simultaneously, along with appropriate screening of the consort for human papillomavirus disease (Fig. 16.41).

For the moment, any recommendation as to the treatment of subclinical human papillomavirus lesions of the vulva must be given with caution. Our knowledge of the natural history, pathophysiology and progression potential of these lesions is incomplete. This includes our understanding of the precise role of human papillomavirus in the carcinogenesis of invasive squamous lesions of the anogenital tract.

Furthermore, there have been recent studies of the prevalence of human papillomavirus infection in the general and apparently well population, using the new, highly sensitive PCR technology for the identification of human papillomavirus DNA. These data suggest that an alarmingly high percentage of women and presumably their consorts may carry the virus. Finally, there is little information to suggest that there is any reasonable hope of eradicating the virus from the entire anogenital epithelium by destroying subclinical papillomavirus infection with any of the available methods.

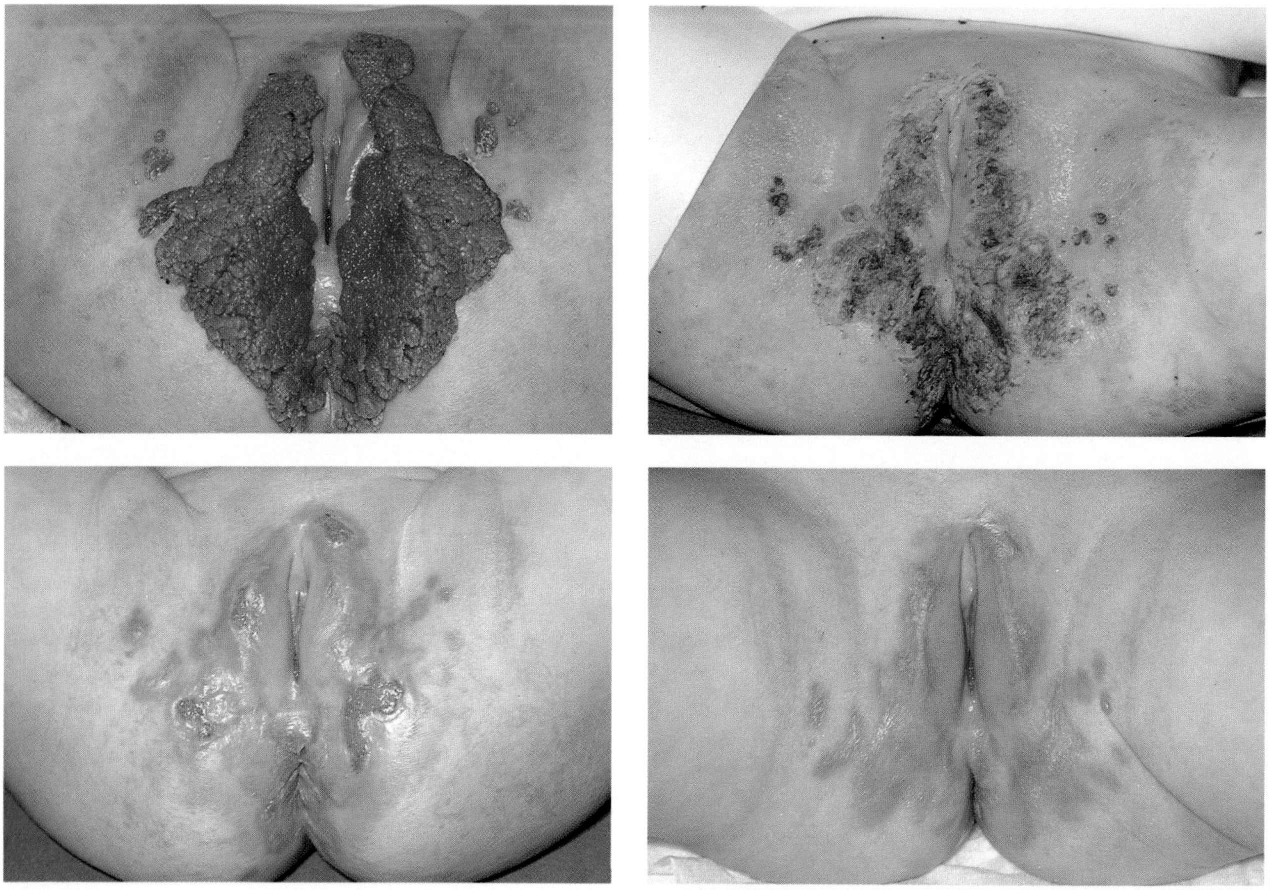

(a)
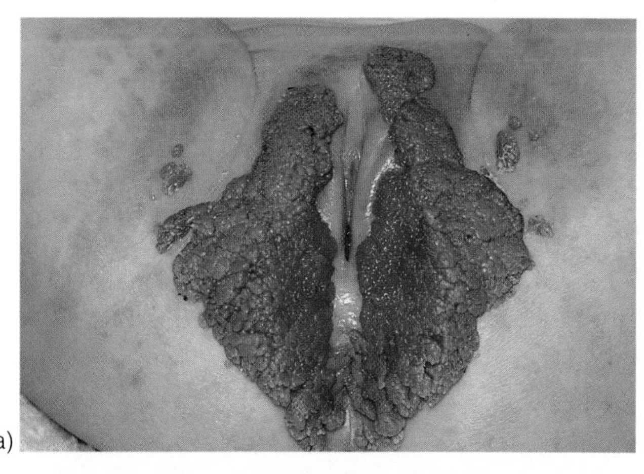

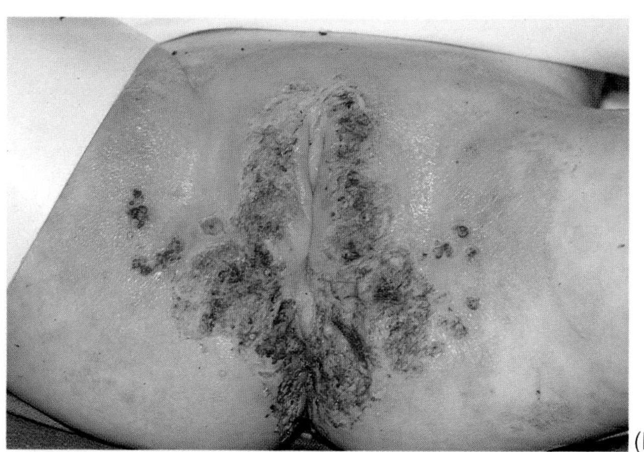
(b)

(c)
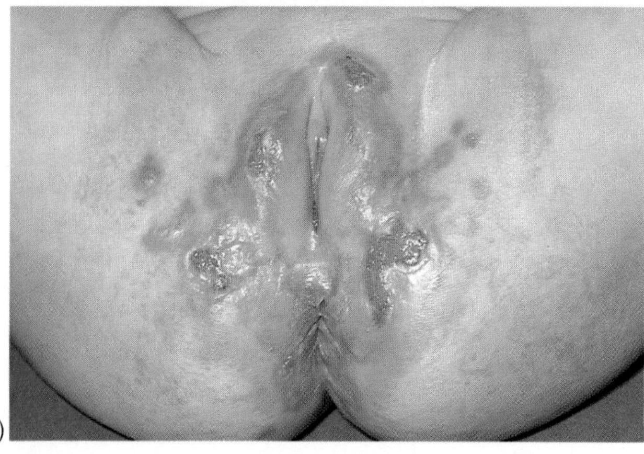

(d)

Fig. 16.40 Gigantic juvenile vulval condylomata (HPV-6/11) in an 18-month-old child. These were recurrent, despite several previous attempts to ablate using diathermy. **(a)** Immediately before treatment. **(b)** Immediately after combination treatment, involving initial excision of main bulk with electrodiathermy loop, followed by laser vaporization. **(c)** Three weeks after treatment; healing is seen to progress well. **(d)** Five weeks after treatment.

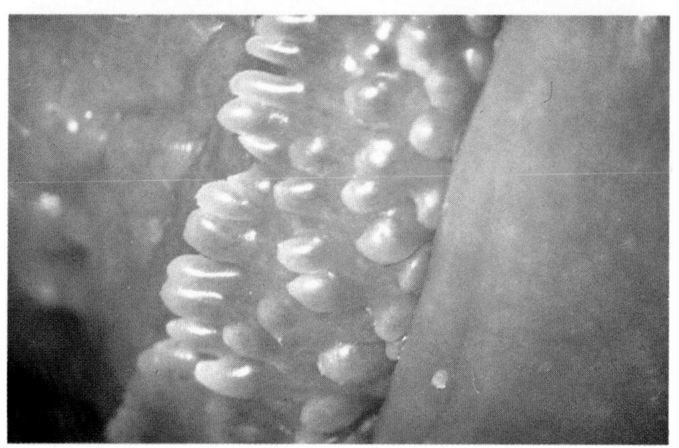

Fig. 16.41 Human papillomavirus-induced papillae in the penile coronal sulcus.

17. *Anal intraepithelial neoplasia and anal colposcopy*

INTRODUCTION

It is recognized that in women, genital intraepithelial neoplasia may be multifocal, and may involve the cervix, vagina and vulva, either singly or in combination. Anal intraepithelial neoplasia (AIN) is a relatively recently recognized clinical problem, whose prevalence is largely unknown and malignant potential uncertain. However, it is now apparent that such anal lesions may from time to time form part of a more general anogenital intraepithelial or invasive neoplastic process, and it is appropriate for them to be considered here.

SUBDIVISIONS OF THE ANAL CANAL

The boundaries of the perianal epithelium and the anal canal are poorly defined. Different anatomical boundaries have been described by a number of authors. Arbitrarily, from the colposcopist's point of view, the perianal skin and lower anal canal are defined as the area which can be readily seen on parting the buttocks widely. The upper anal canal epithelium is above this level, limited cephalad by the rectal mucosa at the anal squamocolumnar junction, and best examined using a proctoscope.

Anatomically, the canal is usually identified as lying between the upper and lower borders of the internal anal sphincter and includes the dentate line, which is identified by the naked eye by the anal valves and the bases of the anal columns (Fig. 17.1) Histologically, the canal is composed of a colorectal zone (lined by columnar epithelium), separated by the squamocolumnar junction from the anal transition zone, which is lined by stratified columnar ('transitional') mucosa (Fig. 17.2). Distal to this level, the lower anal canal is lined by non-keratinizing stratified squamous epithelium; this becomes keratinized at the anal opening and perianal skin.

DEFINITION OF ANAL INTRAEPITHELIAL NEOPLASIA

Anal intraepithelial neoplasia (AIN) is a condition whose histopathological and clinical features have been described in the last decade, characterized by the presence of cellular and nuclear abnormalities in the perianal and anal canal epithelium without breach of the epithelial basement membrane, and similar to its cervical, vaginal and vulval counterparts – CIN, VAIN and VIN.

Prevalence and risk groups

The true prevalence of AIN is unknown. It was initially thought to be a rare condition; the frequency of occurrence of unrecognized intraepithelial neoplasia encountered during minor surgery of the anal canal being reported as between 0.2% and 4.4%. However, in groups thought to be at risk, namely, homosexual men who practise receptive anal intercourse, immunosuppressed HIV-positive individuals, women with high-grade genital intraepithelial and invasive squamous neoplasia, renal allograft recipients, and individuals of both sexes

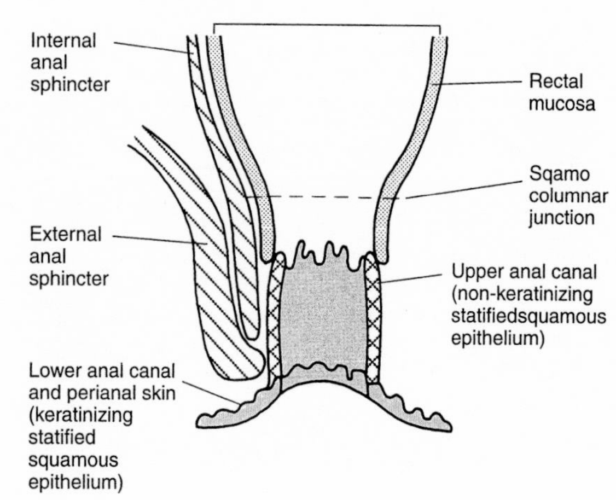

Fig. 17.1 The anatomy of the anal canal. (After Talbot and Price.)

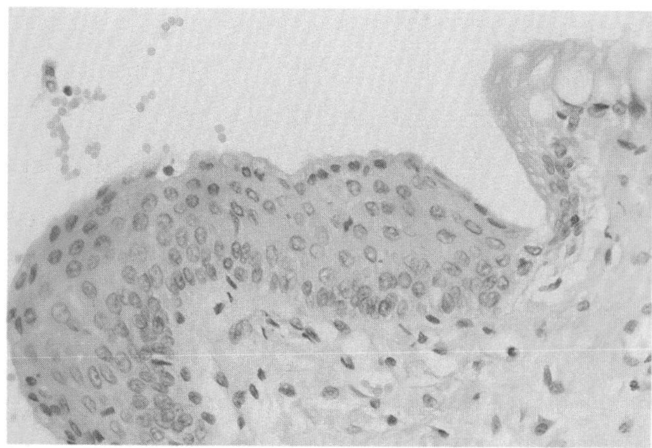

Fig. 17.2 Normal anal transition zone (ATZ). The squamocolumnar junction separates the columnar epithelium of the colorectal zone (right), from the stratified non-keratinized 'transitional'-type epithelium (left).

with anogenital condylomata (warts), the prevalence of AIN is high. This varies from 15% to 53% in immunosuppressed HIV positive individuals, from 19% to 47% in women with high-grade genital intraepithelial or invasive neoplasia, and 24% in renal allograft recipients. In contrast, the prevalence of AIN in control populations is very low, being reported to be less than 1%.

Pathological features

Histologically, AIN is characterized by a loss of epithelial cellular maturation with associated nuclear hyperchromasia, pleomorphism, cellular crowding, and abnormal mitoses within the anal epithelium. These features are identical to those of similar cervical and vulval lesions, and AIN lesions are classified according to the cervical intraepithelial neoplasia (CIN) nomenclature. In AIN 1 (Fig. 17.3), cellular and nuclear abnormalities are restricted to the lower third of the epithelium, in AIN 2 and AIN 3 (Fig. 17.4), the lower two-thirds and the full thickness of the epithelium respectively are affected. The histological features of AIN 3 are consistent with it being the precursor lesion of invasive and squamous cancer.

Aetiology

It is now generally accepted that squamous neoplasia at the various levels of the anogenital region may share common aetiological factors. Current evidence strongly implicates oncogenic human papillomaviruses (HPV), particularly HPV type 16, as a major factor in the aetiology of anogenital neoplasia. It appears that HPV infection of this region occurs in a manner that may result in synchronous or sequential development of anogenital neoplasia. HPV-16 has been identified in 56–80% of squamous cell carcinoma of the anus and AIN lesions. AIN 3 lesions appear to contain HPV-16 more frequently than lower grades of AIN.

Despite the strong causal relationship between HPV and anogenital neoplasia, it is unlikely that HPV on its own is sufficient for the production and maintenance of the neoplastic state. It possible that HPV acts in a synergistic fashion with other factors such as other viruses and smoking, and the interaction between HPV, oncogenes and tumour suppressor genes.

The association between neoplasia and systemic immunosuppression is well established. Studies based primarily on organ transplant recipients have demonstrated an overall risk of 5–6% of developing a neoplasm after transplantation. Although the nature of this predisposition is unknown, immunosuppression in this group may reduce immunosurveillance by the lymphoreticular system. Reports from Cancer Registry data and controlled studies suggest that there is a four- to 14-fold increase in the incidence and prevalence of HPV-associated high-grade intraepithelial and invasive tumours of the cervix. Registry data suggest a similar increase for the prevalence of invasive anal and vulval neoplasia. However, systemic immunosuppression does not appear to be a prerequisite for the development of multifocal HPV-associated neoplasia. In three recent

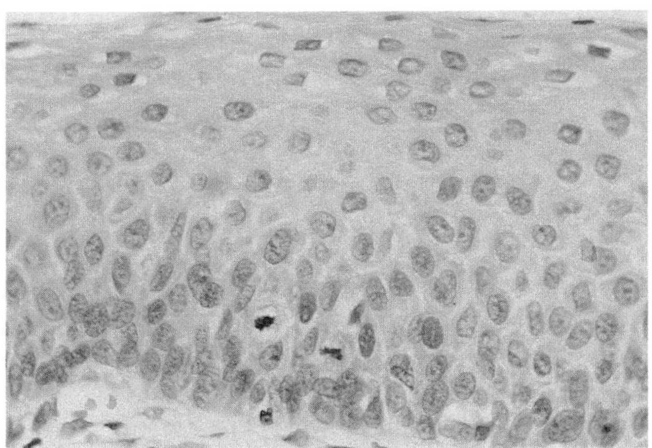

Fig. 17.3 AIN 1. The cellular and nuclear abnormalities are restricted to the lower third of the epithelium.

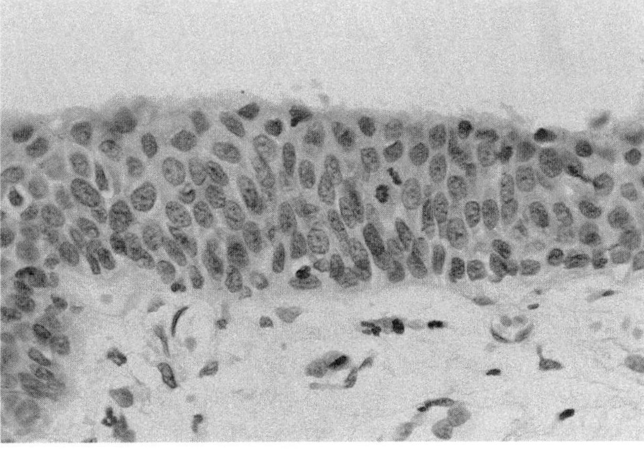

Fig. 17.4 AIN 3. Cellular and nuclear abnormalities extend throughout the full thickness of the epithelium.

clinical studies on apparently immunocompetent women who had high-grade cervical and vulval intraepithelial neoplasia, and invasive vulval cancer, prevalence rates of 50%, 19% and 47% respectively for anal HPV infection and AIN were reported. It is possible that HPV infection of this area produces change in the local cellular immunity which facilitates progression to neoplastic change.

Natural history and epidemiology

The natural history of AIN is unknown. In cervical neoplasia, rates of progression are well documented, but such data are lacking for anal dysplasia. Aetiological parallels with CIN and the histological appearances of AIN 3, suggest that AIN 3 has malignant potential. AIN 3 has been observed in the anal canal mucosa of routinely excised haemorrhoidal tissue. In a mean follow-up period of six years, only one patient developed recurrent disease, and none developed invasive disease. These reports suggest that incidentally discovered AIN 3 is a non-aggressive lesion. However, others have reported the presence of AIN 3 in 81% (13/16) of cases of anal squamous carcinoma. The lesions were found to be situated at the border of the invasive lesions as well as in areas separated from the tumours by normal mucosa.

In Sheffield, a total of 32 patients with AIN 3, including nine anal cancers in a field change of AIN 3, have been identified in prospective clinical studies over a four-year period. Of these, five (15.5%) developed invasive anal disease within a median follow-up period of 18 months (range 0.5–2 years). This suggests strongly that AIN, and particularly AIN 3, has malignant potential. However, the proportion of AIN 3 lesions that may progress to invasive disease, or indeed regress, remains to be determined. Even less is known of the fate of low-grade AIN lesions (AIN 1 and 2). In the Sheffield series regression of low-grade lesions was observed in 13% (3/23) of cases over a median follow-up period of seven months. There is a need for longitudinal studies to determine the rates of progression to high-grade disease in the various risk groups.

Invasive anal cancer is at present an uncommon malignancy constituting 3% of all large bowel tumours, with a male to female ratio of 1:2. Since it is less common than cervical cancer, it is possible that the risk of progression from intraepithelial neoplasia to invasive cancer is lower for the anus than for the cervix. However, a recent epidemiological report from the USA, showed that the incidence of AIN and anal cancer, particularly in the anal canal, is rising. In this study, a three-fold increase in the incidence of anal cancers in both sexes between 1959 and 1986 was observed. This is supported by further data from Scandinavia. This may be partly due to the increasing prevalence of anogenital HPV infections. If the natural history of AIN is similar to that of CIN, then the development of anal cancer may occur several years after the diagnosis of AIN.

Clinical features

Anal HPV infection and AIN are usually asymptomatic. However, some patients may present with perianal and anal canal condylomata (warts), pruritus ani and, very occasionally, bleeding. Although AIN lesions have been identified in the perianal skin, the most frequent site for AIN would appear to be the anal transition zone (ATZ). This suggests that anal HPV infection in the ATZ is more susceptible to dysplastic change than infections in the perianal region. However, AIN lesions may also occur at both sites in some individuals, stressing the importance of examining the perianal skin and anal canal in individuals suspected of having anal HPV infection.

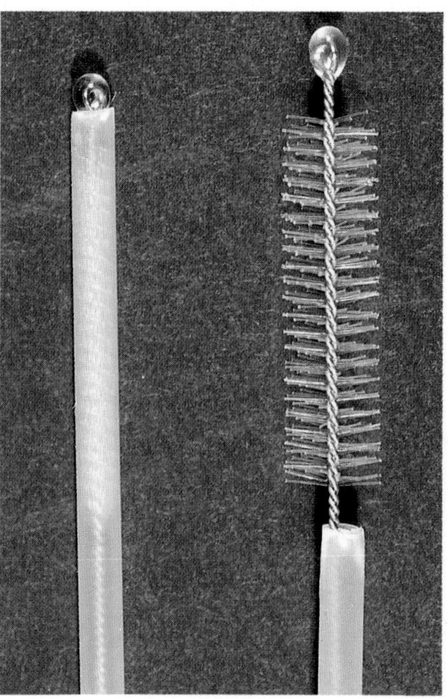

Fig. 17.5 Uterobrush. One of several devices being assessed for cytological sampling of the anal canal. Sampling brush within introducer (left), and extended (right).

Exfoliative cytology of the anal canal

Although some have attempted to use anal cytology in the diagnosis of AIN, the ability of exfoliative cytology to detect anal neoplasia consistently has yet to be determined. A number of collection devices are under appraisal, such as the Cytobrush and the Uterobrush (Fig. 17.5). Furthermore, as AIN lesions may be multifocal, affecting both the perianal skin and anal canal, sampling of the anal canal alone may miss perianal AIN lesions. In addition, difficulty may be experienced in obtaining representative samples as a result of the presence of anal folds, faeces or mucus.

ANOSCOPY

Anoscopy or anal colposcopy is the examination of the anal canal and perianal skin using a colposcope or in conjunction with a proctoscope. Using criteria for the colposcopic diagnosis of CIN or VIN by assessing the colour, vascular pattern and appearance of the anal canal and perianal epithelium before and after the application of 5% aqueous acetic acid, it is possible to make an assessment of the likelihood of the presence of HPV infection or AIN.

Technique of anoscopy

The patient is examined in a modified lithotomy position, using the classical saline and acetic acid techniques. Anal colposcopic examination is performed following genital examination by parting the buttocks to examine the perianal skin. Traction on the perianal skin also permits examination of the lower anal canal. The perianal skin and lower anal canal are examined colposcopically before the application of 5% aqueous acetic acid. The perianal skin is then covered with swabs soaked in acetic acid for three minutes before further examination. The anal canal is then examined using an oblique-viewing Graham Anderson proctoscope (Fig. 17.6), before and after application by spraying of aqueous acetic acid. The Graham Anderson proctoscope provides a good view of the anal canal (Fig. 17.7), but rotation of the instrument within the canal through 180° is necessary to view its whole circumference. Using this instrument, views of the upper anal canal, the transition zone and low rectal mucosa are readily obtained, even in those women being examined without anaesthesia. Spraying the anal canal with acetic acid is adequate as the epithelium in the anal canal is less heavily keratinized than the perianal skin and therefore responds rapidly to the acetic acid spray.

Colposcopically targeted biopsies (Fig. 17.6), under local anaesthesia where appropriate, may be taken of any abnormal epithelium for histological assessment using mini-Tischler punch biopsy forceps.

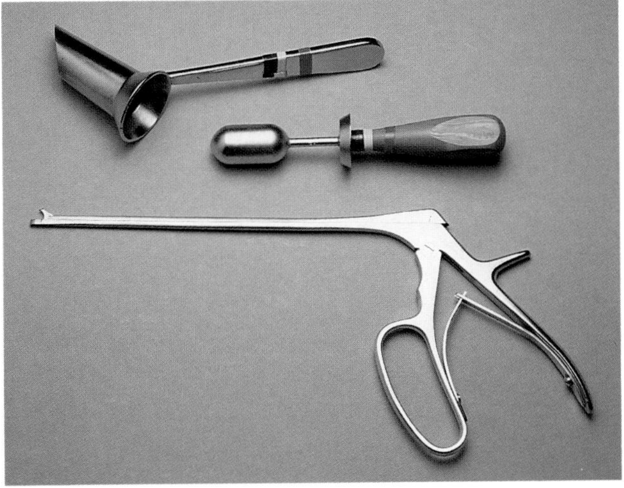

Fig. 17.6 Graham Anderson proctoscope (above) and mini-Tischler biopsy forceps (below).

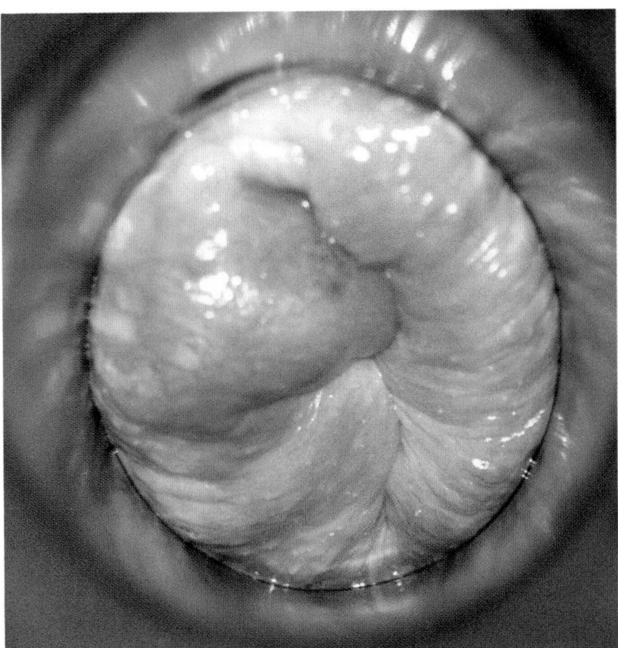

Fig. 17.7 Anoscopy. Preliminary view of the anal transition zone in the upper anal canal, using the Graham Anderson proctoscope. Rotation of the instrument through 180° allows inspection of the full circumference.

Normal perianal skin and anal canal

Normal perianal skin and the lower anal canal (Fig. 17.8) resemble adjacent vulval skin on colposcopy both before and after the application of acetic acid. The application of acetic acid to the perianal skin needs to be of several minutes' duration. Only after such prolonged soaking does any acetowhite area become apparent.

Normal upper anal canal

Colposcopy of the anal canal using an oblique-viewing proctoscope provides an excellent view of the anal cushions, the pectinate line and transition zone (Fig. 17.9). Spraying acetic acid on to the upper anal canal causes the transition zone to become more opaque and hence more obvious. The transition zone is usually located slightly cephalad to the pectinate line, although its position varies from one individual to another. The transition zone becomes more obvious if mucus from the lower rectum is removed via the proctoscope using a cotton swab. Mucus in the anal canal or rectum may be misleading as it readily opacifies due to protein coagulation with the acetic acid. It is therefore essential to remove such mucus during the course of anal colposcopy in order to see the underlying epithelium and its response to acetic acid clearly.

Immature, normal squamous epithelium may show slight acetowhite change, necessitating careful interpretation in patients who have recently undergone any anal surgery or who have anal symptoms such as pruritus ani.

Low-grade AIN and HPV infection

Subclinical papillomavirus infection (SPI), AIN 1 or 2 are usually characterized by mild to moderate acetowhite change on colposcopy. Abnormal vessel patterns are not common. Biopsy is required to differentiate these lesions.

High-grade AIN

In the anal canal high-grade intraepithelial neoplasia is often associated with dense acetowhite change (Fig. 17.10), sometimes occupying the full circumference. In perianal skin, high-grade AIN is at times apparent on naked-eye inspection as patchy, irregular pigmentation (Fig. 17.11). In the absence of pigmentation, a further clue to high-grade anal intraepithelial neoplasia is thickening of the skin, sometimes associated with a papilliferous, warty-looking surface. Such areas may be single or multiple and occasionally extend cephalad to the rectal mucosa or caudad on to the vulva and even the buttocks and thighs. Capillary patterns are unusual on the perianal epithelium even in high-grade disease. By contrast, though uncommon, punctation (Fig. 17.12) and mosaic changes may be noted within high-grade lesions in the anal canal.

Invasive anal carcinoma

These lesions may be characterized colposcopically by heaped-up, irregular, dense acetowhite epithelium, within which lie dilated irregular vessels.

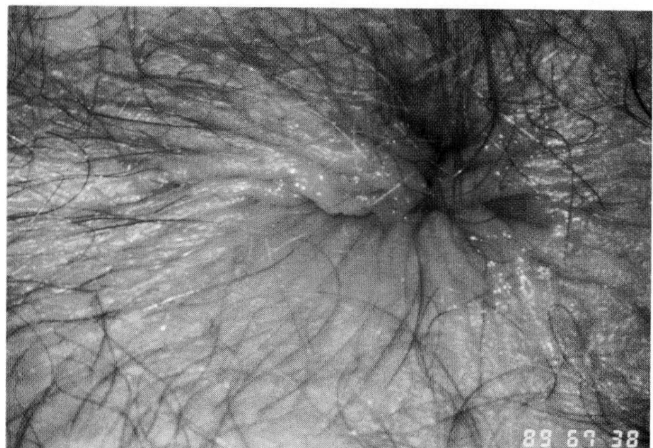

Fig. 17.8 Anoscopy normal perianal skin and lower canal. View obtained by wide retraction of the buttocks. Note similarity to vulval skin.

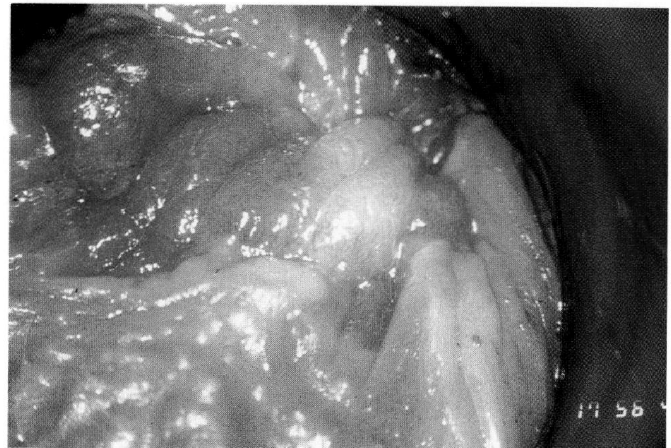

Fig. 17.9 Anoscopy normal anal transition zone (ATZ). Note rectal mucosa at upper limit.

Of considerable importance is the fact that, in some cases of high-grade AIN 3 suspected on colposcopy, unexpected early invasion may be revealed within the field of AIN 3 on histology (Fig. 17.13 (a,b)).

The normal perianal skin is heavily keratinized and responds slowly to acetic acid soaks. Hyperkeratotic perianal epithelium responds to acetic acid even more slowly. In the anal canal, the dysplastic epithelium may appear hyperaemic on examination before the application of acetic acid. However, such areas become more obvious after application of acetic acid spray. The colposcopic appearances of anal canal intraepithelial neoplasia are similar to those seen on the cervix, namely acetowhite areas with punctation and mosaic, although the latter are less common. In keeping with the lack of a clear anatomical distinction between the anal canal and perianal skin, the colposcopic features of papillomavirus infection and dysplasia in the lower anal canal and perianal skin merge into each other. Changes seen in this area by colposcopy are similar to changes described for corresponding vulval disease.

As is the experience with colposcopic assessment of the cervix, anal colposcopy predictions correlate well with the final histological diagnosis, at the normal and high-grade AIN ends of the spectrum. The colposcopic predictive distinction between pure non-condylomatous papillomavirus infection and low-grade AIN (1–2) is less accurate.

Colposcopically targeted biopsy under local anaesthetic is well tolerated using mini-Tischler biopsy forceps. We would recommend biopsy in all cases where colposcopic appearances deviate from normal.

(a) 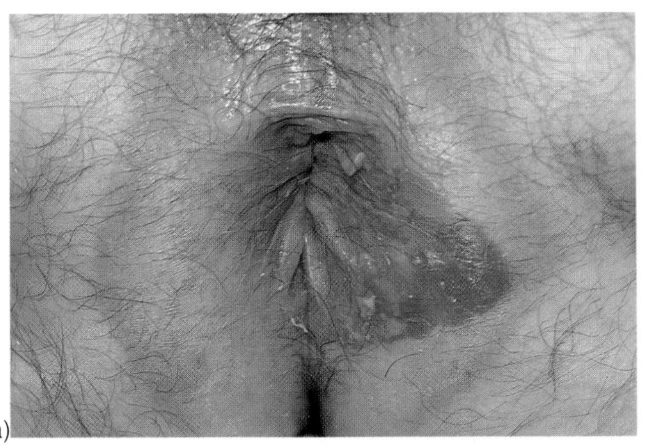

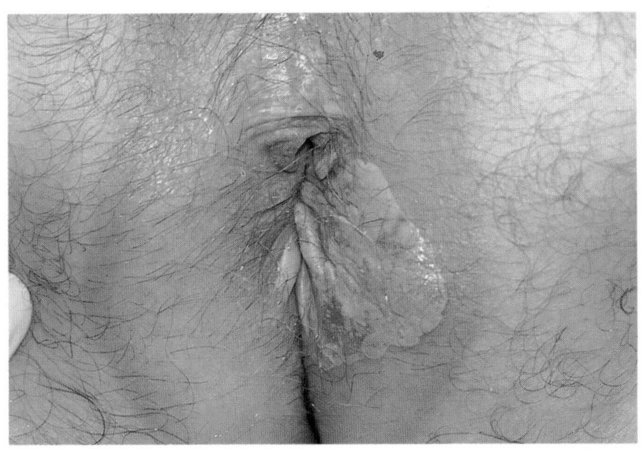 (b)

Fig. 17.10 (a) High-grade AIN showing as raised red lesion in perianal skin. Use of the proctoscope revealed extension in continuity to the upper anal canal. **(b)** Same lesion as in Fig. 17.13(a) after prolonged 5% aqueous acetic acid soak. The lesion is now densely acetowhite. AIN 3 on excision.

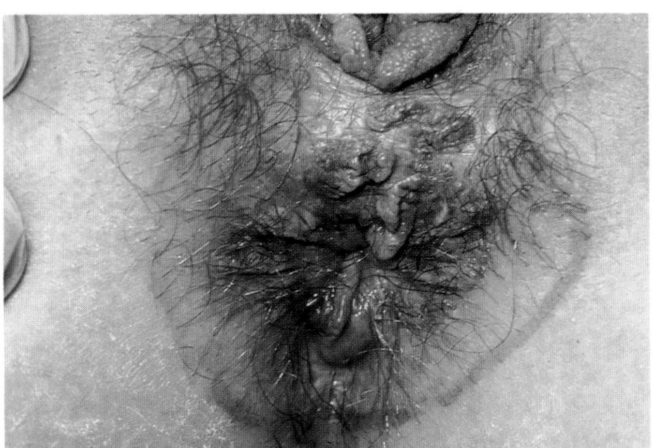

Fig. 17.11 Rosette of multifocal pigmented lesions in perianal skin. AIN 3 on biopsy. Note associated high-grade VIN at fourchette.

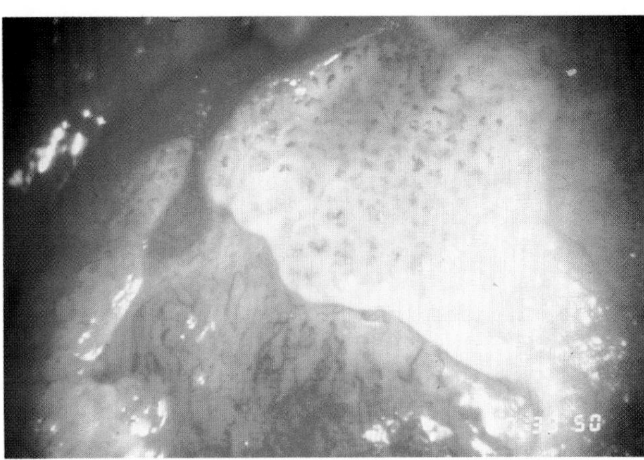

Fig. 17.12 Acetowhite lesion with coarse punctation. Upper anal canal. Note also adjacent epithelial stripping revealing underlying stroma. Indicative of high-grade lesion.

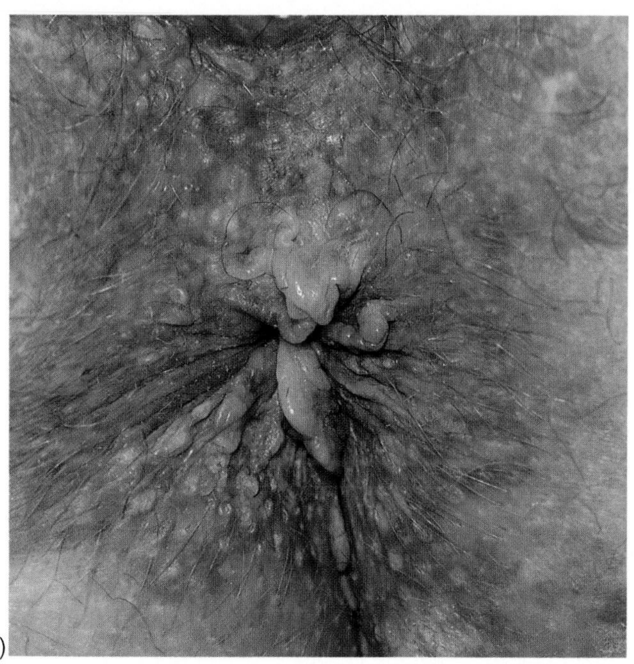

(a)

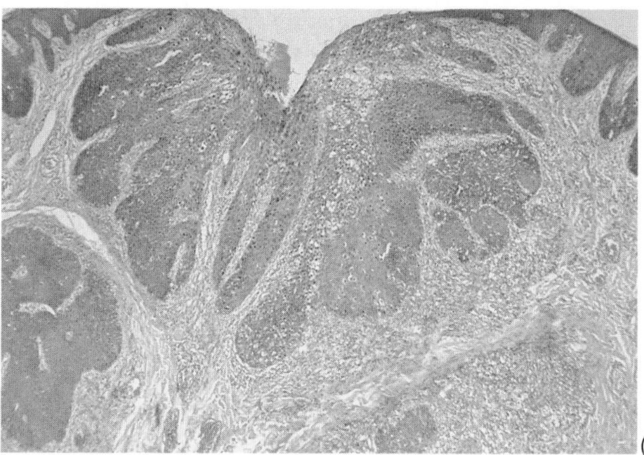

(b)

Fig. 17.13 (a) Widespread multifocal pigmented high-grade lesions in perianal skin. **(b)** Histopathology of full-thickness biopsy of perianal lesions shown in Fig. 17.13(a). Early invasive anal squamous cell carcinoma within a field of AIN 3. The invasive element was not suspected on anoscopy.

MANAGEMENT

The management of AIN presents a dilemma primarily because little is known of its natural history, and anal cancer, the first-line treatment of which is becoming non-surgical, is relatively uncommon. Since it seems unlikely that low-grade lesions will rapidly progress (except possibly in immunosuppressed individuals), it may be better not to actively manage such lesions beyond confirmatory biopsy and monitoring. Management strategies for AIN 3 present a much vexed question. While it is attractive to consider a monitoring-only approach, which would yield invaluable information on the proportion of AIN 3 lesions that might progress to cancer, it is likely that this approach may prove ethically unacceptable due to the small but significant number of cancers observed in association with AIN 3. Conversely, active treatment of immunocompromised individuals may also cause ethical and clinical problems, in view of the possible delays in healing and the risks of infection in this group of patients.

If active management of AIN 3 is deemed appropriate, what modality should be used? While it may be attractive to consider local ablative therapies such as carbon dioxide laser vaporization or cryosurgery, the experience of gynaecologists in the use of these modalities on similar vulval lesions has shown that these methods are often unsuccessful, and rapid disease recurrence is not unusual. In addition there is the risk of overlooking early invasive lesions using these ablative methods. The prevalence of unsuspected early invasion in women who have undergone skinning vulvectomy for VIN 3 is 19%. Furthermore, no quantitative data currently exist for AIN as to the involvement of skin appendages such as hair shafts, sebaceous glands and apocrine sweat glands in the perianal skin, which may act as a reservoir for recurrent disease. Since AIN may be multifocal, affecting large areas of epithelium, and anoscopy in studies to date cannot completely exclude invasive disease, surgical excision may be necessary.

In conclusion, although there is now considerable evidence implicating oncogenic HPV types in the pathogenesis of anogenital neoplasia, and it is likely that high-grade AIN has malignant potential, much remains to be elucidated about the aetiology, pathogenesis and natural history of AIN and its optimum management. Future studies need to focus on the role of other factors such as HIV, Epstein–Barr virus (EBV), HSV-2, immunity (local and systemic) oncogenes and tumour suppressor genes, in the aetiology and pathogenesis of AIN. In addition a widely acceptable screening test needs to be found if routine screening is to be advocated in the high-risk groups. There is an urgent need to determine the natural history of AIN of all grades within high prevalence groups. This will hopefully facilitate the understanding of its role as a cancer precursor, and the formulation of appropriate and effective management strategies.

18. *Oral contraceptive changes*

HISTOLOGY

Microglandular endocervical hyperplasia

Microglandular endocervical hyperplasia (MEH; Figs 18.1–18.4) was first described in 1967. It is a combination of cellular changes in the endocervix, resulting from progestogenic influences on the epithelium. Although this condition is commonly seen in women taking the combined oral contraceptive pill and in pregnancy, it has also been reported in postmenopausal women.

Occasionally, microglandular endocervical hyperplasia is so florid that it presents as cervical polyps that are visible to the naked eye. However, more usually the cervix is macroscopically normal.

Multiple and apparently complex superficial cervical crypts are the most striking microscopical feature. Characteristically, the condition consists of numerous small glandular spaces lined by regular, cuboidal cells. The nuclei are uniform and vesicular, with occasional nucleoli. Mitotic figures may be present, but they are not found in every case. Sometimes vacuoles are prominent; these are often intracellular, although some are extracellular.

The 'microglandular' pattern of the lesion is produced by secondary gland formation, with budding of the endocervical crypts. Between the

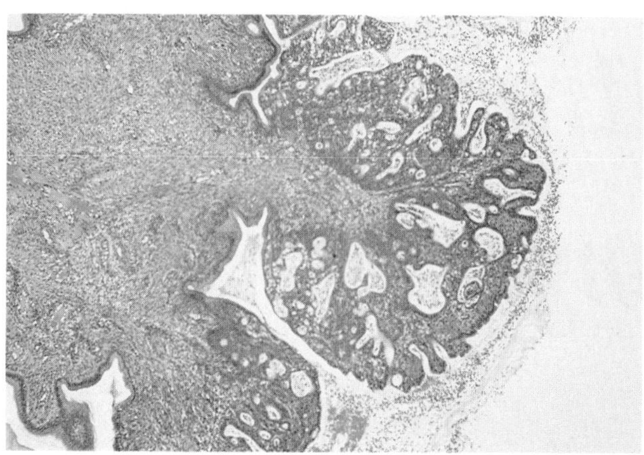

Fig. 18.1 Microglandular endocervical hyperplasia. At low magnification, the surface of the cervix is seen to be polypoid. Reduplication of gland crypts is apparent near the surface.

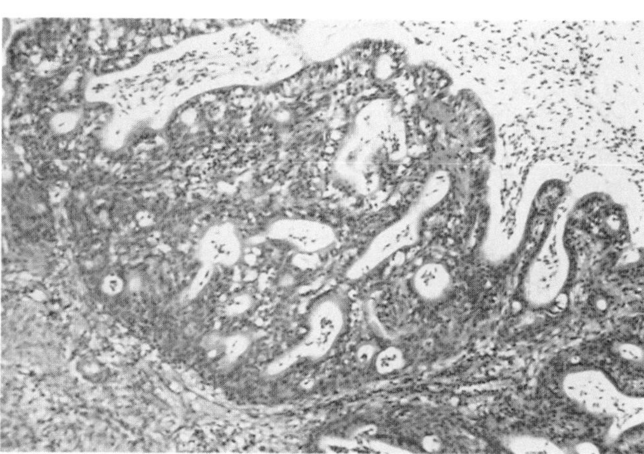

Fig. 18.2 Microglandular endocervical hyperplasia. In addition to glandular reduplication, the more solid background of reserve cell hyperplasia is seen. This example also shows a moderate degree of inflammation.

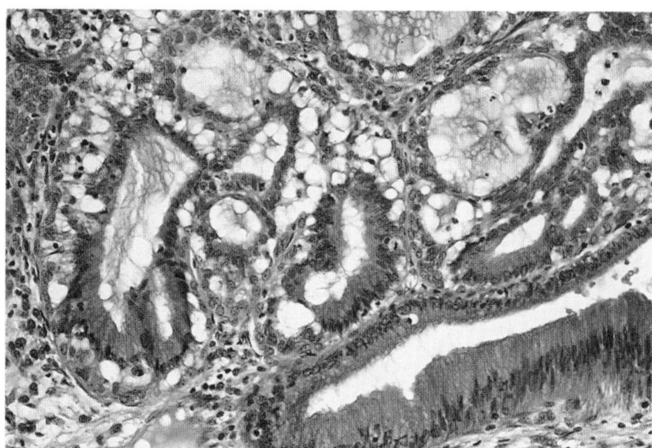

Fig. 18.3 Microglandular endocervical hyperplasia. At higher magnification, 'signet ring' cells and pronounced subnuclear vacuolation are seen.

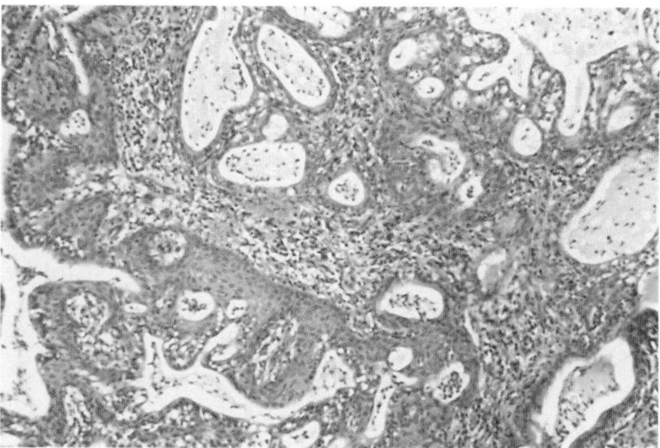

Fig. 18.4 Microglandular endocervical hyperplasia. In this example, maturing squamous metaplasia is mingled with glandular changes.

glandular epithelial elements are cells that have the appearance of reserve cells, and immature squamous metaplastic elements can sometimes also be recognized. This finding suggests that microglandular endocervical hyperplasia may develop when conditions are right for squamous metaplasia, in the presence of a strong progestogenic stimulus. It is most important that the changes produced are not mistaken for malignancy.

Irregular nuclei and virtually absent mitotic figures are the most useful features for distinguishing the condition from carcinoma, but, as with so many other conditions, an awareness of its existence is the best safeguard for a correct diagnosis.

Fig. 18.5 Cytological appearances associated with oral contraception. Mainly intermediate cells are seen, with a few superficial squamous cells showing clumping and numerous Doederlein bacilli.

CYTOLOGY

Cervical smears from women taking oral contraceptives can vary considerably, ranging from smears of an almost atrophic pattern with mainly parabasal cells, to those showing a well-oestrogenized pattern with predominantly superficial squamous cells. However, a significant proportion of women, particularly those on high-dose progestogen pills, present with unsatisfactory smears due to excessive clumping and folding of the cells with large numbers of Döederlein bacilli (Fig. 18.5).

In the first instance, a repeat smear taken between the eighth and twelfth day of the cycle may prove satisfactory, but smears from some women in this group will always be unsatisfactory, irrespective of their timing within the menstrual cycle. It is therefore difficult to offer precise guidelines, and colposcopy may need to be considered in this small but significant group, as dyskaryosis may not be easy to identify.

Microglandular endocervical hyperplasia, although a well-defined histological entity, is difficult to recognize and differentiate cytologically from endocervical cells of normal appearance, and reliable diagnostic features remain elusive.

COLPOSCOPY

At macroscopic examination, the cervix of a woman on combined oral contraception will often be red, friable, and covered with thick mucus, and the area around the external os may be showing an 'erosion'.

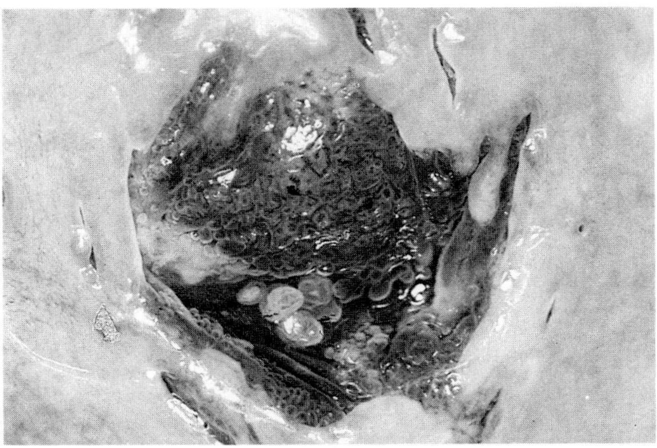

Fig. 18.6 Microglandular endocervical hyperplasia. In the lower part of the endocervical canal, some of the villi have become so enlarged that they have the appearance of small polyps. Reproduced with permission from Jordan and Singer, 1976.

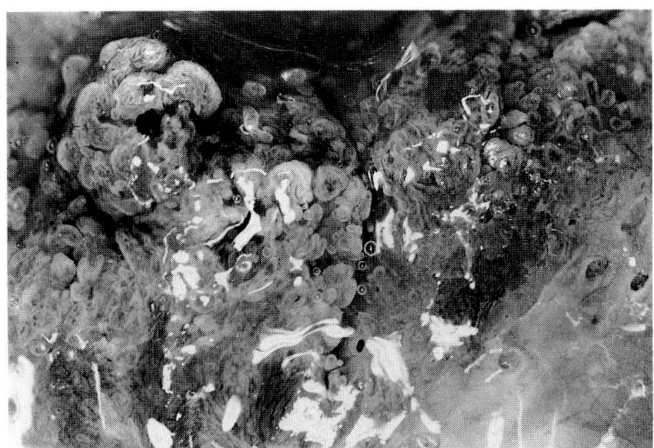

Fig. 18.7 Clumped villi. Sometimes these can produce an irregular polypoidal mass which may appear quite abnormal at naked-eye examination. Reproduced with permission from Jordan and Singer, 1976.

At colposcopic examination, the cervix will often be enlarged because of generalized hyperaemia, such as occurs in early pregnancy. The squamous epithelium is seen to be unaltered in appearance, but changes are recognizable in the columnar epithelium. Individual columnar villi become enlarged and hyperaemic, and the apparent erosion represents nothing but enlargement and hyperaemia occurring in normal villi. In some cases these will increase to become almost polypoidal (Figs 18.6 and 18.7).

Sometimes enlargement of columnar epithelial villi is such that columnar epithelium protrudes from the endocervical canal, resulting in eversion. Occasionally, this may be exaggerated by further eversion of the lower canal, following the insertion of a bivalve speculum. For these reasons, women are often incorrectly referred for treatment of an erosion which colposcopy shows to be perfectly normal epithelium.

19. *Pregnancy*

NORMAL CERVIX IN PREGNANCY

Three changes may be histologically identified in the cervix during pregnancy: decidual change, microglandular endocervical hyperplasia and Arias-Stella change.

Decidual change

Decidual change is an alteration in cervical tissue effected by the action of progestogens. Although usually regarded as a hormonal response of the endometrial stroma, it can also be seen affecting the superficial stroma of the cervix, as well as the lamina propria of the fallopian tubes, the surface of the ovaries, and the peritoneum.

Microscopy shows features similar to decidual change at more familiar sites (Figs 19.1 and 19.2). The cells of the superficial cervical stroma are grossly enlarged and pale, with large, round nuclei and prominent nucleoli. The change is usually quite focal, affecting only a small area of the cervix. It may be situated on the endocervix or ectocervix. Occasionally, cells that are morphologically indistinguishable from endometrial granulocytes may be found among the enlarged stromal cells (Fig. 19.3).

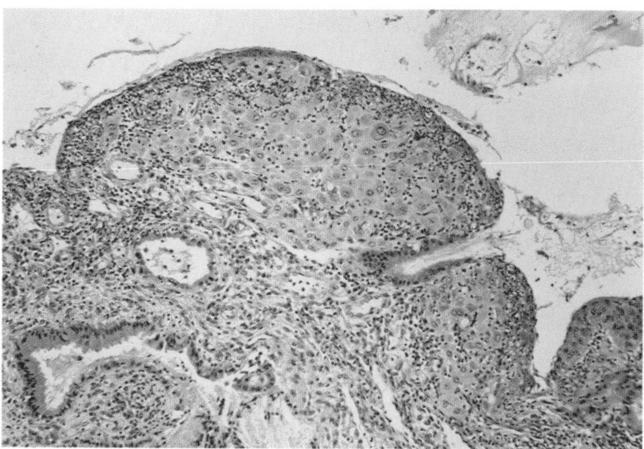

Fig. 19.1 Decidual change in the cervix of a pregnant woman. A group of large, pale, decidualized stromal cells are present beneath the surface epithelium.

Microglandular endocervical hyperplasia

This has been fully described in Chapter 18. There are no recorded differences between microglandular endocervical hyperplasia associated with pregnancy and that associated with oral contraception.

Arias-Stella change

As with decidual change, this phenomenon is more usually associated with the endometrium. However, very rarely, endocervical glands may show features of Arias-Stella change (Fig. 19.4). The most striking histological feature, in the endometrium as well as in the endocervix, is the presence of enlarged, hyperchromatic nuclei of irregular shape. This may or may not be accompanied by increased

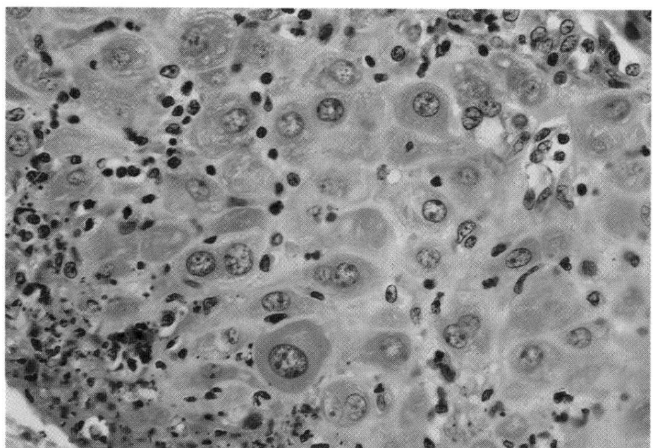

Fig. 19.2 Decidual change. At higher magnification, the large, pale decidualized stromal cells are seen.

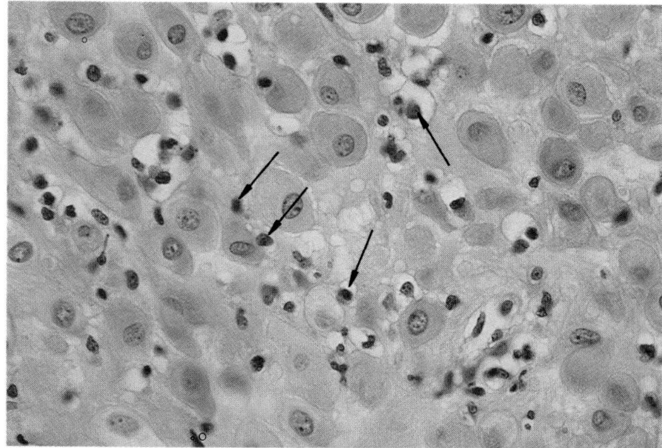

Fig. 19.3 Decidual change. In addition to the decidualized stromal cells, this example also shows endometrial granulocytes (arrows).

secretory activity. Distinction from glandular atypia may be difficult, but the presence of fairly abundant cytoplasm and absence of mitotic figures point towards a benign diagnosis.

CYTOLOGY IN PREGNANCY

The cervical smear pattern in normal pregnancy does not vary significantly from that seen in the normal secretory phase. On most occasions, the smear will be satisfactory for assessment, but in some instances the exaggerated progesterone effect may render the smear unsuitable, with excessive clumping and folding of the cells.

Navicular cells, since they are glycogenated intermediate squamous cells, are an indication of well-marked progesterone response and should not be regarded as diagnostic or even suggestive of pregnancy.

A well-marked oestrogen effect may suggest a deficient progesterone level, and the presence of endometrial cells in a cervical smear during pregnancy is an abnormal finding. Both observations should be reported.

Decidual change

On rare occasions, decidual change occurring in the cervix may give rise to large cells in the cervical smear. These have round, centrally located nuclei, sometimes with prominent nucleoli (Fig. 19.5). Since this finding is unusual, the decidual cells may be mistaken for dyskaryotic cells.

Arias-Stella change

Cytologically, the large cells with irregularly shaped and hyperchromatic nuclei associated with Arias-Stella change may be confused with dyskaryotic cells, particularly since this pattern is rarely seen in cervical smears.

ABNORMAL CERVIX IN PREGNANCY

Histology and cytology

The histological interpretation of material taken from a cervix during pregnancy is often said to be more difficult than that in the non-pregnant state. This is misleading because, once the changes described above are eliminated, there is no difference between the histological appearances of epithelial abnormalities in the pregnant and non-pregnant states.

Cytologically, the features associated with cervical intraepithelial neoplasia in pregnancy do not differ from those seen in the non-pregnant state (see Chapter 2).

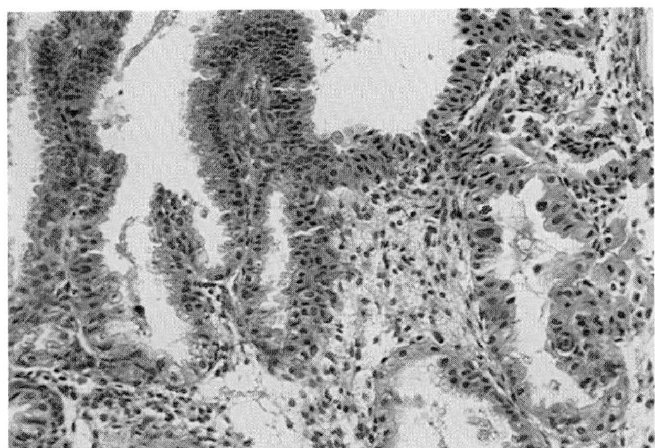

Fig. 19.4 Arias-Stella change in the cervix. The appearances are similar to those frequently seen in the endometrium, with a slight increase in complexity of the glands and a little increase in secretory activity. However, the hallmark of Arias-Stella change is the presence of enlarged and hyperchromatic nuclei. Mitotic figures are not seen.

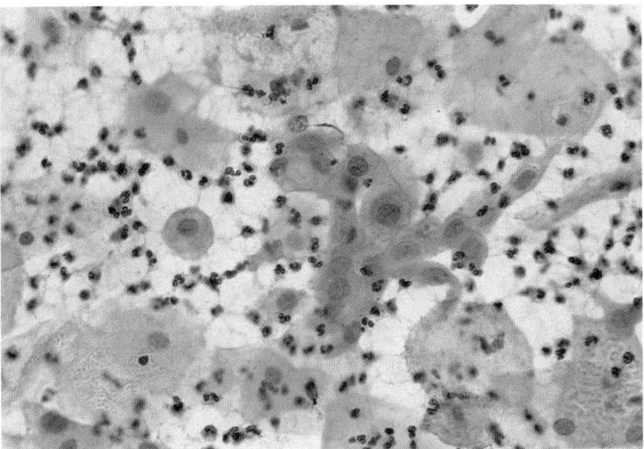

Fig. 19.5 Cytology in pregnancy. The central group of cells have enlarged nuclei and abundant pale cytoplasm, characteristic of decidual change.

GROSS PHYSIOLOGICAL CHANGES

In addition to the gross changes affecting the cervix and cervical epithelium during adolescence, pregnancy has a similar and major effect. At gross level, there are two changes: eversion of the endocervical canal, and gaping of the external os. The effect of these is exposure of previously protected columnar epithelium to the acid pH of the vaginal environment, and a reawakening of the process of squamous metaplasia. Eversion permits this by relocation of columnar epithelium to the vaginal aspect of the cervix, and gaping allows streaming of acidic vaginal secretions into the canal.

In the primigravid woman, eversion is the most important phenomenon, and its highest point is during the latter weeks of the first trimester. By contrast, gaping of the external os is an outstanding feature in the multigravida, and is evident from as early as 12 weeks of gestation.

In addition to these mechanical alterations, squamous metaplasia is observed (Fig. 19.6). Moreover, the exposed endocervical villi become large and hypertrophic, being partly responsible for the vascular appearance of the uterus. The uterus is also affected by alterations in the vascular tree itself, under the influence of pregnancy hormones. As a result, the cervix takes on its typical dusky bluish hue of pregnancy (Fig. 19.7). Glandular secretion increases, and the process of decidualization affects the stromal elements.

Finally, the effects of labour and vaginal delivery on the cervix and cervical epithelium must be considered. The passage of the fetus through a completely or incompletely dilated cervix produces substantial and easily recognizable injury to the epithelial and subepithelial tissues. These include:

1. True erosion or ulceration, with loss of surface epithelium.
2. Laceration, with extension of the tissue damage into the underlying stroma.
3. Bruising or ecchymosis.
4. Necrotic changes, colposcopically identified as yellow, featureless areas, usually associated with the edges of deeper lacerations. These lesions are obviously the direct result of trauma, and as such are more common in the primigravida after delivery, than in the multigravida.

Remarkably, healing is generally complete by approximately six weeks after delivery, at which time it is usual to find that the gross appearance and contour of the cervix bear little resemblance to its predelivery state.

As these active healing processes continue during the puerperium, it is usually best to defer further colposcopic assessment of women with abnormal cytology during pregnancy, until about three months postdelivery (see below); otherwise, confusing cytological and colposcopic appearances may be observed.

COLPOSCOPY OF THE NORMAL GRAVID CERVIX

The colposcopic appearances of physiological changes in the gravid cervix were presented in the 1970s by Singer, and the following account is based on that description.

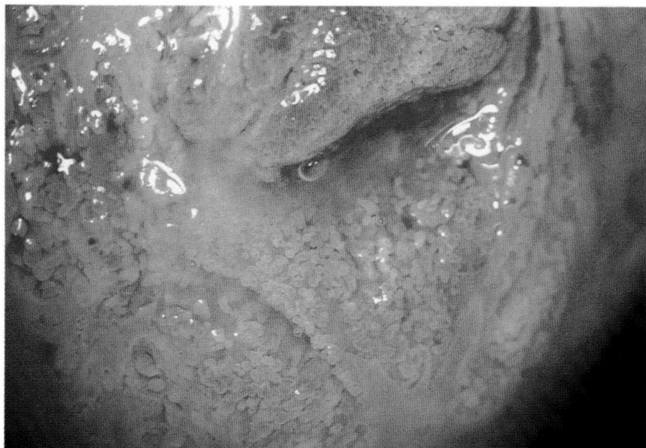

Fig. 19.6 Primigravida: cervix at 12 weeks of gestation. Early squamous metaplasia is seen, with fusion of villi.

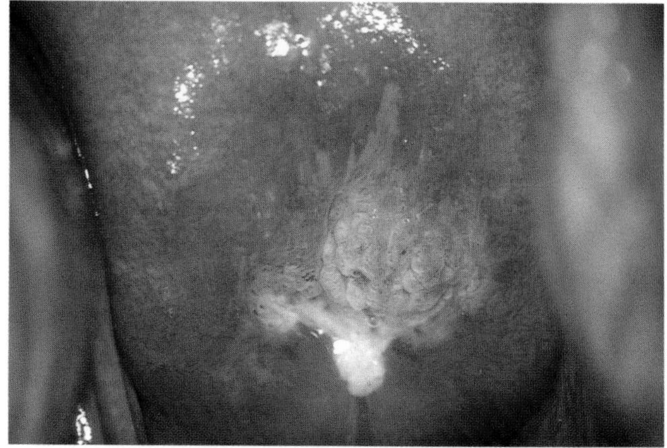

Fig. 19.7 Primigravida: cervix at 16 weeks. Note the dusky blue background of the epithelium due to underlying vascularity.

In the primigravida in the early part of the first trimester the cervix shows large areas of columnar epithelium with little evidence of squamous metaplasia. The latter process commences during the later weeks of the first trimester (see Fig. 19.7), coinciding with eversion. Very rapidly, islands of villous fusion occur, producing islands of immature squamous metaplasia.

This process becomes more active in the second trimester, and maturation occurs in the third trimester. Some metaplastic transformation also occurs within the canal, probably as a result of gaping of the external os.

In the multigravida, similar but more limited changes are observed. Metaplastic change tends to be a feature of the third trimester, accompanying eversion. With gaping of the external os and streaming of acidic vaginal fluid into the canal, metaplastic change develops in the furrows or clefts within the canal.

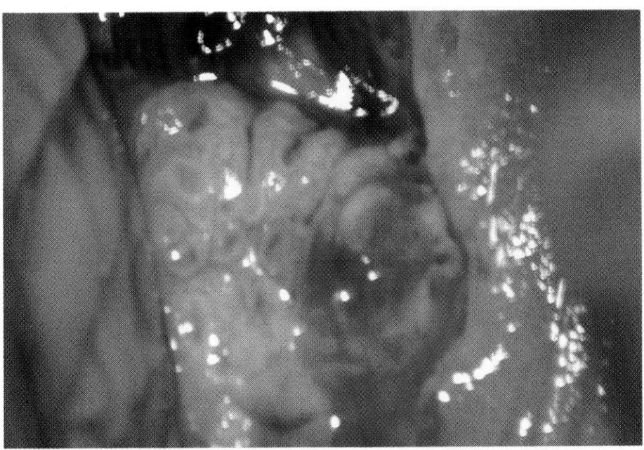

Fig. 19.8 Multipara: cervix at 20 weeks of gestation. Large gland openings with umbilicated rims are seen.

Increased glandular activity is evidenced by profuse mucus secretion from gland openings which may be large and with pronounced rims (Fig. 19.8). Villi are large and hypertrophic, as seen in users of oral contraception. Vascularity produces a dusky bluish hue, and decidualization may present as 'doughnut' rims to the gland openings; in cases of extreme change, these may come to resemble 'mooncraters' (Fig. 19.9). The eversion and gaping effects facilitate visualization of the new squamocolumnar junction. This is a useful and important consideration where colposcopy is performed in the presence of an abnormal smear.

COLPOSCOPY OF THE ABNORMAL CERVIX IN PREGNANCY

The indications for colposcopy in gravid women are more or less the same as those for non-gravid women, namely:

1. Dyskaryosis at cervical cytology: any woman with a positive cervical smear in pregnancy must receive a colposcopic assessment to determine the nature and severity of the underlying lesion.
2. Human papillomavirus changes in the smear: this indication may not be regarded by all gynaecologists as an absolute indication for colposcopy. However, it seems wise to attempt to define the exact nature of the lesion, as in the non-pregnant state, even though active treatment may not be contemplated. The association of human papillomavirus lesions with cervical intraepithelial neoplasia should not be forgotten (see page 147).

(a)

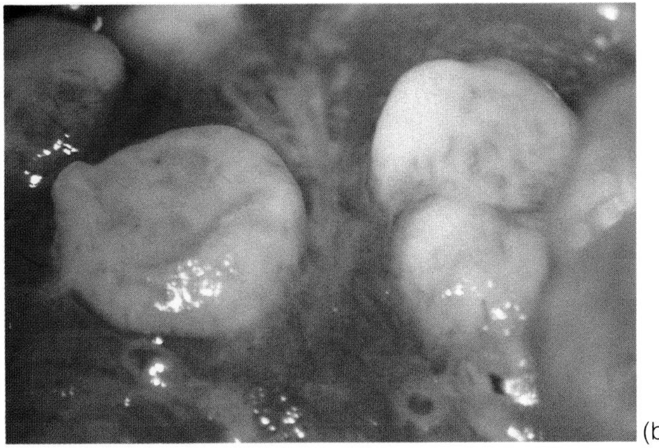

(b)

Fig. 19.9 Gross decidualization of gland openings in pregnancy. (a) At low magnification. **(b)** At high magnification. Courtesy of Miss Rhona Stringer.

3. Clinically suspicious cervix: as in the non-pregnant state, clinical suspicion of possible underlying neoplasia, regardless of normal cytology, is an indication for colposcopy in pregnancy. Abnormality may have been observed through speculum examination in cases of recurrent and otherwise unexplained bleeding at any stage of gestation. Alternatively, naked-eye inspection of the cervix may have taken place during routine cervical cytology screening at an antenatal visit.

Colposcopic technique

During the first 16 weeks of gestation, the technique of colposcopy is basically the same as for the non-gravid woman. Both saline and acetic acid methods can be employed. In general, the appearances associated with underlying cervical intraepithelial neoplasia, invasive disease and the common human papillomavirus lesions are as would be expected.

Active squamous metaplasia in pregnancy, especially of the immature type, presents a difficulty. The condition may be typified by acetowhite change. Excessive mucus secretion may require a little more attention to interpret, before the formal examination.

Furthermore, the vascularity of the uterus may accentuate the patterns of mosaic, punctation and suspect atypical vessels, giving a colposcopist the impression that the existing lesions are of a higher grade than actual. However, because of the physiological eversion and gaping of the external os, the new squamocolumnar junction is often readily visible, rendering colposcopic examination satisfactory or complete in these instances (Fig. 19.10).

During the remaining 24 weeks of gestation, the saline and acetic acid methods may be employed. As pregnancy progresses, access to the cervix may become more difficult: the increasingly lax vaginal walls tend to collapse into the field of view, at times through the gaps in the sides of a bivalve speculum. Moreover, part of the fetus may present deep in the pelvis. The cervix may also be significantly displaced posteriorly towards the sacrum.

Despite these difficulties, it is extremely important that the entire examination is based on gentleness, as the tissues are easily traumatized. Even application of acetic acid needs care, and it requires a most delicate approach during pregnancy. In some colposcopy units, a spray bottle is used for applying the solution in pregnant and non-pregnant women. Sidewall retractors or ensheathing the bivalve speculum in a condom or one 'finger' from a rubber glove, with the end cut off, may help to overcome the problem of lax, bulging vaginal walls, thus facilitating this otherwise very difficult examination.

At this stage in pregnancy, punch biopsy is often accompanied by brisk bleeding, and therefore it should be undertaken only where absolutely necessary. If bleeding is encountered, simple pressure for a few minutes may control it. Monsel's solution, applied to the biopsy site even in pregnancy, almost never fails.

MANAGEMENT OF ABNORMAL CYTOLOGY IN PREGNANCY

A positive smear in the pregnant woman will always be a problem for subsequent management (Table 19.1). Before the advent of colposcopy, there was a

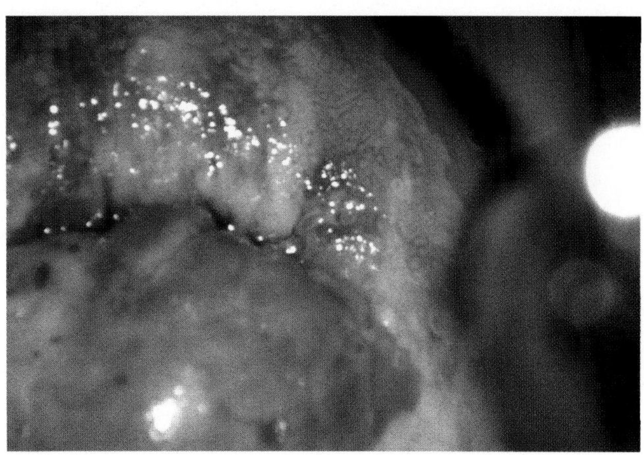
(a)

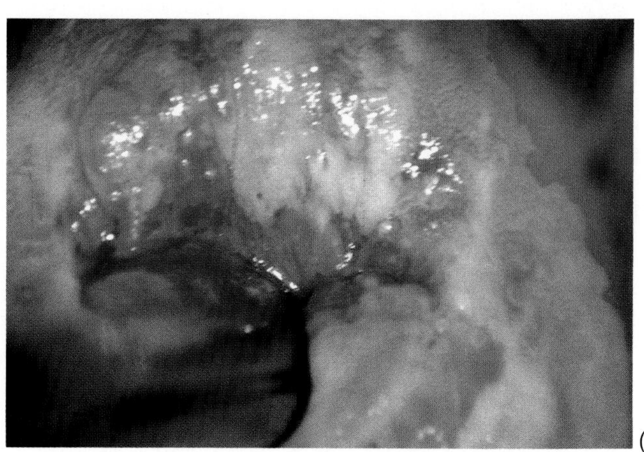
(b)

Fig. 19.10 Dusky blue cervix in pregnancy, with widespread acetowhite change. (a) Initial view, with the squamocolumnar junction not visible. **(b)** Minimal manipulation exposes the junction anteriorly.

Table 19.1 Suggested management protocol. Abnormal smear in pregnancy

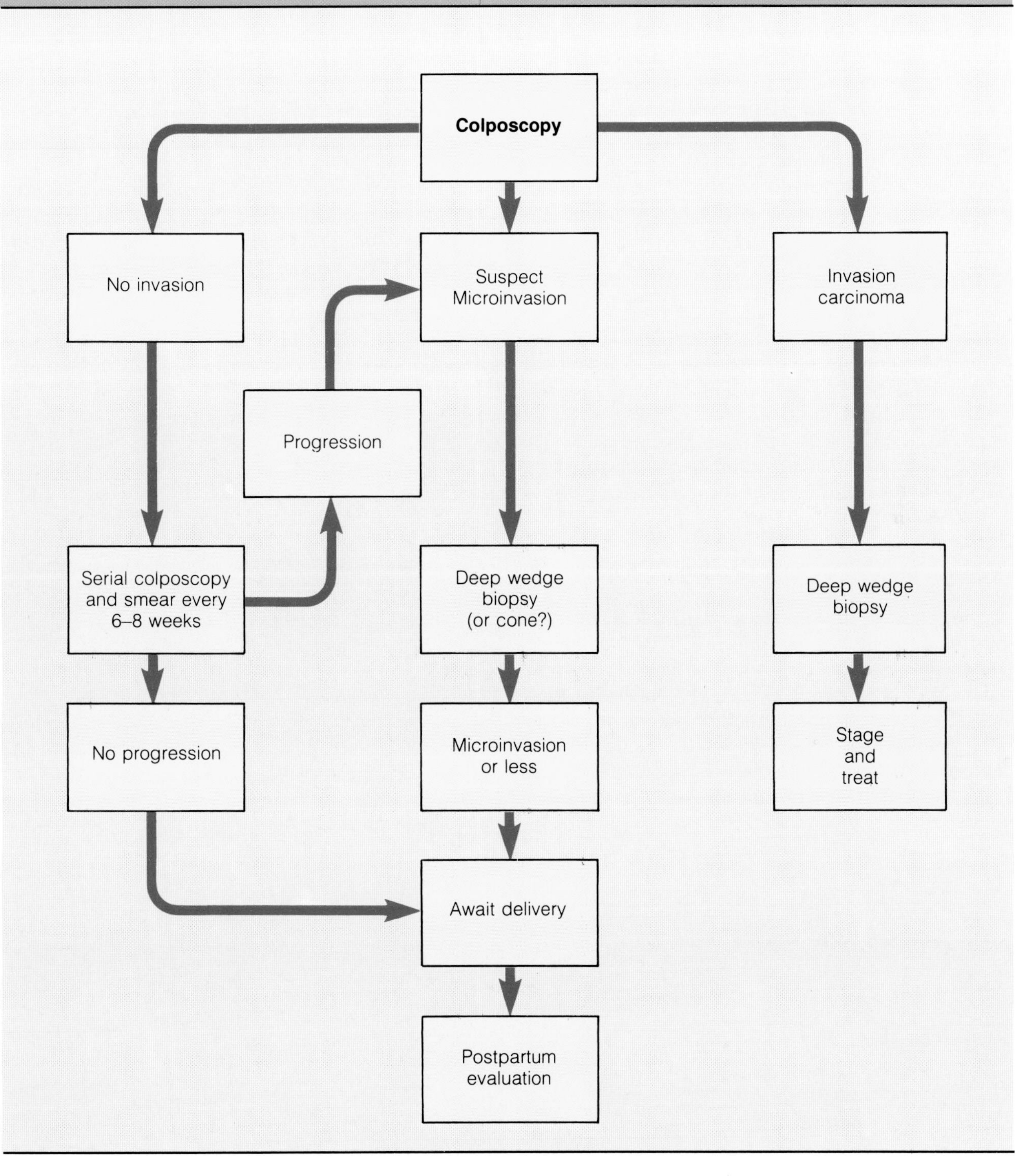

tendency to rush to aggressive methods of diagnosis and treatment, namely knife cone biopsy. If the diagnosis is overt invasive disease, there is good reason for concern. However, this would be unusual, as such lesions are relatively rare and occur only in approximately one in 4000 pregnancies.

Cone biopsy in pregnancy is fraught with complications, including a higher incidence of primary and secondary haemorrhage. Increased perinatal mortality (stillbirth, preterm labour and abortion) has been attributed to this procedure, and is reported in 25–30% of cases. Furthermore, even after cone biopsy, the incidence of residual disease might remain in the order of 50%.

Despite these alarming statistics, two decades ago many gynaecologists would recommend this step in the management of a woman with a positive smear in pregnancy. However, colposcopy has created a much more conservative diagnostic approach, based on skilled, serial colposcopic appraisal in conjunction with parallel exfoliative cytology. Biopsy is thus minimized and limited to highly significant lesions where invasion cannot otherwise be excluded.

Management recommendations

At the outset it should be made clear that if, at any stage during pregnancy, there is colposcopic or cytological suspicion of microinvasive or frankly invasive disease, a large biopsy will be required for diagnosis; this will be either a colposcopically directed, deep wedge biopsy, or a cone biopsy. Obviously, either of these will be carried out under general anaesthesia.

MANAGEMENT OF LOW-GRADE LESIONS

In this context, a low-grade lesion will refer to subclinical papillomavirus infection, CIN 1 or CIN 2. Colposcopic examination should be carried out by an experienced colposcopist. Having established that the lesion falls into one of the above categories (Fig. 19.11; see Table 19.1), a confirmatory biopsy during pregnancy will usually be omitted, provided that the initial and repeat cervical smear reports are in broad agreement.

Colposcopy and cytology should then be repeated in each of the remaining trimesters, and again at approximately three months after delivery, when formal characterization of the lesion would be obtained by an appropriate biopsy. If necessary, treatment would also be selected. At any stage during this conservative management in pregnancy, a biopsy might be indicated if the colposcopic impression or cytology suggests progression of the lesion

Low-grade lesions should not influence normal obstetric management of the patient, and in themselves are not an indication for elective Caesarean section. Proper colposcopic re-evaluation must be carried out at the postpartum examination. It is never appropriate to treat the cervix without this re-evaluation, as over the course of several months some

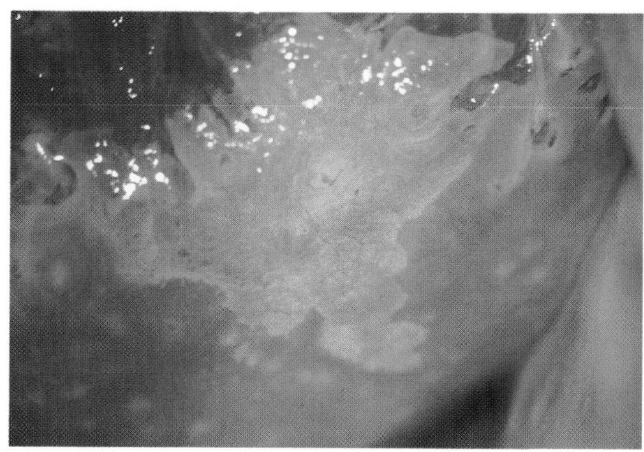

Fig. 19.11 Cervix in pregnancy. This is a low-grade acetowhite lesion with an irregular outline. Subclinical papillomavirus and CIN 1 are present.

(a)

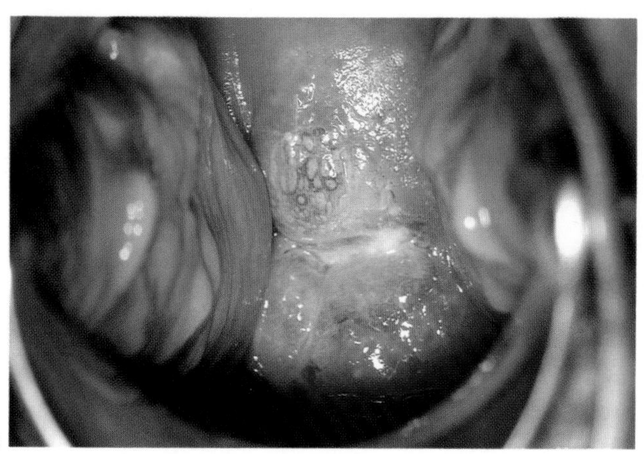

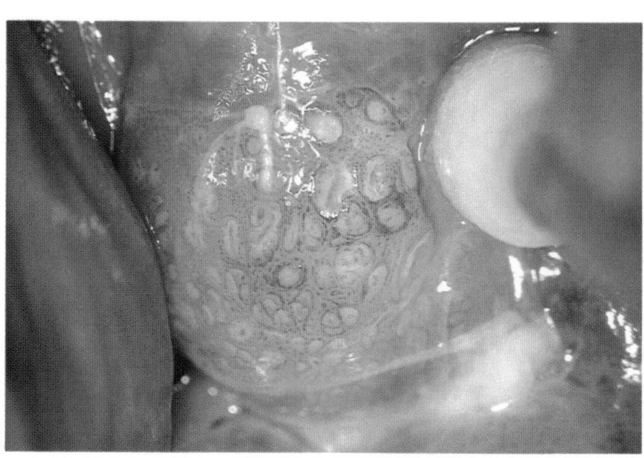

(b)

Fig. 19.12 Cervix in pregnancy. This is a high-grade lesion, with acetowhite change and a coarse mosaic pattern. **(a)** At low magnification; note the laxity of vaginal walls. **(b)** At high magnification.

low-grade lesions may alter, either by regression or indeed progression.

MANAGEMENT OF HIGH-GRADE LESIONS

High-grade lesions imply CIN 3 (Figs 19.12–19.14). In addition, very large lesions of lesser grade would merit the same attention, as it may be more difficult to exclude progressive change occurring within a very large area.

Essentially, the management of these two groups is much the same as that for low-grade lesions. However, as the risk of progression to microinvasive disease, although small, may be greater, re-examination both by colposcopy and cytology must be frequent, approximately every six weeks. The keystone of management is to observe for signs of microinvasion (see Fig. 19.15). These signs are the same as in the non-gravid state, and include the abnormal vascular patterns of markedly dilated vessels, vessels running horizontally in the epithelium, 'corkscrew' and 'comma' vessel configurations, and any significant increase in intercapillary distance.

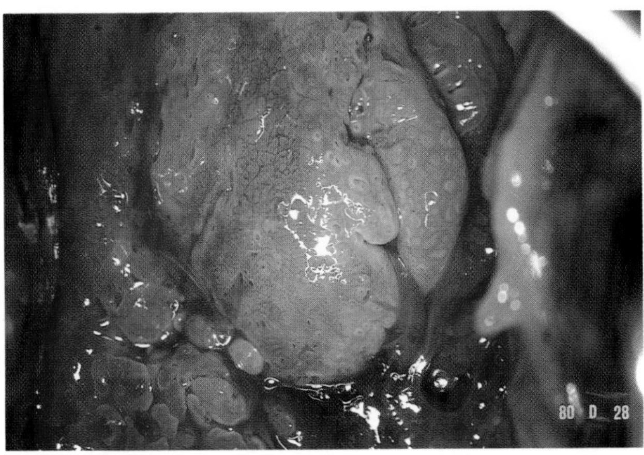

Fig. 19.13 Cervix in pregnancy. This is a high-grade lesion, with acetowhite epithelium and a mosaic pattern. Note the large hypertrophic villi, typical of pregnancy (below left).

It should be stressed that the increased vascularity of the gravid cervix tends to exaggerate vascular patterns, which may cause them to look worse than would be expected for the underlying lesion. Again, provided that the lesion remains intraepithelial, this conservative approach may be continued into the postpartum period and should not influence the obstetric management.

If concerns are expressed about possible breach of the basement membrane, then a large biopsy should not be delayed. This does not have to be a cone biopsy, as a large, deep (10 mm) wedge biopsy performed under general anaesthesia will often suffice to exclude microinvasion. The depth of any invasion present will help the histopathologist to differentiate between stage Ia and stage Ib disease, a point of considerable relevance to subsequent management.

MICROINVASIVE DISEASE IN PREGNANCY

The difficulty of establishing a diagnosis of microinvasion with certainty has already been alluded to, together with the need for a large biopsy in these circumstances to rule out frankly invasive carcinoma. Fortunately, evidence from the literature and local studies supports the view that progression of high-grade lesions in pregnancy is an unusual event, and

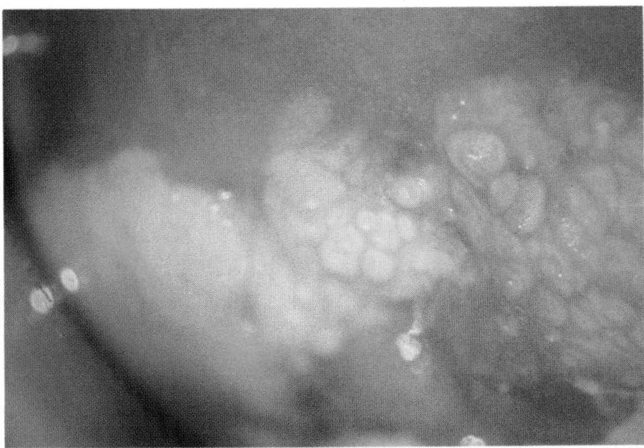

Fig. 19.14 Cervix at 20 weeks of gestation. This is a mixed high-grade lesion, with dense acetowhite epithelium on the left (CIN 3). The lesion on the right proved to be subclinical papillomavirus infection.

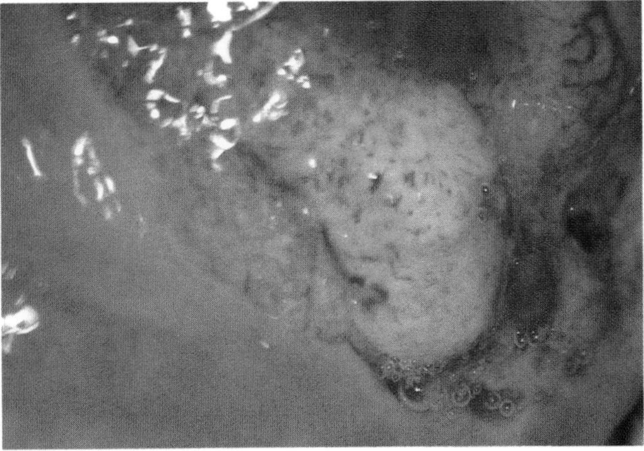

Fig. 19.15 Highly suspicious lesion in early pregnancy. CIN 3 with microinvasion.

management of microinvasion in the gravid woman is uncommon. When it does occur, there are two considerations: maternal well-being and fetal welfare.

In the majority of cases, the maternal well-being will be paramount. For the fetus, the main concern will usually be whether it is sufficiently mature to survive outside the uterus; among other factors, this will depend on the gestational age and quality of available paediatric services. Currently it is possible to expect a reasonable chance of survival for a fetus of 24 or 26 weeks, if delivery is inevitable.

In the presence of an immature fetus, pregnancy may be allowed to continue if the diagnostic biopsy, especially a cone biopsy, shows complete excision of the lesion, provided that it comes within the criteria for microinvasion. Obviously, careful surveillance will be mandatory. There is probably no good reason for elective Caesarean delivery in cases of microinvasion in which the lesion has been completely removed by cone biopsy. Indeed, many gynaecological oncologists believe that Caesarean section need not be performed even in the presence of microinvasion. At later periods of gestation, it is helpful if pregnancy can be allowed to continue until fetal lung maturity is reached. Again, it is not necessary to opt for Caesarean section.

FRANKLY INVASIVE CARCINOMA IN PREGNANCY

In general, pregnant women with a frankly invasive carcinoma of the cervix (Fig. 19.16) will usually be young. Treatment is by radical hysterectomy with lymph node dissection, after referral to a gynaecological oncologist. Treatment of a pregnant woman should proceed without regard for the fetus, unless the lesion is discovered at a stage close to fetal viability, when a delay of a few weeks may be considered justifiable. In all cases, the views of a fully informed patient must be taken into consideration before any decisions are made.

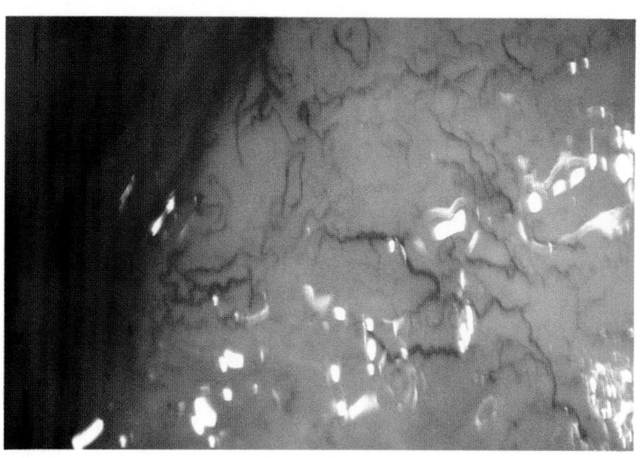

Fig. 19.16 Atypical vascular pattern on clinically overt, raised, densely white, frankly invasive lesion in pregnancy.

20. *Diethylstilboestrol exposure*

VAGINAL ADENOSIS

Vaginal adenosis is a benign condition in which normal columnar epithelium covers not only the cervix, but also part of the upper vagina. This condition reached prominence when it was reported that maternally ingested diethylstilboestrol exposure resulted in vaginal adenosis in approximately 90% of female offspring.

In addition to vaginal adenosis, other benign changes were recognized and have been collectively termed 'cervicovaginal deformities' (Table 20.1). These deformities tend to be called diethylstilboestrol changes, but similar changes can and do occur spontaneously, albeit uncommonly, in babies who have not been exposed to diethylstilboestrol *in utero*. These benign changes usually undergo spontaneous resolution over a period of time following transformation of adenosis to mature squamous epithelium by a process of metaplasia.

Interest developed in this particular cervicovaginal change, because of a theory in the early 1970s that these changes carried a high risk of producing clear cell adenocarcinoma of the vagina and/or cervix. It has been subsequently suggested that such patients have a higher incidence of premalignant squamous disease of the cervix. The cervix and upper vagina may look peculiar, and in young women the changes can appear quite bizarre. In the past, these changes usually went unnoticed; this is due to the fact that, as the young woman develops, the changes tend to disappear so that by the time she is first seen and assessed by a gynaecologist for some other reason, the macroscopically and colposcopically abnormal signs may have disappeared. The appearances of immature metaplasia on large areas of vaginal adenosis may be worrying because they share some of the features of premalignancy. Also, some of the irregularities noted on these cervices can give rise to concern, unless the colposcopist is aware of their significance.

Table 20.1 Relative incidence of cervicovaginal deformities (n = 320)

Cervicovaginal deformity	No. of patients	%
Type I cervix (circular sulcus on face of ectocervix)	117	35.5
Type II cervix (recessed area of perioral tissue)	22	6.9
Type III cervix (complete covering of ectocervix with endocervical epithelium)	22	6.9
Anterior cervical protuberance (smooth or rough)	46	14.4
Pseudopolyp	15	4.7

From Sandberg, E. C. (1976) Benign cervical and vaginal changes associated with exposure to stilbestrol *in utero*. *American Journal of Obstetrics and Gynecology*, **125**, 6, 777.

Vaginal adenosis in a diethylstilboestrol-exposed young woman is seen in Fig. 20.1. The cervix is covered by columnar epithelium which extends on to the posterior fornix and on to the posterior vaginal

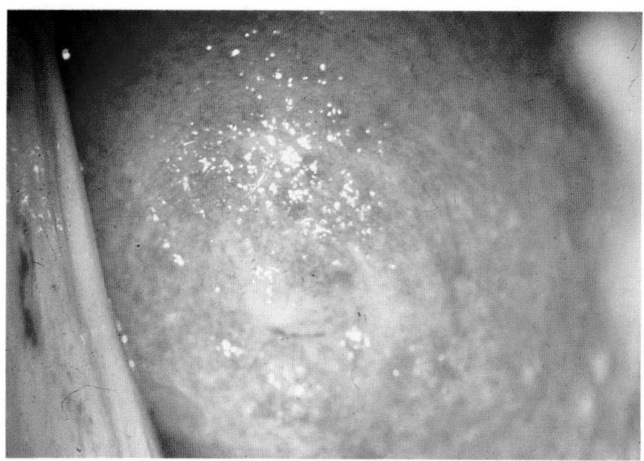

Fig. 20.1 Vaginal adenosis in a diethylstilboestrol-exposed young woman. Courtesy of Mr J M Emens.

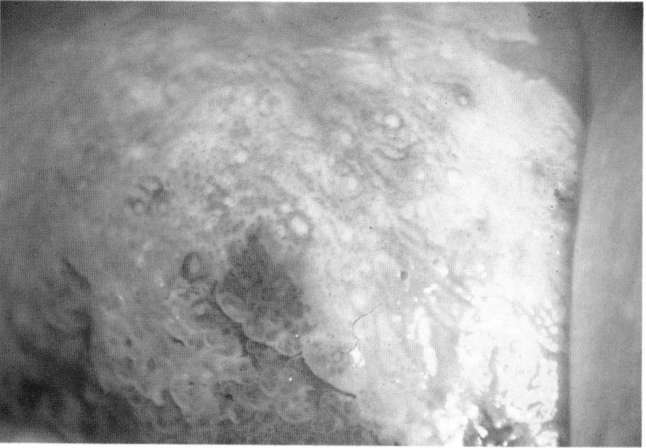

Fig. 20.2 Extensive areas of acetowhite epithelium undergoing metaplasia. Courtesy of Mr J M Emens.

wall. Such areas eventually undergo metaplasia and produce large areas of acetowhite epithelium with some of the characteristics of CIN 1 (Fig. 20.2). It should be remembered that the incidence of vaginal extension of cervical intraepithelial neoplasia occurs in 1.5% of women with cervical intraepithelial neoplasia, who must have started their life with vaginal adenosis.

Multiple sulci on the ectocervix may also be seen (Fig. 20.3). The presence of an anterior cervical protuberance is often called a 'cock's comb', and this can be either smooth (Fig. 20.4) or rough (Fig. 20.5). The pseudopolyp formation is simply columnar epithelium confined to an area around the external os which is vascular and protuberant, giving the appearance of a large cervical polyp (Fig. 20.6).

The cervix of a young woman exposed to diethylstilboestrol is seen in Fig. 20.7. The changes can be easily confused with extensive areas of cervical intraepithelial neoplasia.

On occasion, vaginal smears may be taken where the particular patient is known to have vaginal adenosis. These smears may show squamous metaplasia, together with glandular cells of endocervical type. It is important that a vaginal smear is taken with great care to avoid contamination by metaplastic and glandular cells from the cervix. It is important to remember that all of these changes can occur in non-diethylstilboestrol-exposed young women, and if the colposcopist is examining women under the age of 20 these changes will be seen from time to time.

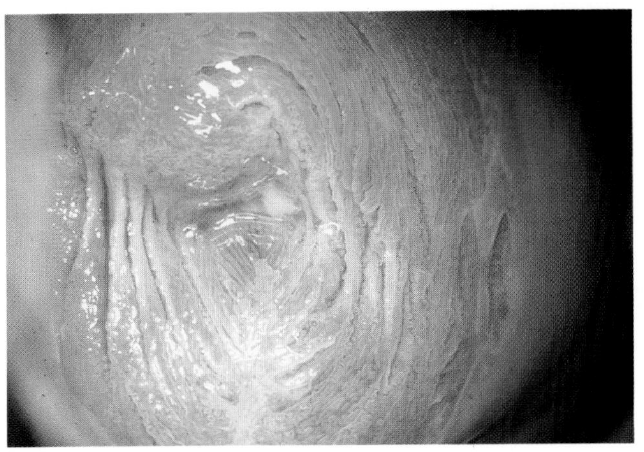

Fig. 20.3 Multiple sulci on the ectocervix. Courtesy of Mr J M Emens.

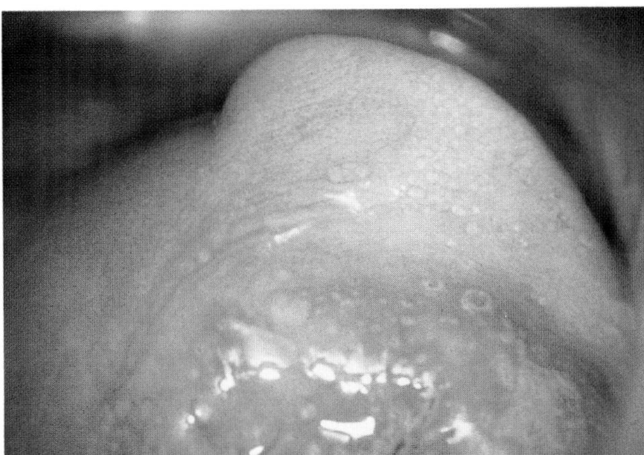

Fig. 20.4 A smooth 'cock's comb'. Courtesy of Mr J M Emens.

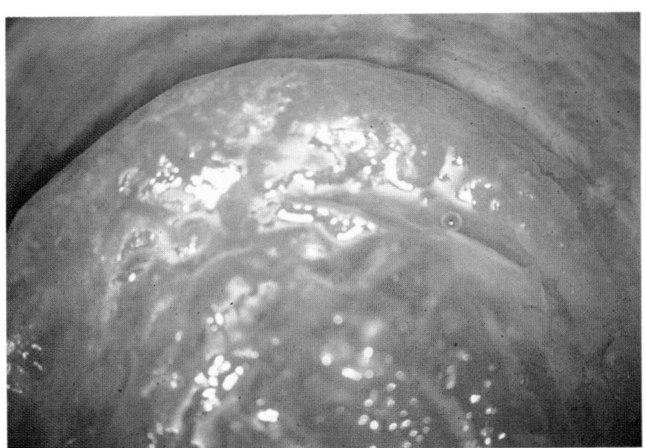

Fig. 20.5 A rough 'cock's comb'. Courtesy of Mr J M Emens.

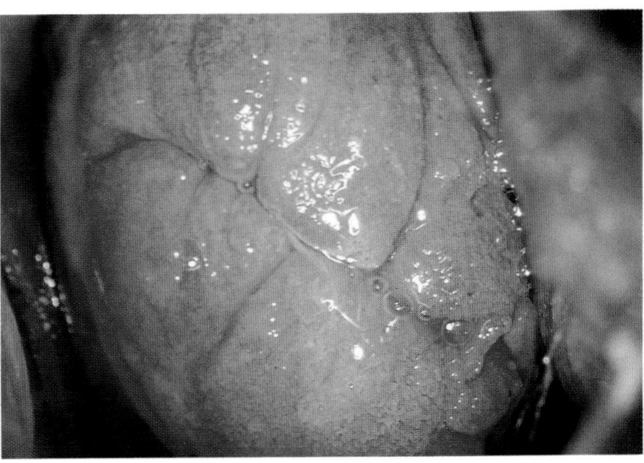

Fig. 20.6 A large pseudopolyp.

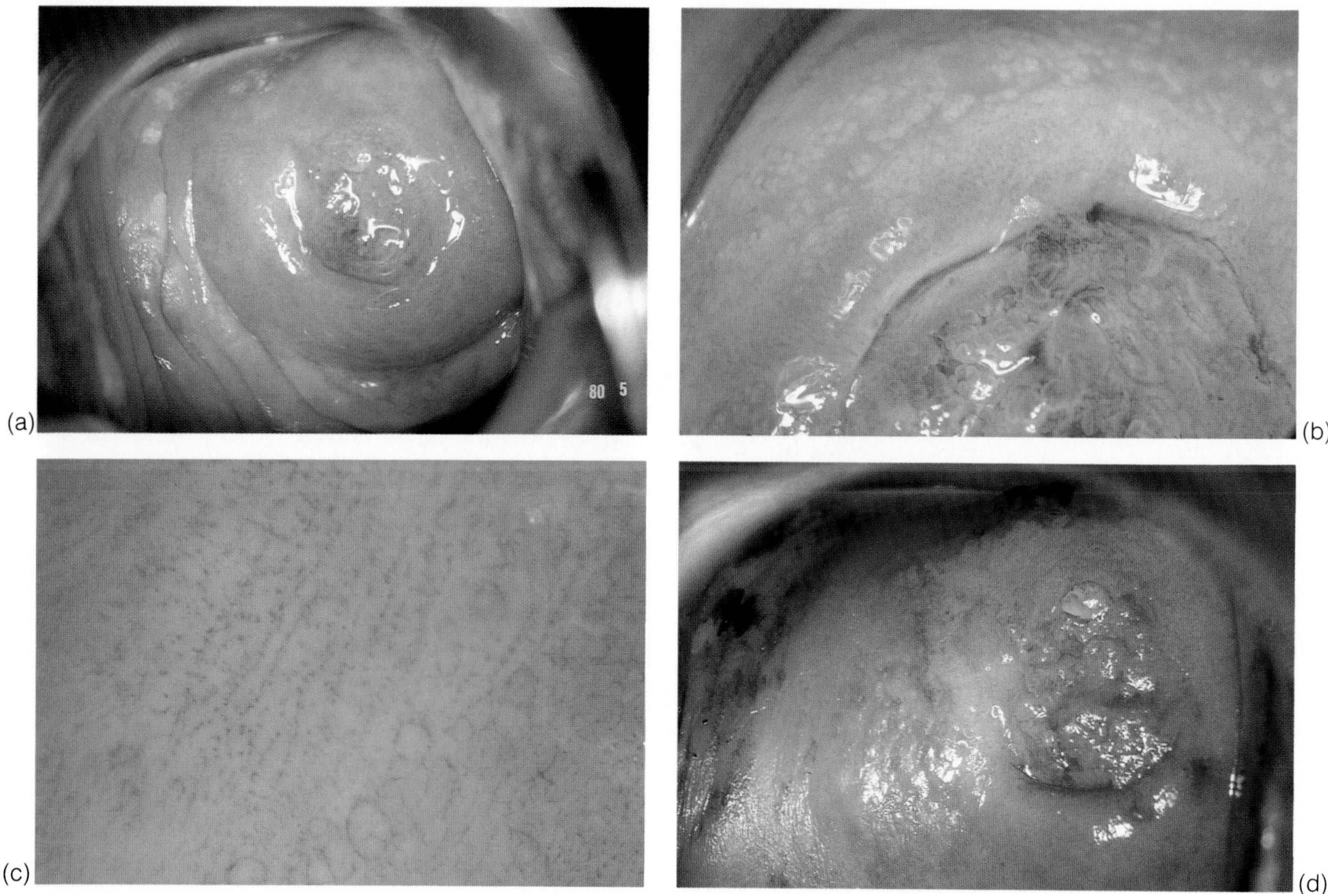

Fig. 20.7 Cervix of a diethylstilboestrol-exposed young woman. (a) At low magnification, a smooth 'cock's comb' can be seen on the anterior lip. In the centre, there is a circular sulcus on the ectocervix. **(b)** Circular sulcus lateral to which there is acetowhite epithelium. **(c)** At high magnification, the acetowhite epithelium gives the appearance of fine punctation and mosaic patterns; the vessels are close together and signify immature metaplasia rather than cervical intraepithelial neoplasia. **(d)** The cervix and upper vagina are covered by non-glycogenated epithelium, clearly demarcating those areas which at one time in the woman's history had been columnar epithelium but at the time of examination were undergoing metaplastic change; in the present case the metaplastic change was complete. The epithelium was completely normal, and it is easy to see how this can be confused with cervical intraepithelial neoplasia.

21. *Cervicography*

INTRODUCTION

There is no doubt that cytology has been the most effective and economical method for cervical cancer detection for many years. Cytology was introduced with the idealistic belief that if every patient was screened by cytology once a year it would be possible to eliminate all cases of cervical neoplasia. This goal, however, has never been accomplished, even where practically 100% of the population was screened, as in British Columbia.

In spite of cytological screening some cases of cervical cancer still occur. The false negative rate of cytology is difficult to determine because, if the cervix is clinically not suspicious and cytology is negative, no further evaluation is undertaken. From mathematical models it has been estimated that the false negative rate of a single cervical smear is 20–42% and it is now well recognized that cytology alone is not a completely satisfactory method for early detection of cervical cancer. Other methods are therefore being evaluated.

In 1958 Navratil *et al* demonstrated that the simultaneous use of cytology and colposcopy increased the accuracy of cervical cancer detection, identifying up to 98% of cases. Navratil's data were confirmed by other investigators but screening colposcopy was never used on a large scale. There are two reasons for this: first, a colposcope is an expensive instrument and it is not possible to have such equipment in every examination room. Secondly, and more importantly, there are not enough experts well trained in colposcopy to undertake the colposcopic screening. Screening colposcopy is more difficult than the colposcopic evaluation of a patient with an abnormal cervical smear because when the smear is abnormal the colposcopist only has to find the area on the cervix that is the most suspicious. On the other hand, most cases are normal on screening colposcopy and it is more difficult for the colposcopist to pick up the few cases that have colposcopic abnormalities. There are some countries, mainly in Europe, where it is claimed that screening colposcopy is a part of routine gynaecological examinations. However, it is doubtful whether the diagnostic accuracy of all the colposcopists doing the examination is of a sufficiently high standard.

In recent years other problems have emerged in the early diagnosis of cervical neoplasia, one of the most important of which was the accurate evaluation of patients with atypical smears. In 1989 the Bethesda System of cytological diagnostic terminology was introduced in the USA (see page 27). It was meant to provide a guide for cytopathologists to report smear results in unambiguous diagnostic terms that have clear implications for patient management. One of the aims of the Bethesda System was to decrease the number of atypical smears (class II Pap smears). Unfortunately the result was quite the reverse. Before the Bethesda system the number of atypical smears was around 5%, but after its introduction the frequency of atypical smears rose on average to 10% and in some institutions up to 20%. The ASCUS (atypical squamous cells of undetermined significance) category was not meant to include benign reactive and reparative changes but the lack of diagnostic criteria has resulted in inconsistency in the diagnosis which has become quite common in some centres. The proper management for these women is still open to debate. It is generally accepted that the most accurate method of evaluation is by colposcopy but the cost of colposcopic evaluation of all patients with ASCUS or borderline nuclear changes would be astronomical.

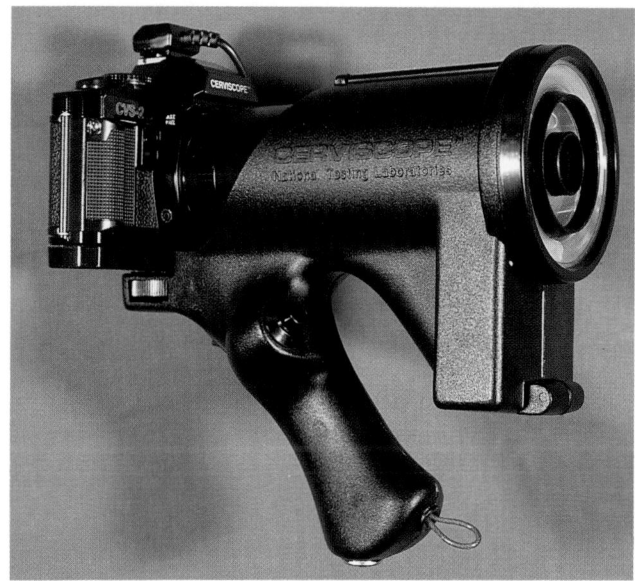

Fig. 21.1 A cerviscope.

To overcome these problems, cervicography was developed by Stafl in 1981.

CERVICOGRAPHY

Cervicography represents a natural development of colposcopy as it evaluates exactly the same features as colposcopy but uses a different instrument. The cervicograph, trade name 'Cerviscope', is produced by National Testing Laboratories, St Louis, Missouri, USA (Fig. 21.1). It is basically a 35-mm camera that has a built-in ring flash and examining light for focusing. Everything on the camera is fixed; it is not possible to change the f-stop or the exposure time, and focusing is done by moving the entire instrument back and forth. Because of this the camera is practically foolproof and the frequency of technically unsatisfactory pictures is very low (2–3%). The main difference between the cervicograph and colpophotographic systems is that the depth of focus in cervicography is 28 mm, which is significantly more than with colpophotographic systems. Therefore, even if the cervix is not focused properly the cervigram is likely to be in focus.

The basic concept behind cervicography is that every healthcare worker, even those with no experience of colposcopy (family physician, nurse, technician), can, after only a short training, take a microscopic picture of the cervix that can then be sent to colposcopic experts for evaluation. It is a non-invasive technique and it adds no more than one minute to a screening gynaecological examination.

For the first time cervicography makes feasible the use of colposcopic principles in cervical cancer screening. With screening colposcopy even an expert can evaluate usually no more than four patients an hour because of the time to prepare the patient for the examination, clean the cervix, etc. However an expert can evaluate 100–200 cervigrams per hour and this makes the use of cervicography in screening practical.

TECHNIQUE OF CERVICOGRAPHY

The technique of the cervicographic examination is very similar to that of colposcopy. The cervix is visualized with a speculum, cervical mucus is cleaned, and 5% acetic acid is applied. Initial inspection with the cervicograph ensures that the entire cervix is in the field with the external os in the centre of the picture. After this a second liberal reapplication of 5% acetic acid is made because it is well known that in some lesions acetowhiteness develops immediately after acetic acid application, whereas in others it takes longer. Using a second application of acetic acid adds consistency to the examination. After the second application of acetic acid the cervix is focused by moving the entire instrument back and forth and a cervicographic picture is obtained. It is recommended that two pictures are taken, using Ektachrome 200. The magnification of the original cervicography picture is actually a reduction 0.6× because the cervix, which is 3–4 cm in diameter, must be squeezed onto a 35-mm slide. The slide is subsequently projected on to a large screen that is at least 1.5 metres in diameter. The projected picture is inspected from a short distance, so that the apparent magnification is similar to the magnification of a colposcope. For evaluators the inspection of the cervicography picture is very similar to or even better than actual examination through the colposcope. The only limitation of cervicography is of course that it is not possible to manipulate the cervix or to use the endocervical speculum as in the colposcopic evaluation.

EVALUATION OF CERVIGRAMS

The results of cervicography will depend on the skill of the evaluators. While taking the picture is very easy, the evaluation of cervigrams is a responsible and difficult task. Therefore the owner of the patent for cervicography, the Medical College of Wisconsin, requires that all the evaluators of cervigrams must be certified by the Medical College. Candidates admitted to the cervicography certification examination need to have at least five years of colposcopic experience. This is necessary because the main aim of colposcopy or cervicography is to rule out invasive cancer.

Microinvasive or small invasive cancers are recognized largely by the presence of atypical vessels but unfortunately these atypical vessels are often less impressive than the mosaic or punctation seen with intraepithelial disease. Missing atypical vessels may mean the failure to diagnose an invasive carcinoma, which is a serious mistake. There are relatively few cases of microinvasive or small invasive cancer and so it can take several years to learn how to recognize atypical vessels unless the colposcopist is working in a cancer referral centre.

Colposcopy and cervicography are techniques that both evaluate the same problem so that experts in colposcopy can very easily become experts in cervicography. However, it is very difficult or impossible to judge expertise in colposcopy, except when working together on a one-to-one basis. On the other hand, using the objectivity of a cervicograph it is possible to achieve a precise measure of colposcopic/cervicographic expertise. Currently there are about 120 certified evaluators in the USA, 30 in the UK and several in most countries worldwide.

TERMINOLOGY

Cervicography terminology differs slightly from colposcopic terminology. Cervicography findings are divided into groups as shown in Table 21.1.

Table 21.1 Cervicography evaluation sheet

☐ **Negative**

☐ N1.____Squamocolumnar junction and transformation zone are fully visible
☐ N2.____Squamocolumnar junction is not fully visible; components of the transformation zone are visible
☐ N3.____Squamocolumnar junction and transformation zone are not visible; an endocervical smear is essential

☐ **Atypical**

☐ A1.____Papilloma/condyloma (HPV infection) outside transformation zone
☐ A2.____Atypical immature squamous metaplasia
☐ A3.____Trivial change of doubtful significance

☐ **Positive**

Compatible with:	Lesion morphology:
☐ P1.____minor grade lesion (CIN 1, HPV)	____acetowhite epithelium
☐ P2.____major grade lesion (CIN 2, CIN 3)	____punctation
☐ P3.____invasive cancer, rule out invasive cancer	____mosaicism
	____atypical vessels

☐ **Technically defective** (Retake cervigram)

☐ ____View of cervix obscured by:
____mucus____blood____speculum____vaginal wall
☐ ____Insufficient acetic acid, or cervigrams taken too late after second application of acetic acid
☐ ____Out of focus____Overexposed/underexposed

Negative findings

Negative findings are subdivided into three groups. In the first group, N1, which corresponds to the colposcopic term 'negative', are cases where the entire squamocolumnar junction is visible and no abnormal colposcopic lesion is present. The possibility that neoplasia exists on the visible portion of the cervix is minimal. A typical negative cervigram is shown in Figure 21.2.

The second group, N2, represents cases where only a portion of the transformation zone is visible but the squamocolumnar junction is not fully visible (Fig. 21.3). Theoretically there is a possibility that some significant lesion might be located higher up in the endocervical canal. From clinical experience, however, this is extremely rare.

The third category, N3, corresponds to the colposcopic term 'unsatisfactory', where the squamocolumnar junction and transformation zone are not visible (Fig. 21.4). In these cases squamous neoplasia located in the endocervical canal cannot be ruled out.

The benefit of the cervicographic examination is that it informs the clinician that an endocervical smear is essential because if some pathology is present it is located in the endocervical canal.

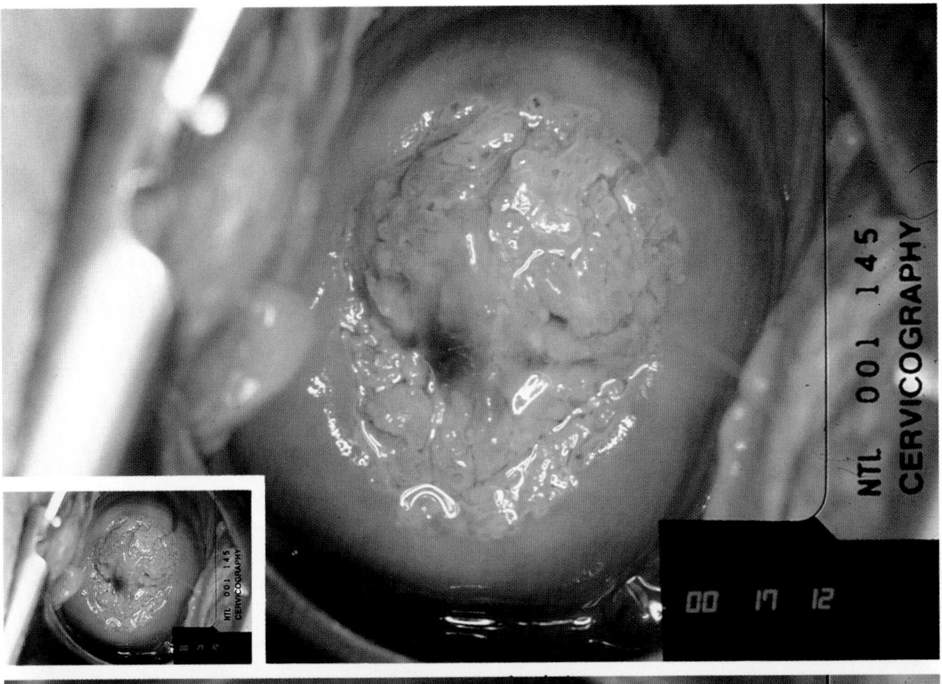

Fig. 21.2 Cervicography category N1. There is eversion of columnar epithelium on both lips. The grape-like structures of the columnar epithelium are visible. At 11 o'clock and 1 o'clock, tongues of squamous metaplasia are present. No abnormal colposcopic lesion is seen and the squamocolumnar junction is fully visible.

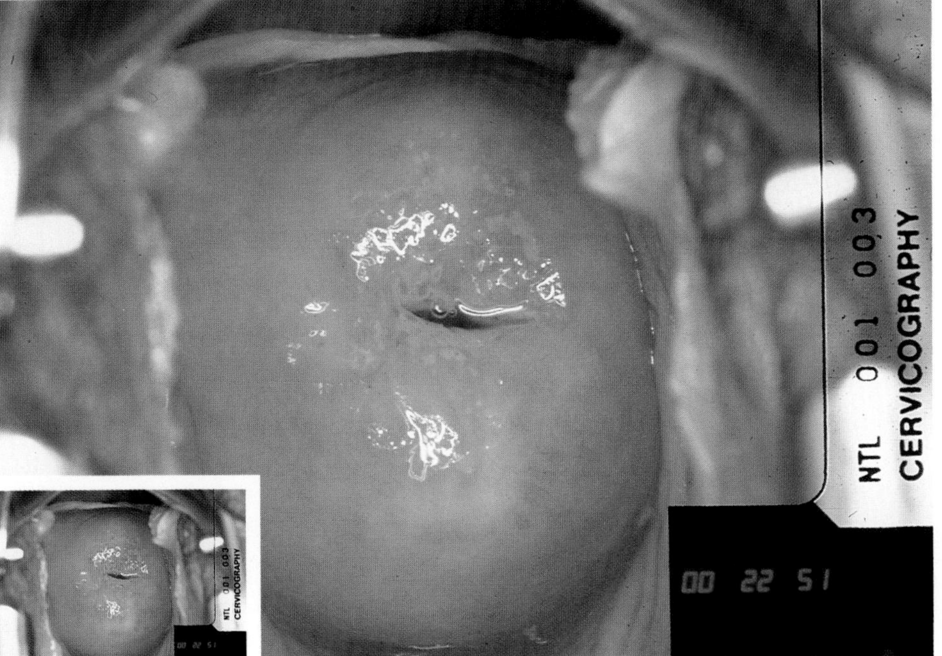

Fig. 21.3 Cervicography category N2. Components of the transformation zone are visible on both lips. Several gland openings are present. No abnormal colposcopic lesion is seen but the squamocolumnar junction is not visible.

Atypical findings

Atypical findings include cases where there are lesions visible on the portio, but the evaluator feels that an immediate biopsy is not necessary. Atypical cases are subdivided into three groups.

A1 includes human papillomavirus (HPV) lesions outside the transformation zone in original squamous epithelium (Fig. 21.5). These lesions have minimal neoplastic potential and often disappear spontaneously, so that immediate biopsy is not necessary.

The second category, A2, is atypical immature squamous metaplasia, which usually occurs in patients below the age of 20. Eversion of columnar epithelium to the portio is visible, and all around this

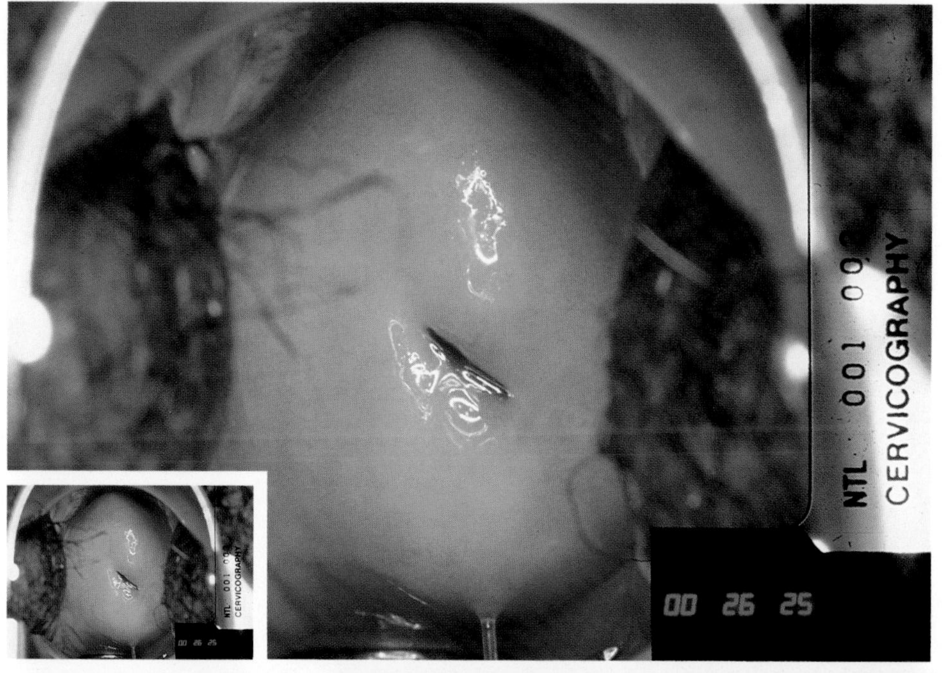

Fig. 21.4 Cervicography category N3. The entire cervix is covered with original squamous epithelium. No transformation zone is seen and the squamocolumnar junction is not visible.

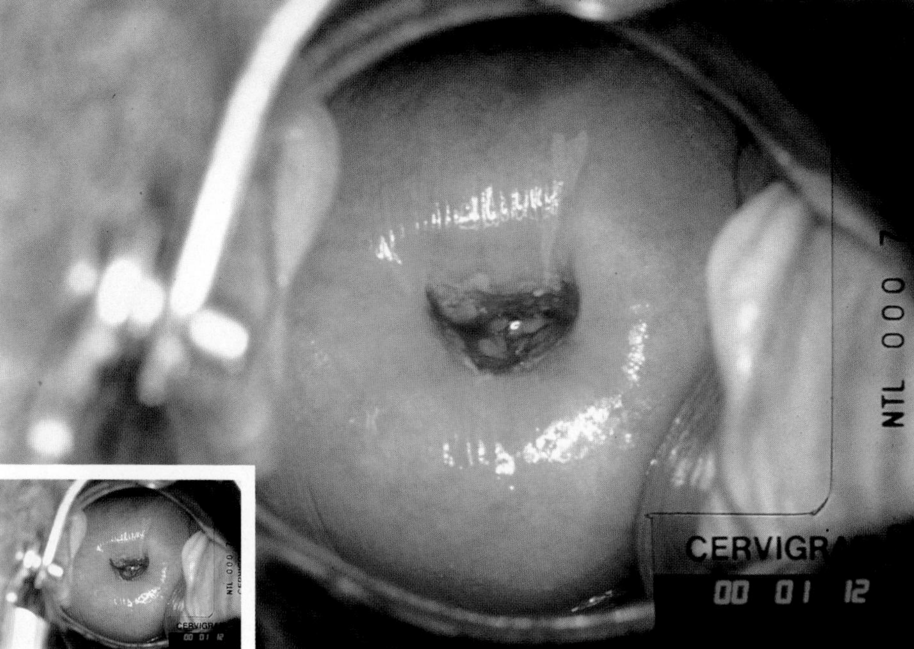

Fig. 21.5 Cervicography category A1. At 1 o'clock a small area of acetowhite epithelium is present within the original squamous epithelium. Impression – flat papilloma.

eversion there is acetowhite epithelium with very vague, ill-defined borders. In some cases a delicate mosaic pattern or punctation can also be present (Fig. 21.6). When a biopsy specimen is taken it is likely that only immature squamous epithelium will be present. However, the cervicographic evaluation cannot predict what will happen to this lesion in the future. It may disappear, leaving well-differentiated squamous epithelium, or a truly abnormal lesion might result. It is recommended that the cervigram and the cervical smear be repeated in six months.

In the third category, A3, are included trivial changes of doubtful significance in which an immediate biopsy is not necessary (Fig. 21.7); follow-up is advised every six to 12 months.

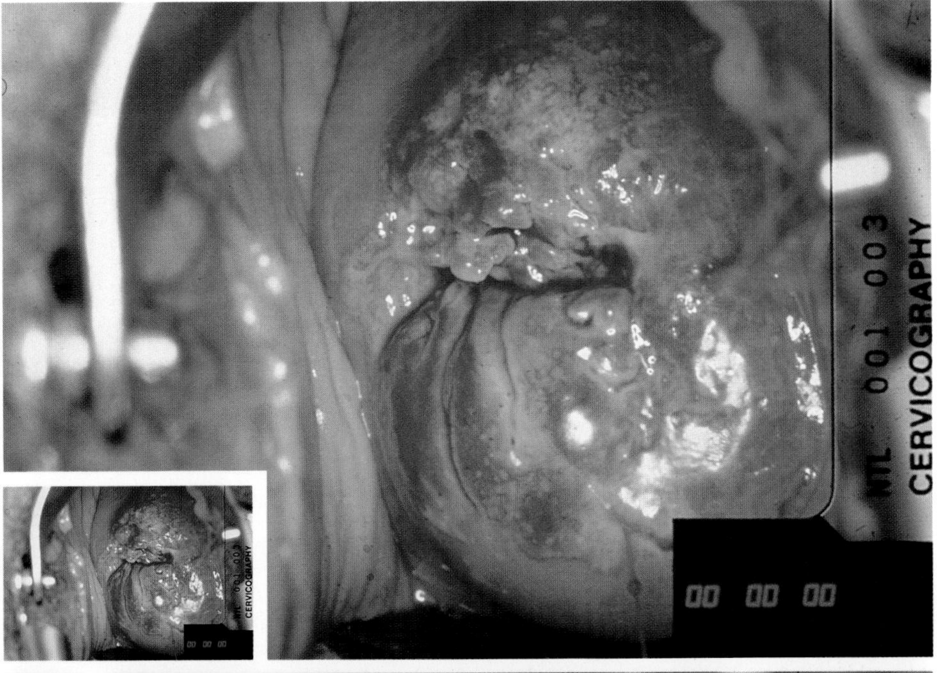

Fig. 21.6 Cervicography category A2. There is eversion of columnar epithelium on both lips around which is an area of acetowhite epithelium. At the margins of this eversion, at 4 o'clock, there is a delicate mosaic pattern. Impression – immature metaplasia.

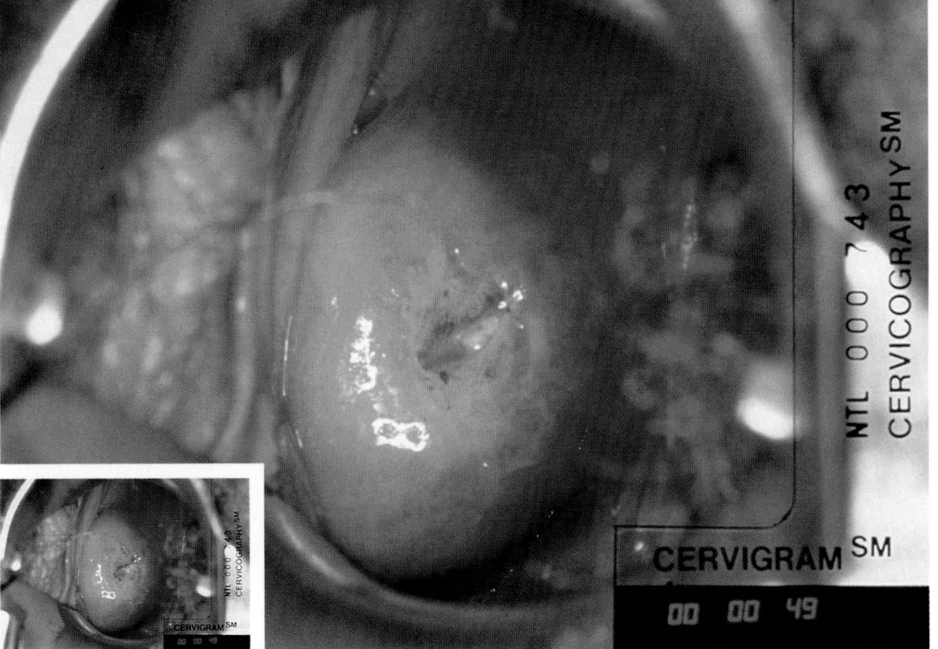

Fig. 21.7 Cervicography category A3. At 11 o'clock there is a small area of acetowhite epithelium with irregular borders, within the transformation zone. This is a typical lesion of doubtful significance.

Positive findings

In cervicographic findings that are classified as positive (Figs 21.8–21.10), colposcopy and colposcopically directed biopsy are indicated. The evaluator documents his or her prediction as to whether it is a minor-grade lesion, major-grade lesion, or lesion suggestive of invasive cancer.

The prediction of histopathological changes is based on five factors: vascular pattern, intercapillary distance, colour tone, surface pattern, and the borders with the normal epithelium (see Chapter 8).

- The **vascular pattern** can distinguish intraepithelial lesions from early invasive lesions. In intraepithelial lesions a vascular pattern of punctation

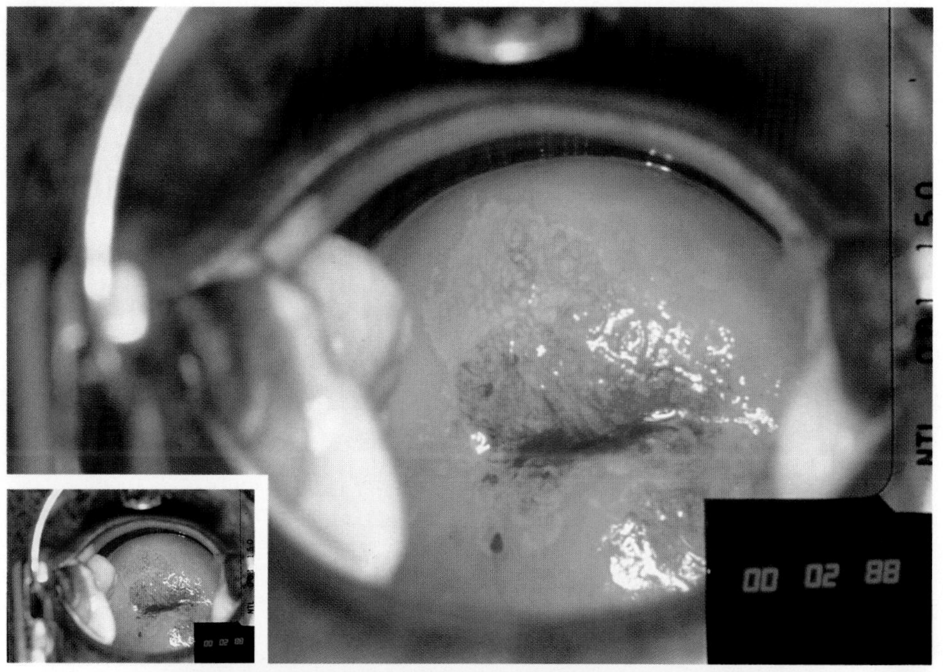

Fig. 21.8 Cervicography category P1. On the anterior lip at the margin of the eversion there is an area of acetowhite epithelium with mosaic with irregular borders. The intercapillary distance is slightly increased in the field of mosaic. Impression – low-grade lesion (wart virus infection or CIN 1).

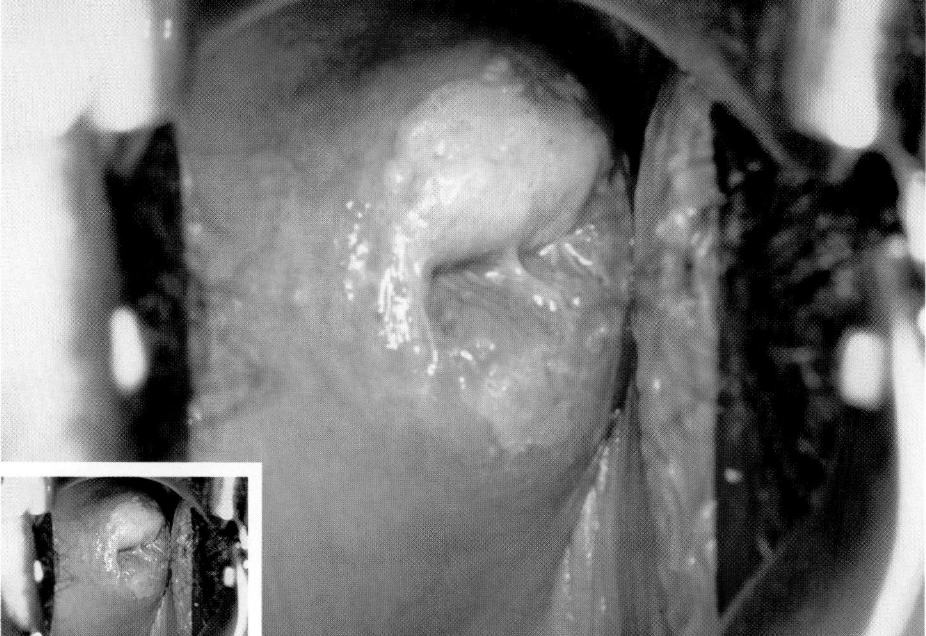

Fig. 21.9 Cervicography category P2. On the anterior lip there is prominent acetowhite epithelium with regular borders. The difference in colour in comparison with the normal epithelium is significant. Prediction – high-grade lesion (CIN 2–CIN 3). On the posterior lip is a small area of acetowhite epithelium with irregular borders. The difference in colour is less significant. This is a P1 lesion compatible with low-grade lesion.

and mosaic may be visible but in microinvasive cancer atypical vessels running parallel with the surface are present. These atypical vessels are suggestive, but not diagnostic, of invasive cancer. They may also be present in some benign conditions such as granulation tissue and decidual reactions. When atypical vessels are found, a directed biopsy is always necessary.

- **Intercapillary distance** relates to the largest distance between the intraepithelial vessels. In punctation it is the distance between the reddish points of punctation. In a mosaic pattern the intercapillary distance relates to the size of the mosaic fields. The normal intercapillary distance is less than 250 μm. With increased intercapillary distance, more significant histopathological

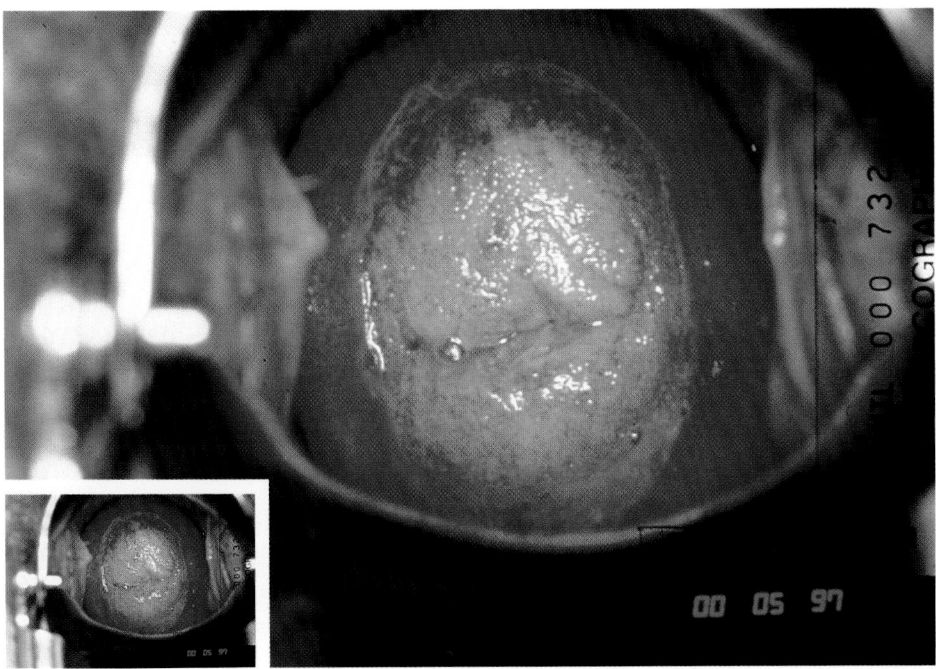

Fig. 21.10 Cervicography category P3. On the anterior lip there is a slightly exophytic lesion with atypical vessels running parallel to the surface. Impression – invasive carcinoma. A directed biopsy from the anterior lip confirmed the diagnosis of invasive carcinoma.

changes can be expected. With colposcopy the intercapillary distance is only estimated but with cervicography exact measurements in microns can be done.

- The **whiteness of epithelium** after application of acetic acid is also related to severity of the abnormality.

- The **surface pattern** can be either smooth or rough. A rough surface pattern is related to a more significant lesion, but an HPV lesion can also greatly influence the surface pattern and might mimic a more significant lesion.

- The appearance of the **borders with the normal tissue** is one of the most important parameters. If the borders are irregular, less significant lesions can be expected. If they are regular, more significant histopathological changes are usually present.

Prediction of the histopathological findings cannot be based on only one parameter but depends on the evaluation of all parameters. The experienced evaluator of cervigrams can predict the histopathological findings within one histological degree in 90% of cases.

Technically defective findings

Technically defective findings are uncommon after initial experience. The picture is very rarely out of focus because the depth of focus in cervicography is 28 mm. Sometimes part of the transformation zone is obscured by the speculum or vaginal wall. Furthermore, mucus or blood may be present on the cervix when it is not properly removed before performing the cervigram. It is very easy for the evaluator to recognize all technically defective findings, and a new cervigram is then recommended.

RESULTS OF CERVICOGRAPHY

In the first published study, Stafl (1981) compared the accuracy of cervicography and colposcopy and found the accuracy of these two methods to be identical, a conclusion based on statistically significant material. In the same study it was also demonstrated that cervicography can detect some cases of CIN missed by cytological screening. The total number of cases, however, was insufficient to draw a statistically valid conclusion. The results of a much larger study were published in 1988 by Tawa and co-workers. This study involved 3271 patients between the ages of 18 and 50 in whom 81 cases of CIN were detected. A cervical smear and cervigram were taken during the same visit. The study was prospective, with blind evaluation of smear and cervigram. If the cervigram or smear was positive, colposcopically directed biopsy was done. From 3271 patients, 81 cases of CIN were diagnosed (2.4%). Fourteen cases of CIN were detected with cytology, and 72 cases were detected with cervicography. The conclusion of the study was that the sensitivity of cervicography is 5.1 times greater than that of cytological screening. The specificity of cervicography in the study was eight times lower than that of cytological screening. Also of significance is that the cervigram is 3.7 times more cost effective than cytological screening when all of the costs related to screening are combined.

This study by Tawa and associates was the first major survey of cervicography screening. Cervicography findings were divided only into positive or negative and when the result was positive, colposcopy and biopsy were automatically carried out. In the more recent cervicographic terminology the term 'atypical' has been introduced. In atypical cases, immediate colposcopic examination and biopsy are not recommended. By introducing the term 'atypical', the false positive rate of cervicography was drastically reduced without reducing sensitivity. Identification of these atypical cases is important but when a biopsy is taken from these atypical lesions that includes the lesion and normal tissue, there is usually no difference in histological appearances from one to the other. Histology is considered to be the final arbiter of cervical changes, but it is possible that colposcopy can detect changes before the morphological changes in the tissue become apparent. It is most likely that atypical cervicographic changes represent subclinical HPV infection, which requires a closer follow-up of the patient. It is possible that in the future the detection of these so-called 'false positive cases' will represent a major contribution of cervicography by identifying patients at risk for eventual development of cervical neoplasia.

Some 1400 patients have been studied for the prevalence of HPV infection (R. Reid, personal communication). Patients were screened by cytology, cervicography and deoxyribonucleic acid (DNA) hybridization. In this study the false negative rate for cytology was 64%, for cervicography 20%, and for DNA hybridization 81%. Spitzer and co-workers (1987) compared the use of cytology, cervicography and colposcopy in the evaluation of patients with atypical smears. The sensitivity of cervicography was much better than that of the smear for both referral (89% compared with 58%) and detection (78% compared with 18%). Cytology was more specific than cervicography (55% compared with 29%).

Kesic and co-workers (1993) studied the sensitivity and specificity of cervical cytology and of cervicography in the detection of CIN and invasive cancer of the cervix in 418 women. Cervicography correctly identified 24 out of 27 women with CIN or invasive cancer, whereas cytology detected only 14 (sensitivity 89% versus 52%) ($P < 0.01$). Cervicography detected CIN in 11 women with negative smears, six having CIN 3. Only one case of CIN 1 was detected by cytology when cervicography was negative. Cervicography was only slightly less specific than cytology, 92% versus 94% (not significant).

Coibion and co-workers (1991) at the Bordet Institute in Brussels, evaluated 1843 patients simultaneously with cytology and cervicography and detected 59 women with CIN 3 (3.4%). The sensitivity of cytology was 19% and of cervicography 93%. The specificity of cytology was 100% and of cervicography 99%.

Presently, cervicography screening is also being evaluated in the developing countries (India, South Africa) where it represents the first economically feasible method of screening for cervical cancer; however, the results of these studies are not yet published.

The results of published studies show that the sensitivity of cervicography is uniformly higher than the sensitivity of cytology. The specificity of cervicography is generally lower than cytology but is still at acceptable levels.

CONCLUSION

Cervicography replaces subjective colposcopic evaluation with objective cervicographic assessment and also provides permanent documentation. Cervicography should always be used in combination with cytology and the cancer detection rate then approaches 100%. Cervicography will replace neither cytology nor colposcopy. If a lesion is found, expert colposcopic evaluation is necessary and a colposcopically directed biopsy specimen should be taken. Present studies demonstrate that cervicography can effectively detect cases of precancer and cancer missed by cytology and thus plays an important role in the detection of cervical cancer.

22. *Planning and management of colposcopy and out-patient treatment services*

INTRODUCTION

All district health authorities in England and Wales have been instructed to introduce computerized call and recall schemes for cervical cytology screening. This also applies to the cytology screening service within the public or private sector of medicine.

It is generally accepted as unethical to introduce a screening programme without being able to offer the necessary supportive diagnostic and treatment facilities. However, often this is not the case, and little consideration may have been given to planning for the consequences, particularly the impact on colposcopy services, of an efficient computerized call and recall scheme.

The minimum essential stages in effective cervical cancer prevention are cytological screening, diagnostic colposcopy and histological diagnosis, appropriate treatment and follow-up, involving further colposcopy and cytological surveillance.

APPROXIMATION OF SERVICE REQUIREMENTS

In order to estimate the requirement for colposcopy and treatment services, there are two possible approaches.

One is to determine the number of women currently screened and the existing level of diagnostic and treatment services provided to meet the demand. An increment may then be added to account for the estimated increase in smears as a result of the introduction of the call and recall scheme. All routinely available statistics from laboratories and family practitioner committees relate to smears processed rather than women screened, and therefore the workload calculation by this method would require an *ad hoc* study.

An alternative method is to estimate likely total demand for the services as a result of introduction of the screening programme. This second method is described here.

Calculation of demand for diagnostic colposcopy

METHOD

The demand for diagnostic colposcopy is dependent, among other things, upon the number of women screened (Table 22.1), the clinical policy for the referral of women with non-negative smears, the rate and category of non-negative smears, and referrals to the service on clinical grounds alone, regardless of a negative smear.

Table 22.1 Population screening factors

Information required	Source
No. of women in the specified age groups in the population to be screened	Local age–sex register
Proportion of women who have had hysterectomy*	Estimated as 12%
Uptake rate for screening	Known or predicted
Recall interval for screening	Agreed local policy
Number of non-resident women screened	Laboratory estimates or *ad hoc* study

*Where previous hysterectomy has been performed in the presence of CIN, ongoing vaginal vault smears are recommended. Therefore, the estimated 12% reduction for the prevalence of hysterectomy may be excessive.

Clinical policy in relation to non-negative smears

Dyskaryosis

There is some evidence in the literature suggesting that an initial cytological description of mild or moderate dyskaryosis may be associated with a more severe grade of cervical intraepithelial neoplasia, as shown by the final histological diagnosis, in a proportion of cases. In addition, mild dyskaryotic change may progress to a more significant grade, as may the underlying histological lesions. For these reasons, in the UK in 1987 an Intercollegiate Working Party on Cervical Cytology Screening recommended that, ideally, all women with dyskaryotic smears of any degree should be investigated by colposcopy as soon as possible. This policy has been adopted in these calculations. However, it is important to point out that more recent opinion has suggested that a repeat smear at an interval of six months is the first line of management, followed by colposcopy in the case of persistent abnormalities (see page 154).

Viral changes only

There is an association, casual or causal, between human papillomavirus infection of the cervix and squamous neoplasia. Human papillomavirus may mask underlying cervical intraepithelial neoplasia and may be associated with an increased risk of progression of the cervical intraepithelial lesion. Human papillomavirus infection also appears to be associated with an increased risk of future development of cervical intraepithelial neoplasia. It has been recommended, therefore, that the latter should be excluded in case of human papillomavirus infection.

Other investigators have suggested that, in such cases, it may be acceptable to repeat the smear in six months, and only if cytological evidence of persistent human papillomavirus change is obtained should colposcopy be indicated. In the calculation to be described, it is assumed that colposcopy will be recommended on the initial smear showing viral changes.

Inflammatory changes only

Inflammatory changes of the cervix, and in turn in the cervical smear, may mask underlying cervical intraepithelial neoplasia. There is some reporting of a high proportion of such changes reverting to normal cytology, if the smear is repeated in three to six months. Of the remainder, approximately 50–75% may have underlying cervical intraepithelial neoplasia.

Detection of inflammatory changes in the initial smear indicates the need to identify and, where appropriate, treat any specific causal organism or agent. If non-specific inflammatory changes persist after six months, colposcopic assessment is indicated. This policy has been assumed in the calculation to be presented.

Non-negative results from population screening

Dyskaryosis

Local data, routine returns and *ad hoc* studies of the prevalence of dyskaryosis may be limited and complicated by a different terminology, inclusion of different degrees of dyskaryosis, and use of combinations of different numerators (smears or women) and denominators (1000 smears and 1000 women). Therefore, for the present purposes, a best working estimate of about 20 cases of dyskaryosis (any degree) per 1000 women screened will be used.

Viral changes only

Information on the prevalence of pure viral cytopathic effects as seen on smears is even more sparse and unreliable, and further complicated by the recently introduced technique, polymerase chain reaction (PCR), being used on a research basis to evaluate genital human papillomavirus infection in relatively small cohorts of the general population (see Chapter 3). The method is apparently ultrasensitive, capable of detecting a single copy of the human papillomavirus genome per 10^5 cells, either in cervical smears or in tissue biopsies. These results are currently being extended in larger studies and their proper evaluation and implications are awaited.

For the moment, in routine clinical practice we must continue to rely on the simple exfoliative cytological approach to uncover subclinical human papillomavirus infection in the asymptomatic population. For a best working estimate, a figure of 10 cases per 1000 women screened will be used. It will be clear that for some populations this will be a substantial underestimate.

Inflammatory changes only

Similar problems to those relating to the prevalence of dyskaryotic changes pertain to inflammatory changes. At least one large study suggests a best working estimate of prevalence of approximately 100 cases per 1000 women screened. After a smear has been reported as showing inflammatory changes, a best estimate of 75% reverting to normal on a repeat smear after six months will be assumed and used in the subsequent calculation.

Clinical referrals

Clinical referrals because of suspicious appearances of the cervix on direct naked-eye visualization, symptomatology suspicious of cervical pathology regardless of naked-eye appearance (e.g. postcoital bleeding), or an overt vulval or vaginal lesion, may account for approximately 2% of the workload of a colposcopy clinic.

DERIVATION OF DEMAND FOR DIAGNOSTIC COLPOSCOPY

On the basis of the above assumptions, if 100 000 women are eligible for cervical screening, the proportion having had a hysterectomy is 12% (but note the comment in Table 22.1); assuming the uptake for screening is 70%, and the recall interval three years, the number of non-resident women screened is 3000, then the total number of women screened per year will be:

$$\frac{[100\,000 - (12\% \times 100\,000)] \times 70\%}{3} + 3000 = 23\,533$$

The predicted number of women with dyskaryosis will be:

23 533 × 20/1000 = 471

The predicted number of women with viral changes only will be:

23 533 × 10/1000 = 235

The predicted number of women with inflammatory changes only on two consecutive smears (assuming 75% revert to normal on the second smear) will be:

23 533 × 100/1000 × 25% = 588

Therefore, the total demand for diagnostic colposcopy from screening is predicted to be:

471 + 235 + 588 = 1294

Assuming 2% of the workload is from clinical referrals, the total demand for diagnostic colposcopy will be:

1294 × 102% = 1320

CALCULATION OF DEMAND FOR TREATMENT

Method

The following assumption will be made: currently, the majority of women with cervical intraepithelial neoplasia receive locally destructive treatment to the transformation zone. Approximately 5% of those requiring treatment have multilevel disease involving the vagina or vulva, or extensive ectocervical or forniceal disease necessitating treatment on an in-patient basis under general anaesthesia. A further 20% of those patients that should be treated will require large excisional cone biopsy, as the lesion extends into the endocervical canal and the whole transformation zone cannot be visualized, or microinvasion/frank invasion is present or suspected.

A number of factors will influence the demand for treatment, including the number of women having diagnostic colposcopy, the proportion discharged after one colposcopic assessment, the proportion discharged after follow-up colposcopy, without treatment, and the average number of attendances per woman for treatment.

PROPORTION DISCHARGED AFTER ONE COLPOSCOPIC ASSESSMENT

Approximately 50% of women with persistent inflammatory cytology can be discharged after initial colposcopy. Women with a negative first colposcopy initiated by dyskaryotic or viral changes in the smear, may have a further interval colposcopy.

PROPORTION DISCHARGED AFTER FOLLOW-UP COLPOSCOPY WITHOUT TREATMENT

It will be assumed, on the basis of published literature, that 25% of women with dyskaryotic smears and 55% of women with viral changes can be discharged without treatment, after negative repeat cytology and with the precaution of follow-up colposcopy.

AVERAGE NUMBER OF ATTENDANCES PER WOMAN FOR TREATMENT

The accepted success rate from one treatment by laser vaporization cone, for example, is 96%, therefore the average number of attendances per woman is 1.04.

Example calculation

Of 471 women with dyskaryotic changes, a predicted 75% will require treatment:

471 × 75% = 353

Of 235 women with viral changes, 45% are predicted to require treatment:

235 × 45% = 106

Of 588 women with inflammatory changes, 50% may require treatment:

588 × 50% = 294

Of 1294 referrals, some 2% or 26 women may be referred on clinical grounds. The total demand for treatment, therefore, may be:

353 + 106 + 294 + 26 = 779

Of these patients, 20% may require cone biopsy:

779 × 20% = 156

Also, 5% may require in-patient laser treatment:

779 × 5% = 39

Another 75% may require out-patient ablative therapy, such as laser vaporization cone:

779 × 75% = 584

If the average number of out-patient laser treatment attendances per woman is 1.04, then the required number of treatment appointments per year will be:

$584 \times 1.04 = 607$

CALCULATION OF DEMAND FOR FOLLOW-UP COLPOSCOPY

Method

The demand for follow-up colposcopy depends on the number of women receiving treatment; the average number of attendances per woman for post-treatment follow-up colposcopy, and the number of women receiving follow-up colposcopy without previous treatment.

AVERAGE NUMBER OF ATTENDANCES PER WOMAN FOR FOLLOW-UP COLPOSCOPY AFTER TREATMENT

From an examination of local data, it will be assumed that the average attendance rate per woman for follow-up colposcopy is 2.4.

Example calculation

Of 779 women to be treated, all will require colposcopic follow-up after treatment. If each of these women has an average of 2.4 attendances, then the number of appointments required after treatment will be:

$779 \times 2.4 = 1870$

If 25% of the 471 women with dyskaryotic changes and 55% of the 235 with viral changes are to have one follow-up colposcopy, then the additional requirement will be:

$(471 \times 25\%) + (235 \times 55\%) = 118 + 129 = 247$

Therefore, the total demand for appointments for follow-up colposcopy per year will be of the order:

$1870 + 247 = 2117$

MEDICAL WORKLOAD IMPLICATIONS

The following are not unreasonable assumptions in trying to assess the medical requirements within the colposcopy clinic dealing with the above hypothetical overall patient numbers: the equivalent of four new patients and eight follow-up patients can be seen per colposcopy table session; six out-patients can be treated per laser table session; five patients can be added to a routine gynaecology operating list for cone biopsy or local destructive treatment of cervical intraepithelial neoplasia under general anaesthesia; and all such out-patient or in-patient sessions will function for 50 working weeks per year.

Table 22.2 Summary of a colposcopy clinic annual workload for a population screening of 100 000 women

Activity	No.
Diagnostic colposcopy appointments	1320
Out-patient laser or other treatments	607
In-patient laser treatments in theatre	39
Excisional cone biopsies	156
Follow-up colposcopy appointments	2117

Based on the estimates and assumptions made, the annual requirements per 100 000 women eligible for population screening would be as shown in Table 22.2.

In the example given, the requirement would be for six colposcopy table sessions per week, two laser table sessions per week, and 0.8 operating sessions per week. These figures can be compared with current provision (if any) and the additional requirements calculated. If the service also acts as a tertiary referral centre, additional capacity will be necessary. Each doctor session will require a matching nurse session, and it is likely that a clinic functioning with the doctor and nurse levels discussed above will demand the services of a full-time secretary and an appointments clerk.

There is a complex relationship between non-attendance rates (which may be of the order of 8% for primary diagnostic colposcopy, 10% for out-patient treatment such as laser, and 21% for follow-up colposcopy), and the number of appointments required. If the non-attendance represents 'never attending', a reduction in the number of appointments would result. However, if the non-attendant eventually comes to the clinic, and the clinic is not deliberately overbooked, then an increase in the number of appointments available would be necessary. In practice, it is likely that non-attendants will be a mix of these two categories, but this is not readily quantifiable from the routinely available statistics used in the calculations presented above.

Large numbers of opportunistic smears, as opposed to 'call and recall' smears in a systematic computerized population screen, will distort the distribution of required capacity. However, assuming that smears are not unnecessarily duplicated out of phase, the total capacity should remain unchanged.

The assumptions upon which the presented model is based vary in the degree of confidence that can be attached to them, but the final result is of the right order of magnitude and is fairly robust. A major determining factor is the uptake rate in the screening programme. These assumptions are based on the available information, which is sparse. Improvements to the population screening data might soon become available if the information from computerized 'call and recall' schemes could be analysed in relation to women rather than smears.

There will be an inevitable increase in the demand for diagnostic and treatment services, arising out of more comprehensive cervical cytology screening programmes. The data provided here should allow those concerned with service provision to plan for the capital and revenue implications of such an increase.

COLPOSCOPY CLINIC LAYOUT

Accommodation requirements at the clinic level are obviously dictated by the overall workload. For a small clinical throughput all that may be required is to have one room within an existing clinic or practice set-up specially adapted to house the colposcope, with or without the facility to undertake out-patient treatment. If the latter is solely the equipment of large loop excision of the transformation zone by diathermy, for instance, then the additional space for treatment will be minimal.

On the other hand, if the technique of choice is the carbon dioxide laser, then space will be taken up by the laser console and smoke evacuation system, an essential requirement from the point of view of health and safety of staff. In addition, even in a smaller facility, it is not uncommon to find the colposcope embellished with a video television camera, with further space demanded by the television monitor. The end result is the need for a fairly commodious room.

The layout shown in Fig. 22.1 is for a purpose-built clinic sited in a large teaching hospital department of gynaecology, functioning within the public sector in the National Health Service in the UK, and offering a major proportion of the colposcopy service for a city of some 600 000 people and its environs, with a throughput of about 1000 new and 3500 follow-up patients per year, along with out-patient treatments thus generated.

The clinic also meets the educational needs of undergraduates and postgraduates, including short introductory courses in practical colposcopy. Currently, the favoured out-patient treatment modalities are carbon dioxide laser excision or vaporization cone and large loop excision of the transformation zone.

Description

Near the entrance, which must allow easy access for the disabled, the patient is welcomed at the reception/appointments office by the clerk. This office has a computer terminal connecting with the hospital patient administration system (PAS). This terminal also connects with the colposcopy patient records and management computer network, allowing direct transfer of basic patient biodata and appointment details between both, which is a time-saving step.

The secretary's office is nearby, with full typing facilities and the main colposcopy computer system (CPU). This office also allows temporary storage of active standard hardcopy hospital case records for current patients.

Proceeding through the clinic, there is the patient waiting area, with comfortable seating, a hot drinks dispenser and piped music. Adequate toilet facilities are essential, which must also cater for males and the disabled.

A small technical maintenance laboratory is provided, allowing a safe area for the servicing of laser equipment by the hospital medical physics department staff. For this reason, this room has an appropriate illuminated laser sign at the entrance. The ability to conduct a minimal level of in-house laser maintenance is essential for the smooth running of the treatment sessions.

A small staff rest room is provided, with a seminar room adjacent to it, reflecting the teaching role of the clinic. This latter room has slide projection facilities and video playback equipment, with a monitor that can also be connected via a network of video cables to any of the video cameras in the four colposcopy examination/treatment rooms.

Finally, a computer terminal as part of the patient records and management system is also located here, both as a work terminal and as a demonstration point during the short practical courses for postgraduates.

The clinical area is designed so that four doctor table sessions can be run simultaneously. There are four colposcopy rooms, with integral patient chang-

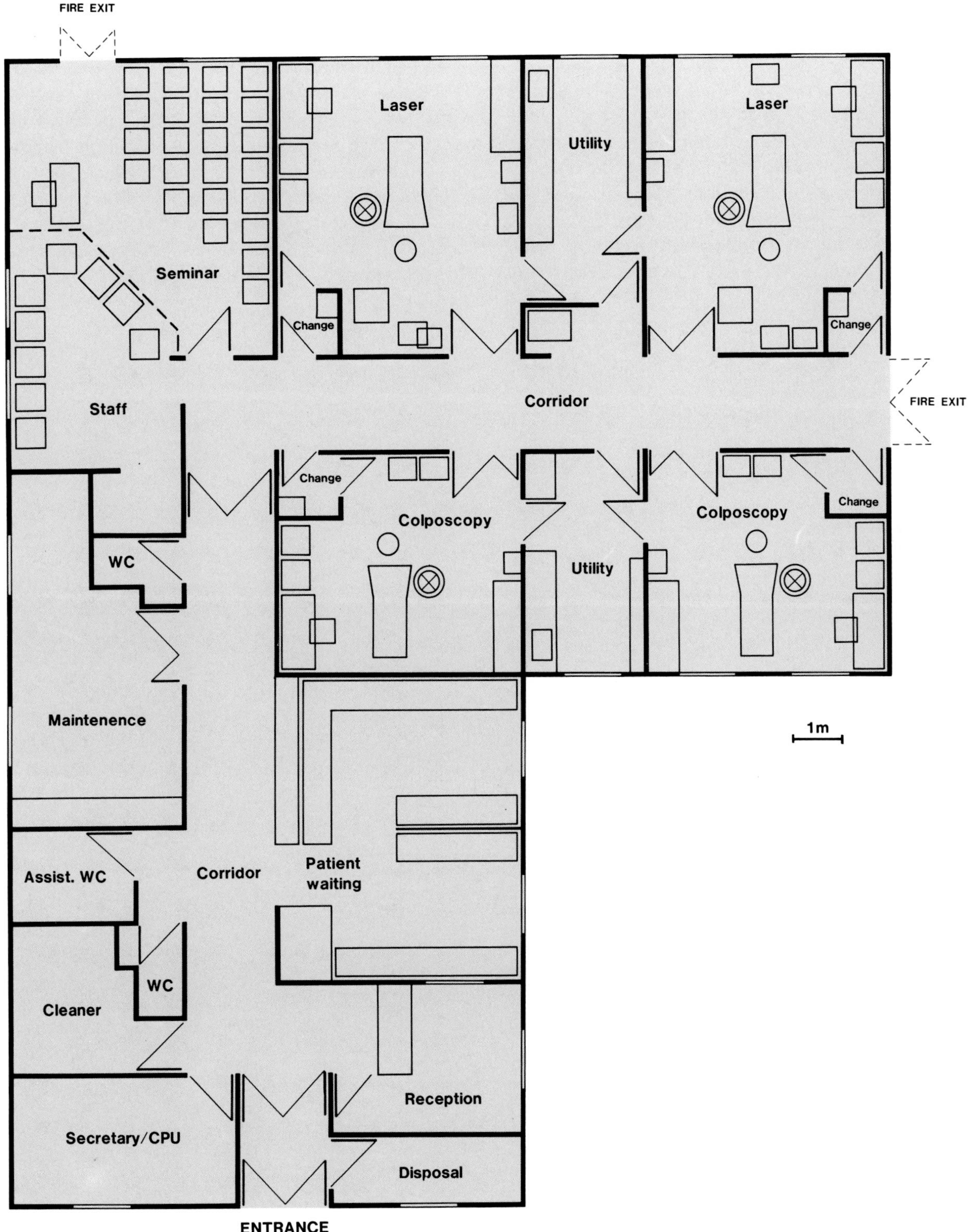

Fig. 22.1 Layout for a large dedicated colposcopy facility, fulfilling diagnostic, treatment and teaching roles. The maintenance room is designated for in-house maintenance of carbon dioxide lasers. Other aspects of the layout are self-explanatory.

ing cubicle. Histories are taken at a desk with a computer terminal consisting of a visual display unit and keyboard linked via a network to the CPU in the secretary's office. Patients details are entered 'real-time'. All four rooms are kitted out for diagnostic colposcopy and biopsy, but two are larger to accommodate the additional equipment for laser surgery.

Each room has a video television option, with the monitor in sight of the patient. This is a useful arrangement for explaining findings and giving an indication of what the treatment involves. Most women are appreciative of this facility, which has been included primarily as a teaching aid both for colposcopists in training and for the nursing staff.

These examination rooms are paired so as to be served by a small utility room where trolleys are set up, waste disposal units are available and CSSD packs, etc., are stored. At a central point of access in the clinical area there is a resuscitation trolley, for the unlikely event of profound vasovagal or other collapse in a patient receiving attention in the clinic. Minor vasovagal episodes are not uncommon in a busy clinic after punch biopsy or even apparently straightforward diagnostic colposcopy.

23. *Epilogue*

EVOLVING TECHNOLOGY

Histopathology

The histological appearances covered in earlier chapters are based on routinely processed material stained with haematoxylin and eosin. These basic techniques have long been the mainstay of histological diagnosis and are likely to remain so for the foreseeable future. Their use, however, is based on the assumption that the morphological features that are capable of analysis by these methods allow some prediction of the biological potential of the tissue under study. In many areas of histopathology this assumption may be acceptable for practical purposes, but its applicability to some areas of lower genital tract pathology is questionable. This is particularly the case for the prediction of the malignant potential of cervical intraepithelial neoplasia, but is also true for glandular abnormalities and microinvasive carcinoma. There is hope that a reappraisal of the histological grading system for squamous intraepithelial lesions combined with a careful redefining of diagnostic criteria may go some way towards improving the predictive value of conventional histology for this condition. Even so, the accuracy of this method of diagnosis is still likely to fall far short of the ideal that should be attained. Attention is therefore being turned to the use of alternative methods, in an attempt to assess the neoplastic and malignant potential of tissues.

Nucleic acid analyses, using nucleic acid probes, are capable of identifying the sequences that make up a segment of a gene. The gene in question may be of any type, those currently of most interest being of viral origin, oncogenes and anti-oncogenes. A variety of techniques is available for applying the nucleic acid probes to the tissue: solid-support hybridization assays include dot/blot/slot hybridization and their variants, and Southern and Northern hybridization. These methods involve digestion of tissue and therefore destruction of its architecture. *In situ* hybridization allows the nucleic acid probe to be applied to a histological section, so that the distribution of the genomic sequences can be determined. These techniques also allow an attempt at quantitation to be made. An amplification procedure, the polymerase chain reaction (PCR), amplifies specific DNA sequences and may be used when the gene to be detected is only present in single copies per cell, or when the amount of sample DNA to be analysed is very small (see page 45).

At present, the practical applications of these DNA techniques, used either individually or in combination, in cervical pathology include the identification of human papillomavirus and its subtypes within the epithelium, and the recognition and quantitation of various oncogenes.

Immunocytochemistry depends upon a reaction in which antibodies (often monoclonal but sometimes polyclonal) raised against selected antigenic determinants bind to that antigen. The site of binding is indicated by a colour change (a peroxidase–antiperoxidase reaction is usually employed, resulting in a brown colour), so that the distribution of the antigen in the tissue can be determined. The reaction is also often considered to be capable of some degree of quantitation. A very wide variety of antigens can be identified with immunocytochemistry such as intermediate filaments (cytokeratins, desmin, vimentin, etc.), growth factor receptors and oncogene protein products.

Finally, mention must be made of flow cytometry, the main application of which has been in cell ploidy analysis. The analysis is carried out on disaggregated tissue and so the origin of the nuclei measured is not always certain. Slide-based image processing technology may well replace flow cytometric instruments for DNA ploidy analysis, because of the increased ability of the operator to control and monitor the process, including selection of the cells for measurement. Flow cytometry may also be used for measuring monoclonal antibody uptake of cells.

This account lists only some of the new techniques which are currently being investigated. The majority of the information available is too preliminary to justify the inclusion of any of these methods in the diagnostic or prognostic evaluation of a particular patient's lesion, and much more investigation is required to ascertain which markers, genetic and otherwise, will be useful in this clinical field. Because these techniques are able to identify an ever-increasing variety of cellular characteristics, which are quite distinct from those recognized by conventional methods, it is hoped that eventually a marker or, more probably, a series of markers, such as nucleic acid sequences or cell surface receptors, will be identified which will allow an accurate assessment of neoplastic state and malignant potential.

Cytology

The DNA hybridization and immunocytochemistry techniques outlined above have already led to great advances in cytology, both in routine diagnosis and research, although at the moment they are used to the greatest benefit in non-gynaecological areas. Many of these techniques are at least as applicable to cytology as to histopathology, and their use results in an even greater blurring of the artificial distinction between the disciplines.

Automated screening offers the greatest potential for radical change in gynaecological cytology. However, despite the immense sums that have been spent over many years of development, the cell counter and flow cytometry methods have still not achieved acceptable levels of reliability or cost effectiveness for widespread use in routine laboratories. Currently, the greatest promise for automated screening lies with imaging techniques. Early attempts were disappointing, but the most recent advances in computer technology, with the emergence of neural network systems, have led to the development of small, mobile prototype systems that could be readily sited in all cytology departments, even the smallest, at a cost of only a few pounds per smear examined.

Neurocomputer imaging systems carry many advantages. The cervical smear is taken and prepared in the standard way, without the need for the special processing that other experimental automated systems have required. The computer automatically analyses a large number of images taken from the slide, and the slide itself is then available for subsequent review by conventional light microscopy, thus eliminating the need for immediate recall of the patient. Furthermore, the images of cells analysed by the computer are presented to the observer in exactly the same way as they appear in the cervical smear, so that minimal additional training is necessary.

The ever-increasing problems of providing and maintaining adequate numbers of trained staff in cytology departments make the idea of developing automated screening systems that are able to identify safely the majority of truly negative cervical smears, more attractive than ever. The neural network automatic computerized imaging system is the most exciting development to date, and has the potential to achieve this aim.

Other screening methods

Many studies are in progress to evaluate the place of HPV DNA typing in screening for CIN, both in conjunction with cytology and as a free-standing test. The development of semi-automated, semi-quantitative PCR testing has enabled relatively large numbers of tests to be performed quite cheaply. Preliminary results show that the identification of high levels of HPV 16 DNA in cervical scrape material correlates closely with the presence of CIN 2 and 3, as demonstrated by the histology of colposcopically directed biopsies. HPV testing was found in one study to be more specific and more sensitive than a cytological diagnosis of moderate dyskaryosis for identifying high-grade disease. Furthermore, HPV-DNA typing and quantitation of material from the cervices of women with mild dyskaryosis has been shown to allow the identification of the subgroup of the women in that category who are harbouring high-grade disease. It remains to be seen whether HPV-DNA typing will eventually replace cytology as the best screening method for the precursors of cervical cancer; at the moment it appears that a combination of the two tests may well turn out to be better than either alone.

A totally different and novel approach to the detection of precancer and cancer of the cervix is the Polarprobe (Coppleson *et al.*, 1994), which is an electronic instrument. A pen-sized probe tip moves systematically across the cervix, stimulating the tissue with one minor electrical pulse and two optical pulses. The response of the tissue to these pulses is picked up by the probe, which is connected to a computer that interprets them with reference to 14 tissue types determined previously by mathematical modelling. Preliminary results using this equipment show a concordance with colposcopy and histology of 85% with low-grade lesions, 90% with high-grade lesions and as much as 99% with invasive cancer. These findings are very encouraging and the results of large independent trials are awaited.

GUIDELINES FOR TRAINING IN COLPOSCOPY

Most authorities accept that colposcopy training can be broken down into two categories, basic and advanced colposcopy, but there is still some disagreement as to when a colposcopist passes from one grade to the next.

Basic colposcopy implies an understanding of the principles of colposcopy and problems which the colposcopist will be asked to assess. It also implies a knowledge of the various treatment options that are available if treatment proves necessary. Ideally, all trainee gynaecologists should receive training in basic colposcopy, in the same way that they are trained in ultrasound scanning, laparoscopy, etc. Many of them will never have to use it, but at least they would have knowledge of it and of its potential.

This form of training will be of an ongoing nature and usually taught on a one-to-one basis. On the other hand, throughout the world there are many specialist gynaecologists with no knowledge of colposcopy, who wish to learn about it. The subject cannot be learned from a book, and the recommended introduction to colposcopy is to attend a two-day theoretical course of instruction, followed by a course of practical work with a tutor.

Both may be extremely difficult in some parts of the world, but nevertheless colposcopy should not be practised unless there has been an opportunity to spend some time with an experienced colposcopist. The aim of basic colposcopy is to demonstrate what the colposcopist looks at and what should be done once the diagnosis has been made. The basic colposcopist should be very wary of relying on destructive methods of treatment, in case unsuspected invasive carcinoma is missed, and should therefore use colposcopy as a guide to planning excisional methods of treatment.

On the other hand, advanced colposcopy cannot be taught simply, quickly or easily. It requires many months of intensive training in a unit that receives many hundreds or even thousands of cases per year. This will allow the student not only to recognize the basic colposcopic patterns, but also to become skilled in the management of lower genital tract premalignancy. The advanced colposcopist also needs to recognize lesions that are not intraepithelial neoplasia, such as immature metaplasia, congenital transformation zone, human papillomavirus infection, changes due to simple atrophy, and changes due to radiotherapy.

All of these can confuse even the most experienced colposcopist, and it is important that lesions are recognized for what they are, rather than committing a patient to a course of surgical treatment that may turn out to be totally unnecessary.

Unfortunately, such training is time consuming and may not be widely available; therefore, the limitations of basic colposcopy need to be clearly defined so that a colposcopist with no more than basic training is not tempted to embark on treatment regimens that are beyond his or her capabilities.

At whatever level colposcopy is to be practised, some knowledge of cytology and histopathology is essential, together with a good working relationship between those specializing in the three disciplines.

As regards the question of who should be trained in colposcopy, traditionally, only gynaecologists have practised it, but clinical gynaecological training is not mandatory. Pathologists interested in the cervix can make excellent colposcopists. In some parts of the world, nurses have been trained to perform basic colposcopy, particularly in countries where there are not enough doctors, or the patients cannot afford the fee of a medically trained colposcopist. There is no reason why a nurse should not be trained in basic colposcopy, and this can be compared with the question: 'Who should deliver babies, midwives or obstetricians?' Throughout the world, midwives carry a great responsibility, but only after a period of very intensive training.

Similarly, in the UK, some colposcopists are general practitioners with no specialist training in gynaecology, but who nevertheless have been trained in the rudiments of colposcopy and do an excellent job: not only does this training provide colposcopists, but it also allows highly trained gynaecologists to be free for other clinical duties.

Colposcopy cannot be learned from a book or by attending a two-day course. It is the responsibility of colposcopy societies in different countries to provide training in their own territories. Members of each national society should have the opportunity to meet on an annual basis and discuss current problems and techniques. The formation of the International Federation of Cervical Pathology and Colposcopy in 1972 made it possible to meet at an international level every third year. Meetings such as these teach us that training is never complete, and new techniques, new drugs and new principles evolve year after year.

Bibliography

General

ANDERSON, M.C. (1991) Female reproductive system, in *Systemic Pathology*, 3rd edn, Vol. 6 (ed. W.St C. Symmers), Churchill Livingstone, Edinburgh.

BURGHARDT, E. (1991) *Colposcopy, Cervical Pathology, Textbook and Atlas*, 2nd edn, George Thième Verlag, Stuttgart.

CARTIER, R. (1984) *Practical Colposcopy*, Laboratoire Cartier, Paris.

COPPLESON, M. (ed.) (1992) Gynaecological Oncology, 2nd edn, Churchill Livingstone, Edinburgh.

COPPLESON, M. and REID, B. (1967) *Pre-Clinical Carcinoma of the Cervix Uteri; Its Origin, Nature and Management*, Pergamon, Oxford.

FLUHMANN, C.F. (1961) *The Cervix Uteri and its Diseases*, W.B. Saunders, Philadelphia.

JORDAN, J.A. and SINGER, A. (eds) (1976) *The Cervix*, W.B. Saunders, Philadelphia.

KOSS, L.G. (1992) *Diagnostic Cytology and its Histopathologic Bases*, 4th edn, Lippincott, Philadelphia.

Chapter 1

ANDERSON, M.C. (1991) The cervix, excluding cancer, in *Female Reproductive System* (ed. M.C. Anderson), Vol. 6 of *Systemic Pathology*, 3rd edn, (ed. W.St C. Symmers), Churchill Livingstone, Edinburgh, pp. 47–65.

KOSS, L.G. (1992) Effects of therapeutic procedures and drugs on epithelia of the female genital tract, in *Diagnostic Cytology and its Histopathologic Bases*, 4th edn, Vol. 1, (ed. L.G. Koss), Lippincott, Philadelphia, pp. 251–94.

Chapter 2

ABDUL-KARIM, F., FU, Y., REAGAN, W. and WENTZ, W. (1982) Morphometric study of intraepithelial neoplasia of the cervix. *Obstetrics and Gynecology*, **60**, 210.

AL-NAFUSSI, A.I., COLQUHOUN, M.K. and WILLIAMS, A.R.W. (1993) Accuracy of cervical smears in predicting the grades of cervical intraepithelial neoplasia. *International Journal of Gynecologic Cancer*, **3**, 89.

ANDERSON, M.C. (1987) Premalignant and malignant disease of the cervix, in *Haines and Taylor: Obstetrical and Gynaecological Pathology* (ed. H. Fox), Churchill Livingstone, Edinburgh, pp. 255–301.

ANDERSON, M.C. (1991) Cervical precancer, in *Female Reproductive System* (ed. M.C. Anderson), Vol. 6 of *Systemic Pathology*, 3rd edn (ed. W.St C. Symmers), Churchill Livingstone, Edinburgh, pp. 92–7.

ANDERSON, M. and HARTLEY, R. (1980) Cervical crypt involvement by intraepithelial neoplasia. *Obstetrics and Gynecology*, **55**, 546.

ANDERSON, M.C., BROWN, C.L., BUCKLEY, C.H. *et al.* (1991) Current views on cervical intraepithelial neoplasia. *Journal of Clinical Pathology*, **44**, 969–78.

BARTON, S., JENKINS, D., HOLLINGSWORTH, A. and SINGER, A. (1989) An explanation for the problems of the false negative cervical smear. *British Journal of Obstetrics and Gynaecology*, **96**, 492.

BOON, M.E., ALONS-VAN-CORDELAAR, J.J.M. and RIETVELD-SCHEFFERS, P.E.M. (1986) Consequences of the introduction of combined spatula and Cytobrush sampling for cervical cytology. Improvements in smear quality and detection rates. *Acta Cytologica*, **30**, 264.

BUCKLEY, C.H., BUTLER, E.B. and FOX, H. (1982) Cervical intraepithelial neoplasia. *Journal of Clinical Pathology*, **35**, 1–13

CUZICK, J., TERRY, G., HO, L., HOLLINGSWORTH, T. and ANDERSON, M. (1992) Human papillomavirus type 16 DNA in cervical smears as a predictor of high grade intraepithelial neoplasia. *Lancet*, **339**, 959.

EVANS, D.M.D., HUDSON, E.A., BROWN, C.L. *et al.* (1986) Terminolgy in gynaecological cytopathology: report of working party of the British Society for Clinical Cytology. *Journal of Clinical Pathology*, **39**, 933–44.

EVANS, D.M.D., HUDSON, E.A., BROWN, C.L. *et al.* (1987) Management of women with abdominal cervical smears: supplement to terminology in gynaecological cytopathology. *Journal of Clinical Pathology*, **40**, 530–1.

GILES, J.A., HUDSON, E. and WALKER, P. (1988) Colposcopic assessment of the accuracy of cervical cytological screening. *British Medical Journal*, **296**, 1099.

JARMULOWICZ, M., JENKINS, D., BARTON, S.E. and SINGER, A. (1989) Cytological status and lesion size: a further dimension in cervical intraepithelial neoplasia. *British Journal of Obstetrics and Gynaecology*, **96**, 1061.

KOSS, L.G. (1992) Epidermoid carcinoma of the uterine cervix and related precancerous lesions. Part II: Cytologic diagnosis and its consequences, in *Diagnostic Cytology and its Histopathologic Bases*, 4th edn, Vol. 1, Lippincott, Philadelphia, pp. 424–512.

LUFF, R., KURMAN, R. and SOLOMON, D. (1992) The Bethesda system for reporting cervical vaginal cytologic diagnoses – report of the 1991 Bethesda workshop. *American Journal of Surgical Pathology*, **16**, 914–16.

National Cancer Institute Workshop: The 1988 Bethesda System for reporting cervical/vaginal cytological diagnoses (1989) *Journal of the American Medical Association*, **262**, 931–4.

National Health Service Cervical Screening Programme (1992) *Guidelines for Clinical Practice and Programme Management* (ed. I.D. Duncan), National Co-ordinating Network, Oxford.

RICHART, R.M. (1990) A modified terminology for cervical intraepithelial neoplasia. *Obstetrics and*

Gynecology, **75**, 131–3.

The Bethesda System for Reporting Cervical/Vaginal Cytological Diagnoses (1993) *Acta Cytologica*, **73**, 115–24.

Wolfendale, M.R., Howe-Guest, R., Usherwood, M.M. and Drape, G.J. (1987) Controlled trial of a new cervical spatula. *British Medical Journal*, **294**, 33.

Chapter 3

Anderson, M.C. (1991) The natural history of cervical intraepithelial neoplasia. *Current Obstetrics and Gynaecology*, **1**, 124–9.

Brinton, L.A. (1992) Epidemiology of cervical cancer – overview, in *The Epidemiology of Cervical Cancer and Human Papillomavirus* (eds N. Munoz, F.X. Bocsh, K.V. Shah and A. Meheus), International Agency for Research on Cancer, Lyons, pp. 3–23.

Farthing, A., Masterson, P., Mason, W.P. *et al.* (1994) Human papillomavirus detection by hybrid capture and its possible clinical use. *Journal of Clinical Pathology*, **47**, 649–52.

Lane, S. and Wells, M. (1994) Human papillomaviruses, p53, and cervical neoplasia. *Journal of Pathology*, **172**, 299–300.

Parazzini, F., La Vecchia, C., Negri, E. *et al.* (1992) Risk factors for cervical intraepithelial neoplasia. *Cancer*, **69**, 2276–82.

Schiffman, M.H., Bauer, H.M., Hoover, R.N. *et al.* (1993) Epidemiologic evidence showing that human papillomavirus infection causes most cervical intraepithelial neoplasia. *Journal of the National Cancer Institute*, **85**, 958–64.

Chapter 4

Simons, A.M., Phillips, D.H. and Coleman, D.V. (1993) Damage to DNA in cervical epithelium related to smoking tobacco. *British Medical Journal*, **306**, 1444–8.

Soutter, W.P., Wisdom, S., Brough, A.K. and Monaghan, J.M. (1986) Should patients with mild atypia in a cervical smear be referred for colposcopy? *British Journal of Obstetrics and Gynaecology*, **93**, 70.

Walker, E.M., Dodgson, J. and Duncan, I.D. (1986) Does mild atypia on a cervical smear warrant further investigation? *Lancet*, **2**, 672.

Chapter 6

Brown, J., Campion, M., Cuzick, J. and Singer, A. (1988) Psychosexual trauma of an abnormal smear. *British Journal of Obstetrics and Gynaecology*, **95**, 175.

Chapter 7

Coppleson, M., Pixley, E. and Reid, B. (1986) *Colposcopy*, 3rd edn, Charles C. Thomas, Springfield.

Kolstad, P. and Stafl, A. (1982) *Atlas of Colposcopy*, 3rd edn, Churchill Livingstone, Edinburgh.

Maddox, P., Szarewski, A., Dyson, J. and Cuzick, J. (1994) Cytokeratin expression and acetowhite change in cervical epithelium. *Journal of Clinical Pathology*, **47**, 15–17.

Schiller, J. (1929) Jodpinselung und Abschabung des Portioepithels. *Zentralblatt für Gynakologie*, **53**, 1056.

Chapter 8

Kolstad, P. (1965) The development of the vascular bed in tumours, as seen in squamous cell carcinoma of the cervix uteri. *British Journal of Radiology*, **38**, 216.

Shafi, M.I., Finn, C.B. and Luesley, D.M. (1991) Lesion size and histology of atypical cervical transformation zone. *British Journal of Obstetrics and Gynaecology*, **98**, 490.

Shafi, M.I., Dunn, J., Finn, C.B., Kettoe, S., Buxton, E. and Jordan, J. (1993) Characterization of high and low grade intraepithelial neoplasia. *International Journal of Gynecologic Cancer*, **3**, 203.

Chapter 10

Anderson, M.C. (1987) Premalignant and malignant disease of the cervix, in *Haines and Taylor: Obstetrical and Gynaecological Pathology* (ed. H. Fox), Churchill Livingstone, Edinburgh, pp. 274–7.

Benedet, J.L., Anderson, G.H. and Boyes, D.A. (1985) Colposcopic accuracy in the diagnosis of microinvasive and occult invasive carcinoma of the cervix. *Obstetrics and Gynecology*, **65**, 557.

Burghardt, E., Girardi, F., Lahousen, M. *et al.* (1991) Microinvasive carcinoma of the uterine cervix (International Federation of Gynecology and Obstetrics Stage Ia). *Cancer*, **67**, 1037–45.

Burghardt, E., Girardi, F., Lahousen, M., Pickel, H. and Tamussino, K. (1991) Microinvasive carcinoma of the uterine cervix (International Federation of Gynaecology and Obstetrics stage Ia). *Cancer*, **67**, 1037.

Creasman, W.T., Fetter, B.F., Clarke-Pearson, D.L., Kaufmann, L. and Parker, R.T. (1985) Management of stage 1a carcinoma of the cervix. *American Journal of Obstetrics and Gynecology*, **153**, 164.

Kolstad, P. (1989) Follow-up study of 232 patients with stage Ia1 and 411 patients with stage Ia2 squamous cell carcinoma of the cervix (microinvasive carcinoma cervix). *Gynecologic Oncology*, **33**, 265

KOSS, L.G. (1992) Epidermoid carcinoma of the uterine cervix and related precancerous lesions. Part II: Cytologic diagnosis and its consequences, in *Diagnostic Cytology and its Histopathologic Bases*, 4th edn, Vol. 1, Lippincott, Philadelphia, pp. 424–512.

MORGAN, P.R., ANDERSON, M., BUCKLEY, H. *et al.* (1993) Royal College of Obstetrics and Gynaecology microinvasive carcinoma of the cervix study. *British Journal of Obstetrics and Gynaecology*, **100**, 664.

TIDBURY, P., SINGER, A. and JENKINS, D. (1992) CIN Ill: the role of lesion size in invasion. *British Journal of Obstetrics and Gynaecology*, **99**, 583.

TWEEDDALE, D.N., LANGENBACH, S.R., RODDRICK, J.K. *et al.* (1969) The cytopathology of microinvasive squamous cancer of the cervix uteri. *Acta Cytologica*, 13, 447–54.

Chapter 11

ANDERSON, M.C. (1991) Invasive carcinoma of the cervix, in *Female Reproductive System* (ed. M.C. Anderson), Vol. 6 of *Systemic Pathology*, 3rd edn, (ed. W.St C. Symmers), Churchill Livingstone, Edinburgh, pp. 105–28.

AYER, B., PACEY, F., GREENBERG, M. and BOUSFIELD, L. (1987) The cytological diagnosis of adenocarcinoma *in situ*. *Acta Cytologica*, **31**, 397–411.

AYER, B., PACEY, F., GREENBERG, M. and BOUSFIELD, L. (1987) The cytologic diagnosis of adenocarcinoma *in situ* of the cervix uteri and related lesions. 1. Adenocarcinoma *in situ*. *Acta Cytologica*, **31**, 397.

BERTRAND, M., LICKRISH, G.M. and COLGAN, T.J. (1987) The anatomic distribution of cervical adenocarcinoma *in situ*: implications for treatment. *American Journal of Obstetrics and Gynecology*, **157**, 21.

BETSILL, W.L. and CLARK, A.H. (1985) Early endocervical glandular neoplasia. 1. Histomorphology and cytomorphology. *Acta Cytologica*, **30**, 115.

BOON, M.E., DE GRAAFF GUILLOD, J.C., KOK, L.P., OLTHOF, P.N. and VAN ERP, E.J. (1987) Efficacy of screening of cervical squamous and adenocarcinoma. The Dutch experience. *Cancer*, **8**, 62.

BROWN, L.J.R. and WELLS, M. (1986) Cervical glandular atypia associated with squamous intraepithelial neoplasia – a premalignant lesion? *Journal of Clinical Pathology*, **39**, 22.

HITCHCOCK, A., JOHNSON, J., MCDOWELL, K. and JOHNSON, I.R. (1993) A retrospective study of the occurrence of cervical glandular atypia in cone biopsy specimens. *International Journal of Gynecologic Cancer*, **3**, 164.

KOSS, L.G. (1992) Adenocarcinoma and related tumours of the uterine cervix, in *Diagnostic Cytology and its Histopathologic Bases*, 4th edn, Vol. 1, Lippincott, Philadelphia, pp. 513–34.

LAVERTY, C.R., FARNSWORTH, A., THURLOE, J. and BOWDITCH, R. (1988) The reliability of a cytological prediction of cervical adenocarcinoma *in situ*. *Australia and New Zealand Journal of Obstetrics and Gynaecology*, **28**, 307.

LUESLEY, D.M., JORDAN, J.A., WOODMAN, C.B., WATSON, N. and WILLIAMS, D.R. (1987) A retrospective review of adenocarcinoma *in situ* and glandular atypia of the uterine cervix. *British Journal of Obstetrics and Gynaecology*, **94**, 699.

OSTOR, A.G., PAGANO, R., DAVOREN, R.A.M. *et al.* (1984) Adenocarcinoma *in situ* of the cervix. *International Journal of Gynecologic Pathology*, **3**, 179.

PACEY, F., AYER, B. and GREENBERG, M. (1988) The cytological diagnosis of adenocarcinoma in situ of the cervix uteri and related lesions III. Pitfalls in diagnosis. *Acta Cytologica*, **32**, 325–30.

PETERS, K., CHAO, A., MACK, T.M. *et al.* (1986) Increased frequency of adenocarcinoma of the uterine cervix in young women in Los Angeles county. *Journal of the National Cancer Institute*, **76**, 423.

WELLS, M. and BROWN, L.J. (1986) Glandular lesions of the uterine cervix: the present state of our knowledge. *Histopathology*, **10**, 777.

Chapter 12

BIBBO, M., KEEBLER, C.M. and WIED, G.L. (1971) The cytologic diagnosis of tissue repair in the female genital tract. *Acta Cytologica*, **15**, 133–7.

BLOCH, B., DEHAECK, K. and SOETERS, R. (eds) (1995) *Manual of Practical Gynecological Oncology*, Chapman & Hall Medical, London.

BUCKLEY, C.H., HERBERT, A., MACKENZIE, E.F.D. et al. (1994) Borderline nuclear changes in cervical smears: quicklines on their recognition and management. *Journal of Clinical Pathology*, **47**, 481–92.

GUPTA, P.K. (1982) Intrauterine contraceptive devices. Vaginal cytology, pathologic changes and clinical implications. *Acta Cytologica*, **26**, 571–613.

KOSS, L.G. (1992) Part I: Inflammatory processes; Part II: Other benign disorders of the cervix and vagina, in *Diagnostic Cytology and its Histopathologic Bases*, 4th edn, Vol. 1, Lippincott, Philadelphia, pp. 314–70.

KOSS, L.G. (1992) Effects of therapeutic procedures and drugs on epithelia of the female genital tract. *Diagnostic Cytology and its Histopathologic Bases*, 4th edn, Vol. 1, Lippincott, Philadelphia, pp. 251–94.

KOSS, L.G. (1992) Effects of therapeutic procedures and drugs on epithelia of the female genital tract. *Diagnostic Cytology and its Histopathologic Bases*, 4th edn, Vol. 1, Lippincott, Philadelphia, pp. 663–6.

KYRIAKOS, M., KEMPSON, R.L. and KONIKOR, N.F. (1968) A clinical and pathologic study of endocervical lesions associated with oral contraceptives. *Cancer*, **22**, 99–100.

McLennan, M.T. and McLennan, C.E. (1975) Significance of cervicovaginal cytology after radiation therapy for cervical carcinoma. *American Journal of Obstetrics and Gynecology*, **121**, 96–100.

Meisels, A. and Fortin, R. (1976) Condylomatous lesions of the cervix and vagina. I. Cytological patterns. *Acta Cytologica*, **20**, 505–9.

Mitchell, H. and Medley, G. (1989) Evidence against diathermy as a beneficial treatment for human papillomavirus infection of the cervix. *Australia and New Zealand Journal of Obstetrics and Gynaecology*, **29**(4), 439.

Rome, R., Chanen, W. and Pagano, R. (1987) The natural history of human papillomavirus (HPV) atypia of the cervix. *Australia and New Zealand Journal of Obstetrics and Gynaecology*, **27**, 287.

Chapter 13

Ali, S.W., Evans, A.S. and Monaghan, J.M. (1986) Results of CO_2 laser cylinder vaporisation of CIN in 1234 patients. An analysis of failures. *British Journal of Obstetrics and Gynaecology*, **93**, 75.

Anderson, D.J.M., Strachan, F. and Parkin, D.E. (1992) Cone biopsy: has endocervical sampling a role? *British Journal of Obstetrics and Gynaecology*, **99**, 668.

Anderson, M.C. (1982) Treatment of cervical intraepithelial neoplasia with carbon dioxide laser: a report of 543 patients. *Obstetrics and Gynecology*, **59**, 720.

Anderson, S.E., Thorup, K. and Larsen, G. (1988) Results of cryosurgery for cervical intraepithelial neoplasia. *Gynecologic Oncology*, **30**, 21.

Benedet, J.L., Miller, D.M. and Nickerson, K.G. (1992) Results of conservative management of cervical intraepithelial neoplasia. *Obstetrics and Gynecology*, **79(1)**, 105.

Bigrigg, A., Haffenden, D.K., Sheehan, A.L., Codling, B.W. and Read, M.D. (1994) Efficacy and safety of large-loop excision of the transformation zone. *Lancet*, **343**, 32.

Buxton, E.J., Luesley, D.M., Shafi, M.I. and Rollason, M. (1991) Colposcopically directed punch biopsy; a potentially misleading investigation. *British Journal of Obstetrics and Gynaecology*, **98(12)**, 1273.

Chanen, W. (1989) The efficacy of electrocoagulation diathermy performed under local anaesthesia for the eradication of precancerous lesions of the cervix. *Australia and New Zealand Journal of Obstetrics and Gynaecology*, **29**, 189.

Chanen, W. and Rome, R. (1983) Electrocoagulation diathermy for cervical dysplasia and carcinoma *in situ*; a fifteen-year survey. *Obstetrics and Gynecology*, **61**, 673.

Creasman, W.T., Hinshaw, W.N. and Clarke-Pearson, D.L. (1984) Cryosurgery in the management of cervical intraepithelial neoplasia. *Obstetrics and Gynecology*, **63**, 145.

de Cristofana, D., Fontana, P. and Pezzoli, C. (1988) Pathological study of the cervix after cold coagulation. *American Journal of Obstetrics and Gynecology*, **159**(5), 1053.

Giles, J.A, Walker, P.C. and Chalk, P.A. (1987) The treatment of CIN by radical electrocoagulation diathermy: five years' experience. *British Journal of Obstetrics and Gynaecology*, **94**, 1089.

Goodman, J. and Sumner, D. (1991) Patient acceptability of laser and cold coagulation for premalignant cervical cancer. *British Journal of Obstetrics and Gynaecology*, **98(11)**, 1168.

Gordon, H.K. and Duncan, I.D. (1991) Effective destruction of cervical intraepithelial neoplasia (CIN III) at 100°C using the Semm cold coagulator: 14 years' experience. *British Journal of Obstetrics and Gynaecology*, **98**(1), 14.

Hamou, J. (1991) *Hysteroscopy and Microcolpohysteroscopy – Text and Atlas*, Appleton and Lange, Norwalk, California.

Jones, J.M., Sweetman, P. and Hibbard, B.N. (1979) The outcome of pregnancy after cone biopsy of the cervix: a case control study. *British Journal of Obstetrics and Gynaecology*, **86**, 813.

Loobuyck, H.A. and Duncan, I. (1993) Destruction of CIN 1 and 2 with the SEMM cold coagulator: 13 years' experience. *British Journal of Obstetrics and Gynaecology*, **100**(5), 465.

Lopez, A., Pearson, S., Mo, R. *et al.* (1989) Is it time for a reconsideration of the criteria for cone biopsy? *British Journal of Obstetrics and Gynaecology*, **96**, 1345–7.

Luesley, D.M., Cullimore, J., Redman, C.W. and Laughton, F.G. (1990) Loop diathermy excision of a cervical transformation zone in patients with abnormal cervical cytology. *British Medical Journal*, **300**, 1690.

McIndoe, A., Robson, M., Tidy, J., Mason, P. and Anderson, M.C. (1989) Laser excision rather than vaporization: the treatment of choice for cervical intraepithelial neoplasia. *Obstetrics and Gynecology*, **74**, 165.

Monaghan, J.M., Kirkup, W., Davis, J.A. and Edington, P. (1982) Treatment of cervical intraepithelial neoplasia by colposcopically directed cryosurgery and subsequent pregnancy experience. *British Journal of Obstetrics and Gynaecology*, **89**, 387.

Murdoch, J.B., Crimshaw, R.N., Morgan, P.R. and Monaghan, J.M. (1992) The impact of loop diathermy on management of early invasive cervical cancer. *International Journal of Gynecologic Cancer*, **2**, 129.

Murdoch, J.B., Morgan, P., Lopes, A. and Monaghan, J.M. (1992) Histological incomplete excision of CIN after large loop excision of the transformation zone (LLETZ) merits careful follow-up, not retreatment. *British Journal of Obstetrics and Gynaecology*, **99**(12), 990.

Paraskevaidis, E., Jandial, L., Mann, E. M., Fisher,

P.M. and KITCHENER, H.C. (1991) Patterns of treatment failure following laser for cervical intraepithelial neoplasia; implication for follow-up of protocol. *Obstetrics and Gynecology*, **78**(1), 80.

PARTINGTON, C., TURNER, M., SOUTTER, P. and GRIFFITHS, M. (1989) Laser vaporization versus laser excision conisation in the treatment of cervical intraepithelial neoplasia. *Obstetrics and Gynecology*, **73**, 775.

PRENDIVILLE, W., CULLIMORE, J. and NORMAN, S. (1989) Large loop excision of the transformation zone (LLETZ). A new method of management for women with cervical intraepithelial neoplasia. *British Journal of Obstetrics and Gynaecology*, **96**, 1054.

SHAFI, M.I., DUNN, J.A., BUXTON, E.J. *et al.* (1993) Abnormal cervical cytology following large loop excision of the transformation zone: a case controlled study. *British Journal of Obstetrics and Gynaecology*, **100**, 145.

SOUTTER, W.P., FENTON, D., GUDGEON, P. and SHARP, F. (1984) Quantitative microcolpohysteroscopic assessment of the extent of endocervical involvement by cervical intraepithelial neoplasia. *British Journal of Obstetrics and Gynaecology*, **91**, 712.

SZE, E., ROSENZWEIG, B., BIRENBAUM, D. *et al.* (1989) Excisional conisation of the cervix-uteri. *Journal of Gynecologic Surgery*, **5**, 325.

TABOR, A. and BERGET, A. (1990) Cold knife and laser conisation for cervical intraepithelial neoplasia. *Obstetrics and Gynecology*, **76**(4), 622.

TOWNSEND, D.E. and RICHART, R.M. (1983) Cryotherapy and carbon dioxide laser management of cervical intraepithelial neoplasia; a controlled comparison. *Obstetrics and Gynecology*, **61**, 75.

TURNER, M.J., RASMUSSEN, M.J.I., FLANNELLY, C.M., MURPHY, J.F. and LENEHAN, P.M. (1992) Outpatients' loop diathermy conisation as an alternative to inpatient knife conisation of the cervix. *Journal of Reproductive Medicine*, **37**, 314.

VERGOTE, I.B., MAKARE, A.P. and KJORSTAD, K.E. (1992) Laser excision of the transformation zone as treatment of cervical intraepithelial neoplasia with satisfactory colposcopy. *Gynecologic Oncology*, **44**(3), 235.

VOLANTE, R., PASERO, L. and SARACENO, L. (1992) Carbon dioxide laser surgery with colposcopy for cervico-vaginal intraepithelial neoplasia treatment: ten years' experience and failure analysis. *European Journal of Gynecologic Oncology*, **13**(Suppl. 1), 78.

WOODMAN, C.B., JORDAN, J.A., MYLOTTE, M.J., GUSTAFESON, R. and WADE-EVANS, T. (1985) The management of cervical intraepithelial neoplasia by coagulation electrodiathermy. *British Journal of Obstetrics and Gynaecology*, **92**, 751.

WRIGHT, V.C., GAGNON, S., RICHART, R.M. and FERENCZY, A. (1992) Treatment of cervical intraepithelial neoplasia using the loop electrosurgical excision procedure. *Obstetrics and Gynecology*, **79**(2), 173.

WRIGHT, V.C., RICHART, R.M., FERENCZY, A. and KOULOS, J. (1992) Comparison of specimens removed by CO_2 laser conisation and the loop electrosurgical excision procedure. *Obstetrics and Gynecology*, **79**(1), 1471.

Chapter 14

ANDERSON, M.C. (1993) Invasive carcinoma of the cervix following local destructive treatment for cervical intraepithelial neoplasia. *British Journal of Obstetrics and Gynaecology*, **100**, 657–63.

HUGHES, R.G., HADDAD, N.G., SMART, C.E. *et al.* (1992) The cytological detection of persistent CIN after local ablative treatment: a comparison of sampling devices. *British Journal of Obstetrics and Gynaecology*, **99**(6), 498.

KOLSTAD, P. and KLEM, V. (1976) Long-term follow-up of 1121 cases of carcinoma-in-situ. *Obstetrics and Gynecology*, **48**, 125.

LOPES, A., MOR-YOSEF, S., PEARSON, S., IRELAND, D. and MONAGHAN, J. (1990) Is routine colposcopic assessment necessary following laser ablation of cervical intraepithelial neoplasia. *British Journal of Obstetrics and Gynaecology*, **97**, 175.

PEARSON, S.E., WHITTAKER, J., IRELAND, D. and MONAGHAN, J.M. (1989) Invasive cancer of the cervix after laser treatment. *British Journal of Obstetrics and Gynaecology*, **96**, 486.

SEVIN, B., FORD, J.H., CIRTANNER, R.D. *et al.* (1979) Invasive cancer of the cervix after cryosurgery. Pitfalls of conservative management. *Obstetrics and Gynecology*, **53**, 465.

Chapter 15

KOSS, L.G. (1992) Disease of the vagina and vulva, in *Diagnostic Cytology and its Histopathologic Bases*, 4th edn, Vol. 1, Lippincott, Philadelphia, pp. 588–617.

Chapter 16

ANDERSON, B.L. and HACKER, N.F. (1983) Psychosexual adjustment after vulvar surgery. *Obstetrics and Gynecology*, **62**, 457.

ANDREASSON, B. and BOCK, J.E. (1985) Intraepithelial neoplasia in the vulvar region. *Gynecologic Oncology*, **21**, 300.

BAGGISH, M.S. (1985) Improved laser techniques for the elimination of genital and extragenital warts. *American Journal of Obstetrics and Gynecology*, **153**, 545.

BAGGISH, M.S. and DORSEY, J.H. (1981) CO_2 laser for the treatment of vulvar carcinoma *in situ*. *Obstetrics and Gynecology*, **57**, 371.

BAGGISH, M., SZE, E., ADELSON, M., COHN, G. and OATES, R. (1989) Quantitative evaluation of the skin and accessory appendages in vulvar carcinoma *in situ*. *Obstetrics and Gynecology*, **74**, 169.

BARBERO, M., MICHELETTI, L., PRETI, M. *et al.* (1990) Vulvar intraepithelial neoplasia. A clinicopathologic study of 60 cases. *Journal of Reproductive Medicine*, **35**(11), 1023.

BECKMANN, A.M., KIVIAT, N.B., DALING, J.R., SHERMAN, K.J. and MCDOUGALL, J.K. (1988) Human papillomavirus type 16 in multifocal neoplasia of the female genital tract. *International Journal of Gynecologic Pathology*, **7**, 39.

BENEDET, J.L. and MURPHY, K.G. (1982) Squamous carcinoma *in situ* of the vulva. *Gynecologic Oncology*, **14**, 213.

BENEDET, J.L., WILSON, P.S. and MATISIC, J. (1991) Epidermal thickness and skin appendage involvement in vulvar intraepithelial neoplasia. *Journal of Reproductive Medicine*, **36**(8), 608.

BERGERON, C., NAGHASHFAR, Z., CANAAN, C. *et al.* (1987) Human papillomavirus type 16 in intraepithelial neoplasia (Bowenoid papulosis) and coexistent invasive carcinoma of the vulva. *International Journal of Gynecologic Pathology*, **6**, 1.

BERGERON, C., FERENCZY, A., RICHART, R. and GURALNICK, M. (1990) Micropapillomatosis labialis appears unrelated to human papillomavirus. *Obstetrics and Gynecology*, **76**(2), 281.

BERNSTEIN, S.G., KOVACS, B.R., TOWNSEND, D.E. and MORROW, C.P. (1983) Vulvar carcinoma-in-situ. *Obstetrics and Gynecology*, **61**, 304.

BHAWAN, J. (1980) Multicentric pigmented Bowen's disease. A clinically benign squamous cell carcinoma *in situ*. *Gynecologic Oncology*, **10**, 201.

BOMSTEIN, J. and KAUFMAN, R.H. (1988) Combination of surgical excision and carbon dioxide laser vaporization for multifocal vulvar intraepithelial neoplasia. *American Journal of Obstetrics and Gynecology*, **158**, 459.

BOMSTEIN, J., KAUFMAN, R.H. and ADAM, E. (1988) Multicentric intraepithelial neoplasia involving the vulva. Clinical features and association with human papillomavirus and herpes simplex virus. *Cancer*, **62**(8), 1601.

BORGENO, B., MICHELETTI, L. and BARBERO, M. (1988) Epithelial alterations adjacent to 111 vulvar carcinomas. *Journal of Reproductive Medicine*, **33**(6), 500.

BRESLOW, A. (1970) Thickness, cross-sectional areas and depth of invasion in the prognosis of cutaneous melanoma. *Annals of Surgery*, **172**, 902.

BUCHLER, D.A. (1975) Multiple primaries and gynecologic malignancies. *American Journal of Obstetrics and Gynecology*, **123**, 376.

BUCKLEY, C.H., BUTTLE, E.B. and FOX, H. (1984) Vulvar intraepithelial neoplasia and microinvasive carcinoma of the vulva. *Journal of Clinical Pathology*, **37**, 1201.

BUSCEMA, J., STEM, J. and WOODRUFF, J.D. (1980) The significance of the histological alterations adjacent to invasive vulvar carcinoma. *American Journal of Obstetrics and Gynecology*, **137**, 902.

BUSCEMA, J., WOODRUFF, J.D., PARMLEY, T.H. and GENADRY, R. (1980) Carcinoma *in situ* of the vulva. *Obstetrics and Gynecology*, **5**, 225.

BUSCEMA, J., NAGHASHFAR, Z., SAWADA, E. *et al.* (1988) The predominance of human papillomavirus type 16 in vulval neoplasia. *Obstetrics and Gynecology*, **71**, 601.

CAGLAR, H., TAMER, S. and HRESHCHYSHYN, M.M. (1982) Vulvar intraepithelial neoplasia. *Obstetrics and Gynecology*, **60**, 346.

CAGLAR, H., DELGADO, G. and HRESHCHYSHYN, M.M. (1986) Partial and total skinning vulvectomy in treatment of carcinoma *in situ* of the vulva. *Obstetrics and Gynecology*, **68**, 504.

CHOO, Y.C. and MORLEY, G.W. (1980) Multiple primary neoplasms of the anogenital region. *Obstetrics and Gynecology*, **56**, 365.

COLLINS, C.G., HANSEN, L.H. and THERIOT, E. (1966) A clinical stain for use in selecting biopsy sites in patients with vulvar disease. *Obstetrics and Gynecology*, **28**, 158.

COLLINS, C.G., ROMAN-LOPEZ, J.J. and LEE, F.Y. (1970) Intraepithelial carcinoma of the vulva. *American Journal of Obstetrics and Gynecology*, **108**, 1187.

COX, S.M., KAUFMAN, R.H. and KAPLAN, A. (1986) Recurrent carcinoma in situ of the vulva in a skin graft. *American Journal of Obstetrics and Gynecology*, **155**, 177.

CRUM, C.P., IGAWA, K., FU, Y.S. *et al.* (1982) Intraepithelial squamous lesions of the vulva: biologic and histological criteria for the distinction of condyloma from vulvar intraepithelial neoplasia. *American Journal of Obstetrics and Gynecology*, **144**, 77.

DALING, J.R., SHERMAN, K.J., HISLOP, T.G., MADEN, C. and WEISS, N.S. (1992) Cigarette smoking and risk of anogenital cancer. *American Journal of Epidemiology*, **135**, 180.

DISAIA, P.J. and RICH, W.M. (1981) Surgical approach to multifocal carcinoma *in situ* of the vulva. *American Journal of Obstetrics and Gynecology*, **140**, 136.

DUDZINSKY, M.R. and RADER, J.S. (1990) The mons pubis, an excellent graft donor site in gynecological surgery. *American Journal of Obstetrics and Gynecology*, **162**(3), 722.

FERENCZY, A. (1983) Using the laser to treat vulvar condylomata acuminata and intraepidermal neoplasia. *Journal of the Canadian Medical Association*, **128**, 135.

FIORICA, J.V., CAVANAGH, D., MARSDEN, D. *et al.* (1988) Carcinoma *in situ* of the vulva; 24 years' experience in south west Florida. *Southern Medical Journal*, **81**(5), 589.

FORNEY, J.P., MORROW, C.P., TOWNSEND, D.E. and DISAIA, P.J. (1977) Management of carcinoma *in situ* of the vulva. *American Journal of Obstetrics and Gynecology*, **127**, 801.

FRIEDRICH, E.G. (ed.) (1983) *Vulvar Diseases*, 2nd edn, W.B. Saunders, Philadelphia.

FRIEDRICH, E.G., WILKINSON, E.J. and FU, Y.S. (1980) Carcinoma *in situ* of the vulva: a continuing challenge. *American Journal of Obstetrics and Gynecology*, **136**, 830.

FU, Y.S., REAGAN, J.W., TOWNSEND, D.E. *et al.* (1981) Nuclear DNA study of vulvar intraepithelial and invasive squamous neoplasms. *Obstetrics and Gynecology*, **57**, 643.

GANJEI, P., GUERALDO, K.A., LAMPE, B. and NADJI, M. (1990) Vulvar Paget's disease. Is immunocytochemistry helpful in assessing the surgical margins? *Journal of Reproductive Medicine*, **35**(11), 1002.

GARDNER, S.H., STOUT, F.E., ARBOGAST, J.L. and HUBER, C.P. (1953) Intraepithelial carcinoma of the vulva. *American Journal of Obstetrics and Gynecology*, **65**, 539.

HELWIG, E.B. and GRAHAM, J.H. (1963) Anogenital (extramammary) Paget's disease. *Cancer*, **16**, 387.

HOFFMAN, J.S., KUMAR, N.B. and MORLEY, G.W. (1983) Microinvasive squamous carcinoma of the vulva: search for definition. *Obstetrics and Gynecology*, **61**, 615.

HOFFMAN, M.S., LA POLLA, J.P., ROBERTS, J.S. and KAUFNER, D. (1990) Use of local flaps for primary anal reconstruction following perianal resection for neoplasia. *Gynecologic Oncology*, **36**(3), 348.

HUSSEINZADEH, N., NEWMAN, N.J. and WESSELER, T.A. (1989) Vulvar intraepithelial neoplasia: a clinicopathological study of carcinoma-in-situ of the vulva. *Gynecologic Oncology*, **33**(2), 157.

JONES, R.W. and MCLEAN, M.R. (1986) Carcinoma *in situ* of the vulva; a review of 31 treated and 5 untreated cases. *Obstetrics and Gynecology*, **68**, 499.

KIMURA, S., FHRAI, A., HARADA, R. and NAGASHIMA, M. (1978) So-called multicentric pigmented Bowen's disease. *Dermatologica*, **157**, 779.

LEE, S.C., ROTH, L.M. and EHRLICH, C. (1977) Extramammary Paget's disease of the vulva. *Cancer*, **39**, 614.

LEUCHTER, R.S., TOWNSEND, D.E., HACKER, N.F. *et al.* (1984) Treatment of vulvar carcinoma in situ with the CO_2 laser. *Gynecologic Oncology*, **19**, 314.

MCADAM, A.J. and KISSNER, R.W. (1958) Relationship of chronic vulvar disease. Leukoplakia and carcinoma-in-situ to carcinoma of the vulva. *Cancer*, **11**, 740.

MCDONALD, T.W., NEUTENS, J.J., FISHER, C.M. and JESSEE, D. (1989) Impact of CIN diagnosis and treatment on self-esteem and body image. *Gynecologic Oncology*, **34**, 345.

MENE, A. and BUCKLEY, C.H. (1985) Involvement of the vulval skin appendages by intraepithelial neoplasia. *British Journal of Obstetrics and Gynaecology*, **92**, 634.

MOLL, I. and MOLL, R. (1985) Cells of extramammary Paget's disease express cytokeratins different from those of epidermal cells. *Journal of Investigative Dermatology*, **84**, 3.

PLANNER, R.S. and HOBBS, J.B. (1987) Human papillomavirus infection and associated intraepithelial neoplasia of the cervix, vagina and vulva. *Obstetrics and Gynecology*, **27**, 132.

PLANNER, R.S. and HOBBS, J.B. (1988) Intraepithelial and invasive neoplasia of the vulva in association with human papillomavirus infection. *Journal of Reproductive Medicine*, **33**, 503.

REID, R. (1985) Superficial laser vulvectomy: a new surgical technique for appendage-conserving ablation of refractory condyloma and vulvar intraepithelial neoplasia. *American Journal of Obstetrics and Gynecology*, **152**(5), 504.

RETTENMAIER, M.A., BERMAN, M.L. and DISAIA, P.J. (1987) Skinning vulvectomy for the treatment of multifocal vulvar intraepithelial neoplasia. *Obstetrics and Gynecology*, **69**, 247.

RIDLEY, C.M. (ed.) (1988) *The Vulva*, Churchill Livingstone, Edinburgh.

RIDLEY, C.M. (1989) ISSVD new nomenclature for vulvar disease. *American Journal of Obstetrics and Gynecology*, **160**, 769.

RIDLEY, C.M., FRANKMAN, Q., JONES, I.S.C. and WILKINSON, E.J. (1989) New nomenclature for vulvar disease. International Society for the Study of Vulvar Disease. *Human Pathology*, **20**, 495.

RIDLEY, C.M., FRANKMAN, O., JONES, I.S.C., PINCUS, S.H. and WILKINSON, E.J. (1989) New nomenclature for vulvar disease. Report of the Committee on Terminology, International Society for the Study of Vulvar Disease. *International Journal of Gynecologic Pathology*, **8**, 83.

RIDLEY, C.M., ORIEL, J.D. and ROBINSON, A.J. (1992) A *Colour Atlas of Diseases of the Vulva*, Chapman & Hall Medical, London.

RUTLEDGE, F. and SINCLAIR, M. (1968) Treatment of intraepithelial carcinoma of the vulva by skin excision and graft. *American Journal of Obstetrics and Gynecology*, **102**, 806.

SCHLAERTH, J.B., MORROW, C.P., NALICK, R.H. and GADDIS, O. (1984) Anal involvement by carcinoma *in situ* of the perineum in women. *Obstetrics and Gynecology*, **64**, 406.

SHATZ, P., BERGERON, C., WILKINSON, E. and FERENCZY, A. (1989) Vulvar intraepithelial neoplasia and skin appendage involvement. *Obstetrics and Gynecology*, **74**, 769.

SILLMAN, F.H. and SEDLIS, A. (1991) Anogenital papillomavirus infection and neoplasia in immunodeficient women; an update. *Dermatology Clinics*, **9**, 353.

SILLMAN, F.H., BOYCE, J.G., MACASET, M.A. and NICASTII, A.D. (1981) 5-Fluorouracil/chemosurgery for intraepithelial neoplasia of the lower genital tract. *Obstetrics and Gynecology*, **58**, 356.

SILLMAN, F.H., SEDLIS, A. and BOYCE, J.C. (1985) 5-FU/chemosurgery for difficult lower genital intraepithelial neoplasia. *Contemporary Obstetrics and Gynecology*, **30**, 79.

SIMONSEN, E.F. (1989) The CO_2 laser used for carcinoma-in-situ/Bowen's disease (VIN) and lichen sclerosus in the vulvar region. *Acta Obstetricia et Gynecologica Scandinavica*, **68**(6), 551.

SINGER, A. and MITCHELL, H. (1990) Treatment of vulvar premalignancy. *Clinical Practice in Gynaecology*, **2**(2), 231.

SKINNER, M.S., STERNBERG, W.H., ICHINOSE, H. and COLLINS, J. (1973) Spontaneous regression of Bowenoid atypia of the vulva. *Obstetrics and Gynecology*, **42**, 40.

STAFFORD, E.M., GREENBERG, H. and MILES, P.A. (1990) Cervical intraepithelial neoplasia III in an adolescent with Bowenoid papulosis. *Journal of Adolescent Health Care*, **11**(6), 523.

THEUSEN, B., ANDREASSON, B. and BOCK, J.E. (1992) Sexual function and somatophysic reactions after local excision of vulvar intraepithelial neoplasia. *Acta Obstetricia et Gynecologica Scandinavica*, **71**(2), 126.

TOWNSEND, D.E., LEVINE, R.U., RICHART, R.M., CRUM, C. and PETRILLI, E.S. (1982) Management of vulvar intraepithelial neoplasia by carbon dioxide laser. *Obstetrics and Gynecology*, **60**, 49.

ULBRIGHT, T.M., STEHMAN, F.B., ROTH, L.M. *et al.* (1982) Bowenoid dysplasia of the vulva. *Cancer*, **50**, 2910.

WADE, T.R., KOPF, A.W. and ACKERMAN, A.B. (1979) Bowenoid papulosis of the genitalia. *Archives of Dermatology*, **115**, 306.

WILKINSON, E.J. (1992) Normal histology and nomenclature of the vulva, and malignant neoplasms, including VIN. *Dermatology Clinics*, **10**, 283.

WILKINSON, E.J., FRIEDRICH, E.G. and FU, Y.S. (1981) Multicentric nature of vulvar carcinoma *in situ*. *Obstetrics and Gynecology*, **58**, 69.

WOLCOTT, H.D. and GALLUP, D.C. (1984) Wide local excision in the treatment of vulvar carcinoma *in situ*: a reappraisal. *American Journal of Obstetrics and Gynecology*, **150**, 695.

WOODRUFF, J.D. (1977) Paget's disease. *Obstetrics and Gynecology*, **49**, 511.

WRIGHT, V.C. and DAVIES, E. (1987) Laser surgery for vulvar intraepithelial neoplasia: principles and results. *American Journal of Obstetrics and Gynecology*, **156**, 374.

ZACHOW, K.R., ASTROW, R.S., BENDER, M. and WATTS, S. (1981) Detection of human papillomavirus DNA in anogenital neoplasias. *Nature*, **300**, 771.

ZAINO, R.J., HUSSEINZADE, N., NAHHAS, W. and MORTEL, R. (1982) Epithelial alterations in proximity to invasive squamous carcinoma of the vulva. *International Journal of Gynecologic Pathology*, **1**, 173.

Chapter 17

ALLOUB, M.I., BARR, B.B.B., MCLAREN, K.M., SMITH, I.W., BUNNEY, M.H. and SMART, G.E. (1989) Human papillomavirus infection and cervical intraepithelial neoplasia in women with renal allografts. *British Medical Journal*, **298**, 153–6.

BECKMANN, A.M., ACKER, R., CHRISTIANSEN, A.E. and SHERMAN, K.J. (1991) Human papillomavirus infection in women with multicentric squamous cell neoplasia. *American Journal of Obstetrics and Gynecology*, **165**, 1431–7.

CAUSSY, D., GOEDERT, J.J., PALEFSKY, J. *et al.* (1990) Interaction of human immunodeficiency and papilloma viruses: association with anal epithelial abnormality in homosexual men. *International Journal of Cancer*, **46**, 214–19.

DALING, J.R., WEISS, N.S., HISLOP, T.G. *et al.* (1987) Sexual practices, sexually transmitted diseases, and the incidence of anal cancer. *New England Journal of Medicine*, **317**, 973–7.

DANIELL, H.W. (1985) Re: causes of anal carcinoma. *Journal of the American Medical Association*, **254**, 358.

Department of Health and Social Security (1979) Sexually transmitted diseases, in *On the State of Public Health: Annual Report of the Chief Medical Officer of the Department of Health and Social Security for the year 1978*. HMSO, London, pp. 1–65.

DYSON, N., HOWLEY, P.M., MUNGER, K. and HARLOW, E. (1989) The human papillomavirus 16 E7 oncoprotein is able to bind to the retinoblastoma gene product. *Science*, **243**, 934–7.

FENGER, C. and NIELSEN, V.T. (1981) Dysplastic changes in the anal canal epithelium in minor surgical specimens. *Acta Pathologica et Microbiologica Scandinavica*, **89**, 463–5.

FENGER, C. and NIELSEN, V. (1986) Precancerous changes in the anal canal epithelium in resection specimens. *Acta Pathologica et Microbiologica Scandinavica*, **94**, 63–9.

FOUST, R.L., DEAN, P.J., STOLER, M.H. and MOINUDDIN, S.M. (1991) Intraepithelial neoplasia of the anal canal in haemorrhoidal tissue: a study of 19 cases. *Human Pathology*, **22**, 528–34.

FRAZER, I.H., MEDLEY, G., CRAPPER, R.M., BROWN, T.C. and MACKAY, I.R. (1986) Association between anorectal dysplasia, human papillomavirus and human immunodeficiency virus infection in homosexual men. *Lancet*, **ii**, 657–60.

FRISCH, M., MELBYE, M. and MOLLER, H. (1993) Trends in the incidence of anal cancer in Denmark. *British Medical Journal*, **306**, 419–22.

GRODSKY, L. (1967) Unsuspected anal cancer discovered after minor anorectal surgery. *Diseases of the Colon and Rectum*, **10**, 471–9.

HALPERT, R., BUTT, K.M.H., SEDLIS, A. *et al.* (1985) Human papillomavirus infection and lower genital neoplasia in female renal allograft recipients. *Transplantation Proceedings*, **17**, 93–5.

HAWTHORN, R.J.S., MURDOCH, J.B., MACLEAN, A.B. and MACKIE, R.M. (1988) Langerhans' cells and subtypes of human papillomavirus in cervical intraepithelial neoplasia. *British Medical Journal*, **297**, 643–6.

HOLMES, F., BOREK, D., OWEN-KUMMER, M. *et al.* (1988) Anal cancer in women. *Gastroenterology*, **95**, 107–11.

HUGHES, R.G., NORVAL, M. and HOWIE, S.E.M. (1988) Expression of major histocompatibility class II antigens by Langerhans' cells in cervical intraepithelial neoplasia. *Journal of Clinical Pathology*, **41**, 253–9.

KIVIAT, N., ROMPALO, A., BOWDEN, R. *et al.* (1990) Anal human papillomavirus infection among human immunodeficiency virus seropositive and seronegative men. *Journal of Infective Diseases*, **162**, 358–61.

KIVIAT, N.B., CRITCHLOW, C.W., HOLMES, K.K. *et al.* (1993) Association of anal dysplasia and human papillomavirus with immunosupression and HIV infection among homosexual men. *AIDS*, **7**, 43–9.

MCINDOE, W.A., MCLEAN, M.A., JONES, R.W. and MULLINS, P.R. (1984) The invasive potential of carcinoma *in situ* of the cervix. *Obstetrics and Gynecology*, **64**, 451–8.

MELBYE, M. and SPROGEL, P. (1991) Aetiological parallel between anal cancer and cervical cancer. *Lancet*, **338**, 657–9.

MELBYE, M., PALEFSKY, J., GONZALES, J. *et al.* (1990) Immune status as a determinant of human papillomavirus detection and its association with anal epithelial abnormalities. *International Journal of Cancer*, **46**, 203–6.

MELBYE, M., COTE, T.R., KESSLER, L. *et al.* (1994) High incidence of anal cancer among AIDS patients. *Lancet*, **343**, 636–9.

MORSON, B.C. (1960) The pathology and results of treatment of squamous cell carcinoma of the anal canal and anal margin. *Proceedings of the Royal Society of Medicine*, **53**, 416–20.

NASH, G., ALLEN, W. and NASH, S. (1986) Atypical lesions of the anal mucosa in homosexual men. *Journal of the American Medical Association*, **256**, 873–6.

NORTHOVER, J.M.A. (1991) Epidermoid cancer of the anus – the surgeon retreats. *Journal of the Royal Society of Medicine*, **84**, 389–90.

OCADIZ, R., SAUCEDA, R., CRUZ, M., GRAEF, A.M. and GRANIGLIO, P. (1987) High correlation between molecular alterations of the c-*myc* oncogene and carcinoma of the uterine cervix. *Cancer Research*, **47**, 4173–17.

Office of Population Censuses and Surveys (1991) *Cancer Statistics and Registrations, 1986*. HMSO, London, Series MB1, No. 19.

OGUNBIYI, O.A., SCHOLEFIELD, J.H., RAFTERY, A.T. *et al.* (1994) Prevalence of anal human papillomavirus infection and intraepithelial neoplasia in renal allograft recipients. *British Journal of Surgery*, **81**, 365–7.

OGUNBIYI, O.A., SCHOLEFIELD, J.H., ROBERTSON, G. *et al.* (1994) Anal human papillomavirus infection and squamous neoplasia in patients with invasive vulvar cancer. *Obstetrics and Gynecology*, **83**(2), 212–16.

PALEFSKY, J.M., GONZALES, J., GREENBLATT, R.M., AHN, D.K. and HOLLANDER, H. (1990) Anal intraepithelial neoplasia and anal papillomavirus infection among homosexual males with Group IV HIV disease. *Journal of the American Medical Association*, **263**, 2911–16.

PALEFSKY, J.M., HOLLY, E.A., GONZALES, J. *et al.* (1991) Detection of human papillomavirus DNA in anal intraepithelial neoplasia and anal cancer. *Cancer Research*, **51**, 1014–19.

PALEFSKY, J.M., HOLLY, E.A., GONZALES, J., LAMBORN, K. and HOLLANDER, H. (1992) Natural history of anal cytologic abnormalities and papillomavirus infection among homosexual men with Group IV HIV disease. *Journal of Acquired Immunodeficiency Syndromes*, **5**, 1258–65.

PALMER, J.G., SCHOLEFIELD, J.H., COATES, P.J. *et al.* (1989) Anal cancer and human papillomaviruses. *Diseases of the Colon and Rectum*, **32**, 1016–22.

PENN, I. (1974) Chemical immunosuppression and human cancer. *Cancer*, **34**, 1474–80.

PENN, I. (1986) Cancer is a complication of severe immunosuppression. *Surgery Gynecology and Obstetrics*, **162**, 603–10.

PENN, I. (1986) Cancers of the anogenital region in renal transplant recipients. Analysis of 65 cases. *Cancer*, **58**, 611–16.

PETERS, R.K., MACK, T.M. and BERNSTEIN, L. (1984) Parallels in the epidemiology of selected anogenital carcinomas. *Journal of the National Cancer Institute*, **72**, 609–15.

PORRECO, R., PENN, I., DROEGEMUELLER, W., GREER, B. and MAKOWSKI, E. (1975) Gynecologic malignancies in immunosuppressed organ homograft recipients. *Obstetrics and Gynecology*, **45**, 359–64.

PRASSAD, M.L. and ABCARIAN, H. (1980) Malignant potential of perianal condyloma acuminatum. *Diseases of the Colon and Rectum*, **23**, 191–7.

RABKIN, C.S., BIGGAR, R.J., MELBYE, M. and CURTIS, R.E. (1992) Second primary cancers following anal and cervical carcinoma: evidence of shared aetiologic factors. *American Journal of Epidemiology*, **136**, 54–8.

RETTENMAIER, M.A., BERMAN, M.L. and DISAIA, P.J. (1987) Skinning vulvectomy for the treatment of multifocal vulvar intraepithelial neoplasia. *Obstetrics and Gynecology*, **69**, 247–50.

SCHOLEFIELD, J.H., SONNEX, C., TALBOT, I.C. *et al.* (1989) Anal and cervical intraepithelial neoplasia: possible parallel. *Lancet*, **ii**, 765–8.

SCHOLEFIELD, J.H., HICKSON, W.G.E., SMITH, J.H.F., ROGERS, K. and SHARP, F. (1992) Anal intraepithelial neoplasia: part of a multifocal disease process. *Lancet*, **340**, 1271–3.

Scholefield, J.H., Ogunbiyi, O.A., Smith, J.H.F., Rogers, K. and Sharp, F. (1994) Anal colposcopy and the diagnosis of anal intraepithelial neoplasia in high risk gynaecological patients. *International Journal of Gynaecological Cancer*, **4**, 119–26.

Sherman, K.J., Daling, J.R., Chu, J., McKnight, B. and Weiss, N.S. (1988) Multiple primary tumours in women with vulvar neoplasms: a case control study. *British Journal of Cancer*, **57**, 423–7.

Siegal, A. (1962) Malignant transformation of condyloma acuminatum: review of the literature and report of a case. *American Journal of Surgery*, **103**, 613–17.

Sixbey, J.W., Lemon, S.M. and Pagano, J.S. (1986) A second site for Epstein–Barr virus shedding: the uterine cervix. *Lancet*, **ii**, 1122–4.

Surawicz, C.M., Kirby, P., Critchlow, C., Sayer, J., Dunphy, C. and Kiviat, N. (1993) Anal dysplasia in homosexual men: role of anoscopy and biopsy. *Gastroenterology*, **105**, 658–66.

Wexner, S.D., Milsom, J.W. and Dailey, T.H. (1987) The demographics of anal cancers are changing: identification of a high risk population. *Diseases of the Colon and Rectum*, **30**, 942–6.

Williams, A.B., Darragh, T.M., Vranzian, K. *et al.* (1994) Anal and cervical human papillomavirus infection and risk of anal and cervical epithelial abnormalities in human immunodeficiency virus-infected women. *Obstetrics and Gynecology*, **83**, 205–11.

Wright, V.C. and Davies, E. (1987) Laser surgery for vulvar intraepithelial neoplasia: principles and results. *American Journal of Obstetrics and Gynecology*, **156**, 374–8.

Chapter 18

Govan, A.D., Black, W.P. and Sharp, J.L. (1969) Aberrant glandular polypi of the uterine cervix associated with contraceptive pills, pathology and pathogenesis. *Journal of Clinical Pathology*, **22**, 84.

Taylor, H.B., Irey, N.S. and Norris, H.J. (1967) Atypical endocervical hyperplasia in women taking oral contraceptives. *Journal of the American Medical Association*, **202**, 637.

Chapter 19

Coppleson, M. and Reid, B. (1966) The colposcopic study of the cervix during pregnancy and the puerperium. *Journal of Obstetrics and Gynaecology of the British Commonwealth*, **73**, 375.

Mikuta, I.J., Enterline, H.T. and Braun, T.E. (1968) Carcinoma-in-situ associated with pregnancy. *Journal of the American Medical Association*, **204**, 763.

Chapter 20

Bonney, V. and Clendinning, B. (1910) Adenomatosis vaginae: a hitherto undescribed condition. *Proceedings of the Royal Society of Medicine*, **4**, 18.

Dieckmann, W.J., Davis, M.D., Rynkiewiez, L.M. and Pottinger, R.E. (1953) Does administration of diethylstilbestrol during pregnancy have therapeutic value? *American Journal of Obstetrics and Gynecology*, **66**, 1062.

Faber, K., Jones, M. and Terraza, H.M. (1990) Invasive squamous cell carcinoma of the vagina in a diethyl stilboestrol-exposed woman. *Gynecologic Oncology*, **37**(1), 125.

Herbst, A.L. and Scully, R.E. (1970) Adenocarcinoma of the vagina in adolescents. Report of seven cases including six clear cell adenocarcinomas (so-called mesonephromas). *Cancer*, **25**, 745.

Herbst, A.L. and Byrne, H.A. (eds) (1981) *Developmental Effects of Diethyl Stilboestrol (DES) in Pregnancy*. Thième-Stratton, New York.

Herbst, A., Ulfeder, H. and Poskanzer, D. (1971) Adenocarcinoma of the vagina: association of maternal stilbestrol therapy with tumor appearance in young women. *New England Journal of Medicine*, **284**, 878.

Herbst, A.L., Cole, P., Colton, T., Robboy, S. and Scully, R.E. (1977) Age incidence and risk of diethylstilbestrol-related clear cell adenocarcinomas of the vagina and cervix. *American Journal of Obstetrics and Gynecology*, **128**, 43.

Herbst, A.L., Cole, P., Norusis, M.J., Welsh, W.R. and Scully, R.E. (1979) Epidemiological aspects and factors related to survival of 384 cases of clear cell adenocarcinoma of the vagina and cervix. *American Journal of Obstetrics and Gynecology*, **135**, 876.

Mattsson, L., Cullberg, G., Eriksson, O. and Knutsson, F. (1989) Vaginal administration of low-dose oestradiol effects on the endometrium and vaginal cytology. *Maturitas*, **11**, 217.

Melnick, S., Cole, P., Anderson, D. and Herbst, A.L. (1987) Rates and risks of diethylstilbestrol-related clear cell adenocarcinoma of the vagina and cervix. *New England Journal of Medicine*, **316**, 514.

Monaghan, J. and Sirisena, L.A.W. (1978) Stilboestrol and vaginal clear cell adenocarcinoma. *British Medical Journal*, **1**, 1588.

Noller, K., Townsend, M., Kaufrnan, R. *et al.* (1983) Maturation of vaginal and cervical epithelium in women exposed to diethylstilbestrol (DESAD project). *American Journal of Obstetrics and Gynecology*, **146**, 279.

Nwabineli, N.J. and Monaghan, J.M. (1991) Vaginal epithelial abnormalities in patients with CIN; clinical and pathological features and management. *British Journal of Obstetrics and Gynaecology*, **98**(1), 25.

ROBBOY, S.J., NOLLER, K.L., O'BRIEN, P. *et al.* (1984) Increased incidence of cervical and vaginal dysplasia in 3980 diethylstilbestrol exposed young women; experience of the National Collaborative DES Adenosis project. *Journal of the American Medical Association*, **252**, 2979.

ROBBOY, S., HILL, E., SANDBERG, E. and CZERNOBLISKY, B. (1986) Vaginal adenosis in women born prior to the diethylstilbestrol era. *Human Pathology*, **17**(5), 488.

SANDBERG, E. (1968) Incidence and distribution of occult vaginal adenosis. *American Journal of Obstetrics and Gynecology*, **101**, 333.

SANDBERG, E., DANIELSON, R., CAUWET, R. and BONAR, B. (1965) Adenosis vaginae. *American Journal of Obstetrics and Gynecology*, **93**, 209.

SCULLY, R.E., ROBBOY, S.J. and WELCH, W.R. (1978) Pathology and pathogenesis in diethylstilbestrol related disorders of the female genital tract, in *Intrauterine Exposure to Diethylstilbestrol in the Human* (ed. A.L. Herbst), American College of Obstetrics and Gynecology, Chicago.

SIDERS, D., PARROT, M. and ABELL, M. (1965) Gland cell prosplasia (adenosis) of the vagina. *American Journal of Obstetrics and Gynecology*, **91**, 191.

STAFL, A., MATTINGLEY, R., FOLEY, D. and FETHERSTON, W. (1974) Clinical diagnosis of vaginal adenosis. *Obstetrics and Gynecology*, **43**, 1.

Chapter 21

COIBION, M., VANDAM, M., ANDRY, A. *et al.* (1991) La cervicographie: le complément de la cytologie dans le dépistage des lésions cervicales. *Gynécologie*, **42**, 393–4.

KESIC, V.I., SOULTER, W.P., SULOVIC, V. *et al.* (1993) A comparison of cytology and cervicography in cervical screening. *International Journal of Gynaecological Cancer*, **3**, 395–8.

NAVRATIL, E., BURGHARDT, E., BAJARD, F. *et al.* (1958) Simultaneous colposcopy and cytology used in the screening for carcinoma *in situ* of the cervix. *American Journal of Obstetrics and Gynecology*, **75**, 1292.

SPITZER, M., KRUMHOLZ, B.A., CHERNYS, A.E. *et al.* (1987) Comparative utility of repeat Papanicolaou smears, cervicography and colposcopy in the evaluation of atypical Papanicolaou smears. *Obstetrics and Gynecology*, **69**, 731.

STAFL, A. (1981) Cervicography: a new method for cervical cancer detection. *American Journal of Obstetrics and Gynecology*, **139**, 815–25.

TAWA, K., FORSYTHE, A., COVE, K. *et al.* (1988) A comparison of the Papanicolaou smear and the cervigram: sensitivity, specificity and cost analysis. *Obstetrics and Gynecology*, **71**, 229.

Chapter 22

SINGER, A., WALKER, P., TAY, S.K. and DYSON, J. (1984) Impact of introduction of colposcopy to a district general hospital. *British Medical Journal*, **289**, 1049.

Chapter 23

COPPLESON, M., REID, B.L., SKLADNEV, V.N. and DALRYMPLE, J.C. (1994) An electronic approach to the detection of pre-cancer and cancer of the uterine cervix, a preliminary evaluation of polarprobe. *International Journal of Gynecological Cancer*, **4**, 79–83.

CUZICK, J., TERRY, G., HO, L., HOLLINGWORTH, T. and ANDERSON, M. (1994) Type-specific human papillomavirus DNA in abnormal smears as a predictor of high-grade cervical intraepithelial neoplasia. *British Journal of Cancer*, **69**, 167–71.

DAVIDSON, M., SCHNITZER, P.C., BULKOW, L.R. *et al.* (1994) The prevalence of cervical infection with human papillomaviruses and cervical dysplasia in Alaskan native women. *Journal of Infectious Diseases*, **169**, 792–800.

ERZEN, M., MARIN, J., URSICVRSCAJ, M. and MOZINA, A. (1994) Detection of human papillomaviruses (HPV) 16 and 18 in cervical smears by *in situ* hybridisation. *European Journal of Obstetrics Gynecology and Reproductive Biology*, **55**, 28.

FARTHING, A., MASTERSON, P., MASON, W.P. and VOUSDEN, K.H. (1994) Human papillomavirus detection by hybrid capture and its possible clinical use. *Journal of Clinical Pathology*, **47**, 649–52.

HORDING, U., DAUGAARD, S. and BOCK, J.E. (1994) Detection of human papillomavirus (HPV) DNA in cervical swabs by the polymerase chain reaction – an evaluation of the sensitivity of the method in patients with HPV 16-harboring cervical lesions. *International Journal of Gynecological Pathology*, **13**, 139–42.

JOHNSON, K. (1995) Periodic health examination, 1995 update: 1. Screening for human papillomavirus infection in asymptomatic women. *Canadian Medical Association Journal*, **152**, 483–93.

SYRJANEN, K.J. (1994) Human papillomavirus in genital carcinogenesis. *Sexaully Transmitted Diseases*, **21**, S86–9.

Index

Page numbers in **bold** type refer to figures and page numbers in *italics* refer to tables.